CLINICAL

in the Rheumatic Diseases

Third Edition

SUSAN J. BARTLETT, PhD, EDITOR

CLIFTON O. BINGHAM, III, MD, ASSOCIATE EDITOR

MICHAEL J. MARICIC, MD, ASSOCIATE EDITOR

MAURA DALY IVERSEN, PT, DPT, MPH, CONSULTING EDITOR

VICTORIA RUFFING, RN, CONSULTING EDITOR

Published by the Association of Rheumatology Health Professionals
A Division of the American College of Rheumatology
1800 Century Place
Suite 250
Atlanta, GA 30345-4300

Library of Congress Control Number: 2006933385
ISBN-10: 0-9654316-2-2
ISBN-13: 978-0-9654316-2-0

The information and the views and opinions contained in this publication are those of the authors and unless clearly specified, do not represent the views or opinions of the American College of Rheumatology. The American College of Rheumatology does not endorse, approve, guarantee, or warrant any particular technique or therapy or product, method of instruction, or recommendation contained in this publication.

Managing Editor: Elizabeth E. Axtell
Executive Director, Association of Rheumatology Health Professionals: David M. Haag

Authors

Aryeh M. Abeles, MD
New York University School of Medicine
New York, NY

Ann Aspnes
Duke Medical Center
Durham, NC

Hammad A. Bajwa, MD
University of Minnesota
Minneapolis, MN

Susan J. Bartlett, PhD
Johns Hopkins Asthma & Allergy
Baltimore, MD

Thomas D. Beardmore, MD, FACP, FACR
Rancho Los Amigos Hospital
Downey, CA

Basia Belza, PhD, RN
University of Washington
Seattle, WA

Francesco Boin, MD
Johns Hopkins University School of Medicine
Baltimore, MD

David Borenstein, MD
Arthritis & Rheumatism Associates, PC
Washington, DC

Michele L. Boutaugh, BSN, MPH
Arthritis Foundation
Atlanta, GA

Teresa J. Brady, PhD
Centers for Disease Control and Prevention
Atlanta, GA

D. J. Brower, BA, DPM, PhD
Temple Univ School of Podiatric Medicine
Philadelphia, PA

David S. Caldwell, MD
Duke Medical Center
Durham, NC

A. Betts Carpenter, MD, PhD
Marshall University School of Medicine
Huntington, WV

John A. Carrino, MD, MPH
Johns Hopkins University School of Medicine
Baltimore, MD

L. Frank Cavaliere, MD
Albany Medical College
Albany, NY

Lisa Christopher-Stine, MD, MPH
Johns Hopkins University School of Medicine
Baltimore, MD

Alarcos Cieza, PhD, MPH
Ludwig-Maximilians-University
Munich, Germany

Angela M. Dahle, MD
University of Minnesota
Minneapolis, MN

Kori Dewing, MN, ARNP
Seattle Rheumatology Associates
Seattle, WA

Mazen Elyan, MD
MetroHealth Medical Center
Cleveland, OH

Kevin R. Fontaine, PhD
Johns Hopkins University School of Medicine
Baltimore, MD

Mary Beth Hansen, MA
Univ Pittsburgh Med Center, Center for Biosecurity
Pittsburgh, PA

Pamela B. Harrell, OTR, CHT
Vanderbilt Orthopaedics - Franklin
Franklin, TN 37064

Donna J. Hawley, EdD, RN
Wichita State University
Wichita, KS

Karen W. Hayes, PT, PhD, FAPTA
Northwestern University Feinberg School
of Medicine
Chicago, IL

Howard J. Hillstrom, PhD
Hospital for Special Surgery
New York, NY

Maura D. Iversen, PT, DPT, SD, MPH,
Mass General Hospital Institute of Health
Professions
Boston, MA

Muhammad Asim Khan, MD, MACP
MetroHealth Medical Center
Cleveland, OH

Francis J. Keefe, PhD
Duke Medical Center
Durham, NC

Cheryl L. Koehn
Arthritis Consumer Experts
Vancouver, BC, Canada

Sharon L. Kolasinski, MD
Hospital of the University of Pennsylvania
Philadelphia, PA

Thomas J. A. Lehman, MD
Hospital for Special Surgery
New York, NY

H. Lemont, DPM
Temple Univ School of Podiatric Medicine
Philadelphia, PA

Kathleen S. Lewis, RN, LPC, CMP
Celebrate Life
Marietta, GA

Shari M. Ling, MD
National Institute on Aging
Baltimore, MD

K. T. Mahan, DPM, MS
Temple Univ School of Podiatric Medicine
Philadelphia, PA

Maren Mahowald, MD
Minneapolis Veterans Administration
Medical Center
Minneapolis, MN

Michael J. Maricic, MD
Catalina Pointe Rheumatology Specialists
Tucson, AZ

Alan K. Matsumoto, MD
Arthritis and Rheumatism Associates
Wheaton, MD

James McGuire, DPM, PT
Temple Univ School of Podiatric Medicine
Philadelphia, PA

Jane McKenzie-White, MAS
Johns Hopkins University School of Medicine
Baltimore, MD

Donald R. Miller, PharmD
North Dakota State University
Fargo, ND

Marian A. Minor, PT, PhD
University of Missouri
Columbia, MO

Carolee Moncur, PT, PhD
Salt Lake City, UT

Larry W. Moreland, MD
University of Alabama at Birmingham
Birmingham, AL

Lisa A. Nichols, MSN, RN, CCRA
Novartis Pharmaceuticals
Bellevue, NE

Stephen A. Paget, MD, FACP, FACR
Hospital for Special Surgery
New York, NY

Ozlem Pala, MD
Albany Medical College
Albany, NY

Jerry C. Parker, PhD
Harry S Truman Memorial Veterans Hospital
Columbia, MO

Rahul K. Patel, MD
Univ of North Texas Health Science Center
Fort Worth, TX

Raymond M. Pertusi, DO
Univ of North Texas Health Science Center
Fort Worth, TX

Michelle A. Petri, MD, MPH
Johns Hopkins University Hospital
Baltimore, MD

Michael H. Pillinger, MD
New York University School of Medicine
New York, NY

Michael S. Puniello, DPT, MS, OCS, FAAOMPT
Biomotion Laboratory
Boston, MA

Michael A. Rapoff, PhD
University of Kansas Medical Center
Chicago, IL

Anthony M. Reginato, MD, PhD
Massachusetts General Hospital
Boston, MA

Cheryl Riegger-Krugh, ScD, PT
University of Colorado Health Science Center
Denver, CO

Laura Robbins, DSW
Hospital for Special Surgery
New York, NY

Pamela B. Rosenthal, MD
New York University School of Medicine
New York, NY

Bernard R. Rubin, DO, MPH
Univ of North Texas Health Science Center
Fort Worth, TX

Katherine Rudolph, PhD, PT
University of Delaware
Newark, DE

Victoria Ruffing, RN
Johns Hopkins University
Baltimore, MD

Pasha Sarraf, MD, PhD
National Institute on Arthritis and
Musculoskeletal and Skin Diseases
Bethesda, MD

H. Ralph Schumacher, Jr., MD
Veterans Administration Medical Center
Philadelphia, PA

Peter Schur, MD, MACR
Harvard University School of Medicine
Boston, MA

Philip Seo, MD, MHS
Johns Hopkins Vasculitis Center
Baltimore, MD

Lee S. Simon, MD
Brigham and Women's Hospital
Boston, MA

Karen L. Smarr, PhD
Harry S Truman Memorial Veterans Hospital
Columbia, MO

David Wayne Smith, DEd
Arizona Arthritis Center
Tucson, AZ

Michael T. Smith, PhD
Johns Hopkins University School of Medicine
Baltimore, MD

Mark J. Soloski, PhD
Johns Hopkins University School of Medicine
Baltimore, MD

Robert F. Spiera, MD, FACP, FACR
Hospital for Special Surgery
New York, NY

Prof. Gerold Stucki, MD, MS
Ludwig-Maximilians-University
Munich, Germany

Sangeeta Sule, MD
Johns Hopkins University School of Medicine
Baltimore, MD

Jessica Tischner, PhD
Duke Medical Center
Durham, NC

Anthony M. Turkiewicz, MD
University of Alabama at Birmingham
Birmingham, AL

Bridget T. Walsh, DO
Catalina Pointe Rheumatology
Tucson, AZ

Stephen T. Wegener, PhD
Johns Hopkins University School of Medicine
Baltimore, MD

Mark H. Wener, MD, FACR
University of Washington
Seattle, WA

Marie D. Westby, BScPT, PhD Candidate
Mary Pack Arthritis Program
Vancouver, BC, Canada

Kendrick Whitney, DPM
Temple Univ School of Podiatric Medicine
Philadelphia, PA

Fredrick Wigley, MD
Johns Hopkins University School of Medicine
Baltimore, MD

Carol M. Ziminski, MD, FACP
Johns Hopkins University School of Medicine
Baltimore, MD

Table of Contents

Foreword

The Association of Rheumatology Health Professionals (ARHP), a division of the American College of Rheumatology, is pleased to present the Third Edition of *Clinical Care in the Rheumatic Diseases*. The ARHP aims to provide a comprehensive range of educational products for arthritis health professionals, and this textbook has earned its place as a fundamental resource in the field. It is a valuable addition to any professional library because it compiles current information on quality care for people living with the consequences of arthritis.

Arthritis encompasses more than 100 different conditions, affecting over 43 million Americans. Although the prevalence varies across the population, arthritis knows no boundaries. It occurs across the life-span from very young children through to the very old, regardless of socioeconomic status, gender, or ethnicity. Arthritis leads to physical limitations ranging from mild impairments to significant disability. As a result, many people with arthritis experience limitations in the most basic of daily living activities, such as walking and dressing, as well as participation in school, work, parenting, leisure, and social activities. A significant proportion of people with arthritis experience subsequent psychosocial issues related to the pain, fatigue, and depression that may accompany this chronic illness. With research in basic and clinical science, public health, rehabilitation, and social sciences, better treatments are discovered and ways of preventing arthritis and its disabling effects are developed. This revised textbook brings this new knowledge together in a format easily accessible to all health care providers engaged in caring for people with arthritis.

The editorial team, led by Dr. Susan Bartlett, is to be commended for assembling a group of authors to contribute their expertise and complete this book on an ambitious timeline, ensuring it is both timely and relevant. Appreciation is extended to each editor, author, reviewer, and staff member who contributed to this effort, and in so doing, enabled the College to maintain its commitment to provide educational resources to improve the quality of arthritis care.

Catherine Backman, PhD
President
Association of Rheumatology Health Professionals

Mary K. Crow, MD
President
American College of Rheumatology

Introduction

In 2005, the Association of Rheumatology Health Professionals (ARHP) celebrated 40 years of advancing the care of patients with rheumatic diseases. In the past few years alone, we have witnessed unprecedented progress in the comprehensive treatment of the rheumatic diseases. Thus, the goal of the third edition of *Clinical Care in the Rheumatic Diseases* (CCRD) is to provide a unique and practical compendium of the latest advances in knowledge and patient care on topics ranging from basic musculoskeletal anatomy to enhancing coping and quality of life. Contained within is a remarkable collection of facts, details, stories, and experiences from luminaries in their respective fields. I am truly grateful and deeply impressed that so many busy individuals generously donated their time, experience, wisdom, and enthusiasm with the sole intention of improving the care of people with arthritis everywhere. Ultimately, we trust that this information will serve to further promote excellence in the care of the millions of people throughout the world with rheumatic and musculoskeletal diseases.

As with earlier editions, CCRD strives to be the premier source of information for the wide range of health care professionals specializing in providing care for patients with rheumatic diseases. It reflects the commitment and long-standing partnership between the American College of Rheumatology and ARHP, emphasizing a multidisciplinary approach to research, patient care, and education.

This edition combines the latest news, practical information, and tools ranging from new therapeutics and modalities to the importance of biological, psychological, and social issues in determining patient outcomes. Practical information that is directly relevant to clinicians has been added, including use of the World Health Organization International Classification of Function and Ability, performing joint counts, and referring patients for disability. Credible and up-to-date Internet resources are given for both providers and patients. We also sought to ensure that CCRD would remain a leading resource for teachers and students in training programs for rheumatology and allied health professions.

Editing this book has been a true pleasure and education. There are more than 100 individuals to whom I wish to express my considerable gratitude for their time and knowledge in providing expert and up-to-date information on a broad range of topics. I am deeply indebted to my Associate Editors, Clifton "Bing" Bingham and Michael Maricic for their insight, depth of knowledge, and commitment to obtaining the authors and information that would make a difference to all health professionals working with arthritis patients. Their ability to call upon leaders in the field to contribute to this book reflects the esteem with which these two individuals are held by their colleagues and peers. Consulting editors Maura Iversen and Vicky Ruffing played a similar role in bringing together experts in physical therapy and nursing to enrich the breadth of information provided. They proved invaluable in holding the editors and authors to the task of providing evidence-based information that was relevant, practical, and applicable to all health professionals.

David Haag, Executive Director of ARHP, was the driving force for evolution and launch of the third edition. The Executive Committee of ARHP, and in particular Drs. Carol Oatis and Catherine Backman, provided enthusiastic support for the expanded direction of this book.

Drs. Stephen Wegener and Laura Robbins, editors of earlier editions, along with Dr. Eric Gall, provided helpful guidance throughout the process. Managing Editor Beth Axtell proved to be an unflagging source of assistance coordinating and integrating the efforts of so many at every stage in the evolution of the third edition of CCRD.

I would also like to acknowledge my colleagues and friends at Hopkins who have enriched my understanding of rheumatic diseases immeasurably and contributed in many ways to this book. It is indeed a privilege and honor to work together with such a remarkable collection of dedicated doctors and scientists. The esteem with which the Division is held largely reflects the vision and wisdom of our Director, Antony Rosen. Drs. Rosen, Joan Bathon, and Cynthia Rand have provided the mentorship and skills that helped to identify ideas and people who make a difference by providing compassionate, informed multidisciplinary care in rheumatology. Finally, I would like to thank my husband Ross and daughters Katie and Nicole for their love, encouragement, and patience throughout this endeavor.

Susan J. Bartlett, PhD, Editor
Clinical Care in the Rheumatic Diseases, Third Edition
Baltimore, MD

Forty Years of Advances in the Rheumatology Health Professions

TERESA J. BRADY, PhD

The 40th anniversary of the Association of Rheumatology Health Professionals in 2005 was a propitious time to examine advances made in the rheumatology health professions during the past 4 decades. Although there have been dramatic advances in the medical and surgical treatment of arthritis, including the discovery and use of new pharmaceutical agents (i.e., nonsteroidal antiinflammatory drugs, methotrexate, and biologic agents) and the advent of total joint replacements, there have been less celebrated, but equally dramatic changes in the rheumatology health professions. This brief review highlights 3 research-driven paradigm shifts in professional practice, an evolution in research that has yet to crystallize into major changes in clinical practice, and finally an evolution in professional role.

To put the advances of the past 40 years in perspective, it is important to note the typical care that was provided by rheumatology health professionals during the 1960s. A 1966 publication outlined the home care program from an Arthritis Foundation-designated model clinic: 1) bed rest during acute exacerbations; 2) education of patient and family to increase understanding of disease process and proposed treatment, and to explain need for rest, positioning, and exercise; 3) exercise, with an emphasis on range of motion; and 4) splints and other self-help devices (1). A 1968 publication described the rehabilitation approach to rheumatoid arthritis (RA) with an emphasis on controlled rest (both general and local joint rest with careful positioning to avoid joint deformity) and careful exercise (specified as 5–10 minutes of bed exercise increasing to 30 minutes once or twice a day). Admission to the hospital for bed rest was recommended, and weight bearing was not permitted until the patient could do so without pain (2).

PARADIGM SHIFTS

Exercise

From the earlier emphasis on conservative strategies of preserving joints through controlled rest and careful exercise, the field of exercise and physical activity has dramatically shifted to an emphasis on enhancing function and quality of life with safe but more challenging conditioning and strengthening. In the 1970s, Ekblom, Nordemar, and other Swedish investigators began examining the effects of physical training in RA and osteoarthritis (OA) in carefully supervised settings (3). Minor and colleagues safely moved aerobic exercise for people with RA and OA out into the community in 1989, paving the way for population-based aerobic exercise programs for people with arthritis (4).

As a result of this extensive body of research, we now know that people with arthritis can participate in moderate-intensity conditioning programs using walking, aquatic exercise, stationary bicycling, low-impact aerobic dance, and resistance training without injury or aggravation of disease (5). Evidence also shows that certain types of exercise have positive effects on arthritis symptoms and joint physiology (6).

This dramatic paradigm shift is reflected in American College of Rheumatology (ACR) guidelines for managing RA and OA of the hip and knee. These guidelines now include not only the traditional range-of-motion exercise, but also aerobic conditioning and strengthening exercise (7,8). The exercise paradigm focusing on enhancing fitness and strength can produce clinically meaningful improvements in function, flexibility, muscle strength and endurance, cardiovascular fitness, psychological status, and ultimately, quality of life (5).

Education

A seismic shift has also occurred in the practice of arthritis education. Education in the 1966 model clinic focused on understanding the disease and explaining the need for the conservative treatments. Since that time, the field has moved from simple information dissemination to enhancing patient self-management by building patients' knowledge, skills, and confidence to manage their arthritis themselves. Lorig and colleagues did much of the seminal work in this arena, demonstrating both the beneficial effects and the health care cost reductions of the Arthritis Self-Management Program (ASMP). During this early work, however, Lorig and colleagues discovered that contrary to assumptions, behavior change was only weakly associated with positive health outcomes, and that patients with positive outcomes felt "more control over their symptoms." This discovery and subsequent theoretical explorations eventually resulted in the introduction of self-efficacy as a possible underlying mechanism for the benefits of self-management education programs (9).

The expanding evidence base for self-management education programs changed our view of patient education from one of merely transferring information to one of building patients' generalizable skills and confidence. Current ACR guidelines incorporate the ASMP as part of nonpharmacologic management of RA and OA (7,8). The ASMP was also pivotal in that it moved patient education beyond the clinical realm and made it available in communities across the country.

Measurement

A monumental paradigm shift has also occurred in the conceptualization, role, and focus of measurement. Even during the early 1980s, when the original methotrexate studies were published, measurement of health status and function were minimal. The early methotrexate studies used proxy measures of disease activity, such as erythrocyte sedimentation rate, joint counts, duration of morning stiffness, and grip strength. Physicians and patients provided subjective assessments of "disease status" (10,11). Although functional impairment is the final common pathway of uncontrolled arthritis and the focus of arthritis interventions, it was not being measured, and the clinical and laboratory parameters that were being measured could not predict function (12).

However, concurrent with the publication of the methotrexate studies, validation studies of new self-report measures of health status or functional status were also being published. The disability index of the Health Assessment Questionnaire (13) and the Arthritis Impact Measurement Scales (14) both provided psychometrically sound reports of health status from the patient's perspective. The field of health status measurement has exploded since these seminal studies. For example, a 1992 special issue of *Arthritis Care and Research* reviewed 9 health status measures; a similar 2003 special issue reviewed 108 measures (15,16). Health status measures have become the cornerstone of the ACR 20 measures for documenting clinical improvement (17), and, with increasing frequency, are being used to guide clinical practice. According to Symmons, "it could be argued that a self report functional questionnaire is the single most useful outcome measure to use in routine care" (18).

EVOLUTIONS IN RESEARCH AND PRACTICE

Several other areas of rheumatology health professions research and practice have experienced significant growth and change, but have not yet matured to reach a research-driven paradigm shift in professional practice. The first of these is an evolution in the focus of research and the second is an evolution of a clinical practice role that is not yet well documented in research.

Evolution in Research

In the 1950s and 1960s, psychology was dominated by psychodynamic theorists who attempted to correlate specific illnesses with specific personality traits. In rheumatology, the focus was on studies of the "rheumatoid personality," described as having conforming, moralistic, and perfectionistic traits accompanied by contained hostility (19). The designs of these psychodynamic studies, however, had significant methodologic flaws and a 1987 meta-analysis concluded that there was no evidence that different diseases have different personality traits associated with them (20).

As the field moved away from a focus on personality traits, more enlightening areas of study emerged. Substantial bodies of research examined the prevalence and impact of psychological symptoms, such as depression and anxiety; association of beliefs, such as helplessness or self-efficacy, to health outcomes; impact of stressful life events and daily hassles on physical and psychological health status; the role of various coping skills and strategies in adaptation to arthritis; and a variety of intervention strategies such as cognitive-behavioral therapy and stress management programs (21,22). A key challenge ahead is to find ways to translate these research findings into practice and into community-based support.

Evolution in Practice

Perhaps due to its very ubiquitiuosness, the role of nursing in rheumatology has not been well documented. Early descriptions of multidisciplinary care provided vague summaries of nursing care. According to Pigg, "the contribution of rheumatology nursing to the care of rheumatic disease patients has not been well understood or clearly defined" (23). As early as 1974, however, nurses were assuming specialized roles, such as taking clinical measurements during drug trials. These responsibilities evolved into operating drug-monitoring clinics and, eventually, supervising the day-to-day management of patients with rheumatic disease (24,25).

The increasingly specialized role of the nurse in rheumatology carries a variety of job titles, including nurse educator, clinical nurse specialist, and nurse clinician. Rarely, however, is there any differentiation among these job titles, or scientific studies to support these roles. The strongest evidence addresses the efficacy of the rheumatology nurse practitioner role. Hill and colleagues demonstrated that patients of a rheumatology nurse practitioner experienced statistically significant improvements in a variety of health status measures (26). We now need to better standardize these specialized nursing roles and evaluate their outcomes.

CONCLUSIONS

During the past 40 years, we have seen dramatic changes in the rheumatology health professions. Substantial research has driven substantive practice paradigm shifts in the areas of exercise, education, and health status measurement. The focus of psychological research has evolved from examining personality traits to understanding a broad range of psychological factors that will hopefully influence practice parameters in the future. The role of nursing in rheumatology has evolved, with a need for role delineation and an evidence base to catch up with the evolving roles. Although these evolutions and practice paradigm shifts are impressive professional achievements, equally impressive is the impact they have made on the millions of Americans with arthritis. Minor summarized these advances succinctly when she said "It is a far better world for people with arthritis today than it was even 20 years ago" (Minor M: personal communication).

The findings and conclusions in this book chapter are those of the author and do not necessarily represent the views of the Centers for Disease Control and Prevention.

REFERENCES

1. Cohen BS, Baum J, Loggins B, Terry E. Home care program in the management of rheumatoid arthritis. J Chron Dis 1966;19:631–6.
2. Harris R. Physical methods in the management of rheumatoid arthritis. Med Clin North Am1968;52:707–16.
3. Minor MA. Physical activity in the management of arthritis. Ann Behav Med 1991;13:117–24.
4. Minor MA, Hewett JE, Webel RR, Anderson SK, Kay DR. Efficacy of physical conditioning exercise in patients with rheumatoid arthritis and osteoarthritis. Arthritis Rheum 1989;32:1396–1405.
5. Minor MA. Exercise and arthritis: the times they are a changing. Arthritis Care Res 1996;9:79–81.
6. Minor MA. 2002 Exercise and Physical Activity Conference, St Louis Missouri: exercise and arthritis: "we know a little about a lot of things…" Arthritis Rheum 2003;49:1–2.
7. American College of Rheumatology Subcommittee on Osteoarthritis Guidelines. Recommendations for the medical management of osteoarthritis of the hip and knee: 2000 update. Arthritis Rheum 2000;43:1905–15.
8. American College of Rheumatology Subcommittee on Rheumatoid Arthritis Guidelines. Guidelines for the management of rheumatoid arthritis: 2002 update. Arthritis Rheum 2002;46:328–46.
9. Lorig K, Holman H. Arthritis self-management studies: a twelve-year review. Health Educ Q 1993;20:17–28.
10. Wilkens RF, Watson MA, Paxson CS. Low dose pulse methotrexate therapy in rheumatoid arthritis. J Rheumatol 1980;7:501–5.
11. Steinsson K, Weinstein A, Korn J, Ables M. Low dose methotrexate in rheumatoid arthritis. J Rheumatol 1982;9:860–6.
12. Liang MH, Jette AM. Measuring functional ability in chronic arthritis. Arthritis Rheum 1981;24:80–6.
13. Fries JF, Spitz P, Kraines G, Holman HR. Measurement of patient outcome in arthritis. Arthritis Rheum 1980;23:137–45.
14. Meenan RF, Gertman PM, Mason JH. Measuring health status in arthritis: the Arthritis Impact Measurement Scales. Arthritis Rheum 1980;23:146–52.
15. Special Issue: Health status assessment. Arthritis Care Res 1992;5:117–91.
16. Association of Rheumatology Health Professionals Outcome Measures Task Force. Patient outcomes in rheumatology: a review of measures. Arthritis Rheum 2003;49(5 Suppl):S1–232.

17. Felson DT, Anderson JJ, Boers M, Bombardier C, Furst D, Goldsmith C, et al. American College of Rheumatology preliminary definition of improvement in rheumatoid arthritis. Arthritis Rheum 1995;38:727–35.
18. Symmons DP. Measuring outcome in rheumatoid arthritis: which measures are suitable for routine clinical use? Br J Rheumatol 1995;34:802–4.
19. Brady TJ. Integration of stress research in rheumatoid arthritis: from Alexander to Zautra and back again. Arthritis Care Res 1998;11:77–9.
20. Friedman HS, Booth-Kewley S. The "disease-prone personality": a meta-analytic view of the construct. Am Psychologist 1987;42:539–55.
21. Freeman JB, Blalock SJ, Holman HR, Liang MH, Meenan RF. Advances brought by health services research to patients with arthritis: summary of the Workshop on Health Services Research in Arthritis: from Research to Practice. Arthritis Care Res 1996;9:142–50.
22. Astin JA, Beckner W, Soeken K, Hochberg MC, Berman B. Psychological interventions for rheumatoid arthritis: a meta-analysis of randomized controlled trials. Arthritis Rheum 2002;47:291–302.
23. Pigg JS. Rheumatology nursing: evolution of a role and function of a subspecialty. Arthritis Care Res 1990;3:109–15.
24. Hill J. The expanding role of the nurse in rheumatology. Br J Rheumatol 1997;36:410–2.
25. Hill J. A nurse practitioner rheumatology clinic. Nursing Standard 1992;7:35–7.
26. Hill J, Bird HA, Harmer R, Wright V, Lawton C. An evaluation of the effectiveness, safety, acceptability of a nurse practitioner in a rheumatology outpatient clinic. Br J Rheumatol 1994;33:283–8.

SECTION A: CLINICAL FOUNDATIONS

CHAPTER
2

Overview of the Musculoskeletal System

CAROLEE MONCUR, PT, PhD

To appreciate the impact of rheumatic disease on the musculoskeletal system, it is important to have some understanding of the anatomic characteristics and biomechanical responses of the tissues at risk for developing arthritis. Muscles, bones, cartilage, tendons, ligaments, aponeuroses, and fascia are all dynamic tissues important to the integrity, stability, and mobility of the musculoskeletal system. This chapter presents a brief overview of these structures.

JOINTS

Joints are needed for differential growth, transmission of tensile, shear, compressive, and torsion forces, and a wide variety of movements (1–3). The dominant function at any given time depends on the location of the joint and age of the individual (4). Classification schemes for joints range from simple to more complex systems that are used by specialists to evaluate the intricacies of human movement. Joints can be assigned to 1 of 2 categories: synarthroses or diarthroses. Diarthrodial or synovial joints, in which each articular surface is composed of specialized hyaline cartilage strongly adherent to the underlying subchondral bones, are of primary interest in joint pathology. Synarthrodial joints are solid, nonsynovial joints. They are grouped either as fibrous joints or cartilaginous joints depending on their mode of ossification. Synarthroses are found in the cranial junctions, epiphyseal plates, and various midline joints of the body, such as the symphysis pubis.

Diarthrodial or Synovial Joints

On the outer surface, the cartilage is macroscopically smooth and free to be lubricated. This provides a near frictionless surface over which to move in concert with another articular surface. A classification scheme for diarthrodial joints is presented in Figure 1.

A typical example of the characteristics of the knee synovial joint is shown in Figure 2. Characteristic structures include 2 bones linked by a fibrous capsule that may have intrinsic ligamentous thickenings to support the joint, the synovial membrane deep to the fibrous capsule, an articular disc and/or meniscus not covered by the synovial membrane, a fibrocartilage labrum (as in the case of the hip), fat pads, and a vascular, neural, and lymphatic supply.

Joint Capsule. The joint capsule ensheathes the 2 ends of the bone. Because the fibrous layer of the joint capsule blends with the periosteum of the bones, meeting some distance away from the articulating ends, it does not impede movement. The fibrous layer is composed of relatively inelastic sheets of collagen, which contributes to joint stability and blood vessels and nerves that perforate the layer.

Ligaments of the joint represent cord-like thickenings of parallel collagen bundles formed intrinsically in the fibrous layer of the capsule. They may be separated from the capsule by bursae formed from outpouchings of the synovial lining. Ligaments are pliant and structured to resist excessive or abnormal movements of the joints; they yield very little to tension. Reflex neural mechanisms protect the ligament from excessive tension and stretch (5). In some joints, such as the knee, the intrinsic ligamentous properties are critical to the arthokinematics of the joint.

Synovial Membrane. The synovial membrane or *synovium* lines the joint everywhere, with the exception of the articular cartilage. The inner surface of the membrane is usually smooth and glistening, and it may be folded into numerous processes called *villi*. Synovium is abundantly supplied with blood vessels, nerves, and lymphatics, and it produces synovial fluid and provides immunologic protection. Synovial tissues are capable of rapid and complete repair when injured or surgically removed (6,7). In the healthy joint, the synovial lining membrane is only 1–2 layers thick but can hypertrophy massively in inflammatory arthritis.

Surface Shape	Surface Topology
Plane = gliding joints spheroid = ball and socket or enarthrosis ellipsoid = condyloid ginglymus = hinge bicondylar = double condyloid trochoid = pivot sellar = saddle joint	Simple (concave and convex surfaces) compound (concave and convex surfaces) sellar (concave and convex surfaces)
Axes of Movement	**Joint Mechanics**
uniaxial biaxial triaxial polyaxial	Movements are related to the concept of the mechanical axis of a bone. Movements are all resolvable as rotations around one, two or three orthogonal axes, i.e., possessing 1-3 degrees of freedom of motion.
Types of Movement	**Types of Movement**
Translation Angulation Rotation Circumduction Examples: flexion/extension abduction/adduction pronation/supination elevation/depression protraction/retraction isometric (neuromuscular) stabilizing (mechanical: close-packing)	Terms refer to one mobile articular surface moving relative to its fixed partner: **Spin:** pure rotation of surface around its mechanical axis. Two varieties of spin: pure and impure. **Roll:** tips of mechanical axis move end over end. **Slide:** tips of mechanical axis trace a transiatory path (like ice on ice).
Fundamental Joint Positions	
Loose Packed: controlled free mobility Close Packed: position of functional rigidity	

Figure 1. Classification of diarthrodial joints.

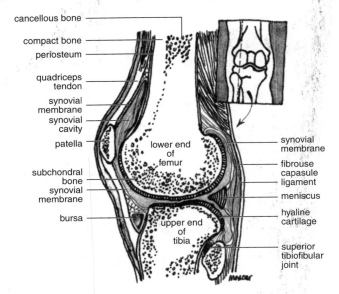

Figure 2. Characteristics of a diarthrodial joint as depicted by the knee joint.

Blood Vessels and Lymphatics. Synovial joints have a relatively rich blood supply. The branches of arteries to a joint commonly supply 3 structures: the epiphysis, the joint capsule, and the synovium. Due to the enriched vasculature of the synovial membrane, injury to the joint may allow blood to escape into the joint space and mix with the synovial fluid.

Nerve Supply. Hilton's law (8), the fundamental statement regarding the nerve supply to joints, postulates that the nerve trunks supplying joint musculature furnish innervation to skin over the muscle and to the tissues of the joint. Arrays of afferent receptors are found in and near the articular capsule. These provide information regarding the position, movement, and stresses that act on the joint. At least 4 types of receptors have been identified (9). Type I endings (Ruffini type), found in the superficial layers of the fibrous capsule, are slowly adapting mechanoreceptors that provide awareness of joint position and movement, particularly in terms of postural control. Type II endings (Pacinian type), which occur in small groups in the deeper structures of the joint capsule, are rapidly adapting, low-threshold mechanoreceptors that are sensitive to movement and pressure changes within the joint capsule. Type III endings (Golgi type), identical to neurotendinous organs in structure and function, are found in the articular ligaments of the joint. They appear to be high-threshold, slowly adapting receptors that prevent excessive tension and stress on the joint by reflex inhibition of the adjacent musculature. Type IV endings are free terminals of myelinated and nonmyelinated fibers located in the articular capsule, the adjacent fat pads, and around blood vessels of the synovial layer. These endings are high-threshold, slowly adapting receptors that respond to excessive motion or injury, potentially providing a basis for articular pain (9).

Articular Cartilage. Healthy hyaline cartilage is a specialized connective tissue characterized by considerable extracellular matrix composed mainly of proteoglycans, collagen, glycoproteins, other proteins, and water. Proteoglycans are hydrophilic and give compressive strength to the cartilage, whereas collagen functions to provide shape and tensile strength. Chondrocytes are responsible for the homeostasis of the extracellular matrix of articular cartilage. Located at a distance from blood vessels, chondrocytes receive their nutrition via diffusion or convection through the matrix. Although hyaline cartilage is avascular, it is thought to receive nutrients from the synovial fluid during movement and loading of the joint, or may receive nutrients from underlying subchondral bone. Hyaline cartilage is also aneural. Collagen, proteoglycans, other proteins, and glycoproteins represent about 20% of the tissue wet weight; water and inorganic salts constitute the remainder. Maintenance of the water content is critical to the continued resilience and function of the cartilage in terms of joint nutrition and lubrication (4,7,10,11).

Synovial Fluid and Lubrication. Synovial fluid is produced by the cells lining the intima of the synovia and is found in the joint space, within bursae, and in tendon sheaths. It provides a liquid environment for joint surfaces; nutrition to chondrocytes, articular discs, and menisci; and lubrication of the joint surfaces and structures. Because synovium has a rich vascular supply that is fenestrated (has openings), diffusion between the plasma and interstitial spaces can occur. A delicate balance exists between the exchange rate of plasma and synovial fluid, particularly in the medical and rehabilitation treatment of the inflammatory arthritides. Severe impairment of this process can create ischemia, effusion, and increased intraarticular temperature (12).

Joint lubrication is an intricate process. Proposed models have followed engineering physics and attempted to equate the human joint with a hydrodynamic function. Considerable data have shown that the human joint is more remarkable than any hydrodynamic system and that the coefficient of friction is very low in a healthy joint (13). The coefficient of friction is defined as a measure of the energy required to move the joint in proportion to the energy available to do the work of moving the joint. That synovial joints possess a highly effective lubrication system is widely appreciated; however, the mechanics are less well understood. Current descriptions include a component called *boundary layer lubrication*, providing protection against wear, and a second component referred to as *hydrodynamic lubrication* (11,14–16), which contributes to the low friction of the joint during motion.

Reaction of Articular Cartilage to Injury. The response of articular cartilage to injury depends on the type and extent of injury. Synovial joints can develop at least 3 types of articular cartilage defects: 1) age-related superficial fibrillation, 2) cartilage degeneration due to osteoarthritis, and 3) focal chondral and osteochondral defects (17). Superficial cartilage fibrillation occurs in joints with increasing age; however, individuals do not usually experience symptoms or have difficulty with joint function. There does not appear to be a progressive loss of articular cartilage (18). In contrast, the joint degeneration that leads to osteoarthritis consists of a progressive loss of proteoglycans, and hence water, resulting in a loss of compressibility that leads to remodeling and sclerosis of articular cartilage. As the cartilage attempts to repair itself, remodeling and sclerosis of subchondral bone, with subchondral bone cysts, may occur and osteophytes may develop due to endochondral ossification (19). It has also been hypothesized that subchondral lining changes may precede cartilage loss. Focal articular cartilage and osteochondral defects appear to result most commonly from trauma. They occur in adolescents and young adults, and some of these individuals may experience joint pain, effusions, and mechanical dysfunction.

Trauma can result in 3 types of articular cartilage injury: chondral damage without visible tissue disruption, disruption of articular cartilage alone, and disruption of articular cartilage and the underlying subchondral bone (20,21). Injury can cause alterations in the matrix of the articular cartilage that may include a decrease in proteoglycan concentration and possible disruption of the collagen framework (22). If the loss of matrix proteoglycans does not exceed what chondrocytes are able to produce, then the matrix can be restored. However, the collagen meshwork needs to remain intact and enough viable chondrocytes must be present (20,21,23). Without a healthy matrix, the chondrocyte can be exposed to excessive loads, and tissue degeneration occurs (12).

Acute or repetitive trauma can cause focal mechanical disruption of articular cartilage including fissures, chondral flaps or tears, and loss of a cartilage segment. The response of articular cartilage to this type of injury is limited by the lack of blood vessels and cells that can repair significant tissue defects (20,21,23). Chondrocytes respond to tissue injury by proliferation and synthesis of the matrix near the injury. The new matrix and proliferating cells may be unable to fill the defect, and soon after the injury the attempt to heal ceases (18).

If the injury extends into the subchondral bone, hemorrhage and fibrin clot formation may occur with an attendant inflammatory response. Vascular invasion and migration of undifferentiated cells into the clot is stimulated, and within 2 weeks of injury some of these cells assume the rounded form of chondrocytes. These cells produce regions of hyaline-like cartilage in the chondral and bone portion of the defect. The repaired chondral tissue typically has a composition and structure intermediate between hyaline and fibrocartilage; it rarely, if ever, has the elaborate structure of normal articular cartilage. Occasionally the repaired cartilage persists unchanged or progressively remodels to form a functional joint surface, but in most large subchondral injuries the chondral repair tissue begins to show degeneration within a year (18).

Intraarticular Menisci. Not all diarthrodial joints have menisci; however, when present, menisci differentiate into fibrocartilage during embryonic development. Menisci may have a free inner border (as in the knee joint) or they may traverse the joint, dividing it into 2 separate synovial cavities (as in the sternoclavicular joint). The functions of intraarticular fibrocartilage include absorbing shock, improving fit between articulating surfaces, improving the mechanics of movement, checking translatory motions of joints, deploying weight over a large surface, and dissipating the synovial fluid throughout the joint space (4).

Surface Shape and Topology. Some synovial joints have 2 articulating surfaces forming simple articulations. In this case, one surface is convex in shape and the other is concave, as in the metacarpophalangeal (MCP) joint. Joints such as the elbow are compound articulations, because there are 2 convex surfaces (capitulum and trochlea) that articulate with 2 concave surfaces (radius and ulna). Furthermore, in the elbow the circumference of the convex radial head articulates with the concave radial notch of the ulna. Joints like the knee, which contain an intracapsular disc or meniscus, are complex articulations (4).

The general shape of synovial joints has been classified into 7 different categories (Figure 1). *Plane or gliding joints* are articulations between almost flat surfaces, such as between the carpal or tarsal bones. *Ginglymi or hinge joints* resemble a hinge and are restricted to one plane of motion, as demonstrated by the interphalangeal joints. *Trochoid or pivot joints* are also uniaxial; however, these rotate around a longitudinal axis, as in the case of the radial head and ulnar notch, or the atlas around the dens of the axis. *Bicondylar joints*, such as the knee, have 2 convex condyles that articulate with 2 concave surfaces. *Ellipsoid joints* are oval and convex. They articulate with an elliptical concave surface, as in the radiocarpal or MCP joints. *Sellar or saddle joints* are concavoconvex surfaces, meaning that both a convex and a concave surface are found on the articulating surfaces. The carpometacarpal joint of the thumb is an example of a sellar joint. *Spheroidal or ball and socket joints* are formed by a spherical surface directed into a cup-like articulating surface, as seen in the hip and shoulder joints (3,4).

TENDONS, LIGMENTS, APONEUROSES, AND FASCIA

Tendons

Tendons, which attach muscles to bones or aponeuroses, are composed largely of collagen fibers. They are somewhat flexible, resist overstretching, and are white in color due to their low density of vascular supply. The anatomic site of tendon attachment to bone is called an *enthesis*, where collagen fibers of the tendon undergo a transition to fibrocartilage and become continuous with the Sharpey's fibers of the bone. Sharpey's fibers anchor tendons, ligaments, and the periodontal membranes of the teeth by becoming buried in bones (7). Entheses can become inflamed in the spondyloarthropathies.

The blood supply to tendons is sparsely provided by small arterioles that run parallel to the adjacent musculature and intercommunicate freely. Vena communicantes and lymphatic vessels accompany these arterioles. Although the metabolism of tendinous tissue is low, it increases in reaction to injury or insult, but repair is almost exclusively due to proliferation of fibroblasts associated with collagen fibers (4,7). Tendons severed in accidents heal very well with proper surgical management and rehabilitation.

The nerve supply to tendons appears to be mostly afferents, and there is no clear evidence of vasomotor control. Specialized neurotendinous endings called Golgi tendon organs are localized, particularly at the myotendinous junction.

Bursae are present where tendons are deflected around bones or pass under a retinaculum near a joint. The bursa is a simple, flattened sac of synovial membrane supported by dense regular connective tissue. It decreases friction by allowing complete freedom of movement over a limited range. Each bursa contains a lubricating film of synovial fluid. Most bursae occur between tendons and bones, tendons and ligaments, or between tendons.

Tendon synovial sheaths occur where tendons would otherwise rub against bone or other friction-generating surfaces. They are arranged in a closed double-walled cylinder, separated by a thin film of synovial fluid. The inner sheath attaches to and encloses the tendon. The external layer attaches to the neighboring connective tissue structures, allowing the surfaces to glide easily past one another in healthy tissues.

The tendon's primary function is to attach muscle to bone and to transmit tensile loads from muscle to bone during joint movement. The tendon guides the muscle belly to maintain optimal distance from the joint center during movement. Viscoelastic properties give tendons a tensile strength that is greater than necessary during normal movement. The tensile strength is similar to that of bone—about half that of steel. A tendon of 1 cm^2 cross-sectional area can support 600–1,000 kg of weight. During muscle contraction, tendons become elastic and can have considerable contractile energy transferred to them during movement (24).

During normal activity, a tendon is subjected to less than one-fourth of its ultimate capacity to handle tension (25). Aging, disease, trauma, medications, mobilization or immobilization, and pregnancy are a few of the factors that can affect the ability of both tendons and ligaments to accomplish their tensile responsibilities.

Ligaments

Ligaments attach one bone to another and often are thickenings of the joint capsule. Like tendons, ligaments are dense, regular connective tissues of sparsely vascularized collagenous tissue. Ligaments also undergo transition into fibrocartilage and attach to the bone, forming an enthesis.

The collagen arrangement in ligaments is aligned parallel and straight, restricting elongation and lending stability and protection from abnormal motion or force. A minor amount of elasticity is present in the collagen fibers of ligaments, which allows some deformation and then return of the fiber to the original position. Excessive or prolonged elongation may impair the ability of the ligament to return to its original position, thus compromising joint stability.

Aponeuroses

Aponeuroses are flat sheets of densely arranged collagen fibers showing a surface iridescence when newly exposed. Aponeuroses usually consist of several layers, with the fasciculi of fibers arranged parallel within one layer but inclined in a different direction in subsequent layers. Typical examples are the aponeurosis forming the sheath of the rectus abdominis muscle and the iliotibial band of the thigh. Smaller aponeuroses are found in the palm of the hand and on the plantar surface of the foot. The aponeurosis of the rectus sheath houses the muscle and serves as a midline attachment for the other abdominal musculature. The iliotibial band lends support laterally to the integrity of the hip and the knee. The palmar aponeurosis is important to the arches of the hand; similarly, the plantar aponeurosis is important to the bony arches of the foot.

Fascia

Fascia can describe a variety of connective tissues large enough to be seen with the unaided eye. Typically, fascia forms the enveloping fibers of muscles, nerves, and tendons, and sheaths between whole muscles, viscera, and skin. Superficial fascia is found below the dermis and serves as an insulator. It also connects the skin to deeper structures. It sometimes contains muscle fibers, for example the muscles of facial expression. It is distinct and of variable thickness over the anterior abdominal wall, the limbs, and the perineum. Fascia tends to be thinnest over the hands and feet, at the side of the neck, around the anus, and over the penis and scrotum. It is particularly dense in the scalp, palms, and soles.

Deep fascia forms intermuscular septa that separate muscles or groups of muscles while connecting extensively to bone. Sometimes the deep fascia becomes specialized into localized transverse thickenings and is attached at both ends to local bony prominences, such as the transverse carpal ligament that helps form the carpal tunnel.

BONE

The skeletal system provides a rigid framework for support and weight bearing. In addition, it forms a lever system to which muscles attach and provides smooth, polished surfaces for joints. Other functions include protection for vulnerable viscera; formation of hematopoietic tissue for production of erythrocytes, granular leukocytes, and platelets; and storage of calcium, phosphorus, magnesium, and sodium.

Cells and the Intercellular Substance of Bone

In order to appreciate how bone develops, it is important to understand the duties and functions of the cells and intercellular substance of bone. Bone is a living tissue. Modeling and remodeling occurs in healthy bone and requires healthy cells and a healthy environment. Osteogenic (bone-producing) cells lie on the deep layers of the periosteum and endosteum of bone. The periosteal membrane covers the outer surface of the bone, except where there is hyaline cartilage. Comprising an outer fibrous coat and an inner cellular coat of osteogenic cells, this membrane is highly vascularized with vessels that enter and leave the nutrient foramen of the bone. Myelinated and nonmyelinated neural fibers accompany the arteries, some of which are nociceptors.

The endosteum lines the inner spaces of the marrow cavity, spaces of cancellous bone, and the canals of compact bone. Large multinucleated cells called *osteoclasts* are scattered along the inner layer of these membranes and function to resorb bone. During growth, the osteoclasts of the endosteum widen the marrow cavity. After growth, the endosteum becomes a resting membrane unless a fracture or change in hormonal levels occur, requiring an increase of osteoclast production.

Osteoblasts, derived from osteogenic cells, synthesize and secrete the organic matrix of bone around their cell processes to form canaliculi and future osteons (the basic unit of bone, also known as a Haversian system). When mature, osteoblasts become osteocytes that reside in the lacunae of bone and maintain bone metabolism. Their osteocyte–osteocyte junctions appear to maintain the integrity of the bone matrix, which is composed of collagen fibers and an amorphous ground substance containing water, glycoproteins, and inorganic materials of calcium, phosphate, fluoride, magnesium, and sodium (4,7).

Bone Remodeling and Healing

Remodeling of bone occurs in response to 1) change in type or amount of physical stress, 2) fractures, or 3) rheumatic disease. The phenomenon of bone deposited in sites subjected to stress and reabsorbed in sites where there is little stress is known as Wolff's Law. This is exemplified by marked cortical thickening on the concave side of a curved bone. The trabeculae align along the lines of weight-bearing stress in the internal architecture of the bone.

Bone healing consists of several phases that occur concurrently: inflammation, soft callus formation, hard callus formation, and remodeling. *Soft callus* is the term given to soft, collagenous, revascularizing, osteogenic tissue that unites the bone fragments and from which bone regenerates. In primary bone healing, new Haversian systems or osteons are regenerated across the site of the fracture. Osteoclasts assemble at ends of the Haversian canals near the fracture site forming spearheads or cutting cones, which advance at a rate of 50–80 μm per day across the fracture, enlarging the canals as they advance. These are closely followed by osteoblasts, which form new Haversian systems in the enlarged canals and cross the fracture site to link bone fragments. The entire process takes about 5 or 6 weeks; however, any major surgical intervention increases the trauma to the tissues and may prolong the healing process (4,7). Excessive motion at the site or an infection may also prolong healing.

Comparison of Cartilage and Bone

Like cartilage, bone consists of cells and an organic intercellular matrix, which in turn consists of collagen fibers embedded in an amorphous component. The osteocytes of bone, like the chondrocytes of cartilage, live in lacunae within a matrix. Just as a cartilage structure is covered with *perichondrium*, the outer surface of bone is covered with a membrane called *periosteum*. Finally, bone tissue, like cartilage, develops from a mesenchymal model (4).

Unlike cartilage, however, bone is a highly vascular, living, constantly changing, and mineralized connective tissue. It is remarkable for its hardness, resilience, characteristic growth mechanisms, regenerative capacity, and its stone-like resistance to bending during weight-bearing. Although all bone consists of cells embedded in an amorphous and fibrous organic matrix permeated by inorganic bone salts, its fine structure varies widely with age, site, and natural history. Thus, bone may develop either by the direct transformation of condensed mesenchyme, or it may be preceded by a cartilaginous model, later replaced by bone. The inorganic matrix may exist as irregular, dense masses with scattered bone cells, or it may be arranged as a series of thin sheets (lamellae) in a variety of patterns, with intervening rows of bone cells. Both lamellar and nonlamellar bone often develop as minute rough cylindrical masses or *osteons*, each with a central vascular canal.

Bone nutrition differs from that of cartilage. If the lacunae in which osteocytes live were solidly calcified, no diffusion of nutrients could occur. The osteocytes would die just as chrondrocytes die if the matrix surrounding them becomes calcified. Microscopic evidence shows that osteocytes in calcified bone are connected to each other and to a canal, or to some other surface where there is tissue fluid, by what appears as fine lines. These lines, called *canaliculi*, are tiny tubular passageways through the calcified matrix. They contain tissue fluid and hair-like cytoplasmic processes of osteocytes that connect osteocytes together. Canaliculi provide the means for nutrients to reach osteocytes, thus keeping them alive within a calcified matrix (7).

SKELETAL MUSCLE

Muscle fibers are the cellular units of skeletal muscle and are bound by a plasma membrane called the *sarcolemma*. This membrane encloses numerous nuclei and a large amount of cytoplasm called *sarcoplasm*. Groupings of muscle fibers (fasciculi) vary in size and pattern depending on the muscle. Connective tissue sheaths surround different components of the muscle, including the delicate network between muscle fibers termed the *endomysium*; a stronger *perimysium* ensheathing individual fascicles of muscle fibers; and *epimysium*, which encases the entire muscle and is continuous with the perimysium and the connective tissue external to the muscle.

Skeletal muscles vary considerably in size, shape, fascicular architecture, type of fiber, and attachment to bone. Each muscle is composed of numerous longitudinal cylindrical myofibrils, which provide range, direction, velocity, and force of action appropriate to the particular joint. Myofilaments of actin and myosin are located on the myofibrils, forming serial units called *sarcomeres* visible only with an electron microscope. Sarcomeres are considered the functional unit of skeletal muscle.

Contraction and Relaxation

Individual muscle fibers demonstrate differences in their rates of contraction, development of tension, and susceptibility to fatigue. All of these are characteristics that classify muscle fibers according to the type of metabolic and contractile properties they display (26–28). Three fiber types have been identified: type I, slow-twitch oxidative fibers; type IIA, fast-twitch oxidative-glycolytic fibers; and type IIB, fast-twitch glycolytic fibers. Type I fibers are characterized by a relatively slow contraction time and have a high potential for aerobic activity. Very difficult to fatigue, type I fibers are capable of prolonged, low-intensity work. Myoglobin content is high in these fibers, giving the muscle a distinct red color.

Type IIA muscle fibers have a fast contraction time, providing a moderately well-developed capacity to do both aerobic and anaerobic work. Possessing a well-developed blood supply, they can maintain contractile activity for relatively long periods as long as the rate of activity does not exceed the ability of the fiber to utilize adenosine triphosphate (ATP). Once exceeded, the muscle will fatigue. Myoglobin content is fairly high in this muscle type; therefore, it is often classified as red muscle.

Type IIB fibers contain very little myoglobin and are often referred to as white muscle. These fibers rely primarily upon glycolytic (anaerobic) activity for ATP production. Very few capillaries appear in the vicinity of these fibers. Although type IIB fibers can produce energy rapidly, they fatigue quickly as their high rate of ATP utilization depletes glycogen needed for their metabolism. These large muscles can produce considerable tension for a short period of time before they fatigue (26–28).

The innervation to the muscle fiber determines the type it will become; thus, each motor unit innervates a single type of muscle fiber. The fiber composition of a muscle depends on the function of that muscle. The soleus muscle of the calf is an example of a muscle with a high percentage of type I fibers, which are necessary in a postural muscle. Muscles that perform both endurance and strength activities are generally composed of a mixture of the 3 fiber types. Controversy exists as to whether fiber types are genetically determined.

The most widely held theory of muscle contraction is the sliding filament theory proposed by Huxley et al (29) and refined by others (30,31). As proposed, muscle contraction requires the sarcomere to actively shorten due to the movement of actin and myosin filaments past one another in response to a variety of stimuli. Wilkie (32) described the activity of the actin and myosin during muscle contraction to be "similar to a man pulling on a rope hand over hand."

Once the motor neuron has initiated an action potential along the sarcolemma, an orderly sequence of events occurs. From the sarcolemma, the action potential proceeds through the T-tubule system to the sarcoplasmic reticulum, resulting in the release of calcium into the sarcoplasm. Calcium concentrations increase, causing release of actin. This allows actin and myosin cross-linkages or bridges to proceed, leading to shortening of the myofilaments. Shortening continues until the calcium source is actively pumped back into the sarcoplasmic reticulum, thus breaking the cross-linkages between actin and myosin and allowing the muscle to relax. Both contraction and relaxation of the muscle are active processes.

Energy Metabolism

Energy for cross-linkage between actin and myosin is provided in the form of hydrolysis of ATP to diphosphate $(ADP+P_1)$ by an ATPase. The splitting of ATP releases energy for the mechanical work of moving the actin filaments along the myosin filaments. Once ATP is hydrolyzed, the remaining ADP and free phosphate leave the binding site on the myosin. ATP provides the energy required to release a contraction of the myofilaments. The muscle relaxes when new ATP is bound to the myosin, promptly disassociating actin from myosin by breaking the cross linkage. Absence of ATP would result in permanent bonding between actin and myosin, as seen in rigor mortis.

JOINT MECHANICS AND MOVEMENT

A classification scheme for the shape of synovial joints is shown in Figure 1. Movement of joints is often taken for granted, and the complexity for accomplishing movement not consciously considered. Kinesiology and biomechanics have become intricate and complex sciences made more intriguing when a joint has been affected by a rheumatic disease. The study of the structure, function, and movement of joints is called *arthrokinesiology*.

Fundamental Joint Positions

Joint surfaces are capable of becoming fully congruent with each other at some point in the movement of the joint. At this juncture, the soft tissues around the joint become elongated, tense, and slightly stretched.

One example occurs during full extension of the knee and is called the *close-packed position* of the knee. No further intrinsic motion can occur and an excessive external force applied to the knee may disrupt tissues. Close-packing is the terminal limiting position of the joint; any further attempt to increase motion will be resisted by reflex protective contraction of the associated muscles around the joint. Excessive close-packing can cause deformation of the ligaments and joint structures, including the articular cartilage.

When the joint capsule is lax and the articular surfaces are not congruent, the joint is said to be in the *loose-packed position*. In mid-position of the range of motion, capsules are lax enough that an external force to the knee may allow separation of the bony surfaces. This concept is the basis for using mobilization techniques to increase the motion of a joint following knee surgery, for example. Furthermore, the loose-packed position allows normal movement to occur in joints. Thus, loose-packed positions are important for joint mobility, whereas close-packed positions are necessary for joint stability (3,4).

Kinematics

The study of the motion within the joint or between bones is called kinematics, without regard for the force that caused the motion. *Osteokinematics* is a subcategory of kinematics that describes the motion of a rotating bone around an axis that is oriented perpendicular to the path of the moving bone. An example of osteokinematics would be a description of the relationship between the femur and the tibia when the knee is flexed or extended. Another way of describing the osteokinematics of bone is by linkages. An open kinematic chain describes the relationship of a moving distal bone to a proximal stable bone (foot and tibia moving on a stable femur). A closed kinematic chain describes the relationship of a proximal moving bone to a distal stable bone (foot and tibia fixed on the floor and femur moving).

Arthrokinematics describes the motions occurring within the joint or between joint surfaces. In the case of the knee, the femoral condyles, tibial plateaus, and patella are related to each other during these motions. Because the femoral condyles are smooth and rounded, while the tibial plateaus are more flattened with a meniscus on each, the arthrokinematics of the motions of flexion and extension require the bones to slide, spin, and roll. These intricate movements require the joint to be in loose-packed position.

Kinetics

Kinetics comprises the unique science of biomechanics and describes the forces and torques necessary to cause the joint to move. Active forces are generally produced by muscle contraction. Passive forces may be generated by the intrinsic structures of the joint, such as the joint capsule, ligaments, or other connective tissues. When evaluating joint motion kinetically, consideration must be given to the ability of the muscle to produce force, the integrity of bone and joint structures, the amount of work the muscle can generate, and the power or rate at which the muscle can perform the work. External forces, such as gravity, body weight, and general health of the person, should also be considered.

Types of Movement

There are a variety of descriptions of the movement of joints (Figure 1); however, most joint movement could be considered to be translation, angulation, rotation, and circumduction. Translation (gliding) is sliding without rotation or angulation of the bone. It is a common arthrokinematic motion, which is frequently combined with other motions, such as a spin or rolling, on the joint surfaces. Angulation describes an osteokinematic movement of bones as seen in flexion/extension or abduction/adduction. Rotation is used to describe rotation around the longitudinal axis of a bone, as seen in pronation/supination of the forearm, or internal/external rotation of the glenohumeral joint. Circumduction is commonly ascribed to ball and socket joints that circumscribe their movements in the shape of a cone, combining all of the above motions (3,4).

Axes of Movement

The type and shape of the synovial joint dictate the axes of movement. Axes of movement are usually perpendicular to the moving bone. However, bones have mechanical axes that run perpendicular to the articular center and allow the bone to rotate or spin in such movements as supination and pronation. Uniaxial joints commonly move in 1 plane of motion (sagittal, frontal, horizontal), such as flexion and extension; biaxial joints move in 2 planes, such as flexion/extension and abduction/adduction; triaxial joints move in 3 planes of motion, such as flexion/extension, abduction/adduction, and internal/external rotation; and multi- or polyaxial joints are capable of moving in all planes of motion, usually resulting in circumduction (4).

SUMMARY

Successful management of the joint impairment caused by rheumatic diseases can be enhanced if the health provider appreciates fully the intricate nature of the structures of the musculoskeletal system. Beyond the effects of rheumatic disease on the musculoskeletal system, considerations should also be given to the effects of age, medications, exercise history, and environment in which the person with arthritis must function. Understanding human movement involves integrating the knowledge of the anatomy, biomechanics, and arthrokinesiology of the musculoskeletal system; the attributes of the specific rheumatic disease and its impact on these structures; and an appreciation of the personal performance attributes and attitudes of the person with arthritis.

REFERENCES

1. Larsen WJ. Development of the limbs. In: Larsen WJ, editor. Human embryology. New York: Churchill-Livingstone; 1993. p.281–307.
2. Viidik A. Biomechanics and functional adaptation of tendons and joint ligaments. In: Evans FG, editor. Studies on the anatomy and function of bones and joints. Berlin: Springer-Verlag; 1966. p. 17–39.
3. Norkin C, LeVange P. Biomechanics. In Norkin C, LeVange P, editors. Joint structure and function: a comprehensive analysis. Philadelphia: FA Davis; 1992. p. 3–51.
4. Williams PL, Warwick R, Dyson M, et al. Skeletal system. In: Williams PL, Warwick R, Dyson M, Bannister LH, editors. Gray's anatomy. 38th ed. Edinburgh: Churchill-Livingstone; 1995. p. 425–736.
5. Smith JW. Muscular control of the arches of the foot in standing: an electromyographic assessment. J Anat 1954;88:152–63.
6. Key JA. The reformation of synovial membrane in knees of rabbits after synovectomy. J Bone Joint Surg 1925;7:793–813.
7. Ham AW, Cormack DH. Histophysiology of cartilage, bone and joints. Philadelphia: JB Lippincott; 1979.
8. Hilton J. Lecture VII. In: Jacobson WHA, editor. On rest and pain: a course of lectures on the influence of mechanical and physiological rest in the treatment of accidents and surgical diseases, and the diagnostic value of pain. New York: William Wood; 1879. p. 96.
9. Wyke B. The neurology of joints: a review of general principles. Clin Rheum Dis 1981;7:223–39.

10. Myers ER, Mow VC. Biomechanics of cartilage and its response to biomechanical stimuli. In: Hall BK, editor. Cartilage. Vol. 1. Structure, function and biochemistry. New York: Academic Press; 1983. p. 313–41.

11. Mow VC, Proctor CS, Kelly MA. Biomechanics of articular cartilage. In: Nordin M, Frankel VH, editors. Basic biomechanics of the musculoskeletal system. 2nd ed. Philadelphia: Lea & Febiger; 1989. p. 5–8.

12. Simkin PA. The musculoskeletal system. A. Joints. In: Schumacher HR, Klippel JH, Koopman WF, editors. Primer on the rheumatic diseases. 10th ed. Atlanta: Arthritis Foundation; 1993. p. 5–8.

13. Charnley J. The lubrication of animal joints. In: Proceedings of the Symposium on Biomechanics. London: Institution of Mechanical Engineers; 1959. p. 12–9.

14. McCutcheon CW. Boundary lubrication by synovial fluid: demonstration and possible osmotic explanation. Fed Proc 1966;25:1061–8.

15. Swann DA, Radin EL, Hendren RB. The lubrication of articular cartilage by synovial fluid glycoproteins [abstract]. Arthritis Rheum 1979;22:665–6.

16. Swann DA, Silver FH, Slayter HS, Stafford W, Shore E. The molecular structure and lubricating activity of lubricin isolated from bovine and human synovial fluids. Biochem J 1985;225:195–201.

17. Mankin JH, Buckwalter JA. Restoring the osteoarthritis joint. J Bone Joint Surg Am 1996;78:1–2.

18. Buckwalter JA. Articular cartilage: injuries and potential for healing. J Orthop Sports Phys Ther 1998;28:192–202.

19. Buckwalter JA, Mankin HJ. Articular cartilage. II. Degeneration and osteoarthrosis, repair, regeneration and transplantation. J Bone Joint Surg Am 1997;79:612–32.

20. Buckwalter JA, Rosenberg LA, Hunziker EB. Articular cartilage: composition, structure, response to injury, and methods of facilitation of repair. In: Ewing JW, editor. Articular cartilage and knee joint: basic science and arthroscopy. New York: Raven Press; 1996. p. 19–56.

21. Buckwalter JA, Rosenberg LC, Coutts R, et al. Articular cartilage: injury and repair. In: Woo SL, Buckwalter JA, editors. Injury and repair of the musculoskeletal soft tissue. Park Ridge (IL): American Academy of Orthopaedic Surgeons Symposium; 1988.

22. Buckwalter JA. Mechanical injuries of articular cartilage. In: Finerman G, editor. Biology and biomechanics of the traumatized synovial joint: the knee as a model. Rosemont (IL): American Academy of Orthopaedic Surgions Symposium; 1992. p. 83–96.

23. Buckwalter JA, Mow VC. Cartilage repair in osteoarthritis. In: Moskowitz RW, Howell DS, Goldberg VM, Mankin HJ, editors. Osteoarthritis: diagnosis, medical and surgical management. Philadelphia: WB Saunders; 1992. p. 71–107.

24. Carlstedt CA, Nordin M. Biomechanics of tendons and ligaments. In: Nordin M, Frankel VH, editors. Basic biomechanics of the musculoskeletal system. 2nd ed. Philadelphia: Lea & Febiger; 1989. p. 59–74.

25. Kear M, Smith RN. A method for recording tendon strain in sheep during locomotion. Acta Orthop Scand 1975;46:896–905.

26. Astrand P-O, Rodahl K. Textbook of work physiology: physiological basis for exercise. 2nd ed. New York: McGraw Hill; 1977.

27. Engel WK. Fiber-type nomenclature of human skeletal muscle for histochemical purposes. Neurology 1974;25:344–8.

28. Huxley AF. Muscular contraction. J Physiol 1974;243:1–43.

29. Huxley AF, Huxley HE. Organizers of a discussion of the physical and chemical basis of muscular contraction. Proc R Soc Lond B Biol Sci 1964;160:433–7.

30. Huxley HE. The mechanism of muscular contraction. Science 1969;164:1356–66.

31. Weber A, Murray JM. Molecular control mechanisms in muscular contraction. Physiol Rev 1973;53:612–73.

32. Wilkie DR. The mechanical properties of muscle. Br Med Bull 1956;12:177–82.

Immunity: Recognition, Response, and Recall

A. BETTS CARPENTER, MD, PhD; as updated by MARK J. SOLOSKI, PhD

The immune system evolved to recognize and respond to a wide array of pathogens, including viruses, bacteria, fungi, protozoans, and helminthes. To do this, a complex set of molecules and cells evolved that are capable of specifically recognizing foreign pathogens and then evoking a response that will limit pathogen growth and spread, as well as ensure pathogen clearance. In addition, this first exposure to the foreign pathogen is remembered so that subsequent encounters evoke a quicker and more robust response. The immune system is crucial to our survival because defects in immunity lead to significant morbidity and mortality.

The immune response has 2 major components: innate and adaptive immunity. Innate immunity is the general rapid-response arm (minutes to hours) that serves to provide an immediate limit to the growth and spread of pathogens. In contrast, the adaptive immune response usually takes days to emerge, is highly specific, and is responsible for the complete (sterile) clearance of the pathogen.

The adaptive immune system involves 2 major cell types, B and T lymphocytes that mediate *humoral* and *cellular immunity*, respectively. B lymphocytes produce antibodies that serve to bind and neutralize foreign substances called *antigens*. Antibodies can be found in the serum following antigen exposure, and one can transfer antibody-mediated immunity from one individual to another through serum or plasma. T lymphocytes carry out several functions, including the release of soluble mediators that "help" B cells produce antibody and cytotoxicity toward pathogen-infected cells. Cellular responses are transferred via cells, and are mainly involved with immunity against fungi, parasites, and intracellular bacteria (1–4).

INNATE IMMUNITY

Pattern Recognition Receptors, Neutrophils, and Macrophages

The elements that make up the innate response include natural barriers, such as epithelium, secretions, and respiratory cilia, all of which serve to prevent pathogens from entering the host. When these barriers are breeched, cellular elements of the innate immune system become activated. These cells include neutrophils and macrophages that express a unique class of surface molecules called *pattern recognition receptors* (PRRs).

Monocytes/macrophages and neutrophils are the major phagocytic cell types (1,3). *Monocytes* circulate in the peripheral blood and once they localize to the tissues, they are called *macrophages* or histiocytes. Neutrophils are the other major phagocytic cell (2,5). They comprise the major population of white cells in the peripheral blood (up to 80%). Neutrophils are formed in the bone marrow from myelocytic precursors and are terminally differentiated, living only 1–2 days after reaching the peripheral blood. They have a multilobed nucleus and a variety of storage cytoplasmic granules containing digestive enzymes that break down phagocytized particles. Neutrophils and macrophages provide one of the first lines of defense against foreign invaders, and they are one of the first cell populations present in tissues with an acute infection. They mediate their effects via phagocytosis and the release of granules (5–8).

PRRs are surface proteins that bind to and recognize structures uniquely expressed by pathogens but not present on host cells (9). The unique structures are referred to as *patterns associated with microbial pathogens* (PAMPs) and frequently are molecules essential for pathogen survival. For example, lipopolysaccharide (LPS) found as a major component of the cell wall of gram-negative bacteria is recognized by toll-like receptor 4, a PRR expressed on macrophages and neutrophils. Several families of PRRs recognize a wide range of PAMPs, including bacterial flagellin, glycolipid components of cell walls, double-stranded RNAs found during viral infection, and novel carbohydrate structures. These PRRs serve as early sensors of the presence of a pathogen and trigger the activation of macrophages and neutrophils. Once activated, these cells actively phagocytize pathogens and release granule contents. These events lead to the destruction of the pathogen through the action of antimicrobial substances and lysosomal enzymes.

The Complement System

The complement system is composed of a complex group of serum proteins and is important to both innate and adaptive immunity (1,3). Complement proteins are found in the serum and are normally inactive. When these proteins are activated through proteolysis, they mediate a number of immunologically relevant effects, which include 1) the disruption of cellular membranes where complement proteins have been deposited; 2) the generation of inflammatory mediators that recruit inflammatory cells (neutrophils and macrophages) to the sites of infection or tissue damage; and 3) the aid in removal of foreign pathogens by increasing the efficiency of phagocytosis through opsonization.

The complement system can be activated by 3 different mechanisms, all of which involve the recognition of foreign structures on cell surfaces (10). The 2 systems most relevant for the innate response are the specific binding of the mannose binding lectin (MBL) or the serum protein factor B to bacterial cell surfaces through the recognition of novel carbohydrate structures found only on bacterial surfaces. Once MBL binds, other serum complement proteins (C2 and C4) are attracted, activated via proteolysis, and interact with protein C3 to form an enzymatic complex, which leads to the deposition in the cell membrane of the terminal components of the system (C5–C9) and the formation of the membrane attack complex (MAC). The MAC mediates target cell lysis by intercalating into the lipid bilayer membrane and forming lytic pores allowing for the passage of water into the cell and subsequent cell lysis. The deposition of factor B on the cell surface likewise leads to the formation of a MAC through a different pathway that does not involve C4 or C2. Instead, factor B interacts with other serum factors (D, H, and P) that leads to C3 activation, the deposition of C5–C9, and the formation the MAC. The activation of complement through factor B has been termed the alternative complement pathway.

The specific binding of antibody to cell surfaces can also activate complement. This has been referred to as the classical pathway since it was the first discovered. The classical pathway is activated when IgG and IgM antibodies bind an antigen-forming immune complex. This frequently occurs at the surface of foreign cells and leads to the binding of the unique classical pathway component, C1. C1 and MBL are structurally similar and both lead to the activation of C2 and C4, which, as described above, leads to the formation of the MAC. The classical complement pathway is a major effector mechanism of antibody-mediated immunity because it allows the destruction of antibody-coated microbes and the recruitment of inflammatory cells to sites of inflammation.

The process that leads to the formation of the MAC involves a series of proteolytic steps that generates protein fragments that have potent immunologic effects. Fragments C5a and C3a are anaphylatoxins that cause release of histamine and other vasoactive inflammatory mediators from mast cells. In addition, C5a attracts and activates neutrophils. C3b—bound to the surface of microorganisms—binds to receptors on macrophages and neutrophils and promotes phagocytosis. Complement also improves clearance of immune complexes by enhancing the action of phagocytic cells.

Activation of the complement system plays an important role in the host response to infection (10). The complement system also plays a role in the initiation and progression of several rheumatic diseases (11). For example, >50% of patients with deficiencies of the complement proteins C2 and C4 have systemic lupus erythematosus (SLE). Also, serum levels of complement components can be decreased in individuals with persistent immune activation or inflammation. Serum levels of C3 and C4 often correlate with disease activity in SLE, with lower levels indicating immune complex activation and consumption of complement proteins.

THE ADAPTIVE IMMUNE SYSTEM

B Lymphocytes and Antibody Production

Antibodies (also called immunoglobulins) are produced by a specialized population of bone-marrow–derived cells called B lymphocytes (1–4). Antibodies recognize a wide variety of foreign antigens, including proteins, carbohydrates, lipids, and nucleic acids, and are a critical component of the adaptive immune response to foreign pathogens.

All immunoglobulins have a basic overall structure consisting of least 2 heavy chains (with a molecular weight of 50,000–70,000) and 2 light chains (with a molecular weight of 23,000) that form a Y-shaped divalent structure (Figure 1). Part of each chain is highly conserved from molecule to molecule and is referred to as the *constant (C) region.* In contrast, the amino-terminus (~100 amino acids) can vary considerably from molecule to molecule and is called the *variable (V) region.* Within the variable region, there are areas with high amino-acid variability, the *hypervariable regions.* The variable region is the part of the immunoglobulin molecule involved in antigen binding and the hypervariable regions frequently dictate binding specificity. The carboxy terminus of the heavy and light chains is the highly conserved C region and is involved in other activities of the immune system, such as binding complement component C1 or interacting with immunoglobulin-binding receptors.

The expression of surface immunoglobulin is acquired during the development of B cells in the bone marrow (12). The full-length heavy and light chains are generated by piecing together several mini-gene segments to generate a single functional gene that encodes the full-length heavy and light chains with V and C regions. The process by which these mini-gene segments are pieced together involves the breaking and rejoining of chromosomal segments, which is called gene rearrangement. This *immunoglobulin gene rearrangement* process is tightly regulated, only occurring during B-cell development and can generate a diverse (10^6–10^9) array of immunoglobulins with different

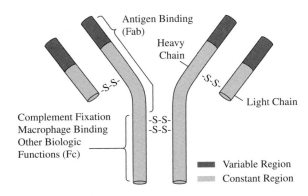

Figure 1. Antibody structure. Reprinted from the Clinical Slide Collection on the Rheumatic Diseases, copyright 1995 by the American College of Rheumatology.

antigen-binding potentials. The rearrangement process is regulated so that only 1 immunoglobulin receptor is expressed on a mature B lymphocyte. This arrangement ensures that only those B cells with the ability to bind antigen will become activated following an encounter with foreign antigen. This is called antigen-driven *clonal selection* (see Figure 2).

There are 5 major classes of immunoglobulins: IgM, IgG, IgA, IgE, and IgD, each with distinctive structures and functions. The major structural feature that distinguishes the immunoglobulin classes is the sequence of the heavy-chain C region. Thus, the heavy chain of all IgMs will have identical heavy-chain C regions but will be different from the C regions found in others classes (IgG, etc.). IgM has a pentameric structure containing 5 individual antibody molecules held together by a J (joining) chain. IgM is the first antibody produced upon exposure to foreign antigen and can interact with complement components most efficiently. IgG is the most abundant immunoglobulin in the serum. In the initial encounter with antigen, IgG antibody levels lag behind IgM but upon a secondary exposure, IgG is the dominant form of antibody produced. IgG can engage immunoglobulin receptors on phagocytes and mediate the uptake of bound antigen. IgA is found in highest levels in mucosal compartments and is highly concentrated in tears, saliva, bronchial secretions, breast milk, intestinal fluids, and other body fluids. IgA is predominantly produced by B cells located within mucosal compartments. IgE is important in triggering allergic reactions and is thought to play a role in responding to parasitic infections. IgD is the least well-understood form of immunoglobulin. IgD has the lowest serum concentration and is predominately coexpressed with IgM on the mature B-cell surface and may have a role in regulating B-cell activation.

Upon first exposure to an antigen, a mature resting B cell responds by proliferating and differentiating into an antibody-producing *plasma cell* that synthesizes a soluble form of its immunoglobulin receptor. Plasma cells are the primary source of antibodies found in serum and other bodily fluids. Upon the first exposure to antigen (primary response), antigen-activated B cells differentiate to produce soluble IgM. This initial activation requires T lymphocytes (discussed below) that "help" B cells become activated. Following activation, some B cells will change the type of immunoglobulin they produce from IgM to another form (IgG, IgA, etc.). This is called *immunoglobulin class switching* and involves a DNA rearrangement in which the genetic information encoding the antigen-binding heavy-chain V region is translocated adjacent to the genetic information encoding a different heavy-chain C region. This process allows for the synthesis of a new heavy chain that has the same antigen-binding features of the initial

Clonal Selection

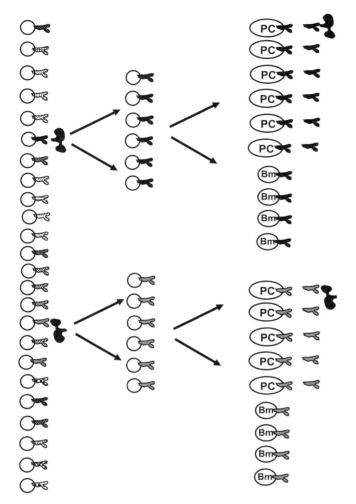

Figure 2. Antigen-driven clonal selection. B Lymphocyte development generates numerous receptor-bearing clones. Those clones with antigen binding receptors are stimulated to expand and differentiate into antibody secreting plasma cells (PCs) or memory B cells (Bm). T cells also undergo a similar antigen-driven clonal selection, differentiating into effector T cells (helper or cytotoxic) and memory T cells.

IgM (V-region identical) but different immunologic properties due to the presence of a new C region.

Upon antigen exposure, some B cells differentiate into antibody-producing plasma cells and others differentiate to form memory cells. These are long-lived cells that allow the immune system to recall and respond quickly to antigen upon repeat exposure. These memory B cells are responsible for the long-term efficacy of vaccines.

T Lymphocytes

T lymphocytes compose the other major lymphocyte population of the adaptive immune system (1–4). T-cell precursors are initially produced in the bone marrow and then fully develop in the thymus, thus the term **T** lymphocytes. Mature T cells produce soluble factors termed *cytokines*, which are important mediators. T cells serve a number of important functions, including providing "help" to B cells, but also display cytotoxic activity toward pathogen-infected cells and tumor cells.

T cells express a surface-antigen receptor that resembles immunoglobulin, but it differs in several features. First, the T-cell antigen receptor is monovalent—consisting of disulfide-bonded alpha and beta chains. The alpha and beta chains each have an amino-terminal V region and a carboxy-terminal C region; as with immunoglobulin, the V region is involved in antigen recognition. As with the immunoglobulin receptors on B cells, the T-cell antigen receptor is clonally distributed, and expression is acquired during development in the thymus. The T-cell antigen receptor is built using a gene rearrangement process analogous to that used in B cells, but the genetic elements used are separate and distinct. Also, analogous to B cells, T-cell receptor genes are rearranged only during thymic T-cell development. T-cell antigen receptors do not undergo class switching nor is there a soluble secreted form of the T-cell antigen receptor.

Antigen recognition by T cells is distinct from that of B cells. First, although binding native antigen can activate B cells, T-cell activation requires the presence of another cell type to properly display the antigen on its cell surface for recognition. This cell type is termed an *antigen presenting cell* (APC) and several cell types can serve as APCs, including dendritic cells, macrophages, and B cells. Second, T cells do not recognize native antigen, instead they recognize short 8–20 amino-acid peptide fragments. These peptides are generated from the intact antigen after it is internalized by the APC. Inside the APC, the antigen undergoes processing that involves proteolytic breakdown of the whole antigen into fragments. These peptide fragments are then displayed on the surface of the APC bound to a protein product of the major histocompatibility complex (MHC) (Figure 3). The MHC is a complex set of genes that encodes protein products involved in the presentation of peptide antigens to T cells. It is the complex of peptide bound to an MHC protein product that is recognized by the T-cell antigen receptor. Because of this novel recognition feature, T-cell recognition is frequently referred to as "*dual-specific*" (recognizing 2 elements) or *MHC restricted* (13).

T cells, Antigen Presentation, and Function

T cells perform several functions, including cytotoxicity and providing help to B cells. It turns out that these 2 distinct functions are carried out by separate subpopulations of T cells and these subsets can be identified by the expression of cell-surface structures recognized by monoclonal antibodies. All mature T cells express the CD3 molecule. T cells involved in B-cell help express CD4, whereas cytotoxic T cells express CD8. Both CD4 and CD8 T cells are crucial in the body's defense against infectious agents. The role of CD4 cells is especially highlighted in acquired immunodeficiency syndrome, in which depleted CD4 cells cause a profound immunodeficiency. CD8 cells have an important role in lysis of pathogen-infected cells and in killing of tumor cells. Both CD4 and CD8 cells produce soluble factors called *cytokines*, which are important mediators (1,3).

The human MHC is a group of closely related genes on human chromosome 6, which encodes proteins important in the immune system (14–16). The protein products of these loci are called human leukocyte antigens (HLA); there are 2 types of MHC proteins involved in T-cell recognition, termed class I and class II molecules. Class I molecules are expressed on the surface of virtually all nucleated cells and present peptide antigens to CD8-cytolytic T cells. Class II antigens are more limited in their cellular distribution to B cells, macrophages, dendritic cells, and other professional APCs. Class II molecules present peptide antigens to CD4 T cells. Class I and class II molecules are expressed on the surface of cells associated with peptides. In the absence of a pathogen or foreign antigen, the MHC-bound peptides are derived from self-proteins, and this may be important in the maintenance of

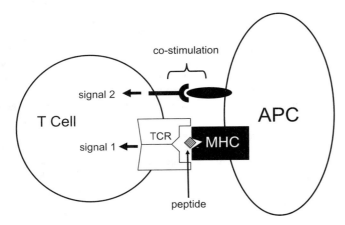

Figure 3. T-cell recognition. The T-cell antigen receptor (TCR) recognizes a complex of peptide antigen bound to a major histocompatibility complex (MHC) molecule. T-cell activation requires 2 signals, one through the TCR and the other through the interaction of costimulatory molecules.

self-tolerance (see below). However, when foreign proteins gain access to APCs (i.e., during an infection), peptides from these molecules are presented on the cell surface (1,3).

T cells are only activated when they encounter the proper peptide/ MHC complex expressed on mature APCs, usually located in the lymph node or spleen. For a T cell to become fully activated, there are 2 signals that need to be received. Signal 1 is generated through the T-cell receptor by recognition of the peptide/MHC complex and signal 2 involves the interaction of a receptor on the T cell (CD28) with a ligand (CD80/86) expressed on the APC. This second signal is frequently called the *costimulatory signal* and is only provided by mature APCs. This is an important site of regulation for a T-cell response, because if a T cell receives only signal 1, the T cell will shut down into an inactive state called *anergy* (17).

Dendritic cells (DCs) are considered the most potent APC and can be found in an immature and mature state. Immature DCs reside in peripheral tissues where they sample the environment through active phagocytosis and express PRRs on their surface (18). When a pathogen enters the tissue, immature DCs actively internalize the pathogen and become activated via signals generated through the PRRs. When activated, the immature DC begins a maturation process involving cessation of phagocytosis, increased processing and presentation of internalized antigens, trafficking to T-cell rich areas in the draining lymph nodes, and upregulation of genes encoding costimulatory molecules. The result is the arrival in the lymph node of a mature DC expressing processed pathogen-derived antigens in the context of MHC and capable of providing signals 1 and 2 to antigen-specific T cells.

Genetics of the MHC and Autoimmune Disease

The HLA-encoded class I and class II molecules are highly polymorphic, meaning that there are many allelic variants within the population. Interestingly, there are no mutant or wild-type forms of class I or II molecules (19). Instead, this variation evolved in response to pressure exerted by pathogens. The region of MHC molecules that exhibits amino-acid sequence polymorphisms are clustered toward the amino-terminus in the part of the molecule involved in binding peptide antigens. As a result, each MHC molecule has the ability to bind a unique set or group of peptides. For example, if a large protein is processed into 20 peptides, only 1 or 2 will bind to one MHC molecule, whereas

different sets will bind to other MHC molecules. Because humans are heterozygotes, we have a maternal and paternal MHC and within each MHC are several class I and II genes. The result is that each individual displays a number of different MHC proteins, all of which are capable of binding different set of peptides, thus allowing a wide range of peptide antigens to be seen by CD4 and CD8 T cells. This natural polymorphism of MHC molecules is thought to offer the host a great advantage in responding to foreign pathogens.

The natural polymorphism of MHC proteins has other important medical implications. In fact, the MHC was initially described as driving graft rejection and it is the MHC difference between donor and recipients that are major barriers in tissue and organ transplantation. In addition, several MHC alleles have been associated with disease. As a result, typing individuals for the MHC class I and II alleles they carry is a very common test in modern medicine. *HLA typing* is now accomplished using molecular approaches from patient DNA samples employing specific DNA probes or using polymerase chain reaction-based technology.

We now know that there are a variety of autoimmune diseases associated with MHC. One of the strongest links is between the autoimmune disease ankylosing spondylitis and the HLA class I allele HLA–B27. Although >90% of Caucasian patients with ankylosing spondylitis have HLA–B27, only a small percentage of individuals with HLA–B27 actually have ankylosing spondylitis. The remainder of disease associations are with class II molecules, primarily with the HLA–DR. Associations with various rheumatic diseases are listed in Table 1. The significance of an HLA disease association is generally expressed using relative risk, which is defined as the risk of an individual with the particular HLA allele of developing the disease as compared with the risk for an individual without the allele. For example, an individual with HLA–B27 is 90 times more likely than someone who is HLA–B27 negative to develop ankylosing spondylitis. The relative risks listed in Table 1 are reported as a range of figures representing data from numerous studies. HLA–B27 is also associated with Reiter syndrome; however, the association is not as strong (16).

Molecular DNA typing of the class II molecule HLA–DR4 has led to the identification of a common amino-acid sequence among rheumatoid arthritis (RA) patients, termed the *shared epitope* (20). Studies have shown that patients who receive 2 copies of the epitope (one from each parent) have more severe disease (20).

When examining the association of HLA and disease, there are several caveats. First, HLA disease associations are neither sufficient nor necessary for the development of a particular disease. Autoimmune disease causation is multifactorial and involves HLA genes, non-HLA genes, and environmental factors. For example, a mouse model of lupus found >20 non-HLA genes important in disease susceptibility and in human lupus, 9 non-HLA loci have been linked to disease development (21). Association with a particular HLA antigen may not be with the gene itself, but the actual disease-associated gene could be a non-HLA locus that is closely linked to the MHC. It must be emphasized that possession of a particular HLA allele is not diagnostic of a particular disease; it simply means that an individual has an increased risk for developing a particular disease. Many of the HLA associations are based on epidemiologic data from large groups of individuals, and they may not significantly affect individual patients. With the mapping of the human genome and the explosion of our knowledge of genetics, information that is more definitive will be available in the near future. Routine DNA typing of patients with rheumatic diseases is controversial at present. As additional information is gained, this type of testing could become part of routine clinical practice to confirm diagnosis and provide additional information regarding prognosis.

Table 1. Association of human leukocyte antigens with rheumatic diseases.*

Disease	HLA antigen	Relative risk
AS	HLA–B27	69–90
RS	HLA–B27	37
RA	HLA–DR4	2.7–6
SS	HLA–DR2	5.2–9.7
	HLA–DR3	3.6
SLE	HLA–DR2	2.3
	HLA–DR3	2.5–5.8

* Data compiled from references 1–3 and 19–21. AS = ankylosing spondylitis; RS = Reiter syndrome; RA = rheumatoid arthritis; SS = Sjögren syndrome; SLE = systemic lupus erythematosus.

Natural Killer Cells

Natural killer (NK) cells are a lymphocyte population distinct from T or B cells (22). They have large cytoplasmic granules and are thus called large-granular lymphocytes. These cells were originally identified based on their ability to kill tumor cells and virus-infected cells. In contrast to the killing by cytotoxic $CD8^+$ T cells, killing mediated by NK cells does not require previous exposure or products of the MHC. NK cells do not express immunoglobulin or T-cell antigen receptors; instead they express activating NK receptors. Activating NK receptors recognize gene products that are silent in normal cells but become expressed when a cell reaches an abnormal state, either due to neoplastic transformation or vial infection. In this manner, NK cells can recognize abnormal cells and exhibit cytotoxicity toward them. In addition, NK cells can interact with antibody-coated tumor cells and kill them in a process called *antibody-dependent cellular cytotoxicity*. The exact role of NK cells in normal immunity has not been unequivocally established. Rare individuals with a deficiency of NK cells have been shown to develop severe viral infections, and genetic evidence has implicated NK cells and their receptors in autoimmune disease.

THE EFFECTOR FUNCTIONS OF IMMUNE CELLS

When an immune cell becomes activated, it turns on a number of new genes and among them are genes encoding cytokines. Cytokines are soluble mediators produced by a variety of cell types (1–4). Most of these substances are produced in very small amounts and either act locally on the cell that produces it, adjacent cells, or distally on other cells and tissues. Cytokines have a wide variety of effects on many cellular functions and cell populations. Their major roles include regulating lymphocyte growth and differentiation, and mediating inflammatory reactions. One major group of cytokines are the interleukins (IL), which are presently numbered 1–33. Some additional cytokines include tumor necrosis factor (TNF) and the interferons. Only some of the cytokines with special relevance to the rheumatic diseases will be discussed.

IL-2 is a crucial growth factor for T cells. Activated T cells produce IL-2, which then acts on the same cell that produced it to further stimulate its growth. It also stimulates the growth of nearby cells. IL-2 has been utilized to grow T cells in the laboratory, furthering our knowledge of cellular interactions. It has also been used therapeutically in some cancers.

Interleukins 4 and 6 are cytokines released by CD4 T cells that function to promote B-cell activation, proliferation, and differentiation into plasma cells. These cytokines play an important role in the ability of CD4 T cells to help B cells.

IL-1 and TNFα are cytokines that differ structurally but have many overlapping physiologic effects. These cytokines are produced by many cell types, including activated phagocytic cells (macrophages). IL-1 and TNFα function as important mediators of the inflammatory response through their ability to increase vascular permeability, leading to increases in fluid and cellular infiltrates in tissue. These cytokines also mediate local tissue destruction and, along with IL-6, can have systemic effects causing fever and inducing the synthesis of plasma proteins called *acute phase reactants*. Acute phase reactants include the third component of complement (C3), C-reactive protein, serum amyloid protein, and haptoglobin. They are increased in a number of circumstances, including infection, neoplasia, burns, trauma, and during immune-mediated tissue damage. Frequently the levels of these proteins are measured to determine whether a patient is undergoing an inflammatory response.

IL-1 and TNFα are particularly important in the pathogenesis of several rheumatic diseases, including RA, causing bone loss, affecting joint cartilage, and inducing changes to joint tissues (1–4,9). As a result, TNFα and IL-1 have been targeted for immunotherapeutic strategies to control immune-mediated tissue destruction. Three TNF antagonists—etanercept, infliximab, and adalimumab—have been approved to treat adults and children with RA and other rheumatic diseases (23,24) (see also Chapter 35, Pharmacologic Interventions: Biologic Agents). Anakinra is a receptor antagonist of IL-1 that blocks signaling through the IL-1 receptor, and has demonstrated efficacy in RA. A number of other cytokines, including IL-6, IL-12, IL-15, and IL-18, are also involved in the inflammatory response and are potential therapeutic targets.

INFLAMMATION

Inflammation is the response of the body to injury or invasion (1–4,25). It is characterized by the movement of vascular fluid and cells from the vessels into the extravascular spaces. The inflammatory response is a complex process initiated by a variety of foreign insults (microbes, altered cells, and foreign particles) and involving a variety of cells and soluble inflammatory mediators. It can be acute or chronic. Acute inflammation often occurs as a byproduct of the initial innate and adaptive immune response to pathogens and can result in tissue injury or damage. It is characterized by a cellular infiltrate, primarily of neutrophils, and subsides when the pathogen is cleared. Chronic inflammatory responses occur later in the immune response, largely in the context of an overwhelming or persistent infection or tissue damage. It is characterized by complex infiltrates of lymphocytes and macrophages.

The classic signs of inflammation include redness, heat, swelling, and pain. These features are due to changes in the endothelial cells lining the vessel walls, allowing for movement of fluid and cells into the extravascular spaces and to the site of injury. The inflammatory cells (neutrophils, platelets, mast cells, eosinophils, basophils, and lymphocytes) release mediators with myriad effects, including an increase in vascular permeability, recruitment of additional cells, contraction of some smooth muscles, and release of additional mediators. Thus, from the initial injurious stimuli, the body responds with an amplifying cascade of events. In most cases, the initial inflammatory response resolves and restores the tissue to normal. However, in a number of pathologic situations, resolution can be slow and chronic, resulting in severe tissue injury. The inflammatory response may become chronic due to characteristics of the inciting agent (persistent, intracellular) or due to host genetic factors (26).

At the core of the inflammatory response are the mediators released from the infiltrating cells. Cytokines play a key role and have been discussed above. Other mediators are preformed and packaged in cytoplasmic granules, and some are formed from the metabolism of membrane phospholipids, such as prostaglandins and leukotrienes. Prostaglandins and leukotrienes have diverse proinflammatory actions, including chemotaxis, smooth-muscle constriction, and vasoactive properties; as such, they are important pharmacologic targets in the control of inflammation. Arachidonic acid is a precursor in the generation of prostaglandins and leukotrienes that is predominantly generated from membrane phospholipids by phospholipase A2 enzymes. Arachidonic acid can then proceed either by the cyclooxygenase pathway to form prostaglandins and thromboxanes or via the lipoxygenase pathway to yield leukotrienes. Nonsteroidal anti-inflammatory drugs (NSAIDs) directly inhibit the cyclooxygenase pathway, thus inhibiting the formation of prostaglandins and thromboxanes.

The cyclooxgenase pathway has been targeted in the design of antiinflammatory drugs. There are 2 distinct enzymes involved in the cyclooxygenase pathway, cyclooxygenase 1 (COX-1) and cyclooxygenase 2 (COX-2); NSAIDs inhibit both of these enzymes (26). A common side effect of NSAID use is gastrointestinal toxicity, which has been found to be mediated primarily by the inhibition of COX-1. Selective COX-2 inhibitors (celecoxib and rofecoxib) have been developed; they have similar antiinflammatory effects, but fewer gastrointestinal side effects (ulceration) than nonspecific COX inhibitors. COX-2 inhibitors have been widely used to treat many rheumatic diseases but their use has been curtailed due to an apparent increased risk of thrombotic cardiovascular events (see Chapter 34, Pharmacologic Interventions: Small Molecules).

AUTOIMMUNITY, THE LOSS OF SELF-TOLERANCE

Autoimmunity is defined as pathologic changes that arise following an immune reaction against autologous (self) antigens (1–4). This loss of self-tolerance results in the production of autoantibodies, the generation of self-reactive T cells, and tissue damage. In many rheumatic diseases, the detection of circulating levels of autoantibodies are useful in diagnosis, following disease activity, and determining prognosis (27). For example, the presence of antibody against double-stranded DNA (anti-dsDNA) in SLE is used for initial diagnosis and may reflect disease activity. Anti-dsDNA immune complexes may be deposited along the glomerular basement membrane in the kidney and along the dermal-epidermal junction in the skin. In some cases, autoantibodies are believed to be an important factor in disease pathology, but in others it is unclear if they initiate disease or develop as a consequence of tissue damage.

Self-reactive B cells are the source of autoantibodies. Consequently, a number of therapies have been developed that selectively deplete or inactivate B cells. For example, CD20 is a cell-surface marker expressed through most of the stages of a B cell's life, lost only after differentiation into a plasma cell. Rituximab is an antibody against CD20 originally developed to treat B-cell lymphomas. Recently, rituximab therapy has been found to be effective in the treatment of RA and is now being examined for its effectiveness in a variety of autoimmune diseases (28). B-cell activating factor (BAFF, also called BlyS) and APRIL are 2 recently discovered soluble factors that play a role in B-cell survival and proliferation. Belimumab is an anti-BAFF monoclonal antibody that has shown promising results in early clinical trials for RA and SLE. BAFF and APRIL mediate their effects by binding to surface receptors. Consequently, soluble forms of these receptors are being tested for their clinical effectiveness. Interestingly, the receptor TACI can bind both BAFF and APRIL; an Ig-fusion protein (TACI-Ig) is being tested for clinical effectiveness because it is predicted to block both activities. For additional information on targeted treatment of autoimmune diseases see Chapter 35, Pharmacologic Intervention: Biologic Agents.

The autoimmune state represents a loss of self-tolerance. During B-cell and T-cell development, a large variety of antigen receptors are generated via the recombination process, some of which react to self-antigens. To prevent self-reactive T and B cells from reaching maturity, each receptor is "tested" for reactivity to self-antigens encountered during cell maturation. For B cells, if surface immunoglobulin expressed by developing B cells recognizes antigens encountered in the bone marrow, the cell dies. In T cells, this occurs during development in the thymus and involves testing T-cell antigen receptors for their ability to recognize self-peptide presented by MHC molecules expressed in the thymus. If receptor engagement occurs, indicating self-reactivity, the developing B or T cell is signaled to undergo cell death. This form of tolerance is termed *central tolerance*, occurring in immature lymphocytes and resulting in the deletion of cells bearing self-reactive antigen receptors (29–31).

A second form of tolerance is termed *peripheral tolerance*. Peripheral tolerance eliminates self-reactive lymphocytes that escaped deletion in the bone marrow or thymus, a necessary mechanism because the bone marrow or thymus does not express the entire repertoire of self-antigens, and thus self-reactive clones would escape central tolerance. Peripheral tolerance occurs among B and T cells, but T-cell peripheral tolerance is best understood. The mechanism of T-cell peripheral tolerance is via the requirement for a second costimulatory signal in addition to the engagement of the T-cell receptor with MHC and antigen. Signals 1 and 2 are provided only by professional APCs. A T cell that receives only signal 1 leads to clonal anergy. In the absence of a foreign antigen, MHC molecules display self-peptides on the surface of non-APCs (epithelial cells, fibroblasts, muscle cells, etc.). Since these cells do not express costimulatory molecules (signal 2), an encounter with a T cell that recognizes self-peptide will result in T-cell inactivation. In this manner, tolerance to tissue-specific self-antigens can be achieved. It is thought that central and peripheral tolerance provide the major mechanisms for preventing self-reactivity. Also, because signal 2 is a major point for control of the T-cell response, molecules involved in this process are targets for immunomodulatory therapy that can potentially lead to downregulation of self-reactive T cells. For example, the interaction between CD28 and CD80/86 is interrupted by a targeted therapeutic agent, abatacept, a compound approved for the treatment of RA. Other second signals may also be engaged that enhance T-cell activation, including the interaction between T-cell CD40 ligand and CD40 expressed on B cells and between leukocyte function antigen-3 on T cells and CD2 expressed on APCs. Agents that act through blockade of these and other costimulatory pathways have been used for other inflammatory diseases.

Autoimmune diseases occur when there is a breakdown of this normally elegant system that controls reactivity against self. An immune response normally designed to control foreign invaders and infected or malignant cells becomes activated toward normally silent self antigens. Given the mechanisms in place to maintain self-tolerance, it is thus unclear by which mechanisms autoimmunity occurs. One explanation is that individuals who develop autoimmune disease have a defect in central or peripheral tolerance mechanisms, allowing self-reactive cells to emerge. Another model proposes that self-tolerance is incomplete, with self-reactive B cells emerging but T-cell tolerance intact. In this case, a self-reactive antibody is not made due to a lack of functional self-reactive T cells to provide B-cell help. In this scenario, autoimmunity occurs when potentially self-reactive T cells, which were initially rendered anergic, are reactivated to provide help to the self-responsive B cells. It has been hypothesized that pathogen-derived polyclonal activators (viral superantigens, bacterial LPS) may contribute to this process. Another model, termed molecular mimicry, predicts that self-reactive T cells arise following stimulation with microbial antigens that structurally resemble self-molecules or modify self-antigens so that they are perceived as foreign (20). Models involving infectious agents are supported by the finding that some forms of inflammatory arthritis (reactive arthritis) develop following infection (32). Also, there are models proposing that tissue injury or inflammation causes the release of normally hidden self-antigens or generation of unique immunogenic fragments of tolerized antigens (such as proposed to occur through peptide citrullination in the pathogenesis of rheumatoid arthritis) (33). Lastly, as discussed in the section on the HLA system, a variety of genetic factors plays a role in the autoimmune system. In summary, no one theory explains all autoimmune diseases; rather, it is likely a complex interplay between environmental factors, including exposure to microbial antigens, in a genetically susceptible host that determines the development of autoimmune disease.

REFERENCES

1. Janeway CA, Travers P, Walport M, Shlomick MJ. Immunobiology: the immune system in health and disease. 6th ed. New York: Garland Science; 2005.
2. Rosen FS, Raif Geha. Case studies in immunology: a clinical companion. 4th ed. New York: Garland Science; 2004.
3. Abbas AK, Lichtman AH, Pober JS. Cellular and molecular immunology. 5th ed. Philadelphia: WB Saunders; 2005.
4. Abbas AK, Lichtman AH. Basic immunology: functions and disorders of the immune system. 2nd ed. Philadelphia: WB Saunders; 2006.
5. Bogdan C, Rollinghoff M, Diefenbach A. Reactive oxygen and reactive nitrogen intermediates in innate and specific immunity. Curr Opin Immunol 2000;12:64–76.
6. Aderem A, Underhill DM. Mechanisms of phagocytosos in macrophages. Annu Rev Immunol 1999;17:593–623.
7. Gompertz S, Stockley RA. Inflammation: role of the neutrophil and the eosinophil. Semin Respir Infect 2000;15:14–23.
8. Dahlgren C, Karlsson A. Respiratory burst in human neutrophils. J Immunol Methods 1999;232:3–14.
9. Janeway CA Jr, Medzhitov R. Innate immune recognition. Annu Rev Immunol 2002;20:197–216
10. Walport MJ. Complement. N Engl J Med 2001;344:1058–66, 1140–4.
11. Manderson AP, Botto M, Walport MJ. The role of complement in the development of systemic lupus erythematosus. Annu Rev Immunol 2004;22:431–56.
12. Schlissel MS. Regulating antigen-receptor gene assembly. Nat Rev Immunol 2003;3:890–9.
13. Hennecke J, Wiley DC. T cell receptor-MHC interactions up close. Cell 2001;104:1–4.
14. Salazar M, Yunis EJ. MHC: gene structure and function. In: Frank MM, Austen KF, Claman HN, Unanue ER, editors. Samter's immunologic diseases. 5th ed. Boston: Little, Brown; 1995. p. 101–16.
15. McDevitt HO. Discovering the role of the major histocompatibility complex in the immune response. Annu Rev Immunol 2000;18:1–17.
16. Kwok WW, Nepon GT. Genetic influences: major histocompatibility complex. In: The autoimmune diseases. 3rd ed. New York: Academic Press; 1998. p. 75–84.
17. Schwartz RH. T cell anergy. Annu Rev Immunol 2003;21:305–34.
18. Mellman I, Steinman RM. Dendritic cells: specialized and regulated antigen processing machines. Cell 2001;106:255–8.
19. ParhamP, Adams EJ, Arnett KL. The origins of HLA-A,B,C polymorphism. Immunol Rev 1995;143:141–80.
20. Rose NR. Infection, mimics, and autoimmune disease. J Clin Invest 2001;107:943–4.
21. Wakeland EK, Liu K, Graham RR, Behrens TW. Delineating the genetic basis of systemic lupus erythematosus. Immunity 2001;15:397–408.
22. Yokoyama WM, Kim S, French AR. The dynamic life of natural killer cells. Annu Rev Immunol 2004;22:405–29.
23. Hehlgans T, Pfeffer K. The intriguing biology of the tumour necrosis factor/tumour necrosis factor receptor superfamily: players, rules and the games. Immunology 2005;115:1–20.
24. Zwerina J, Redlich K, Schett G, Smolen JS. Pathogenesis of rheumatoid arthritis: targeting cytokines. Ann N Y Acad Sci 2005;1051:716–29.
25. Kupper TS. Immunity and inflammation in cutaneous tissues. In: Frank MM, Austen KF, Claman HN, Unanue ER, editors. Samter's immunologic diseases. 5th ed. Boston: Little, Brown; 1995 p. 353–62.
26. Robinson DR. Inflammation. In: Hochberg MC, Silman AI, Smolen JS, Weinblatt MH, editors. Rheumatology. 3rd ed. New York: Mosby; 2003. p. 147–158.
27. Plotz PH. The autoantibody repertoire: searching for order. Nat Rev Immunol 2003;3:73–8.
28 Browning JL. B cells move to the centre stage: novel opportunities for autoimmune disease treatment. Nat Rev Drug Discov 2006;5:564–76.
29. Basten A. Basis and mechanisms of self-tolerance. In: Rose NR, MacKay IR, editors. Autoimmune diseases. 3rd ed. New York: Academic Press; 1998:9–28.
30. Goodnow CC. Balancing immunity and tolerance: deleting and tuning lymphocyte repertoires. Proc Natl Acad Sci U S A 1996;93:2264–71.
31 Hogquist KA, Baldwin TA, Jameson SC. Central tolerance: learning self-control in the thymus. Nat Rev Immunol 2005;5:772–82.
32 Kim TH, Uhm WS, Inman RD. Pathogenesis of ankylosing spondylitis and reactive arthritis. Curr Opin Rheumatol 2005;17:400–5.
33. Duan-Porter WD, Casciola-Rosen L, Rosen A. Autoantigens: the critical partner in initiating and propagating systemic autoimmunity. Ann N Y Acad Sci 2005;1062:127–36.

Effective Patient–Provider Communication for Rheumatic Diseases: The First Step in Providing Patient-Centered Care

MAURA D. IVERSEN, PT, DPT, SD, MPH

The study of provider–patient communication began around the turn of the century by medical sociologists who posited that the provider–patient relationship can and should be viewed through a social system framework (1) wherein expectations, perceptions, social roles, and awareness of social factors (e.g., culture, education) influence the dynamics of the interaction (1–3). Later, application of a social-psychological perspective was adapted to analyze interactions and recommend behaviors to improve communication (3).

From the 1930s to 1970s, analysis of the patient–provider relationship focused on the physician–patient interaction. Research has since expanded to include all health care provider communication. What we have learned over the past 90 years is that provider–patient communication is complex and it influences adherence and health outcomes (see Figure 1). We recognize that language conveys content, describes reality, and informs clinical decision making. In this chapter, I review the functions and models of communication in the clinical encounter, discuss what is known about the impact of communication on health outcomes in arthritis, address issues related to specific populations, and present strategies for effective communication.

FUNCTIONS OF COMMUNICATION IN CLINICAL ENCOUNTERS

Communication is the process by which we educate patients and identify and achieve health care goals. Effective provider–patient communication helps providers establish rapport (4), collect information to formulate an accurate diagnosis and prognosis (5,6), elicit patient preferences for treatment and outcomes (7,8), and obtain informed consent (9). Communication aids in mutual decision making (10), improves patient understanding of their disease and treatment (11), increases satisfaction with care (12,13), impacts adherence (14), and improves health outcomes (5,15). Research demonstrates that aspects of verbal communication, such as the tone, content, word emphasis, and pattern of talk, influence the manner in which information is conveyed and received (15–17).

Although most providers recognize that communication and counseling are essential components of patient care, many feel unprepared for or uncomfortable providing patient counseling (18,19). Successful communication is achieved when providers understand patients' need for information, their expectations of and preferences for care, and desire for involvement in decision making (20,21).

MODELS OF PROVIDER–PATIENT COMMUNICATION

Models of provider–patient communication reflect the social context of our society and advancements in medicine (1–3). These models are based on 4 essential tasks of the clinical encounter: cognition and information processing, interpersonal interaction, conflict resolution, and identification of social influences (15,22,23). The paternalistic model views the provider as the expert who makes decisions on behalf of the patient. This model ignores the autonomy of the patient and the patient's nonhealth issues and values. This model is considered outdated (10) because patients are now presented with an array of interventions, and society stresses patient autonomy and participation in decision making.

Other models have emerged. In the contractual model, the doctor and patient "contract" for each other's mutual benefit. This model emphasizes patient and provider autonomy and mutual decision making but ignores the relationship aspect of the provider–patient encounter (15). The shared decision-making model describes the patient and provider as partners in the development of a plan of care. This model shares many similarities with the patient-centered approach to medical care, but also emphasizes active patient participation in decision making (10). In this model, providers are expected to elicit patient preferences for treatments, share information, build consensus, and mutually develop goals for care. Although decision-making preferences vary by patient (24), patients report greater satisfaction and are more likely to adhere to treatments when they engage in decision making and express their concerns (8,10,17,25).

WHAT IS KNOWN ABOUT PROVIDER–PATIENT COMMUNICATION?

Provider Factors

A variety of provider factors influence the provider–patient interaction, such as interpersonal style, clinical training, sex, personality, race, and cultural background. These factors combine to influence the clinician's verbal and nonverbal communication (15).

Interpersonal style influences the frequency and type of nonverbal behaviors expressed by providers. Nonverbal behaviors convey emotions and can reinforce or hinder communication (15,26). Encouraging nonverbal behaviors include sitting with arms open, making eye contact, leaning toward patient, and head nodding. Examples of hindering behaviors include sitting with arms crossed across the chest, leaning away from the patient, looking at the clock, and taking calls during the visit (16). To determine physicians' ability to detect and interpret nonverbal behaviors, DiMatteo and colleagues gave physicians a standardized test of ability to interpret nonverbal cues (26). Physicians' ability to interpret nonverbal cues varied. Patients of physicians who scored higher on the test were more satisfied with their care and more adherent with their appointment schedules.

Clinical training influences verbal communication. Emphasis is placed on developing clinical information rather than teaching interpersonal behaviors that promote empathy, establish rapport, and show

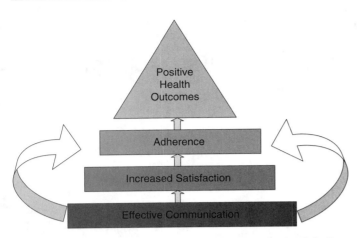

Figure 1. Influence of effective communication on patient satisfaction, adherence and improved health outcomes.

respect for patient values (27). Students are taught to ask questions and mentally categorize information to form clinical decisions. This process emphasizes more provider talk rather than active listening in the encounter (27–29). Studies show that patients are frequently interrupted during the clinic visit (29,30). Marvel and colleagues noted that 72% of the physicians they studied interrupted their patients within the first 23 seconds of the interview (28). Yet, when patients were allowed to express their concerns without interruption, they only required 6 additional seconds. Providers who interrupt patients develop less accurate clinical diagnoses (29) and report more patients who present clinical concerns as they exit the office (28). Training also reinforces the use of medical jargon, which can alienate patients and lead to misunderstandings and poor adherence (31). Clinicians who use a paternalistic model of communication have less satisfied patients and patients who are less adherent (15,18,22,31).

Sex, a frequently studied factor, influences discussion. On average, female clinicians provide more counseling (15,22) and use more behaviors that demonstrate sensitivity than men (32). For example, female providers are more likely to talk about emotional and psychosocial topics, spend more time with their patients, engage in partnership building, and use more positive verbal and nonverbal behaviors than male doctors (33,34). The use of these behaviors is associated with greater satisfaction and adherence and improved health outcomes (15,22,32,33,34).

Another factor influencing communication is the extent to which the provider likes the patient (13,15). Rheumatology health care providers are human and naturally have preferences for different personality characteristics. They do not like all their patients to the same degree. Research demonstrates that patients, in turn, are quite accurate in determining if they are liked. Furthermore, patient satisfaction and patient's desire to change physicians correlate with the degree to which the physician likes the patient (13).

Patient Factors

Health status, attributions, ethnicity and social factors, expectations and preferences, literacy, self-efficacy, age, and sex are some of the patient factors that influence the clinical discussion (15). Unfortunately, the likelihood a provider stereotypes a patient increases when the provider is stressed, under time constraints, and multitasking—typical features of a clinic visit (35).

Research indicates that sicker patients are less satisfied with their physicians than their healthier counterparts (36). Patient dissatisfaction may result from the patient's poor health status and negative outlook on life, leading to more negative discussion and impacting the provider–patient relationship. Alternatively, Hall and colleagues tested the hypothesis that physician styles of communication differ with sicker patients (36). Their study supports the hypothesis that patient dissatisfaction results from the provider's use of negative behaviors, such as engaging in less social conversation with sicker patients.

Patients' attributions, or models of disease that are developed to help explain symptoms, affect their clinical discussions. Attributions help patients understand and describe their disease and symptoms, aid in their understanding of how their bodies work, and are influenced by ethnic and cultural beliefs, social networks, and the mass media (18,36). These beliefs influence how information is interpreted, what they recall from the discussion, and how they respond to clinical advice (18).

Ethnicity and culture influence the manner in which patients present and emphasize symptoms (15,36,37). Some ethnic groups are very vocal about their pain symptoms and use this as a means of dissipating anxiety associated with pain. Other ethnic groups tend to minimize pain reporting in an effort perhaps to cope with or deny pain, or because discussing pain is not deemed culturally acceptable (15,36,38). Unless providers are aware of the impact of cultural, ethnic, and social influences on the presentation of symptoms, clinical symptoms may be misinterpreted, particularly when these issues are compounded by language barriers (15,36–38). Sleath and Rubin described the influence of patient sex and ethnicity on physician—patient communication about depression (39). A total of 383 primary care patient visits were audiotaped and transcribed. Physicians were more likely to ask Hispanic patients and those patients who rated their health as poor about anxiety (39). Cultural and ethnic factors also influence disease management strategies and adherence (37,40,41). In a study among Chinese immigrants diagnosed with arthritis, Chinese medicine was viewed as more effective than Western medicine for chronic conditions such as arthritis (42).

Literacy impacts clinical communication and health outcomes (42). A recent study of literacy in patients with rheumatoid arthritis indicated that 1 in 6 patients was illiterate and had significantly more hospital visits (43). Patients with low literacy tend to have poor health, poor understanding of treatment, greater use of health services, and low adherence to treatment regimens (42–44). Patients with low literacy rely heavily on oral explanations, visual clues, demonstrations of tasks, or a friend or family member to interpret and learn material (18). To increase patient comprehension during the visit, providers should use simple language and avoid medical jargon (42,44). Research indicates that the provision of written information and instructions that are culturally sensitive and relevant (written at the 5th to 8th grade reading level with illustrations to convey culturally sensitive issues) are most effective (18,36,42,43). Providers should also be aware that the presence of a third person (e.g., significant other or family member) or interpreter can sometimes reduce discordance but it could also increase discordance between the provider and patient (45).

Self-efficacy, an individual's situation-specific confidence in carrying out a task, is an important patient characteristic affecting clinical discussions (18). Self-efficacy has been strongly correlated with health behavior and positive health outcomes (22). Therefore, it is important to elicit a patient's self-efficacy for undertaking the plan of care.

The explosion in technologic advances has impacted provider–patient communication and adherence to treatments. Patients receive health information from a variety of sources and may not be able to distinguish the quality of the information (46). One in 4 patients with arthritis reported they searched the Internet for information about their diagnosis, medications, and alternative treatments; and nearly one-third stated the process was easier than seeking information from the health care provider (18). Rheumatology health care providers need to recognize the influence of electronic information and assist patients in

Table 1. Suggestions for effective communication with older adults

- Reduce or minimize background noise and maintain visual contact.
- Keep language simple and avoid medical jargon.
- Rephrase rather than repeat sentences—this will help you determine whether the problem is a conduction issue or comprehension issue.
- Pause at the end of a topic before beginning a new topic.
- Elicit patient preference for participation in decision making.
- Evaluate role of caregiver in interview—if obstructionist then conduct interview independently.

evaluating this information. A recent pilot study evaluating the use of e-mail communication between primary care providers and patients found patients allocated to the e-mail group were more satisfied with their care than the group that did not use e-mail; furthermore, they felt this mode of communication was more convenient (47).

Communication between health care providers and older adults differs from communication with young persons and may be complicated by a variety of factors, including the presence of multiple comorbidities, preferred models of discussions, health literacy, and ageist attitudes (15). Visual changes, such as reduced acuity, contrast sensitivity, visual fields, and glare intolerance, increase with age and sensorineural hearing loss is present in 70–80% of adults aged 70 years and older (48). To increase comprehension, providers should increase the volume of their voice, allow pauses between topics, and rephrase rather than repeat statements to reduce patient frustration and enhance understanding (49) (Table 1).Health literacy decreases with age in patients who are 65 years and older, so written materials should be clear, concise, and written in plain English (42,44). In addition, font sizes of 14–16 are easier to read given the visual changes these patients experience.

Older adults tend to be less consumeristic (interested in seeking information and questioning medical advice) than younger patients and providers, leading to differing interactions in the clinical encounter (15,49). Concordance between patients and providers on the disease progression, symptom presentation, and impact of impairments is necessary for effective decision making and selecting appropriate interventions (10). Unfortunately, research indicates there is less concordance between providers and patients on topics and goals of the clinical discussion, and older patients, on average, are less involved in decision making (4,49,50).

Ageist attitudes may not be overt. For example, providers may trivialize problems presented by older patients or may recommend less aggressive interventions because they unconsciously attribute these symptoms to the natural aging process (49). Finally, ~20–50% of older adults have another person or caregiver present during the clinical encounter (50). Although the presence of a third person may facilitate communication, there is a chance this person may also inhibit information sharing. It is important to evaluate the role of the third person in the interview and determine whether the presence of this person is a help or hindrance.

Interaction of Provider and Patient Factors

Studies indicate that the female–female dyad in the provider–patient relationship tends to correlate with more positive discussion, greater use of open-ended questions, and discussion of psychosocial issues, whereas the male–male dyad is the least likely to demonstrate these behaviors (15,33). Why do these differences occur? Some speculate that patient expectations of communication styles in male and female providers influence the manner in which they communicate in the clinical encounter. The providers then react to this pattern of behavior, producing these sex-based differences in discussion (33).

Communication is a dynamic process, so the manner in which each participant behaves will, in turn, influence the other's response. For example, when prescribing steroids, the provider may approach the discussion by listing the side effects and benefits of the drug. Alternatively, the provider may initiate the discussion with a question such as, "I am recommending you start taking a steroid, what do you think this about drug?" The latter approach will result in quite a different discussion from the first approach because the provider is attempting to elicit patient understanding and attributions of the drug, which are factors known to influence adherence.

Patients' needs for information and participation in decision making are not always recognized (15,18,51). Failure to elicit patient expectations, beliefs, and attitudes toward treatments and to negotiate treatment alternatives impacts satisfaction and outcomes of care (5,22,28,51,52). Even patients who would rather be passive are more satisfied with their physician when they participate more fully in negotiations about treatments (10).

COMMUNICATION STUDIES IN PERSONS WITH ARTHRITIS

Most studies of provider–patient communication have been conducted in primary medicine and oncology practices. In this section, I highlight some recent work conducted in the arthritis field.

Research demonstrates that patients often do not state their expectations in the clinic visit without rheumatology health care providers actively exploring these issues (53,54). Research also shows that providers may be unaware of the psychosocial issues impacting their patients (22,55). As a result, patients' expectations are not always met (54,55). Rao et al conducted a survey of rheumatology patients to examine whether patients' expectations were met during their clinical encounter (21). In this study, 58% of patients reported unmet expectations. Forty-seven percent stated their expectations for general information were not met and 31% stated their expectations for new medications were not met. Patients were 5.6 times more likely to report unmet expectations if they had shorter visits. Expectations of treatment also impact functional outcomes. In a study examining patient expectations of surgery for lumbar spinal stenosis, patients' expectations were found to be significant predictors of self-reported pain relief and function 6 months postoperatively (56). When patient expectations for pain relief and function were not met, they reported poorer outcomes. Patient perspectives and attitudes align with their satisfaction with care (57).

Patients seek reassurance from their rheumatology health care providers to alleviate fears. A qualitative study of 35 patients seen at a rheumatology clinic was conducted to determine which techniques providers use to reassure their patients, patients' perceptions of reassurance, and how these techniques impacted patients (53). Researchers interviewed patients prior to their visit, audiotaped clinical discussions, and conducted followup interviews. Patients interpreted physician reassurances in the context of their own views and perceptions of illness and did not always interpret doctors' statements about the nonserious nature of the disease correctly. When patients perceived their concerns were properly addressed, they felt more reassured. A recent qualitative study of patients with inflammatory and noninflammatory disease identified 2 major themes as important to these patients: to be seen and to be heard. Among patients with noninflammatory disease, this meant they wished to receive an explanation for their symptoms. Among patients with inflammatory arthritis, these themes referred to the need to be seen as an individual and for their doctors to believe their reports of pain and suffering (58).

Patients and providers often hold differing preferences and opinions about treatments and need for referrals (22,56,59). In a study examining how rheumatologists and their patients discuss exercise in the clinical encounter, 25 rheumatologists and 132 patients were enrolled and their discussions audiotaped. Seventy patients discussed exercise with their rheumatologist and 18 received an exercise prescription. When the rheumatologist initiated the exercise discussion, patients were 4 times more likely to receive a prescription for exercise (60).

Physicians may not be aware of their patients' lack of understanding regarding treatments and how to adhere to the plan of care. Patients not only need to know why they are taking medications, they require information on how to take it properly and whether a latency period exists before the drug takes effect. In a study of patients who were new to a rheumatology clinic, 15% failed to understand the purpose of their prescriptions (22). Patients forget about half the instructions provided in the clinical encounter (18). Actively engaging patients in clinical discussions can improve adherence and may impact morbidity (21,47,61).

Communicating with Parents and Children with Arthritis

Confronting chronic illness at an early age affects development. Clinical discussions in the context of treating a child with arthritis are complex (62). Rheumatology health care providers are confronted with patients' perspectives and roles in the discussion, the child's agenda (which may or may not be aligned with that of the parents), and their own perspectives on treatment and role (63) (Figure 2). Often, providers are uncertain regarding their ability to manage shared decision making with parents and the child, especially in the face of the changing needs of the child and parents over time (64–66). The clinical discussion is driven by developmental issues, the child's competency, and such social determinants as organizational and legal influences (62).

Children with chronic illness differ from their healthy counterparts. These children report more age-related concerns (e.g., weight issues) than their healthy counterparts, participate in exercise less frequently, and report higher levels of fatigue (67). In a prospective study designed to assess perceptions of quality of life in children with chronic disease, 181 parents and children and their doctors were enrolled. The children were admitted to the hospital with complications from cystic fibrosis, acute lymphatic leukemia, asthma, or juvenile arthritis. The study

demonstrated that pediatricians and parents differed in their perceptions of the child's health and wellbeing at diagnosis and at followup. The greatest differences were found in reports of emotions (range 28–85% agreement) and child's pain and discomfort (range 11–33% agreement). In this study, pediatricians repeatedly under-reported the child's pain and discomfort compared with parents' reports, despite a prolonged parent–provider relationship (68).

A number of strategies have been developed to improve communication with and assessment of a child during the clinical encounter. A few are presented here. Drawing and writing activities are helpful to ascertain the child's understanding of the disease, particularly in young children (69). Collective versus individual models of shared decision making and information sharing can improve communication. When children are allowed to set the agenda, information sharing is enhanced (70). Another option to help children formulate their thoughts and share information is the use of group discussions (62). These techniques combined with strategies discussed earlier can result in improved information sharing, adherence, and satisfaction with care.

CAN COMMUNICATION SKILLS BE LEARNED?

Communication styles can be learned (Table 2). In a review of provider–patient communication studies in chronic disease, including arthritis, Suarez-Almazor found providers can be trained, irrespective

Table 2. Tips for effective communication

DO:
- Remember, communication issues are not the result of poor patient communication but reflect relationship issues between the patient and provider.
- Encourage patients to write down their concerns prior to the visit and bring the list to the visit.
- Elicit fears and concerns about treatments and assess patient's understanding of the treatment plan.
- Ask the patient about their preferred role in decision making.
- Elicit patient understanding of the disease, their expectations, and confidence in managing symptoms and adhering to the plan of care.
- Explore social supports, physical environment, and family influence; identify whether these factors promote or hinder patient adherence; and develop plans to address these factors.
- Negotiate and develop an individualized plan of care.
- Tailor education to specific needs of the patient (and family in the case of a child with juvenile arthritis).
- Set achievable and measurable goals with the patient.
- Ask the patient about adherence to the intervention; do not assume the patient plans to adhere.
- Provide patients with external resources (Arthritis Foundation, self-help programs, etc).
- Provide a written plan for behavior change and reinforcements.
- Ask patients to describe for you what they believe is causing their symptoms and how their medication helps control symptoms.
- Explain the purpose, dosage, side effects, and how to judge effectiveness of treatments.
- Summarize information; allow patients to correct misinterpretation.
- Model problem-solving skills.

DON'T:
- Forget patients value communication skills and technical skills.
- Offer advice and reassurance before the main problems have been identified.
- Attend only to physical symptoms.
- Forget that patients forget about half of the information you provide.
- Switch topics on the patient.
- Allow interruptions during the visit.
- Forget to ask about adherence; don't assume patients will adhere.
- Forget to set achievable measurable goals.
- Forget to pay attention to your nonverbal behaviors.

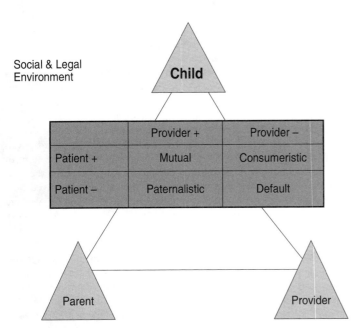

Figure 2. Models of information sharing in the child–parent–provider relationship. Adapted from reference 15.

of years in practice, to provide patient-centered care (71). A variety of techniques have been used to train providers to enhance their communication skills. For example, Fallowfield et al enrolled physicians with variable communication competency levels in a study to evaluate the impact of a training program on communication skills (72). Physicians were videotaped before and 3 days following the training. Trained coders reviewed the tapes and found that communication skills improved, especially with respect to expressions of empathy, responses to patient cues, and use of leading questions (50).

The best method for teaching and learning communication skills is based on the tenants of social cognitive theory (73). A program should include cognitive input, modeling, and practice of communication skills. Detailed information on the communication deficiencies in the clinical encounter, reasons for deficiencies, adverse effects, and how to address prevailing negative attitudes about the use of these strategies should be addressed. Interactive demonstrations, audiotapes, and videotapes all assist in modeling good and bad communication skills (74). Practice with simulated patients is necessary to adopt new skills. Feedback on these simulations should be immediate, constructive, and detailed to highlight activities that may be blocking or encouraging in the clinical discussion.

REFERENCES

1. Henderson LJ. The order of nature. Cambridge (MA): Harvard University Press; 1917.
2. Parsons T. The social system. New York: Free Press; 1951.
3. Szasz TS, Hollender MH. A contribution to the philosophy of medicine: the basic models of doctor-patient relationship. In: Stoeckle, JD, editor. Encounters between patients and doctors: an anthology. Cambridge (MA): The MIT Press; 1987.
4. Charon R., Narrative medicine: a model for empathy, reflection, professionalism, and trust. JAMA 2001;286:1897–1902.
5. Du Pre A. Communicating about health: current issues and perspectives. Mountain View (CA): Mayfield Publishing Co; 2000.
6. Maguire P, Pitceathly C. Key communication skills and how to acquire them. BMJ 2002;325:697–700.
7. Lee SJ, Back AL, Block SD, Stewart SK. Enhancing physician-patient communication. Hematology 2002;1:464–83.
8. Stewart M, Brown JB, Weston WW. Patient-centered medicine. Thousand Oaks (CA): Sage; 1995.
9. Albrecht TL, Franks MM, Ruckdeschel JC. Communication and informed consent. Curr Opin Oncol 2005;17:336–9.
10. Stevenson FA, Barry CA, Britten N, Barber N, Bradley CP. Doctor-patient communication about drugs: the evidence for shared decision making. Soc Sci Med 2000;50:829–40.
11. Morris LA, Kanouse DE. Informing patients about drug side effects. J Behav Med 1982;5:363–73.
12. Bidaut-Russell M, Gabriel SE, Scott CG, Zinsmeister AR, Luthra HS, Yawn B. Determinants of patient satisfaction in chronic illness. Arthritis Rheum 2002;47:494–500.
13. Beck RS, Daughtridge R, Sloane PD. Physician-patient communication in the primary care office: a systematic review. J Am Board Fam Practi 2002;15:25–38.
14. Heidenreich PA. Patient adherence: the next frontier in quality improvement. Am J Med 2004;117:130–2.
15. Roter D, Hall J. Doctors talking with patients, patients talking with doctors: improving communication in medical visits. Westport (CT): Auburn House; 1992.
16. Minden P. The importance of words: suggesting comfort rather than pain. Holist Nurs Pract 2005;19:267–71.
17. Iversen MD, Eaton HM, Daltroy LH. How rheumatologists and patients with rheumatoid arthritis discuss exercise and the influence of discussions on exercise prescriptions. Arthritis Rheum 2004;51:63–72.
18. Daltroy LH, Barclay GR. Health promotion and patient education for people with arthritis. In: Hochberg MC, Silman AJ, Smolen JS, Weinblatt ME, Weisman MH, editors. Rheumatology, 3rd ed. St Louis: Mosby; 2003. p. 361–8.
19. Merkel WT, Margolis RB, Smith RC. Teaching humanistic and psychosocial aspects of care: current practices and attitudes. J Gen Intern Med 1990;5:34–41.
20. Neame R, Hammond A, Deighton C. Need for information and for involvement in decision making among patients with rheumatoid arthritis: a questionnaire survey. Arthritis Rheum 2005;53:249–55.
21. Rao JK, Winberger M, Anderson LA, Kroenke K. Predicting reports of unmet expectations among rheumatology patients. Arthritis Rheum 2004;51:215–21.
22. Daltroy LH. Doctor-patient communication in rheumatological disorders. Baillières Clin Rheumatol 1993;7:221–39.
23. Joos SK, Hickam DH. How health professionals influence health behavior: patient-provider interaction and health care outcomes. In: Glanz K, Levis FM, Rimer BK, editors. Health behavior, health education, 2nd ed. San Francisco: Jossey-Bass; 1990. p. 216–41.
24. McKinstry B. Do patients wish to be involved in decision making in the consultation? A cross sectional study with video vignettes. BMJ 2000;321:867–71.
25. Bauman AE, Fardy JH, Harris PG. Getting it right: why bother with patient-centered care? Med J Aust 2003;179:253–6.
26. DiMatteo RM, Friedman HS, Taranta A. Sensitivity to bodily nonverbal communication as a factor in practitioner-patient rapport. J Nonverbal Behav 1979;4:18–26.
27. Branch WTJ, Kern D, Haidet P, Weissemann P, Gracey C, Mitchell G, et al. Teaching the human dimensions of care in clinical settings. JAMA 2001;286:1067–74.
28. Marvel MK, Epstein RM, Flowers K, Beckman HB. Soliciting the patient's agenda: have we improved? JAMA 1999;281:283–7.
29. Sanson-Fisher R, Fairbairn S, Maguire P. Teaching skills in communication to medical students–a critical review of the methodology. Med Educ 1981;15:33–7.
30. Waitzkin H. Doctor-patient communication: clinical implications of social scientific research. JAMA 1984;252:2441–6.
31. Beckman HB, Frankel RM. The effect of physician behavior on the collection of data. Ann Intern Med 1984;101:692–6.
32. Sleath B, Rubin RH. Gender, ethnicity, and physician-patient communication about depression and anxiety in primary care. Patient Educ Couns 2002;48:243–52.
33. Roter D, Lipkin M Jr, Korsgaard A. Sex differences in patients' and physicians' communication during primary care medical visits. Med Care 1991;29:1083–93.
34. Roter DL, Hall JA, Aoki Y. Physician gender effects in medical communication: a meta-analytic review. JAMA 2002;288:756–64.
35. Committee on Understanding and Eliminating Racial and Ethnic Disparities in Health Care. Institute of Medicine's report. Unequal treatment: confronting racial and ethnic disparities in health care. Washington DC: National Academies Press; 2006.
36. Hall JA, Roter DL, Milburn MA, Daltroy LH. Why are sicker patients less satisfied with their medical care? Tests of two explanatory models. Health Psychol 1998;17:70–5.
37. Betancourt JR, Carrillo JE, Green AR. Hyeprtension in multicultural and minority populations: linking communication to compliance. Curr Hypertens Rep 1999;1:482–8.
38. Baker L, Wagner TH, Singer S, Bundorf MK. Use of the internet and e-mail for health care information: result from a national survey. JAMA 2003;289:2400–06.
39. Cooper LA, Powe NR. Disparities in patient experiences, health care processes, and outcomes: the role of the patient-provider racial, ethnic, and language concordance. The Commonwealth Fund. Accessed June 14, 2006. URL: www.cmwf.org.
40. Kramer BJ, Harker JO, Wong AL. Arthritis beliefs and self-care in an urban American Indian population. Arthritis Rheum 2002;47:588–94.
41. Wong AL, Harker JO, Lau VP, Shatzel S, Port LH. Spanish Arthritis Empowerment Program: a dissemination and effectiveness study. Arthritis Rheum 2004;51:332–6.
42. Zhang J, Verhoef MJ. Illness management strategies among Chinese immigrants living with arthritis. Soc Sci Med 2002;55:1795–802.
43. Rudd RE, Moeykens B, Colton T. Health and literacy: a review of the medical and public health literature. In: Comings J, Garner B, Smith C, eds. Annual review of adult learning and literacy. San Francisco: Jossey-Bass; 2000.
44. Gordon MM, Hampson R, Capell HA, Madhok R. Illiteracy in rheumatoid arthritis patients as determined by the Rapid Estimate of Adult Literacy in Medicine (REALM) score. Rheumatology 2002;41:750–4.
45. Health literacy: report of the Council on Scientific Affairs. Ad Hoc Committee on Health Literacy for the Council on Scientific Affairs, American Medical Association. JAMA 1999;281:552–7.
46. Prochaska TR, Glasser M. Patients' views of family involvement in medical care decisions and encounters. Res Aging 1996;18:52–69.

47. Leong SL, Gingrich D, Lewis PR, Mauger DT, George JH. Enhancing doctor-patient communication using email: a pilot study. J Am Board Fam Pract 2005;18:180–8.

48. Cobbs EL, Duthie EH, Murphy JB, editors. Geriatrics review syllabus, 4th ed: a core curriculum in geriatric medicine. Dubuqe (IA): Kendall/Hunt; 1999.

49. Adelman RD, Greene MG, Ory MG. Communication between older patients and their physicians. Clin Geriatr Med 2000;16:1–24.

50. Greene MB, Majerovitz SD, Adelman RD, Rizzo C. The effects of a presence of a third person on the physician medical interview. J Am Geriartr Soc 1994;42:413–9.

51. Lambert BL, Butin DN, Moran D, Zhao SZ, Carr BC, Chen C. Arthritis care: comparison of physicians' and patients' view. Semin Arthritis Rheum 2000;30:100–10.

52. Iversen MD, Fossel AH, Daltroy LH. Rheumatologist-patient communication about exercise and physical therapy in rheumatoid arthritis. Arthritis Care Res 1999;12:180–92.

53. Dovovan JL, Blake DR. Qualitative study of interpretation of reassurance among patients attending rheumatology clinics: "just a touch of arthritis, doctor?". BMJ 2000;320:541–4.

54. Lang F, Flyod MR, Beine KL. Clues to patients' explanations and concerns about their illnesses. A call for active listening. Arch Fam Med 2000;9:222–7.

55. Neville C, Fortin PR, Fitzcharles MA, Baron M, Abrahamowitz M, Du Berger R. The needs of patients with arthritis: the patient's perspective. Arthritis Care Res 1999;12:85–95.

56. Simpson M, Buckman R, Stuart M, Maguire P, Buckman R, Lipkin M, et al. Doctor-patient communication: the Toronto consensus statement. BMJ 1991;303:1385–7.

57. Iversen MD, Daltroy LH, Fossel AH, Katz JN. The prognostic importance of patient pre-operative expectations of surgery for lumbar spinal stenosis. Patient Educ Couns 1998;34:169–78.

58. Leeb BF, Andel I, Leder S, Leeb A, Rintelen B. The patient's perspective and rheumatoid arthritis disease activity indexes. Rheumatology 2005;44:360–5.

59. Haugli L, Strand E, Finset A. How do patients with rheumatic disease experience their relationship with their doctors? A qualitative study of experiences of stress and support in the doctor-patient relationship. Patient Educ Couns 2004;52:169–74.

60. Fraenkel L, Bogardus ST, Concato J, Felson DT, Wittnik DR. Patients preferences for treatment of rheumatoid arthritis. Ann Rheum Dis 2004;63:1372–8.

61. Iversen MD, Eaton HM, Daltroy LH. How rheumatologists and patients with rheumatoid arthritis discuss exercise and the influence of discussions on exercise prescriptions. Arthritis Rheum 2004:51:63–72.

62. Ward MM, Sundaranurthy S, Lotstein D, Bush TM, Neuwelt CM, Street RL. Participatory patient-physician communication and morbidity in patients with systemic lupus erythematosus. Arthritis Rheum 2003;49:810–8.

63. Gabe J, Olumide G, Bury M. "It takes three to tango": a framework for understanding patient partnership in paediatric clinics. Soc Sci Med 2004;59:1071–9.

64. Heneghan AM, Mercer M, DeLeone NL. Will mothers discuss parenting stress and depressive symptoms with their child's pediatrician? Pediatrics 2004;113:460–7.

65. Dixon-Woods M, Young B, Heney D. Partnerships with children. BMJ 1999;319:778–80.

66. Britto MT, DeVellis RF, Hornung RW, DeFriese GH, Atherton HD. Health care preferences and priorities of adolescents with chronic illness. Paediatrics 2004;114:1271–80.

67. Swallow VM, Jacoby A. Mothers' evolving relationships with doctors and nurses during the chronic childhood illness trajectory. J Adv Nurs 2002;36:755–64.

68. Ford CA, Millstein SG, Halpern-Felsher BL, Irwin CE Jr. Influence of physician confidentiality assurances on adolescents' willingness to disclose information and seek future health care: a randomized controlled trial. JAMA 1997;278:1029–34.

69. Janse AJ, Sinnema G, Uiterwaal CS, Kimpen JL, Gemke RJ. Quality of life in chronic illness: perceptions of parents and paediatricians. Arch Dis Child 2005;90:486–91.

70. Oakley A, Benedelow G, Barnes J, Buchanan M, Hussain OA. Health and cancer prevention: knowledge and beliefs of children and young children. BMJ 1995;310:1029–33.

71. Tates K, Meeuwesen L. Doctor-parent-child communication: a review of the literature. Soc Sci Med 2001;53:839–85.

72. Suarez-Almazor ME. Patient-physician communication. Curr Opin Rheumatol 2004;16:91–5.

73. Fallowfield L, Jenkins V, Farewell V, Saul J, Duffy A, Eves R. Efficacy of a cancer research UK communication skills training model for oncologists: a randomized controlled trial. Lancet 2002;359:650–6.

74. Bandura A. Social foundations of thought and action: a social cognitive theory. Upper Saddle River (NJ): Prentice-Hall; 1986.

75. Gordon T, Edwards WS. Making the patient your partner: communication skills for doctors and other caregivers. Westport (CT): Auburn House; 1995.

History and Physical Assessment

CAROL M. ZIMINSKI, MD, FACP, and LISA A. NICHOLS, MSN, RN, CCRA

More than 100 rheumatic diseases are classified by the American College of Rheumatology. Although this number is, at first glance, daunting, one of the unique aspects of rheumatology is that careful history and physical examination, especially the former, provide most of the important information required for diagnosis, assessment, and treatment. Laboratory tests remain useful aids to confirm a diagnosis or narrow a differential diagnosis already derived. The history provides much information about the disease process and the impact of the condition on the patient, while the examination allows the sorting-out of anatomic structures involved. Thus, together, the careful history and comprehensive physical examination remain the most important elements leading to diagnosis in most cases (1–10).

THE RHEUMATOLOGIC HISTORY

Obtaining a complete rheumatologic history involves the art of medicine as much as the science. In some circumstances the only need may be to establish the presence or absence of major musculoskeletal disorders. In most cases, however, it is both necessary and rewarding to obtain a complete history and physical examination, particularly since an apparently simple regional problem may be a manifestation of a more generalized condition.

The history should be obtained in a private setting, before the physical examination is conducted. Attending to the patient's comfort at the outset will help establish a positive patient-provider relationship. A non-threatening environment can aid in gaining the patient's trust and help allay fears and, when possible, the interviewer should face the patient without intervening barriers. If the patient is in pain or has difficulty sitting without support, he or she can sit in a chair with arms, or perhaps recline rather than sit on the examining table, or even remain in his or her wheelchair.

Comprehensive history taking may be considered in 2 phases: an initial "open" phase in which the examiner listens, followed by a second "specific" phase in which more direct questioning elicits additional information. The interview should begin with a general open-ended question such as "What brings you in to see me today?" This will help elicit the chief complaint. The interviewer must be prepared to wait, and to encourage the patient with nonverbal signals, such as leaning forward, establishing eye contact, and looking interested, as the patient focuses on the issues that are of concern. The interviewer should resist the temptation to hurry the process along by suggesting language to describe the problem. It is important to listen to the exact words the patient uses to describe the symptoms, to encourage the patient to describe what they mean if they complain of specific processes such as "inflammation" in some symptomatic site, as well as to note any nonverbal clues. If the patient is reluctant to give information spontaneously, or has difficulty describing symptoms, more coaxing and encouragement by the interviewer may be needed. The loquacious, anxious, or distracted patient may need help and direction to get to the point. When assessing the pediatric patient, both the child and the child's parent or guardian should be questioned about current complaints and past examination findings (1,6).

The second, more specific, phase of history taking should elicit information including demographic data (age, occupation, etc.), the presenting problem, history of presenting complaint, past history, family and psychosocial history, past and current therapy, and review of systems. In patients with chronic rheumatic diseases, it may be useful to order the information in a slightly different way to emphasize 3 issues: current symptoms, chronology of the condition (including the effect of any treatments), and the impact of the disorder in both physical and psychosocial terms. Once that information is obtained, review other features. Although the pattern of symptoms is most key in the differential diagnosis, the selective process really begins with the patient in demographic terms (Table 1).

Assessing the Chief Complaint

The most important presenting symptoms in rheumatology include pain, stiffness or locking, swelling, weakness, limitation of movement, fatigue, and emotional lability (such as anxiety and depression). The pain associated with rheumatic conditions most frequently causes patients to seek medical attention. Analysis of these symptoms helps the examiner to consider the rheumatic complaint as articular versus nonarticular, inflammatory versus noninflammatory or mechanical, symmetric versus asymmetric, peripheral versus central, articular only versus articular plus extraarticular, systemic rheumatic disease versus nonrheumatic disease causing musculoskeletal symptoms, or another process.

A stepwise approach should be used for eliciting explicit information. Evaluation of particular symptom details can provide significant diagnostic clues: location, quality, intensity, course, aggravating and relieving factors, setting, and associated features (1,3,4,6).

Pain. The specific *location* of pain helps determine whether the pain is articular or nonarticular. Regional disorders, with pain in one area,

Table 1. Demography and diagnosis

Characteristic	Diagnostic considerations
Age	
The very young (<20 years)	Juvenile chronic polyarthritis ("JRA")
	Acute rheumatic fever
The young (20–50 years)	Almost all inflammatory joint diseases
The older (>50 years)	Osteoarthritis
	Pseudogout
	Polymyalgia rheumatica
	Giant cell arteritis
	Tumor-related syndromes
Sex	
Male (ratio men:women)	Anklylosing spondylitis (9:1)
	Reiter's syndrome (9:1)
	Polyarthritis (3:1)
	Primary gout (almost all)
Women (ratio women:men)	Rheumatoid arthritis (2:1)
	Primary Sjögren's (9:1)
	Systemic lupus erythematosus (8:1)
	Gonococcal arthritis (almost all)

must be distinguished from systemic conditions in which there is generalized pain. In addition, pain may be referred to areas of the body distal to the primary lesion. Pain described as "deep" or difficult to pinpoint with 1 finger is more likely to be articular, whereas pain described as "superficial" or easily pinpointed along tendons or adjacent to joint structures is more likely to be extraarticular. Establishing the pattern of involvement is key in the differential diagnosis (Table 2).

The *quality* of the pain may be described by the patient in comparison to another type of pain, such as "like a toothache" or "similar to labor pains." The origin of the pain can often be inferred from the patient's description. Muscular pain or myalgia is usually described as "crampy" or "throbbing," whereas neurologic pain is described as "pins and needles" or "electric shocks."

The *intensity* of pain is sometimes difficult to assess, as patients have different pain thresholds. Some patients, because of a need to convince the provider of the severity of the pain, may actually inflate the pain intensity. Use of a visual analog pain scale (0 = no pain, 10 = severe pain) may be beneficial in assessing the level of pain. Children may best express their perception of pain by use of a cartoon pain assessment scale with several faces ranging from smiling to crying. The child chooses the face that best represents how he or she feels (10).

The *course* of the pain, including onset and character with time, may be of diagnostic importance. For example, patients with gout may have sudden onset of symptoms, typically intensely painful, and may be able to identify the date (and even time) of onset. In contrast, patients with osteoarthritis (OA) or rheumatoid arthritis (RA) have more insidious onset of symptoms, and typically present with chronic symptoms (greater than 6 weeks duration). Joint pain may be episodic (as in gout), additive (RA or OA), or migratory. Migratory articular pain implies a rapidly changing pattern of joint involvement and should suggest rheumatic fever, viral arthritis, or gonococcal arthritis. Nocturnal pain in a child may suggest growing pains, osteoid osteoma, or an emerging inflammatory condition.

Aggravating or relieving factors, such as rest or activity, heat or cold, should be identified. It is useful to inquire about what activities induce pain—such as repetitive motion, climbing stairs, arising from a low chair. Musculoskeletal pain in a child that occurs only during the school week may suggest a school-related stressor. Associated features, whether local (bony enlargements), constitutional (weight loss), or emotional (depression), can help determine the nature of the underlying process.

Stiffness. The feeling of discomfort or restriction of movement after a period of inactivity is stiffness, or *gelling*. Morning stiffness of >1 hour is a hallmark of inflammatory arthritis, such as RA. Patients with inflammatory joint disease typically feel worse in the morning and improve over the course of the day and with activity. Stiffness that occurs after brief periods of inactivity and lasts <60 minutes may occur in noninflammatory conditions, such as OA. Patients with noninflammatory or mechanical conditions typically feel better in the morning or after rest, and become more uncomfortable over the course of the day, with increased use of involved joints. Patients may be unclear what the interviewer means by stiffness, and may have difficulty quantifying the sensation. Some patients liken stiffness to pain, soreness, tightness, weakness, or fatigue. It may be useful to ask if the individual feels stiff upon awakening in the morning and the time stiffness is first noted. Then inquire about when the patient is most limber. The duration of stiffness is the time elapsed. Because patients may feel more stiff on some days and less on others, it is best to have them give an average of morning stiffness for the past week, rather than just on the day of the interview.

Swelling. Joint swelling is an important component of many rheumatic diseases, and implies inflammation of a joint or periarticular structure. Swelling may be subjective (i.e., perceived by the patient) or objective. As with pain, patients should be questioned about the location, pattern of onset, and aggravating or relieving factors related to

Table 2. Pattern of arthritis and diagnosis*

Characteristic	Diagnostic considerations
Number of joints	
Polyarticular	RA
	SLE
	Serum sickness
	Psoriatic arthritis
	ARF
	JRA
Oligoarticular	Reactive arthritis
	IBD
	Gonococcal arthritis
	Psoriatic arthritis
	ARF
	JRA
Monoarticular	Infection
	Trauma
	Gonococcal arthritis
	Gout
	Pseudogout
	JRA
Onset	
Acute	Infectious
	Serum sickness
	Hepatitis B
	Gout
	Psuedogout
	RA
	SLE
	Reactive arthritis
Insidious	Gout (tophaceous)
	CPPD deposition
	RA
	SLE
	Reactive arthritis
Character with time	
Episodic	Gout
	Pseudogout
Evanescent	SLE
Additive	RA
Migratory	SLE
	ARF
	Gonococcal arthritis (early)
Symmetry	
Symmetric	RA
	Serum sickness
	SLE
Asymmetric	Psoriatic
	Reactive arthritis
	IBD
	OA
	Gout
Distribution	
Axial/central	AS
	Reactive arthritis
	Psoriatic
	IBD
Peripheral	RA
	SLE
	Psoriatic
	IBD

* RA = rheumatoid arthritis; SLE = systemic lupus erythematosus; ARF = acute rheumatic fever; JRA = juvenile rheumatoid arthritis; IBD = inflammatory bowel disease; CPPD = calcium pyrophosphate dihydrate; OA = osteoarthritis; AS = ankylosing spondylitis.

the swelling. The pattern of onset may give clues to the acuteness of the problem, such as a traumatic injury. Aggravating and relieving factors may include activity, rest, and response to medications. Additional specific questions regarding, for example, ease in putting on rings or shoes may provide additional information regarding swelling.

Limitation of Movement. Interruption in activities of daily living may reflect loss of range of motion. The patient's ability to bathe, toilet, feed, dress, ambulate at home, and perform normal work or play activities should be addressed. The length of time the limitation has persisted and how the patient has adapted are important. Assessment of the use of ambulatory aids (such as canes or crutches) and assistive devices (such as jar openers and dressing aids) is important. The timing of onset may have diagnostic importance. Sudden limitation of motion may be related to a tendon rupture, whereas more gradual limitation, with attendant contracture formation, may be caused by a chronic inflammatory condition.

Weakness. A decrease in, or loss of, muscle strength is weakness. It may coexist with other symptoms, such as pain, stiffness, and fatigue; therefore, it is sometimes difficult for patients to separate weakness from other symptoms. Actual muscle weakness is noted only when muscles are being used, and it is frequently noted by an inability to carry out activities of daily living, such as walking, gripping, chewing, swallowing, and toileting. The pattern of asymmetric or symmetric muscle weakness, and its central or peripheral distribution may provide key clues to diagnosis. The weakness manifested in inflammatory myopathies is usually present in proximal muscles, with difficulty rising from a chair or getting upright from bed, whereas neuropathies cause distal muscle weakness. Patients with true myopathies have little trouble distinguishing between muscle weakness and generalized fatigue.

Fatigue. Fatigue is one of the most common constitutional complaints associated with rheumatic disease (see Chapter 44, Fatigue). It may be quite disabling, with a general sense of overwhelming tiredness making it virtually impossible for the patient to perform activities of daily living or participate in life activities. Fatigue is assessed by determining the time of onset, frequency, degree of severity, and impact on activities of daily living. Accompanying psychosocial stressors, diet, sleep patterns, and activity level should be determined. Fatigue is often prominent in inflammatory and noninflammatory conditions (e.g., RA and fibromyalgia, respectively).

Emotional Lability. Anxiety and fear are present in many patients, particularly with the first consultation for a possible rheumatic disease. Pain is a potent cause of anxiety because it tends to signal damage to the body. It is important for the examiner to recognize patient fears and to address them honestly, rather than concentrating solely on physical diagnosis. Emotional lability, depression, and other psychiatric disturbances may also be the result of a rheumatic disease, for example depression and the less-common onset of psychosis in a patient with systemic lupus erythematosus (SLE).

Other Pertinent History

A history of previous therapy for the current problem should be sought. Previous use of prescription or nonprescription medications, physical therapies, natural or home remedies, and other nontraditional treatments should be elicited. Questions might encompass length of previous therapy, adherence, presence of side effects, acceptability of cost, and the patient's perception of success or failure of these modalities. In addition, all of the patient's current medications should be reviewed to rule out potential drug interactions or the possibility of drug-induced rheumatic symptoms, such as drug-induced lupus.

Exploring the patient's medical and sexual history can help determine previous serious illnesses and surgeries, as well as identify conditions pertinent to the current illness. For example, urethritis that predates the onset of heel pain may be a significant clue to a diagnosis of reactive arthritis. The family history may also reveal information of diagnostic importance. Some rheumatic diseases have a genetic basis. For example, the HLA–B27-associated spondyloarthropathies (ankylosing

spondylitis, reactive arthritis, psoriatic arthritis, and enteropathic arthritis) can occur in several family members, even children. A family history of lupus in a child with SLE is not unusual, although chronic rheumatic diseases of childhood are seldom familial. A negative family history should also be noted. Potential environmental triggers, occupational exposure, travel, or recent viral or bacterial infection in the patient and family members should not be overlooked. Finally, a careful developmental history should be obtained, especially in children.

Review of Systems

The final part of the history is the review of systems. Because many rheumatic diseases are systemic in nature, a complete review of all body systems is another opportunity to identify important diagnostic symptoms or comorbid conditions. Extraarticular features that may provide key clues to diagnosis are included in Table 3.

THE PHYSICAL EXAMINATION

As with the history, the physical examination should take place in a private setting. Often patients are unable to seat themselves on the examination table without assistance. Conventional tables may have too high a step for the patient with muscle weakness or lower extremity disease. If necessary, the majority of the physical examination can be performed with the patient seated in a chair.

Physical examination of the child is similar to an adult, with two notable exceptions (see Chapter 6, Evaluating Children). First, a developmental assessment of the child should be made to determine whether the child is maturing at an age-appropriate pace. Second, it is wise to modify the order of the examination, saving potentially painful or distressing aspects of the examination until last. Most of the examination can be conducted with the child sitting on the parent or guardian's lap.

The General Physical Examination

The physical examination complements the history and with it completes the clinical assessment. Examination of the patient with rheumatic disease should not encompass only the musculoskeletal system, but should include a complete clinical examination.

The examination should begin with vital signs, including temperature, respirations, pulse, blood pressure, and weight. Measurement of height allows calculation of body mass index, which may be an important influence on symptoms related to weight-bearing joints. Unintentional weight loss may be a feature of neoplasia, chronic infection, or systemic inflammatory disorders. Weight loss may be insidious early in the disease course, and is often only noted through serial evaluation. To allow the maximum yield of clinical information, the adult patient should change into a gown and remove shoes and socks to allow for complete inspection and evaluation. It may not be necessary to thoroughly undress a child. Exposing small areas as they are assessed helps keep the child warm and feeling more in control.

The skin, hair, scalp, and nails are usually examined first. Special attention should be paid to the presence of any nodules, tophi, rashes, ulcerations, telangiectasias, alopecia, or Raynaud's phenomena. Thorough pulmonary and cardiac examinations are of particular importance when systemic sclerosis, SLE, or vasculitis are suspected. Careful neurologic examination, including assessment of muscle strength, is necessary when assessing for inflammatory myopathy, SLE, vasculitis, or nerve entrapment syndromes (Table 3).

Table 3. Extraarticular features and diagnosis*

Clinical feature	Diagnostic considerations
Subcutaneous nodules	RA
	SLE
	Tophaceous gout
	Calcinosis
	Multicentric nodular reticulohistiocytosis
Skin	
Photosensitivity	SLE
	SCLE
	Discoid lesions
Erythema nodosum	Sarcoidosis
	IBD
	Drug-induced
	Infection
Nail changes	Psoriatic
	Reactive arthritis
	SLE
Ocular disease	
Uveitis	AS, Reactive arthritis
	Sarcoidosis
	Arteritis
	Behcet's disease
	Relapsing polychondritis
Episcleritis	RA
	Arteritis
	Behcet's disease
	Relapsing polychondritis
Keratoconjunctivitis	RA
	SLE
	Sjögren's syndrome
Cardiac disease	
Pericarditis	SLE
	RA
Myocarditis	SLE
	Myositis
	Arteritis
Murmurs	
Aortic regurgitation	AS, Reactive arthritis
Mitral regurgitation	ARF
or stenosis	
Pulmonary disease	
Pleuritis	SLE
Fibrosis	RA
	Myopathy/synthetase syndrome
Nodules, infiltrates,	RA
adenopathy	Arteritis
	Sarcoidosis

* Any organ system plus arthritis helps narrow a diagnosis. SCLE = subacute cutaneous lupus erythematosus. For other acronym definitions, see Table 2.

The Musculoskeletal Examination

Examination of the musculoskeletal system is best undertaken in a systematic manner. Many examiners begin at the head and move downward, while others begin with the upper extremities, move toward the trunk and then downward to the feet. The latter approach may be less threatening to the patient because the examination begins in a socially neutral location—the hands. Throughout the examination, the patient should be as comfortable as possible. A relaxed patient is better able to tolerate a thorough examination, thus allowing a more accurate assessment. Informing the patient what maneuvers the examiner is about to perform can assure a relaxed and cooperative patient. Support should be provided above or below an inflamed joint when moving it through range of motion, rather than directly holding the joint itself. Movements should be slow and fluid, rather than sudden or forceful.

The techniques of the examination process include: *inspection, palpation, range of motion,* and *assessment of function.* Inspection and palpation are usually performed simultaneously. Similarly, range of motion and assessment of function can often be assessed together. For example, while a patient is demonstrating active range of motion of the shoulder, the examiner can ask if the patient is able to style her hair.

Joint Findings

The most common joint abnormalities are swelling, tenderness, warmth, crepitus, limitation of motion, and sometimes deformity. *Swelling* can result from several causes, such as bony overgrowth, joint effusion, or synovial proliferation, and is assessed by inspection and direct palpation of the joint. *Tenderness* is assessed by gentle, yet firm, joint palpation. Using both hands, the examiner should palpate joints in all planes, anterior to posterior and medial to lateral. (For an explanation of formal joint counts in patients with inflammatory arthritis, see Chapter 7). Enough pressure is exerted when the nail beds of the examiner's fingers or thumbs blanch. Observing a patient's facial expressions, such as a wince or grimace, as well as listening to verbal cues, is often useful in assessing tenderness. *Warmth* of the joint is best confirmed by comparison with the opposite joint. Skin *color changes,* such as erythema over an inflamed joint, may also be present.

Crepitus is the palpable or audible grating sensation produced by roughened articular or extraarticular surfaces rubbing against each other. Some crepitus may be appreciated in normal joints, but severe cracking or grating is usually indicative of chronic degenerative processes. When assessing *limitation of motion,* it is helpful to appreciate the normal ranges of joint motion. Range of motion should be assessed actively as well as passively. The only exception is the cervical spine, which should not be passively moved in patients with inflammatory arthritis because of the risk of cervical spine instability and neurologic compromise with extreme extension. Limitation of motion can occur either actively or passively; however, because patients are limited by their own pain, passive range of motion is usually greater especially when the patient is distracted, and therefore is a more accurate measure. *Deformity* denotes malalignment, which may result from various causes, such as bony enlargement, joint subluxation, contracture, or destruction of ligamentous support.

Examination of Specific Joints

The Small Joints. The temporomandibular (TM), acromioclavicular (AC), sternoclavicular (SC), and sternomanubrial (SM) joints are important to include in the examination. These joints can exhibit pain, swelling, and crepitus. The TM joint is at the junction of the articular tubercle of the temporal bone and mandibular condyle. Direct palpation over the joint just anterior to the tragus allows assessment of warmth, pain, and swelling. Crepitus can be discerned by inserting the index fingers just inside the external ear canal and gently pulling forward while the patient opens and closes the mouth. Range of motion is adequate if the patient is able to insert the width of 2 fingers inside the mouth. The AC joint is located by tracing the clavicle laterally to the acromion process. The SC joint is medial, where the clavicle meets the sternum. These joints are assessed for tenderness, swelling, and crepitus. Motion may be assessed by firmly pulling down on the forearm. The SC joint has minimal motion, but can be assessed by having the patient shrug the shoulders. The SM joint is located where the manubrium articulates with the body of the sternum, and although this joint has no motion, it may be tender or swollen.

Shoulder. The shoulder is a ball and socket joint formed by the head of the humerus and the glenoid fossa of the scapula. Knowledge of shoulder anatomy is essential to assess the origin of symptoms. Pathology can occur in the glenohumeral joint, rotator cuff, subacromial bursae, bicipital tendon, or axillae. The shoulder is best examined from the front, so both shoulders can be compared. The shoulder is inspected and palpated for warmth, swelling, tenderness, muscle spasm, or atrophy. Range of motion is assessed by having the patient perform the following maneuvers: raise arms forward in a wide arc and touch palms together above the head; with elbows flexed and hands on head, move arms posteriorly; raise arms extended in a sideways arc and touch palms together above head; and rotate the arm internally behind the back and touch between the scapulae. Normal ranges of motion are as follows: forward flexion, 90°; backward extension, 45°; abduction, 180°; adduction, 45°; internal rotation, 55°; and external rotation, 40–45° (3).

Elbow. The elbow is a hinge joint formed by 3 bony articulations: the humeroulnar, radiohumeral, and the proximal radioulnar. The elbow is surrounded by 1 large (the olecranon) and several small bursae. This joint should be inspected for subcutaneous nodules, tophi, and the presence of olecranon bursitis. Palpation is conducted with the elbow flexed to ~70°. Synovitis is best appreciated in the medial paraolecranon groove. Normal elbow extension is 0–5°, and flexion is 135° or greater. Synovitis can cause loss of full extension, and if chronic, may result in flexion contracture (inability to fully extend to 0°).

Wrist and Hand. The wrist contains 8 carpal bones arranged in 2 rows; the proximal row articulates with the radius. The wrist normally has 60–70° of extension and 80–90° of flexion. Ulnar and radial deviation at the wrist is 30° and 20°, respectively. The wrist is inspected and palpated for synovitis, warmth, thickened tendons, cystic swelling, and deformity. Mild synovitis may manifest as pain on movement. Dorsal/ventral instability with or without bogginess of the ulnar styloid is known as the *piano key sign*. Compression of the median nerve in the carpal tunnel is tested by placing the wrist in severe flexion (60°) for at least 1 minute. When numbness or paresthesias are noted along the distribution of the median nerve (first 3 digits and medial half of the fourth), it is known as a positive *Phalen's sign*. This maneuver may be difficult for the patient with acute synovitis. An alternative maneuver is to percuss repeatedly along the volar aspect of the wrist. A tingling or feeling of electric shock in the same median nerve distribution is known as *Tinel's sign*.

Prolonged median nerve compression in the carpal tunnel may produce thenar muscle atrophy, noted on the palm at the base of the thumb. *Dupuytren's contracture* may be noted as thickening and contracture of the palmar aponeurosis, causing severe flexion of the fourth and fifth fingers. *De Quervain's tenosynovitis* is a common cause of wrist pain due to inflammation and stenosing of the tendon sheaths at the base of the thumb near the radial styloid. It is assessed by having the patient flex the thumb into the palm, then grip the fingers over the thumb and move the hand downward (ulnar deviated). If tenosynovitis is present, this movement (*Finkelstein's maneuver*) may produce exquisite tenderness on the radial side of the wrist.

The metacarpophalangeal (MCP), proximal interphalangeal (PIP), and distal interphalangeal (DIP) joints comprise the small joints of the hands. They are hinge joints held in place by tendons and ligaments. Range of motion of these joints is most easily assessed by having the patient slowly flex the fingers to form a fist. Loss of extension in any single digit is best expressed as the number of degrees lacking full extension. Hands should be inspected for swelling, deformity, and skin and nail changes. Rheumatoid arthritis predominantly affects the MCP and PIP joints. Common deformities include *swan neck deformity*, involving hyperextension of the PIP joint and flexion of the DIP joint, and *boutonniere deformity*, or flexion contracture of the PIP joint with hyperextension of the DIP joint. Osteoarthritis predominantly affects the first carpometacarpal joint and the DIP joints. Osteophytic nodules that form on the PIP and DIP joints are known as *Bouchard's nodes* and *Heberden's nodes*, respectively (Figure 1). Scleroderma

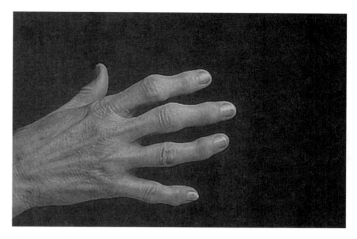

Figure 1. Bony enlargement of the distal interphalangeal joints (Heberden's nodes) and proximal interphalangeal joints (Bouchard's nodes) are common findings in osteoarthritis. These changes are more frequent in postmenopausal women and show some genetic predisposition. Reprinted from The Teaching Slide Collection for Clinicians and Educators: Assessment and Management of the Rheumatic Diseases, third edition.

can cause the skin over the fingers to have a tight, shiny, atrophic appearance (*sclerodactyly*). Pitting of the nails and dystrophic changes (*onycholysis*) may be seen in psoriatic arthritis.

Hip. The hip is a major weight-bearing ball and socket joint, formed by the head of the femur and the pelvic acetabulum. It is surrounded by strong ligaments and bursae. Inspection of the hip begins with gait assessment. Before palpating the hip, instruct the patient to indicate where pain is located. Often patients will point to the lateral side and describe the pain as being in the "hip joint," when in reality they are pointing over the trochanteric bursa. True hip joint pain is typically manifested anteriorly in the groin fold. The hip has a wide range of motions. Extension (normal 30°) can be measured several ways, including having the patient drop the leg off the table; or from a standing position moving one leg backward; or lifting the leg off the table while lying prone. Flexion (normal 120°) is assessed with the patient supine and drawing one knee up to the chest without bending the back. While in this position, the opposite hip can be checked for a flexion contracture. Abduction (normal 45°) is moving the leg away from the midline. Adduction (normal 20° to 30°) is moving the leg across the midline. Internal and external rotation are performed with the knee and hip flexed to 90°. Rotating the heel medially causes external rotation (normal 45°) and outwardly causes internal rotation (normal 35°). Hip movement can be quickly measured by placing the heel medially to the opposite knee and slowly lowering the flexed knee toward the table.

Knee. The knee is a large diarthrodial joint supported by a series of ligaments and surrounded by several bursae. Normal knee extension is 0°; normal flexion is 135°. The knee is inspected for swelling, deformity such as *genu varum* (bow legs) or *genu valgum* (knock knees), flexion contracture, locking or buckling, Baker's or popliteal cysts, and skin changes. The knee is palpated with the patient supine and leg in full extension. The patella should move easily medially and laterally, and may ballot if a large effusion is present. Minor knee effusions are best palpated after milking the fluid away from the medial side and then tapping the lateral aspect of the knee with the other hand. If an effusion is present, a small wave or bulge of fluid will reappear on the medial aspect (*bulge sign*).

Stability of the collateral ligaments is tested by placing the patient supine with the knee at full extension. One hand stabilizes the femur on either side of the knee and acts as a fulcrum, while the other hand grasps the ankle and moves the lower extremity in the direction of the braced hand to assess the contralateral collateral ligament. Excess movement may indicate collateral ligament laxity or damage. The cruciate ligaments are tested by having the patient flex the hip to 45° and the knee to 90°. The examiner fixes the foot position. The fingers are then placed posteriorly in the popliteal space behind the knee, with the thumbs anteriorly over the joint line. The lower extremity is pulled forward or pushed backward to assess the cruciate ligaments. Increased forward motion denotes pathology with the anterior cruciate ligament. Increased posterior motion may indicate posterior cruciate damage. A positive finding is known as a *drawer sign.* Other findings related to knee pathology are quadriceps atrophy, crepitation on movement secondary to cartilage degeneration, and tenderness over the anserine bursa on the anteromedial tibial plateau below the knee.

Ankle and Foot. The ankle is a hinge joint formed by the distal ends of the tibia and fibula and the proximal talus. This joint is limited in motion to plantar flexion (50°) and dorsiflexion (20°). The subtalar joint (articulation of the talus and the calcaneus) is responsible for inversion and eversion (5° each direction). The foot includes the intertarsal joints (midfoot), and the metatarsophalangeal (MTP) and interphalangeal (IP) joints of the toes. The metatarsal heads and the calcaneus are the weight-bearing portions of the foot. Midfoot range of motion is assessed by stabilizing the calcaneus and inverting and everting the forefoot (MTP and IP joints). Forefoot range of motion can be checked by having the patient flex and extend the toes.

The foot and ankle should be inspected in weight-bearing and non–weight-bearing positions, both with and without footwear. Assessment should include swelling, deformity, nodules, tophi, nail changes, and calluses. Swelling of the ankle joint is sometimes difficult to differentiate from generalized edema. True ankle joint effusions are noted as a nonpitting fullness anteriorly and/or posteriorly around the malleoli. Ankle synovitis causes tenderness on movement. The feet and toes are commonly affected in RA, OA, and gout; deformities may include lateral deviation of the great toe (*hallux valgus*), hyperextension of the MTP joint (*hammer toe*), and dorsal subluxation of the MTP joint (*cockup deformity*) (Figure 2). Calluses and abnormal patterns of shoe wear can be important clues in assessing foot problems.

Spine. The spine supports the upright posture of the body and provides protection for the spinal column. Spinal range of motion provides flexibility for the trunk. The vertebral column as a whole produces 90° of flexion. The trunk (minus the cervical spine) extends to 30° posteriorly, and 50° laterally in either direction. The cervical spine provides 45° of flexion, 50–60° of extension, 60–80° of rotation, and 40° of lateral bending. In the RA patient, cervical range of motion is always done actively, as there is a possibility for subluxation of C1 and C2. The spine should be inspected first as a whole and then by section. A thorough examination requires the patient to be standing, with the entire back, shoulders, hips, legs, and feet visible. The spine is inspected for symmetry, abnormal curvature (scoliosis, kyphosis, lordosis), and paravertebral spasm. Palpation is performed systematically from the top down and from side to side. Ankylosing spondylitis commonly affects the thoracic and lumbar spine, causing forward protrusion of the head, decreased chest expansion, thoracic kyphosis, and loss of lumbar lordosis. The *Wright-Schöber test* measures forward flexion of the lumbar spine. A line is drawn at the level of the posterior-superior iliac crests, with a second line 10 cm above the first. The distance between the two marks increases ≥5 cm with normal lumbar mobility and <4 cm in the case of decreased lumbar mobility.

The sacrum is a triangular bone formed by the union of 5 sacral vertebrae. The lateral aspect of the sacrum has a large surface for articulating with the ileum of the pelvis. These sacroiliac joints are assessed with the patient lying on his or her side. The examiner exerts steady

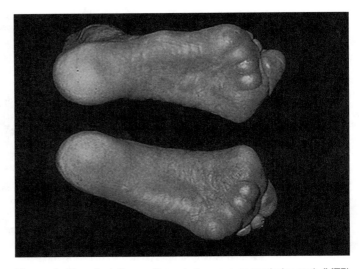

Figure 2. Chronic inflammation at the metatarsophalangeal (MTP) joints causes damage resulting in subluxation of the toes upwards. With the MTP joints displaced, weight bearing is not shared through the toes, but falls directly on the prominent metatarsal heads. This results in pain on weight bearing and difficulty in walking, and can cause the metatarsal heads to erode through the skin on the sole of the foot. The Teaching Slide Collection for Clinicians and Educators: Assessment and Management of the Rheumatic Diseases, third edition.

downward pressure over the upper iliac crest. While localization of pain to the sacroiliac area is a positive sign of sacroiliitis, the diagnostic sensitivity and specificity are poor. The *straight-leg raising test* is a screening tool for neurologic or muscular low back pain. This is done with the patient supine and one knee in full extension. The leg is gradually raised until symptoms occur, reproducing radicular radiation rather than solely back pain, usually within 30–80° of flexion. Pain is aggravated by forced dorsiflexion of the foot and relieved with flexion of the knee.

SUMMARY

A comprehensive history and physical examination are the most important components of the evaluation of rheumatic complaints. In the majority of patients who present with a diagnosable rheumatic problem, the diagnosis will be made primarily on clinical grounds. Over-reliance on or inappropriate interpretation of laboratory testing and radiographic procedures may cloud the diagnostic picture, rather than guide the evaluation and plan of care. Early assessment and intervention can positively impact the morbidity and mortality of patients with rheumatic diseases. A careful history and physical examination can also yield the economic benefits of better utilization of clinician time and resources, and decreased costs to patients.

REFERENCES

1. Bickley LS. The musculoskeletal system. In: Bickley LA, Szilagyi PG, editors. Bates' guide to physical examination and history taking. Philadelphia: Lippincott Williams & Wilkins; 2003. p. 465–533.
2. Cush JJ, Lipsky PE. Approach to articular and musculoskeletal disorders. In: Kasper DL, Braunwald E, Fauci AS, Hauser SL, Longo DL, Jameson JL, editors. Harrison's principles of internal medicine. 16th ed. New York: McGraw Hill; 2005. p. 2029–36.
3. Dieppe P, Sergent H. History. In: Klippel JH, Dieppe PA, editors. Rheumatology. 2nd ed. London, Philadelphia: Mosby; 1998. p. 2.1.1–6.

4. Grahame R. Examination of the patient. In: Klippel JH, Dieppe PA, editors. Rheumatology. 2nd ed. London, Philadelphia: Mosby; 1998. p. 2.2.1–16.

5. Hoppenfeld S. Physical examination of the spine and extremities. New York: Appleton-Century-Crofts; 1976.

6. The history and interviewing process. In: Seidel HM, Ball JW, Dains JE, Benedict GW, editors. Mosby's guide to physical examination. Edinburgh: Elsevier Mosby; 2006. p. 1–37.

7. Musculoskeletal system. In: Seidel HM, Ball JW, Dains JE, Benedict GW, editors. Mosby's guide to physical examination. Edinburgh: Elsevier Mosby; 2006. p. 688–757.

8. Moder KG, Hunder GG. History and physical examination. In: Harris ED, Budd RC, Firestein GS, Genovese MC, Sergent JS, Ruddy S, et al., editors. Kelley's textbook of rheumatology. 7th ed. Philadelphia: Elsevier Saunders; 2005. p. 483–500.

9. American College of Rheumatology Ad Hoc Committee on Clinical Guidelines. Guidelines for the initial evaluation of the adult patient with acute musculoskeletal symptoms. Arthritis Rheum 1996;39:1–8.

10. Cassidy JT, Petty RE. Textbook of pediatric rheumatology. 4th ed. Philadelphia: WB Saunders; 2000.

Evaluating Children with Muscle, Bone, or Joint Complaints

THOMAS J. A. LEHMAN, MD

The clinician evaluating a child with muscle, bone, or joint complaints must always be aware they are dealing with a wide variety of possible diagnoses while confronted with parents and children whose initial thought is always "I/he/she must have injured it." As a result, it is important to ask probing questions and carefully and fully evaluate the child with musculoskeletal complaints, even when your attempts to do so are being dismissed as unnecessary by the family.

Many authors would write this as a detailed chapter of exactly what questions to ask, which joints to examine, and what tests to order. Those answers can be found in chapters dealing with specific diseases. Instead, this chapter is intended to teach you how to go about getting the right answer. But remember, there are no 100% rules in medicine. No rule will be correct in every instance, but those who believe their case is the exception to the rule are more likely wrong.

Dealing with children and their families is not a dry checklist proposition. You need to be watching both the family members and the child while you are collecting information and performing your examination. Sometimes I get to the end of all my questions and my examination without "finding anything." However, watching and listening let me know who is probably okay and who needs additional evaluation.

Many courses on physical diagnosis begin with a discussion of the "chief complaint" or "presenting problem," but for the clinician in practice, the evaluation really begins as you walk into the room. Stop at the doorway for a moment and look to see what the child is doing while waiting for you. If it's a small child, are they running around playful and happy, or clinging fearfully to their mother's lap? Is the child simply lying down or sitting quietly on the exam table? Are they relaxed or fearful as you approach? There are different diagnoses that go with the varied answers to each of those questions. The child with an unrecognized fracture, an infected joint, or an unsuspected malignancy is almost never happy and playing when you come into the room, but the child with juvenile arthritis or a variety of other conditions might well be.

TAKING A HISTORY

When you begin to ask questions, it is always important to take a moment to speak with the child first. This often requires politely stopping the parents by informing them that they will get their turn in a minute. Parents are happy to tell you what they think, but their vision is colored by their assumptions. If you carefully ask a child what hurts, you may find out it's the knee, the ankle, and the wrist even though the parents' have informed the secretary that they are "here for a knee injury that just won't go away." Knowing that the ankle and wrist also hurt gives you a completely different list of diseases to consider. Parents are often unaware of exactly what hurts, where it hurts, and what may be stiff or difficult to move in the morning. Not every child of every age will give you reliable or valuable answers to your questions, but you will never know if you don't ask.

Once you begin asking questions of the child or parent (or both, as appropriate), you want to develop a clear picture in your mind of what's happening. When evaluating any medical problem, there is a simple list you must keep repeating to yourself, "location, quality, duration, time course, exacerbation, and relief." There are characteristic answers to these questions for the majority of diseases.

In evaluating musculoskeletal complaints, the first thing you want to know is where does it hurt. If it's several different places, you will need to ask the same series of questions for each of the different places. Don't settle for answers like, "My leg hurts." There are an awful lot of significant problems that can occur between the tip of the toes and the inguinal crease. All of them might be considered by a child as part of "my leg hurts." Don't be afraid to ask people to point to exactly where it hurts. Don't be afraid to ask them to be more exact. "One finger, one place; show me exactly where it hurts the worst." It's surprising how often "my leg hurts," becomes "my knee hurts," and then becomes "right here!" "Right here" is often the anterior tibial plateau at the insertion of the patellar tendon and the classic location for Osgood-Schlatter disease.

After the location of the pain has become clear, you need to know what the pain is like. Is it a dull ache that is present all the time or is it a sharp stabbing pain? Or, what??? You want to know how long it hurts or has hurt. Does the pain come and go in 5 seconds, 5 minutes, 5 hours, or 5 days? These are very different problems, yet each could be described as a pain that "comes and goes." You also want to know when it hurts. Arthritis often produces stiffness and pain in the morning and evening, with an increase whenever the child sits for a long time. This is the classic for: "Johnny limps in the morning, but looks fine in the afternoon." Johnny may "look fine" in the afternoon, but he usually doesn't have normal exam results, if done carefully. In contrast, a pain that doesn't seem very severe most of the time, but wakes the child up crying in the middle of the night should make the examiner consider growing pains, but this also might be an osteoid osteoma or a slow-growing tumor, or…. These types of details won't always give you the exact answer, but they'll often give you a much clearer sense of where to look and when to keep looking if you don't initially find an answer.

The next important thing to know is what makes the pain better, and what will make the pain worse. Holding still would make a fracture or an infected joint feel better, whereas a child with arthritis will report that they have a hard time moving after sitting still for a long period. A child with a mechanical problem may tire while walking and so might a child with arthritis. But after a period of 20–30 minutes rest, the child with a mechanical problem might be ready to go. In contrast, the child with arthritis might feel better, but report they "stiffened up" and have a hard time getting going again.

Most people will have tried something to make the problem go away before they sought medical care. Does heat make the problem better or worse? What about ice? Ibuprofen-containing products? Acetaminophen? Have they been using any homeopathic or herbal remedies?

The next thing to know is how did it start? It's one thing if the problem started after sliding into second base during the baseball game, and another if the answer is "we're not sure." Injuries and infections are often dramatic in onset. The parents and child can often say he or she "was fine until Friday 2 weeks ago when…." In contrast, malignancies, arthritic conditions, and storage diseases sneak up on people. "It's been going on for a while and at first we weren't too concerned, but now it's getting worse and…."

Keep your eyes on all the participants at this stage of questioning, especially if there was sudden onset of the problem. The explanation may be unreported trauma because a child was doing something he or she wasn't supposed to and has denied it (e.g., the child with a fractured fibula who was jumping on the bed and fell; since they'd been told repeatedly not to jump on the bed, they deny the injury). Trauma may also be the result of sibling-sibling interaction, parent-child interaction, or other caregiver-child interaction and may not always be admitted to the evaluator.

Once you get done asking a careful series of questions, you should have a clear sense of whether the problem is mechanical (an injury or some type of ligamentous or cartilage damage) or inflammatory (arthritis, infection, tumor, etc.). You might think you know exactly what's wrong. Remember to be careful. Sometimes people are confused and they give incorrect answers. Sometimes we subconsciously lead people to give the answers they think we want to hear. Even when you think you've been extremely careful about those issues, you may get the classic description of problem A, only to find it's clearly problem B when you examine the patient. That's never an excuse for doing a bad job of taking the history.

At this point, many people think they've finished taking the history, but they've really just turned one corner. It is very important when evaluating a child that you take a full medical history. That means you need to ask about past medical problems, other medical problems in family members and relatives, a travel history, a social history, and a full review of systems looking for other medical problems. Families often look bored when you are doing this, and medical students often look bored when I make them do it. I would strongly encourage you not to use a form the family fills out in the waiting room. We all know how much attention we pay to all those check boxes. You might see a checked box and remember to ask about something you wouldn't have, but it's far more likely that you'll see no boxes checked and move on without asking any questions. You may never know what you've missed. I've solved many a "mystery case" simply by asking the routine questions carefully and following up on the "funny look on someone's face" when I asked the question.

Here are some examples of what you can learn through careful questioning:

- A child with eye disease and joint pains who didn't have juvenile rheumatoid arthritis (JRA) was quickly diagnosed by the gastroenterologist with Crohn's disease after I sent him for endoscopy. His mother's father and brother were known to have Crohn's, and I knew the joint and eye problems could begin before the stomach complaints were evident; his mother was "shocked."
- A child presented with fevers, chills, and joint pains but didn't have systemic-onset JRA. It was easy to suspect malaria when he told me he spent his entire summer in the mountains of Central America and didn't take any medication.
- A child with tubercular arthritis had never been out of the country and lived in "just the right part of town" and was "never exposed to such things." The child's nanny was from a third-world country and had a chronic cough.
- A child with fever, negative cultures, a high erythrocyte sedimentation rate, and pulmonary infiltrates had psittacosis, not Churg-Strauss syndrome. The father raised pigeons, but no one had asked.
- A child presented with vague complaints and "didn't feel well." He'd been dismissed by several doctors after examination and laboratory test results were normal, but no one noted that he had a complicated

neonatal course and spent 6 weeks in the neonatal intensive care unit requiring several transfusions. He had hepatitis C.

Each of these cases was easy to diagnose because asking the "routine questions" got me answers that made me think of the right diagnosis.

Taking a good history is like painting a picture. Not everyone will be equally smooth or equally good at it, but everyone can learn to do a competent job in a reasonable amount of time if they simply practice. If you are a physician, you should be doing it right, but are you? If you are an allied health professional, it is likely you know many things about the family that the doctor doesn't. If you think you've learned something that might be important, make sure to tell the doctor. The physician caring for the patient should always be interested in what you have to say.

PHYSICAL EXAMINATION

Often people think it is difficult to do a good physical examination of a small child. "They just won't hold still." To my mind that's basically a good thing. When I walk into the room to see a small child and they are lying very still on the examination table, either they are asleep or very sick. I prefer asleep. The key to a good examination of anyone at any age is observation. Watch how the child moves, watch how the child walks, and watch what the child does when reaching for things or given things to play with. You can often get a very clear sense of what hurts and where, simply from watching.

There are many textbooks that will tell you exactly how many degrees of motion children are supposed to have at each individual joint, but that isn't what we want to know in making a diagnosis of rheumatic disease. What we want to know is what hurts and what's swollen. Limitation of motion without pain or swelling is far more likely to be a mechanical problem than a rheumatic disease.

The most important thing to understand when you are evaluating a child's joints is that guarding is not a voluntary response. If you were to put your hand down on a very hot surface you would quickly find yourself looking down at your hand, which you had moved close to your chest. There would not have been a moment when you thought to yourself, "Uh oh, that's hot. I'd better move my hand." By the time you noticed that you had put your hand on something hot, you had already moved your hand. That's because we are protected by spinal reflex arcs. Your hand moved as soon as the nerve centers in your spinal cord recognized pain. You didn't have the opportunity to think about whether or not to move. Similarly when a joint is inflamed, the muscles around that joint tighten up (spasm) to protect the joint and limit its movement. Muscles will also spasm to protect a fractured bone or other injury.

Muscle spasm is easy to evaluate even in the smallest of children. You simply have to have your hand on the muscle group you are evaluating and you can feel the spasm when it occurs. You can feel the quadriceps muscles spasm when you move a painful knee. You can feel the flexors of the forearm tighten when you move a painful wrist. You can feel the gluteal muscles tighten when you rotate a painful hip.

The ease with which muscles spasm can be evaluated is very important in taking care of children. Since the muscle spasm is (almost entirely) involuntary, you can judge how much something hurts. Sometimes in teenagers I hear loud complaints of pain—with no muscle spasm. At other times, they assure me that their wrist doesn't hurt, it's only their knee that's a problem, as I note the muscle spasm and withdrawal. Either way I've gained valuable information.

The key to a good musculoskeletal evaluation in children is noting where there is swelling and where there is guarding. Pain and guarding go together, so do pain and limitation. You also want to know if any of the joints feel hot and inflamed. An arthritic joint may feel hot and inflamed, but an infected joint almost always will. Do remember to differentiate pain in a joint from pain around the joint or in the bone. A child with a tumor may complain of pain in his leg, but the muscle spasm and warmth often will be away from the joint, not at it. Osteomyelitis also typically presents with pain in the bone, not the joint.

A complete physical examination is very important. Just as completing the history requires a lot of questions about things that aren't obviously part of the problem, completing the physical examination does too. Every day someone will ask me why I'm looking in the child's ears or eyes when his knee hurts. Hopefully everyone reading this will recognize that children with arthritis may get uveitis and have unsuspected eye findings. They aren't really likely to have ear problems related to arthritis, but I carefully evaluate everything. Scarred ear drums indicate chronic infections and may be my first clue to IgA deficiency, which predisposes to arthritis. Tongue lesions can be part of Behcet's disease, Crohn's disease, or systemic lupus erythematosus. Difficulty opening the mouth might be my first hint that a child has scleroderma. Purple spots on the lips may indicate unsuspected Peutz-Jeghers syndrome. That's not a rheumatic disease, but it needs to be recognized and treated if the child has it (and yes, that has happened to me).

Every child referred for rheumatic disease evaluation needs to be fully examined. It may lead to a discovery as common as the knee problem is really a hip problem. Or a complete exam may lead to recognition of other problems. A child sent to me with knee pain was diagnosed as having leukemia when I palpated a "rock hard" spleen. A child with hip pain and a limp on the right side had a ruptured appendix that had become a chronic abscess and was causing the limp.

Don't listen to anyone who tells you, "You don't need to do that. There aren't any joints in the abdomen." The key to doing a good job is thoroughness. That means that you look at everything from the top of the head to the bottom of the toes (note: in routine rheumatologic practice that does not include genital or rectal exams unless specifically indicated). Nail fold capillary abnormalities, fingernail pitting, carotid artery bruits, distal fingertip infarcts, café au lait spots, and telangiectasias are all examples of minor findings away from the joints that may lead to the diagnosis.

Looking in the eyes is probably one of the most important and least obvious parts of doing a good physical examination of a child with joint complaints. Many times a young child has been sent to me after months of being treated for an "injury" and I've been able to make an immediate diagnosis of juvenile idiopathic arthritis by looking not at the joint, but at the eyes. Young children with juvenile idiopathic arthritis are at risk for the development of eye inflammation called anterior uveitis. Untreated it can lead to permanent visual damage and even blindness. The problem is that it is not painful and comes on gradually, so the child may not be complaining about it. In the early stages, it can only be detected by an ophthalmologist doing a slit-lamp exam. More advanced disease may be detectable by looking at the child's eye and realizing the pupil isn't round or doesn't expand as well as the pupil of the other eye. Any child with these findings needs immediate ophthalmologic evaluation.

Just as no part of taking a good history should be left out in evaluating a child with musculoskeletal complaints, there is no part of a good physical examination that might not reveal a previously unsuspected diagnosis. This includes doing a complete musculoskeletal examination. Many children with chronic "weak ankles" turn out to have limited back motion or wrist pain or heel pain that hasn't been previously noted by physicians. These findings might not mean anything, but often they make it obvious to a careful examiner that the child has a rheumatic disease and not a chronic injury. The most famous example is the child with early psoriatic arthritis whose first symptom is a swollen finger (dactylitis). Typically they have been sent to a hand

specialist when the finger didn't get better. They often have a tender toe on the foot on the same side and in the same position as the tender finger. (Note: This is also a group that often has eye disease, but hand surgeons don't typically look at eyes or feet.)

LABORATORY TESTS

Laboratory tests may be very misleading in children with rheumatic disease. It's easy if the child's routine laboratory test results are abnormal. Everyone will recognize the importance of a low hemoglobin level or a high erythrocyte sedimentation rate or abnormal muscle enzymes. The specific abnormalities related to individual diseases are discussed in the appropriate chapters. It is important to remember that tests for rheumatoid factor are usually negative in children with arthritis. Tests for antinuclear antibodies (ANA) are often positive. If the ANA is positive, it increases the risk of the child having eye disease (no one is sure why). Every ANA-positive child with joint pain should see an ophthalmologist, even if the routine eye examination is normal. Most children won't have eye disease, but we have to find all the ones that do as early as possible.

Of greater importance is the approach to a child whose laboratory test results are "all normal." It is very unlikely that any patient you see will have been tested for everything. Patients with persistent complaints but normal laboratory tests may have growing pains or fibromyalgia. They may be people who are depressed or complain all the time. But they may also be people with diseases the doctors didn't think to test for. We've all seen depressed people with lots of complaints we can't explain, but I've had patients who were undergoing treatment for chronic depression who suddenly didn't need that therapy when we did the proper tests and made the right diagnosis. Being in pain for a long time and being told by your health care provider "there is nothing wrong with you," or "there's nothing that can be done for you," will make people depressed.

Syndromes like mucopolysaccharidosis type I, Fabre's disease, and celiac disease are easy to recognize and diagnose in their late stages, but they (and many other diseases) may cause muscle and joint pains long before the other symptoms are obvious and long before the routine laboratory test results are abnormal. Children with Fabre's disease or mucopolysaccharidosis type I often give a history of vague hand pains that went on for many years before the proper diagnosis was made.

When a child seems to have very real complaints and "no one can find an answer," it is important to remember that everyone caring for that child has the obligation to assure that a complete evaluation has been done. Occasionally when I'm lecturing to general physicians, some one will stand up in the audience and exclaim that I'm talking about very rare conditions that they've never seen. In turn, I point out that you can never diagnose these conditions if you don't test for them. All the children in my care with these diagnoses were previously seen by physicians who didn't make the diagnosis because they didn't think to do the proper test. Some of the tests that need to be done may not be available in the local laboratory. Children with chronic unexplained complaints may need to be evaluated at a major medical center for all the appropriate testing to get done.

The key for everyone involved in caring for children is to think about what you first saw when you walked into the room and what you heard and saw when you were taking the history and doing the physical examination. These are key in deciding how far to push the laboratory evaluation in search of unusual diagnoses. If the parents keep coming back to the doctor complaining about a problem or have gone from doctor to doctor because "no one will listen," then it is clear something more needs to be done. It may be a psychological problem, not a medical

> ### Nursing Considerations in Pediatric Evaluation
>
> - Educate child as well as family on medications and their side effects. Children should learn the names of any medications used in the long-term.
> - Nurses in the pediatric setting are often called upon to provide support to schools: in-services, letters of medical necessity, Individualized Education Program input.

illness, but a very thorough evaluation should be completed before that decision is made. Many of the children I care for with unusual diseases were initially told there was nothing wrong or they had fibromyalgia. The proper diagnoses were made only after carefully listening to the families convinced me that more testing was needed. Sometimes even then it took months to years for the underlying disease to become obvious.

OTHER DIAGNOSTIC MODALITIES

Many diagnostic modalities are available for the evaluation of a child with musculoskeletal pain. Almost every child with persistent pain has had a radiograph to look for problems. If it's never been done, it should be because it may immediately make the cause of the problem obvious. Infections, such as osteomyelitis, tumors (both benign, e.g., osteoid osteoma; or malignant, e.g., osteosarcomas), and many other bone problems may begin with musculoskeletal complaints. These are often easily seen on radiographs. Do remember that knee pain can be referred from the hip, and a knee radiograph may not show the problem in the hip.

Magnetic resonance imaging (MRI) may show abnormalities that are not visible on routine radiographs. MRIs can demonstrate soft-tissue damage, muscle inflammation, and many other important findings. The test is expensive and time consuming. In addition, for small children it may require anesthesia so they can hold still long enough. When to do an MRI is a matter of clinical judgment. We should not be doing MRIs on every child with complaints, but I will get an MRI on children without an obvious problem if the family's concern is enough to make me worried that there might be something I'm missing or if the clinical picture isn't making sense to me.

Bone scans are done less often than MRIs, but are much less expensive and have the advantage of looking at the entire body. They will pick up evidence of infection before the radiograph. An MRI will also provide an early indication of infection, but you can't image the whole body. It's easy to bone scan the whole body, looking for unsuspected problems or to simultaneously evaluate several areas that hurt.

Musculoskeletal ultrasound is a relatively new technique that it rapidly gaining favor. In the hands of an experienced operator, the ultrasound can provide information about muscles, tendons, synovium, and bone. Good musculoskeletal ultrasound is not widely available yet, but I expect the use and utility of this technique to expand rapidly in the next few years.

CONCLUSIONS

Care of the child with musculoskeletal complaints requires careful evaluation by everyone on the health care team. Even the most conscientious physician may miss a piece of information or an abnormality in the examination that may be noticed by the nurse, physical therapist, occupational therapist, or another health care provider. Everyone on the health care team should be working together, sharing information, observations, and impressions. By working together the members of the health care team can provide the support needed for those with mild problems while assuring that continued and thorough investigation is carried out for those with ongoing complaints. It is not only the initial evaluation of the child that is important, but the ongoing evaluation as well.

Joint Counts

OZLEM PALA, MD, and L. FRANK CAVALIERE, MD

Rheumatoid arthritis (RA) is a chronic systemic inflammatory disease, the presentation and course of which are highly variable in the same patient and between patients. No single quantitative measure is a gold standard to assess and monitor the clinical status in patients with RA. A variety of measures have been used in clinical care and clinical research, including formal joint counts, laboratory and radiographic evaluations, measures of functional status, global measures, and patient self-report questionnaires (1).

Swollen and tender joints are the most characteristic features of RA, and disease severity is directly related to the number of swollen and tender joints. A joint count assessment is the most specific quantitative clinical measure to assess the status of the patient with inflammatory arthropathies, particularly RA. Joint counts are the major part of the Disease Activity Score (DAS) (2,3), the American College of Rheumatology (ACR) Core Data Set for the clinical trials in RA (4), and the ACR remission criteria (5).

COMPONENTS OF AN ARTICULAR EXAMINATION

Abnormalities assessed in formal joint counts include swelling, tenderness, pain on motion, limitation of motion, and occasionally deformity (6). Generally, the examiner may serve as the normal control for range of motion (ROM); similarly, comparison to an unaffected joint on the opposite side of the body can identify individual variations.

Joint swelling is soft tissue swelling that is detectable along the joint margins. The presence of synovial proliferation, joint effusion, and fluctuance are characteristic features of swollen joints, but neither bony enlargement nor joint deformity constitutes swelling. Joint swelling is assessed by inspection and direct palpation of the joint. A thickened synovial membrane in inflammatory arthritis may have a doughy consistency. The examiner should palpate the joint in all planes, medial to lateral and anterior to posterior. Limitation of ROM may also point to the presence of swelling.

Joint tenderness is the presence of pain in a joint at rest with pressure or upon movement of the joint. It is assessed by gentle, yet firm, palpation over the joint. Pressure to elicit tenderness should be exerted by the examiner's thumb and index finger sufficient to cause whitening of the examiner's nail bed. The patient is instructed to notify the examiner if pain is elicited, and observing the patient's facial expressions is often helpful. Pain on motion is highly correlated with tenderness (7) and may be substituted for tenderness in joints in which tenderness is difficult to assess, such as the cervical spine, shoulders, hips (8), and tarsal joints.

Joint deformity is very common in the small joints of the hands and feet of patients with long-standing RA. Deformity is graded as absent or present. Limited ROM is also of value to be assessed in each joint.

FORMAL JOINT COUNTS

A number of joint counts have been developed over the past several decades (Table 1). There is no existing consensus on a single standardized method of counting the number of joints involved in RA. The methods available vary in number of joints assessed and as to whether the joint is scored on a graded scale or simply rated normal or abnormal (9). Commonly preferred and validated methods include the extended ACR Core Data Set 66/68-joint count (10), the Ritchie articular index (11), 44-joint count (3,12), and the reduced 28-joint count (7). There is also a NOAR-DJC (Norfolk Arthritis Register-Damaged Joint Count) that uses a simple binary scoring system evaluating deformity, restricted ROM, and surgical alteration in 51 synovial joints (13). Counts with 36 and 42 joints are used less frequently (14,15).

The 66/68-joint count (10) evaluates 66 joint for swelling and 68 joints for tenderness and pain on motion. The hip joints can be assessed for tenderness, but not for swelling. The following joints are included, **upper**: temporomandibular, sternoclavicular, acromioclavicular, shoulder, elbow, wrist, metacarpophalangeal (MCP), proximal interphalangeal (PIP), and distal interphalangeal; and **lower**: hip, knee, ankle, tarsus, metatarsophalangeal (MTP), and interphalangeal (IP) joints of the feet.

The Ritchie articular index (11) evaluates 52 joints, including the shoulder, elbow, wrist, hip, ankle, talocalcaneal, tarsus, and cervical spine, which are assessed only for tenderness. The MCP and PIP joints are assessed in groups, and the right and left joints are assessed together in the temporomandibular, sternoclavicular, and acromioclavicular joints. Assessment includes grading: 0 = nontender, 1 = tender, 2 = tender with wincing, and 3 = tender with wincing and withdrawal. Total scores range from 0 to 78.

A 44-swollen joint count is included in the original DAS (3,12) and includes the following joints: sternoclavicular, acromioclavicular, shoulder, elbow, wrist, MCP, PIP, knee, ankle, and MTP.

The 28-joint count, used in the DAS28, includes shoulders, elbows, wrists, MCPs, PIPs, and knees, but excludes joints of the feet (Figure 1). This exclusion is based on recognition that feet abnormalities may often result from processes other than arthritis, including fluid retention, venous insufficiency, and effects of footwear. Exclusion of ankle and feet joints in no way denies their importance in routine clinical care because they may be a major source of discomfort and disability (7).

These joint counts, except Ritchie articular index, calculate the number of abnormal joints without grading the extent of swelling or tenderness. That information has not been found to be useful, possibly due to intraobserver variation (7).

Although quantitative joint examination methods are quite useful to record results in clinical trials, some have stated that their complexity makes incorporation into routine clinical practice difficult. However, joint counts are recognized to be useful in the prediction of morbidity (16) and mortality (17). Moreover, joint counts are part of the core set of measurements recommended by the ACR for clinical care.

Various articular indices have been compared and found to have similar validity and reliability (18,19). Joints included in the 28-joint count are more commonly involved than other joints, and findings from the 28-joint count correlated highly with those from 66/68-joint count (20). As a result, the 28-joint count has been advocated as an easier count to perform.

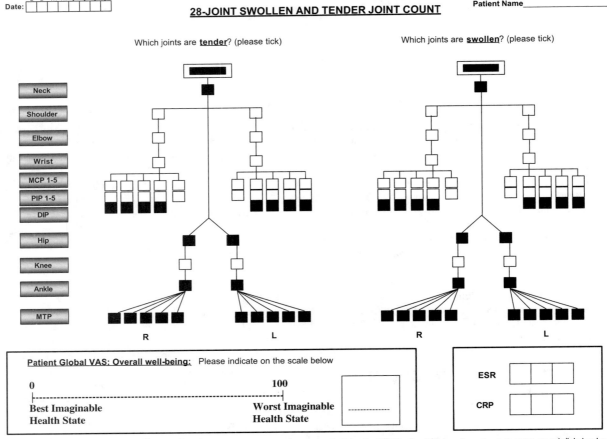

Figure 1. Sample of form to use when performing a 28-joint count. Accessed July 2, 2006. Available at www.arc.man.ac.uk/biologics/pdfs/manikin.pdf.

EXAMINATION OF INDIVIDUAL JOINTS

Swelling and tenderness are assessed as present or absent; no scoring is given for deformities or ROM of the joints. *Soft tissue swelling* is assessed along the joint margins; bony swelling and joint deformities do not constitute joint swelling for the purpose of the joint examination. *Joint tenderness* is performed by applying firm pressure on the joints with enough force that the examiner's nail beds blanche.

The joints that are examined are

- Shoulders
- Elbows
- Wrists
- MCPs
- PIPs
- IPs
- Knees

Shoulder: Evaluation for pain is performed by assessing tenderness through a passive range of motion; joint swelling is assessed by visual inspection.

Elbow: The elbow is flexed to about 80° and palpated for swelling and tenderness between the epicondyles and the olecranon process.

Wrist: The wrist is examined in the neutral position, placing both of the examiner's thumbs on the dorsal aspect and the fingers on the palmar aspect and palpating the wrist. Tenderness is also assessed by performing flexion and extension of the wrist.

MCP: The examiner's thumb and index finger are placed on a slightly flexed MCP joint to palpate the anterior lateral joint margins. Note the first MCP may be examined as a PIP/IP joint.

PIP and IP: Both the examiner's thumb and index finger are placed on the medial/lateral aspect and the superior/inferior aspect, respectively, of the fully extended joint. A slight modification of this would be to place the index and thumb slightly above the medial and lateral portion to assess swelling and tenderness.

Knee: With the knee fully extended, assess the joint for bulge or ballottment signs and evidence of tenderness.

JOINT COUNTS IN CLINICAL TRIALS AND PRACTICE

Although assessments of all joints may be performed in a patient evaluation, formal joint counts include a defined number of joints for comparison from one visit to the next. The ACR Core Data Set includes 7 measures: swollen joint count, tender joint count, patient assessment of global status, an acute phase reactant measure (erythrocyte sedimentation rate [ESR] or C-reactive protein), physical function, pain, and health professional assessment of global status. The first 4 of these measures are included in the DAS. An improvement of at least 20% in both swollen and tender joint scores, along with improvement in 3 of

Table 1. Comparison of joints assessed in various joint counts

Joint	66/68	Ritchie index	44	28
Cervical spine	♦	♦		
Temporomandibular	♦	♦*		
Sternoclavicular	♦	♦*	♦	
Acromioclavicular	♦	♦*	♦	
Shoulder	♦	♦	♦	♦
Elbow	♦	♦	♦	♦
Wrist	♦	♦	♦	♦
Metocarpophalangeal	♦	♦†	♦	♦
Proximal interphalangeal	♦	♦†	♦	♦
Distal interphalangeal	♦			
Hip (evaluates tenderness only)	♦	♦		
Knee	♦	♦	♦	♦
Ankle	♦	♦	♦	
Talocalcaneal		♦		
Tarsus		♦		
Metatarsophalangeal		♦†		
Proximal interphalangeal (toe)				

*Right and left joint assessed as a pair
†Assessed as a group

5 additional measures, is required to meet ACR improvement criteria (21), known as the ACR 20. Higher thresholds for improvement, such as the ACR 50 and the ACR 70, have also been described. The original DAS used the Ritchie articular index, 44-swollen-joint count, ESR, and general health assessment on a visual analog scale. The DAS28 has subsequently been modified for ease of use to assess 28 joints for swelling and tenderness in a nongraded manner. Serial measurements of DAS28 predict physical disability and radiographic disease progression. The DAS28 can also discriminate between patients with high and low disease activity.

Indices, such as ACR criteria and DAS, are used in clinical trials because it is difficult to objectively measure underlying inflammation. Even though ACR improvement criteria and DAS-based European League Against Rheumatism response criteria use different approaches, both perform very well in differentiating between 2 types of active treatment and in differentiating placebo from active treatment.

The CORRONA (The Consortium of Rheumatology Researchers of North America) database (22) is an example for clinical use of joint counts. It was founded by a group of academic rheumatologists in 2000 and is the largest independent database in North America that collects data from both rheumatologists and patients with RA and psoriatic arthritis.

CORRONA uses a 28-joint count for both swelling and tenderness at the time of patient visit and records other relevant clinical, laboratory, hospitalization, disability (assessed by Health Assessment Questionnaire), and medication data. The data collected provide chart documentation of patient progress and also are used for outcomes research on large numbers of patients. Most physicians who have incorporated formal joint counts into their clinical practices have found them useful in more accurately evaluating their patients over time.

Objective clinical measurement, including the routine use of joint counts, can be an important tool to provide high-quality clinical care for RA patients. Whether such documentation will translate into improved clinical outcomes is an area of active interest and research.

REFERENCES

1. Pincus T, Sokka T. Quantitative measures for assessing rheumatoid arthritis in clinical trials and clinical care. Rheum Dis Clin North Am 2004;30: 725–51.
2. van der Heijde DM, van 't Hof MA, van Riel PL, Theunisse LA, Lubberts EW, van Leeuwen MA, et al. Judging disease activity in clinical practice in rheumatoid arthritis: first step in the development of a disease activity score. Ann Rheum Dis 1990;49:916–20.
3. van Der Heijde DMFM, van't Hof MA, van Riel PLCM, van de Putte LB. Development of a disease activity score based on judgments in clinical practice by rheumatologist. J Rheumtol 1993;20:579–81.
4. Felson DT, Anderson JJ, Boers M, Bombardier C, Chernoff M, Fried B, et al., The Committee on Outcome Measures in Rheumatoid Arthritis Clinical Trials. The American College of Rheumatology preliminary core set of disease activity measure for rheumatoid arthritis clinical trials. Arthritis Rheum 1993;36:729–40.
5. Pinals RS, Masi AT, Larsen RA. Preliminary criteria for clinical remission in rheumatoid arthritis. Arthritis Rheum 1981;24:1308–15.
6. American Rheumatism Association Glossary Committee. Dictionary of the rheumatic diseases, volume I. Signs and symptoms. New York: American Rheumatism Association; 1982.
7. Fuchs HA, Brooks RH, Callahan LF, Pincus T. A simplified twenty-eight-joint quantitative articular index in rheumatoid arthritis. Arthritis Rheum 1989;32:531–7.
8. Ritchie DM, Boyle JA, McInnes JM, Jasani MK, Dalakos TG, Grieveson P, et al. Clinical studies with an articular index for the assessment of joint tenderness in patients with rheumatoid arthritis. Q J Med 1968;37:393–406.
9. Pincus T, Callahan LF. Quantitative measures to assess, monitor and predict morbidity and mortality in rheumatoid arthritis. Clin Rheumatol 1992;6:161–91.
10. Cooperating clinics committee of the American Rheumatism Association. A seven day variability study of 499 patients with peripheral rheumatoid arthritis. Arthritis Rheum 1965;8:302–35.
11. Ritchie DM, Boyle JA, McInnes JM, Jasani MK, Dalakos TG, Grieveson P, et al. Clinical studies with articular index for the assessment of joint tenderness in patients with rheumatoid arthritis. Q J Med 1968;37:393–406.
12. van der Heijde D, Klareskog L, Boers M, Landewe R, Codreanu C, Bolosiu HD, et al. Comparison of different definitions to classify remission and sustained remission: one year TEMPO results. Ann Rheum Dis 2005;64:1582–7.
13. Bunn DK, Shepstone L, Galpin LM, Wiles NJ, Symmons DPM, et al. The NOAR-DJC: a clinical measure for assessing articular damage in patients with early inflammatory polyarthritis including RA. Rheumatology (Oxford) 2004;43:1519–25.
14. Egger MJ, Huth DA, Ward JR, Reading JC, Williams HJ. Reduced joint count indices in the evaluation of rheumatoid arthritis. Arthritis Rheum 1985;28:6613–9.
15. Pincus T, Brooks RH, Callahan LF. A proposed Standard Protocol to Evaluate Rheumatoid Arthritis (SPERA) that includes measures of inflammatory activity, joint damage, and longterm outcomes. J Rheumatol 1999;26:473–80.
16. Masi AT, Feigenbaum SL, Kaplan SB. Articular pattern in early course of rheumatoid arthritis. Am J Med 1983;75:16–26.
17. Pincus T, Callahan LF, Vaughn WK. Questionnaire, walking time and button test measures of functional capacity as predictive markers for mortality in rheumatoid arthritis. J Rheumatol 1987;14:240–51.
18. Prevoo ML, van Riel PL, van 't Hof MA, van Rijswijk MH, van Leeuwen MA, Kuper HH, et al. Validity and reliability of joint indices: a longitudinal study in patients with recent onset rheumatoid arthritis. Br J Rheumatol 1993;37:598–94.
19. Fuchs HA, Pincus T. Reduced joint counts in controlled clinical trials in rheumatoid arthritis. Arthritis Rheum 1994;37:470–5.
20. Smolen JS, Breedveld FC, Eberl G, Jones I, Leeming M, Wylie GL, et al. Validity and reliability of twenty-eight-joint count for the assessment of rheumatoid arthritis activity. Arthritis Rheum 1995;38:38–43.
21. Felson DT, Anderson JJ, Boers M, Bombardier C, Furst D, Goldsmith C, et al. American College of Rheumatology: preliminary definition of improvement in rheumatoid arthritis. Arthritis Rheum 1995;38:727–35.
22. Kremer JM. The CORRONA database. Clin Exp Rheumatol 2005; 23(5 Suppl 39):S172–7.

Diagnostic Laboratory Testing

THOMAS D. BEARDMORE, MD, FACP, FACR, and MARK H. WENER, MD, FACR;
as updated by PETER SCHUR, MD, MACR

Laboratory tests have great importance in the diagnosis and assessment of rheumatic diseases. They are an integral part of the American College of Rheumatology (ACR) classification criteria for many of the common rheumatic diseases, including rheumatoid arthritis (RA), systemic lupus erythematosus (SLE), and degenerative joint disease, and are widely used in routine clinical diagnosis. Sometimes negative test results are useful, as in the diagnosis of fibromyalgia and exclusion of inflammatory joint disease. Despite the usefulness of diagnostic tests, it is important to remember that no rheumatic disease is established by tests alone. The careful integration of history, physical examination, laboratory tests, and imaging is necessary to establish diagnosis.

Health care providers and patients benefit when testing is utilized and understood. These tests assist in disease management in several ways: 1) establishing a diagnosis; 2) determining prognosis; 3) monitoring disease activity, progression, or damage; 4) monitoring drug or therapeutic toxicities; 5) establishing complications of the underlying disease process; and 6) excluding alternative diagnoses or complications. The optimal diagnostic test should be *sensitive* (able to identify a disease when present) and *specific* (able to identify that the disease is not present). An evaluative or monitoring test should be sensitive to change in the disease state over time. Ideally, tests should be inexpensive, standardized, easily performed, and readily available. Diagnostic testing is of great importance in establishing treatment modalities, whether these are medicines, exercises, or lifestyle adjustments. Testing is closely associated with prognosis, including the development of disability.

GENERAL LABORATORY TESTING

Rheumatic disorders and treatments can affect major body systems. General laboratory testing reveals multisystem organ involvement and specific organ function. It is important to test the patient at baseline and periodically during the course of treatment to detect disease improvement, progression, and medication toxicity. A flow sheet for laboratory data is a valuable tool for the health care provider to monitor the overall disease state and toxicity.

Hematology

A complete blood count including hemoglobin, hematocrit, white blood cell count with differential, and platelet count is one of the most common baseline tests in systemic rheumatic diseases. It is used not only for rheumatic disease diagnosis and monitoring, but also for detection of anemia or other blood disorders.

Understanding the cause or mechanism of anemia is important for characterizing the disease and for selecting and monitoring treatment. For example, anemia due to accelerated hemolysis is caused by autoantibodies directed against red cells in many patients with SLE. Similarly, leukopenia and thrombocytopenia caused by autoimmunity are common in SLE and may occasionally be seen as part of the underlying disease process in RA. Many rheumatic diseases, such as RA, SLE, and

systemic sclerosis, are associated with a modest anemia (hemoglobin levels as low as 10 gm/dl) called **anemia of chronic disease** or **anemia of chronic inflammation**. In this anemia, the red cells typically have normal shape and hemoglobin content (normocytic and normochromic). The anemia does not respond to administration of iron; in fact, the problem is caused by inflammation, which alters the availability of iron for the developing red blood cell in the bone marrow. This is in contrast to the anemia that develops as a consequence of gastrointestinal bleeding from nonsteroidal antiinflammatory drugs, in which the cells are small, the hemoglobin content low, and the serum iron level is low, which typically responds to iron therapy. Therapy with drugs such as methotrexate may result in folate deficiency and a macrocytic anemia, where red cells are large. More severe anemia should always be investigated to determine whether it is related to drug toxicity, serious complications of the underlying rheumatic diseases, or some other mechanism.

Knowledge of hematologic abnormalities is important in designing exercise programs, education, activities of daily living, and medical treatment. For example, the provider needs to be aware when prescribing medications that bleeding may occur when platelet counts are low or infections may occur when white cell counts are low. When the patient has anemia, he or she may experience general loss of energy and endurance.

Urinalysis

Urinalysis is one of the most informative, easy to perform, and cost-effective laboratory tests. Analysis for protein and microscopic presence of cells and cellular casts is important as a diagnostic aid in SLE, which has a high incidence of nephritis. Proteinuria is one of the ACR classification criteria for SLE. Nephritis can be reflected as increased urinary protein, white cells, or red cells; and the presence of casts on microscopic analysis. When present, proteinuria should be quantitated by a timed collection (typically 24 hours).

Although rarely used, the medications gold and penicillamine require periodic assessment of urine to monitor for associated renal toxicity manifested by proteinuria (both drugs) and hematuria (gold). Trace and modest proteinuria can be managed by reducing dosages, but a large amount of proteinuria requires drug discontinuation.

Chemical Analysis of Blood

Routine blood chemistries are commonly measured as a panel of tests. Serum electrolytes, renal function tests (blood urea nitrogen and creatinine), liver damage and function tests, and mineral metabolism tests are often included. Most medications are metabolized by the liver and excreted by the kidneys, and the possibility of drug toxicity may be monitored with such tests. Toxicity may be reflected as a decrease in serum albumin, a rise in liver damage indicators such as alanine aminotransferase (ALT) and aspartate aminotransferase (AST), or an increase in blood urea nitrogen or creatinine (renal function). For example, an increase in ALT or AST in a patient taking methotrexate or other drugs for RA is an indication of potentially significant liver toxicity, which may require reduction or cessation of the drug.

Elevated serum uric acid is useful in the diagnosis of gout, although the diagnosis can be established with certainty only if sodium urate crystals are seen in tissue or synovial fluid. The higher the level of serum uric acid above the normal range (2–7 mg/dl), the greater is the risk of development of gout. Nevertheless, there are limitations to using serum uric acid as a diagnostic test. Transient and persistent hyperuricemia is common, and not all hyperuricemic patients develop gout. Furthermore, a normal uric acid level may be seen in patients at the time of their acute gout attacks. Once a diagnosis of gout is established, monitoring serum uric acid levels is helpful in determining the appropriate dosages of medications.

Serum measures of muscle damage, including creatine kinase (CK, previously known as creatine phosphokinase or CPK) and aldolase, are used to diagnose and monitor patients with polymyositis and dermatomyositis. The highest and most persistent levels of these muscle damage markers are seen in the inflammatory myopathies and can be used as therapeutic indicators because they will decrease with disease improvement. These measures can be elevated in conditions involving muscle breakdown or necrosis, such as intramuscular injections, extreme exercise, or myocardial infarction. Lactate dehydrogenase and AST may be elevated in muscle disease and mistaken for abnormalities of liver function. A serum CK-MB, while appropriate as a sensitive measurement of heart damage, is not a sensitive measure of skeletal muscle damage, such as occurs in patients with myositis.

Viral Screening Tests

Many of the drugs used to treat rheumatic diseases can cause liver damage; it is thus common to screen for preexisting liver disease before starting these drugs. In addition, various forms of vasculitis and other rheumatic conditions are associated with hepatitis infections. Tests for hepatitis B commonly include measurement of hepatitis B surface antibody (HBsAb) and surface antigen (HBsAg). A positive test result for HBsAb indicates that the patient is protected from hepatitis B, either because of previous infection or previous immunization. A positive test result for HBsAg indicates that the patient is infected with hepatitis B, and followup tests are indicated.

Hepatitis C infection is relatively common, affecting about 1% of the US population. The screening test for hepatitis C virus is performed by testing for antibodies to hepatitis C. If the antibody test result is positive, followup testing is performed to detect circulating hepatitis C RNA, which confirms active infection. In patients with positive antibody test results but negative RNA test results, the infection could be cured or the virus may still be present in the liver. Sometimes, repeat testing for hepatitis C RNA is performed to determine if a negative test result becomes positive, or to quantify the concentration of virus in patients known to be infected.

COMMON SEROLOGIC TESTS

Autoantibodies

An autoantibody is an immunoglobulin that is directed against a normally occurring protein or cellular component (see Chapter 3, Immunity). Autoantibodies may react with soluble serum proteins, such as antibodies directed against gamma globulin (rheumatoid factor), or they may be directed against cell components, such as cytoplasmic or nuclear antigens (antinuclear antibody). Autoantibodies are common in RA, SLE, Sjögren's syndrome, scleroderma, polymyositis,

dermatomyositis, and diffuse connective-tissue diseases. Tests for autoantibodies are commonly performed in patients with musculoskeletal complaints.

Rheumatoid Factor

The commonly observed rheumatoid factor (RF) in RA is an IgM antibody that is directed against the constant portion of IgG. In some laboratories, it is detected by an agglutination test using latex particles. In this test, the latex particles are coated with IgG and reacted with the patient's serum. If IgM rheumatoid factor is present, the latex particles clump or agglutinate. The test is quantified by serial 2-fold dilution of the serum, and the titer (the highest serum dilution at which visible agglutination occurs) is determined. A typical significant positive result of this test would be 1:160, indicating that the serum test had visible agglutination at a 1:160 dilution of serum, but no agglutination at the next dilution (i.e., 1:320). In larger laboratories, RF is more commonly measured on an instrument called a nephelometer, which measures the scatter of a beam of light passing through a solution. Nephelometric techniques provide better quantification and may be automated. Results are typically reported in international units per milliliter, where a typical significant positive result might be 50 IU/ml. Some laboratories measure RF by enzyme-linked immunosorbent assay (ELISA). This technique is also quantitative and can differentiate between IgM, IgA, and IgG rheumatoid factors. Many laboratories in Europe prefer this method.

No matter how it is measured, RF is not diagnostic of RA. In early or mild RA, many patients will test negative for rheumatoid factor. However, up to 90% of patients with RA will become RF positive (1,2). The test cannot be used alone to diagnose RA, but it is one of the ACR classification criteria. A positive RF is also a prognostic test, since high titers of RF are associated with increased disease severity, the development of erosions, extra-articular manifestations, and greater disability (2,3). Rheumatoid factor does not change rapidly with treatment, so there is little reason to repeat this test once a high positive result is found. Rheumatoid factors are also found in some patients with SLE and in a form of vasculitis known as mixed cryoglobulinemia syndrome, which is usually caused by hepatitis C.

False-positive results for RF also limit the diagnostic specificity of this test. The incidence and titer of RF increase somewhat with age until patients reach the age of 70 or 80 years (4). Many other rheumatic diseases, as well bacterial endocarditis, tuberculosis, osteomyelitis, and chronic viral and parasitic infections, may be associated with positive test results for rheumatoid factor (Table 1).

Antibodies to Citrullinated Proteins

There has been considerable interest in developing a better test for the diagnosis of RA; one that has greater sensitivity and specificity than the tests that detect RFs. Within the last decade, as a an outgrowth of determining the molecular specificity of antifilaggrin, antikeratin, and antiperinuclear antibodies, it was recognized that many patients with RA have antibodies to citrullinated proteins. Proteins that are citrullinated have had an arginine replaced by citrulline, a minor amino acid. A number of peptides containing citrulline were created, and a cyclic peptide was used to develop an assay to detect antibodies thereto. This test has now been studied extensively, especially in Europe, for its sensitivity and specificity for diagnosing RA. In a review of the literature, it was concluded that tests for the detection of anti-cyclic citrullinated peptide (CCP) antibodies had better sensitivity and specificity than tests that detect RF for the diagnosis of RA (5). This is summarized in Table 2.

Table 1. Conditions associated with positive tests for rheumatoid factor

Rheumatic diseases
  Rheumatoid arthritis (~70%)
  Sjögren's syndrome (~90%)
  Systemic lupus erythematosus (~20%)
  Cryoglobulinemia syndrome (90%)
Lung diseases
  Interstitial fibrosis
  Silicosis
  Asbestosis
Infections
  Hepatitis B and C virus infection
  Acute viral infections
  Bacterial endocarditis
  Tuberculosis
  Syphilis
  Leprosy
Miscellaneous
  Sarcoidosis
  Malignancies
  Primary biliary cirrhosis
  Aging

In addition, antibodies to CCP are rarely found in patients with spondyloarthopathy, infectious diseases, polymyositis/dermatomyositis, reactive arthritis, or vasculitis, whereas RF is more frequently found. Anti-CCP is even found frequently before the diagnosis of RA. These observations suggest that the anti-CCP test may be more useful for the diagnosis of RA than are RF tests, or at least should be part of the diagnostic algorithm.

Antinuclear Antibodies

Antinuclear antibodies (ANA) are commonly seen in autoimmune rheumatic diseases. A positive ANA test is not diagnostic of connective-tissue disease, but ANA are seen with a high frequency in SLE, systemic sclerosis, Sjögren's syndrome, polymyositis, and RA. Approximately 99% of patients with SLE will be ANA positive over the course of their disease (6–8).

The ANA test is usually performed as an indirect immunofluorescence test using the patient's serum overlaid onto a substrate. The human cell line HEp-2 (an immortalized cancer cell line) is commonly used as the substrate. After the serum is allowed to react with the

Table 2.

	Anti-CCP		RF	
	Sensitivity	Specificity	Sensitivity	Specificity
Healthy controls	0.79			
Rheumatoid arthritis	64	94	60	79
Juvenile arthritis	7.8		13.4	
Osteoarthritis	0			
Palindromic rheumatism	55		42	
Polymyalgia rheumatica	0			
Psoriatic arthritis	11.6			
Sjögren's syndrome	5.4		48.5	
Systemic lupus erythematosus	2.8		21.2	
Hepatitis C	0.5		30	

* CCP = cyclic citrullinated peptide; RF = rheumatoid factor. Reprinted with permission from Reference 5.

substrate cells, the extra serum is washed off. Next, a fluorescent-labeled antibody to normal human IgG is allowed to react with the substrate. The fluorescent-labeled antibody binds to the serum antibody, which has bound to the substrate. This can be detected by looking at the reacted substrate with a fluorescence microscope.

The ANA test is a screening test with a high degree of sensitivity for the diagnosis of SLE. Unfortunately, it is also associated with many false-positive test results, particularly when the ANA is present at low titer. In general, ANA titers of <1/80 have less clinical significance than do higher titers. However, positive test results must always be interpreted in light of the history, physical examination, and other laboratory tests to establish a diagnosis of SLE or related rheumatic diseases.

The ANA patterns as seen under the fluorescence microscope have some importance, but are rarely diagnostically specific. The pattern with the greatest diagnostic significance is the anticentromere pattern, which is typically associated with systemic sclerosis, and most often with limited cutaneous systemic sclerosis. The nucleolar pattern is also associated with systemic sclerosis and Raynaud's phenomenon. The diffuse and speckled patterns have little direct diagnostic significance because they are seen in patients with SLE or a variety of other conditions. When present in low titer, the diffuse and the speckled patterns are most commonly seen in patients without an underlying rheumatic disorder. The peripheral, also called rim, pattern is usually associated with antibodies to DNA and SLE.

If ANA are present and the patient has clinical features that suggest an autoimmune rheumatic syndrome, more specific testing is indicated (7,9) (Table 3). Tests for these specific antigens are generally performed by quantitative ELISA, although antibodies to double-stranded DNA (dsDNA) can also be detected by the immunofluorescent crithidia assay. The antibody against double-stranded or native DNA (anti-dsDNA) has high specificity for the diagnosis of SLE (10). Approximately 70% of patients with SLE will develop anti-dsDNA at some time during their disease course. When present in large amounts, anti-dsDNA is typically associated with diffuse proliferative lupus nephritis and a risk for more severe SLE. Measurements of anti-dsDNA tend to change with disease activity, so this measure is often repeated to help monitor disease activity.

Another antibody, anti-Sm (named for a lupus patient, Mrs. Smith, from whom the antibody was originally obtained) also has high specificity for SLE, but it is present in only ~30% of SLE patients (11). Anti-Sm leads to a speckled ANA pattern. Another important antibody with a speckled ANA pattern is the RNP antibody, seen in sera of patients with SLE or an overlap disease known as mixed connective-tissue disease. Antibodies to SSA (anti-Ro) and SSB (anti-La) are associated with primary Sjögren's syndrome and with SLE, particularly forms of SLE with prominent skin involvement but without prominent renal disease (12). Other diagnostically useful autoantibodies associated with positive ANA tests include antihistone antibodies, associated with drug-induced lupus and spontaneous SLE, and anti–Scl-70 (anti–topoisomerase I), associated with diffuse cutaneous systemic sclerosis (or scleroderma), and anti–Jo-1 (an antisynthesase antibody) and anti–Mi-2 with dermatomyositis.

Antineutrophil Cytoplasmic Antibodies

Antibodies to neutrophil cytoplasmic antigens (ANCA) occur in 2 immunofluorescent patterns: a cytoplasmic (cANCA) distribution, and a perinuclear (pANCA) pattern (13). The cANCA pattern is associated strongly with the form of vasculitis known as Wegener's granulomatosis (WG), and it may be seen in related forms of vasculitis. In general, the greater the severity and extent of clinical involvement, the higher the titer of cANCA. About 90% of patients with active generalized

Table 3. Sensitivity, specificity, and predictive value of different antinuclear antibodies*

Disease	Antibody							
	dsDNA	**ssDNA**	**Histone**	**Nucleoprotein**	**Sm**	**RNP**	**Ro**	**La**
SLE								
Sen	70	80	30–80	58	25–30	50	25–35	15
Spec	95		50	Mod	Mod	99	87–94	
Pre	95	50	Mod	Mod	97	46–85		
Drug LE								
Sen		80	95	50	1		Low	low
Spec	1–5	50	High	Mod				
Pre	1–5	50	High	Mod				
RA								
Sen		Mod	Low	25	1	47	Low	Low
Spec	1	Mod		Low				
Pre	1	Mod		Low				
Scleroderma								
Sen			<1	<1	<1	20		
Spec	<1	Low						
Pre	<1	Low						
PM/DM								
Sen			<1	<1	<1		Low	
Spec	<1	Low						
Pre	<1	Low						
Sjögren's								
Sen		Mod	Low	Mod	1–5	5–60	8–70	14–60
Spec	1–5	Mod	Low	Mod			87	94
Pre	1–5	Mod	Low	Mod			5–48	26–41

Disease	Antibody							
	PCNA	**Scl-70**	**PM-1**	**Mi-1**	**Jo-1**	**Ku**	**Nucleoli**	**Centromere**
SLE								
Sen	5				Low		26	
Spec	95							
Pre	95							
Drug LE								
Sen	Low				Low			
Spec								
Pre								
RA								
Sen	Low				Low			
Spec								
Pre								
Scleroderma								
Sen	Low	15–20	Low		Low		54	25–30
Spec		High						
Pre		High						
PM/DM								
Sen	Low	Low	30–50	Low	30–50			
Spec								
Pre								
Sjögren's								
Sen		5			Low			
Spec								
Pre								

*Values are percentages unless otherwise noted. dsDNA = double-stranded DNA; ssDNA = single-stranded DNA; PCNA = proliferating cell nuclear antigen; SLE = systemic lupus erythematosus; Sen = sensitivity; Spec = specificity; Pre = predictive value; Drug LE = drug-induced lupus; RA = rheumatoid arthritis; PM/DM = polymyositis/dermatomyositis. Other associations are RNP: mixed connective tissue disease; Ro: subacute cutaneous lupus erythematosus, primary biliary cirrhosis, vasculitis, congenital heart block; centromere: calcinosis, Raynaud's phenomenon, esophageal dysmotility, sclerodactyly telangiectasias. Reprinted with permission from reference 7.

WG have a positive ANCA, versus about 60% of patients with inactive generalized WG and 40% of active limited (localized) WG. Also, antibody titers may fall in response to treatment and rise in association with clinical deterioration. The cANCA pattern is highly specific for these clinical entities, although there are a few cases of cANCAs reported in patients with other diagnoses. The cANCA immunofluorescence pattern is almost always caused by antibodies to a neutrophil granule enzyme known as proteinase 3 (PR3); these antibodies can be identified by an ELISA test. Eighty percent to 90% of patients with WG have antibodies to PR3.

The pANCA pattern has been observed in association with a variety of diseases, including various forms of vasculitis, inflammatory bowel disease, SLE, RA, and juvenile rheumatoid arthritis. Several different antigens are recognized by pANCA; however, antibodies directed against the neutrophil myeloperoxidase enzyme (MPO) are those most closely linked to vasculitis. For instance, 70% of patients with microscopic polyangitis are ANCA positive, with most having antibodies to PR3; 50% of patients with the Churg-Strauss syndrome are ANCA positive. Drug-induced vasculitis after treatment with either propylthiouracil, hydralazine, or minocycline is usually associated with a positive ANCA test. Sixty percent to 80% of patients with ulcerative colitis and 10–27% of patients with Crohn's disease have a positive pANCA, usually with antibodies to a 50-kd nuclear envelope protein.

Antiphospholipid (APL) Antibodies

Antibodies directed against phospholipids have received considerable attention in the last few years because of new appreciation of clinical associations and development of newer techniques for their measurement (14). The VDRL test and other serologic tests for syphilis employ reagents containing the phospholipid cardiolipin in the antigen mixture, and for decades, patients with SLE have been known to have false-positive test results for syphilis. Use of more specific assays led to the recognition that ~40% of patients with SLE have antibodies to cardiolipin. Another phenomenon seen in some patients with SLE is the presence of lupus inhibitor or lupus anticoagulant, which is a type of autoantibody that causes a prolonged activated partial thromboplastin time (PTT, clotting test). Studies have demonstrated that the lupus anticoagulant is also an antibody directed against phospholipids and phospholipid-binding proteins. In those laboratory tests, lupus inhibitors led to a prolonged PTT, and therefore might be predicted to lead to bleeding. In contrast, patients with these autoantibodies have an enhanced risk of thrombosis, including arterial and venous thromboses, and an increased risk of pregnancy loss after 10 weeks of gestation. In recognition of the increasing importance of the antiphospholipid syndrome in patients with lupus, the ACR classification criteria for SLE were modified to include the presence of APL as part of the epidemiologic classification criteria (15).

In considering a patient with possible antiphospholipid syndrome, measurement of both the lupus anticoagulant and anticardiolipin antibodies is appropriate, since the presence of one APL does not correlate well with the presence of another. In general, IgG anticardiolipin has a higher predictive value than IgM or IgA anticardiolipin, and the higher the elevation, the greater the positive predictive value for an association with the antiphospholipid syndrome. It has been shown that most of the anticardiolipin activity may be caused by antibodies to one or more protein cofactors that bind to cardiolipin or other phospholipids. The most important of these protein cofactors is a phospholipid-binding protein known as beta-2-glycoprotein I (β2GPI). Because of both biologic and technical variation in APL assays, the presence of antibodies in high titer and the detection of more than one antibody (e.g., anticardiolipin and anti-β2GPI) gives greater credence to the clinical significance of these antibodies in a given patient. However, to make the diagnosis, it is important to demonstrate that at least one test remains positive when the test is repeated at least 12 weeks later (16).

COMPLEMENT

The complement system is a system of proteins that play an important role in fighting infection and enhancing the inflammatory process (17,18). Complement is thought to be involved in disorders that involve immune complexes, such as SLE or certain forms of vasculitis. When immune complexes are formed and cleared from the body, the complement level is decreased.

There are 3 common measurements for serum complement, the protein components C3 and C4, and CH_{50} (total hemolytic complement),

which is a biologic measure of the entire complement pathway. In the rheumatic diseases, low levels of CH_{50}, C3, and C4 are usually related to consumption of complement by immune complex activation of the classical pathway (17,19). Rarely, reductions are related to a genetic absence of one of the complement proteins. Complement measurement is particularly useful in SLE, due to its association with active disease. A decrease in complement level may precede the development of a disease flare, particularly renal disease. Serial measurement of complement levels is frequently performed to assess disease activity in patients with SLE.

HUMAN LEUKOCYTE ANTIGENS

Human leukocyte antigens (HLA) are present on the surface of nucleated cells and play a central role in determining the genetic predisposition to a variety of immune-mediated processes, including autoimmune diseases. Currently, only HLA–B27 is commonly measured in the diagnosis of rheumatic diseases. This antigen is found in 5–10% of the US population, but it is present in 95% of patients with ankylosing spondylitis, 80% of patients with reactive arthritis, and a high percentage of patients with other spondyloarthropathies and acute anterior uveitis (20). The presence of HLA–B27 is not diagnostic for ankylosing spondylitis, but it may provide helpful clinical information in early disease when x-ray changes have not yet occurred. Testing for HLA–B27 may be misleading, because the antigen is also seen in patients without disease. Detection of HLA–B27 has also been used in family counseling. In families where one individual has HLA–B27 and a spondyloarthropathy, the presence of HLA–B27 in another family member suggests they are at high risk for developing a spondyloarthopathy.

There is also considerable interest in assessing HLA genetic markers in patients with RA. A strong association exists between RA and HLA–DR4. Some have advocated routine assessment of HLA–DR4 in patients with RA, especially those who have antibodies to CCP (see above) because the presence of both has a very strong predictive probability for the diagnosis of RA. In the future, HLA typing of patients with other disorders may be useful in establishing the diagnosis or prognosis, and in selecting specific therapies.

SYNOVIAL FLUID ANALYSIS

Aspiration and examination of synovial fluid can be important in the diagnosis of joint swelling. Synovial fluid is usually clear, acellular, viscous, and low in volume. Alterations in the appearance, volume, and cellular content of synovial fluid are useful in diagnosis.

Based on clinical and laboratory findings, the synovial fluid is classified into 1 of 4 groups (21,22). Group I fluids are noninflammatory, with a low white blood cell count (<2,000/µl), and are usually associated with such conditions as osteoarthritis. Group II fluids are inflammatory, with an intermediate white blood count (in the range of 2,000–10,000/µl), and are associated with such diseases as RA. Group III fluids are purulent, with high white blood cell counts (in the range of 100,000/µl), and are typically associated with infections. Group IV fluids are hemorrhagic, with blood typically arising from trauma or bleeding disorders (Table 4). This grouping is a continuum. Depending on the severity of the disorder and the timing of the aspiration, a patient with a given diagnosis may have fluids in different groups. For example, during a quiescent period in a patient with gout, the synovial fluid could be in Group I; at the beginning of a flare, the patient could have a Group II fluid; and with severe gout attacks, the same patient could have synovial fluid which is opaque due to cell counts as high as 100,000/µl (Group III).

Table 4. Categories of synovial fluid based on clinical and laboratory findings*

Measure	Normal	Noninflammatory	Inflammatory	Septic	Hemorrhagic
Volume, ml (knee)	<3.5	Often >3.5	Often >3.5	Often >3.5	Usually >3.5
Clarity	Transparent	Transparent	Translucent–opaque	Opaque	Bloody
Color	Clear	Yellow	Yellow to opalescent	Yellow to green	Red
Viscosity	High	High	Low	Variable	Variable
WBC, per μl	<200	200–2,000	2,000–100,000	>100,000†	200–2,000
PMN, %	<25	<25	≥50	≥75	50–75
Culture	Negative	Negative	Negative	Often positive	Negative
Total protein, g/dl	1–2	1–3	3–5	3–5	4–6
LDH (compared with blood)	Very low	Very low	High	Variable	Similar
Glucose, mg/dl	Nearly equal to blood	Nearly equal to blood	>25, lower than blood	<25, much lower than blood	Nearly equal to blood

*WBC = white blood cells; PMN = polymorphonuclear leukocytes; LDH = lactate dehydrogenase. Reprinted with permission from reference 22.
† Lower with infections caused by partially treated or low-virulence organisms.

The microscopic examination and culture of synovial fluid is extremely important. All synovial fluids in Groups II, III, and IV should be cultured when the diagnosis is unknown and infection is suspected. The culturing of organisms from synovial fluid establishes a diagnosis of infectious arthritis and allows treatment (specific antibiotics), which can result in cure.

In addition to cell counts and differentials, synovial fluid should be examined for crystals. Gout and calcium pyrophosphate dihydrate (CPPD) crystal deposition disease, two naturally occurring crystalline arthropathies, are diagnosed by the demonstration of birefringent crystals, using polarized light microscopy. In each of these conditions, the crystals may be ingested by a polymorphonuclear leukocyte. The CPPD crystal will have a rhomboid or rectangular shape and be weakly birefringent. If a first-order red compensator is used, CPPD crystals will show positive birefringence, demonstrating blue color when the long axis of the crystal is parallel to the "slow" direction noted on the housing of the compensator. Gouty crystals (monosodium urate) are needle-shaped and show strong negative birefringence, having a bright yellow appearance when the needle is parallel to the "slow" direction of the red compensator.

ACUTE PHASE REACTANTS

Among the body's internal responses to inflammation, infection, or other major injuries is a signal to change the production of proteins in the liver and other protein-synthesizing tissues. Proteins whose serum concentrations change in response to inflammation are called acute phase reactants (23,24). Many acute phase reactants demonstrate increased synthesis by the liver, including fibrinogen, prothrombin, haptoglobin, C-reactive protein (CRP), serum amyloid A protein, ceruloplasmin, complement, α-1 antitrypsin, ferritin, and others. Some of the acute phase proteins (e.g., fibrinogen) are normal serum components and may increase modestly. Others (e.g., CRP) may increase in concentration by factors of up to 100 or more. Acute phase reactants are a common component of acute inflammation, but they also accompany chronic inflammation seen in the rheumatic diseases. These reactants can be measured directly, through measurement of CRP, and indirectly, through measurement of the erythrocyte sedimentation rate (ESR).

The ESR is the most common measurement of acute phase proteins in the rheumatic diseases. This simple test can be performed in the office with minimal equipment and requires only 1 hour for the red cells to sediment in a measured tube. The Westergren ESR uses a 100-mm tube to measure the sedimentation rate of cells over the 1-hour period. Sedimentation of the red cells is directly related to the quantity of acute phase proteins that are synthesized by the liver, particularly those with an asymmetric shape, such as fibrinogen. However, this test is nonspecific, and positive findings may be seen in people who have no illness or who have illnesses such as anemia, which is not related to development of acute phase proteins. In addition, incorrect storage of the blood for more than a few hours may lead to errors in measurement.

Another measure of the acute phase response is the quantitation of serum CRP. The changes in CRP occur more quickly and return to normal more quickly than changes in ESR. Unlike the ESR, the CRP is not affected by anemia, nor is it very susceptible to incorrect results caused by specimen handling.

The measurement of acute phase reactants is important in rheumatic diseases, because elevations are generally consistent with the presence of an inflammatory process, and normal values suggest that an inflammatory process is not present. Serial measurement of acute phase reactants may be used to monitor the disease course, particularly for patients with RA, polymyalgia rheumatica, or giant cell arteritis.

The upper limits of the reference normal ranges for both the ESR and CRP are influenced by age and sex. Patients with values above the upper limit of normal for young adults but below the upper limit of normal for their age range may have an inflammatory process, or may have mildly elevated acute phase reactants based on age and sex alone. Simple bedside formulae for the upper limit of normal for the ESR are, for women, (age + 10)/2; and for men, age/2 (25). For CRP, the upper limit of the reference range is age/50 for men, and age/50 + 0.6 for women (26).

There has been considerable interest in sensitive assays that detect low levels of CRP. These have been called high-sensitivity CRP assays (hsCRP). Such assays have detected slight but statistically elevated levels of hsCRP (still within the normal range, however) in patients with coronary artery disease, confirming the inflammatory nature of atherosclerosis. However, such minor elevations are found in a great many diverse conditions (27).

REFERENCES

1. Arnett FC, Edworthy SM, Bloch DA, McShane DJ, Fries JF, Cooper NS, et al. The American Rheumatism Association 1987 revised criteria for the classification of rheumatoid arthritis. Arthritis Rheum 1988;31:315–324.
2. Shmerling RH. Origin and utility of measurement of rheumatoid factors. In: Rose B, Schur PH, editors. UpToDate. Waltham (MA): UpToDate; 2006.
3. Harris ED Jr. Clinical features of rheumatoid arthritis. In: Ruddy S, Harris ED Jr, Sledge CB, editors. Kelley's textbook of rheumatology. 6th ed. Philadelphia: WB Saunders; 2000. p. 967–1000.

4. Tighe H, Carson DA. Rheumatoid factors. In: Ruddy S, Harris ED Jr, Sledge CB, editors. Kelley's textbook of rheumatology. 6th ed. Philadelphia: WB Saunders; 2000. p. 151–160.
5. Schur PH. Anti-cyclic citrullinated peptide antibodies: diagnostic, predictive, and monitoring value in RA. Int J Adv Rheumatol 2006;3:77–83.
6. Tan EM, Cohen AS, Fries JF, Masi AT, McShane DJ, Rothfield NF, et al. The 1982 revised criteria for the classification of systemic lupus erythematosus. Arthritis Rheum 1982;25:1271–1277.
7. Reichlin M. Measurement and clinical significance of antinuclear antibodies. In: Rose B, Schur PH, editors. UpToDate. Waltham (MA): UpToDate; 2006.
8. Solomon DH, Kavanaugh AJ, Schur PH. Evidence-based guidelines for the use of immunologic tests: antinuclear antibody testing. Arthritis Rheum 2002;47:434–44.
9. Von Muhlen CA, Tan EM. Autoantibodies in the diagnosis of systemic rheumatic diseases. Semin Arthritis Rheum 1995;24:323–58.
10. Kavanaugh AF, Solomon DH. Guidelines for immunologic laboratory testing in the rheumatic diseases: anti-DNA antibody tests. Arthritis Rheum 2002;47:546–55.
11. Benito-Garcia E, Schur PH, Lahita R. Guidelines for immunologic laboratory testing in the rheumatic diseases: anti-Sm and anti-RNP antibody tests. Arthritis Rheum 2004;51:1030–44.
12. Reveille JD, Sherrer YRS, Solomon DH, Schur PH, Kavanuagh. Evidenced based guidelines for the use of immunologic laboratory tests: Anti-Ro (SS-A) and La (SS-B). In press.
13. Stone JH, Rose BD. Clinical spectrum of antineutrophil cytoplasmic antibodies. In: Rose B, Schur PH, editors. UpToDate. Waltham (MA): UpToDate; 2006.
14. Bermas BL, Erkan D, Schur PH. Clinical manifestations and diagnosis of antiphospholipid syndrome. In: Rose B, Schur PH, editors. UpToDate. Waltham (MA): UpToDate; 2006.
15. Hochberg MC. Updating the American College of Rheumatology revised criteria for the classification of systemic lupus erythematosus (letter). Arthritis Rheum 1997;40:1725.
16. Miyakis S, Lockshin MD, Atsumi T, Branch DW, Brey RL, Cervera R, et al. International consensus statement on an update of the classification criteria for definite antiphospholipid syndrome (APS). J Thromb Haemost 2006;4:295–306.
17. Piessens W, Ruddy S. Immune complexes and complement. In: Ruddy S, Harris ED Jr, Sledge CB, editors. Kelley's textbook of rheumatology. 6th ed. Philadelphia: WB Saunders; 2001. p. 175–193.
18. Liszewski MK, Atkinson JP. Complement pathways. In: Rose B, Schur PH, editors. UpToDate. Waltham (MA): UpToDate; 2006.
19. Liszewski MK, Atkinson JP. Overview and clinical assessment of the complement system. In: Rose B, Schur PH, editors. UpToDate. Waltham (MA): UpToDate; 2006.
20. Arnett FC. Histocompatibility typing in the rheumatic diseases: diagnostic and prognostic implications. Rheum Dis Clin North Am 1994;20: 371–390.
21. McCarty D. Synovial fluid. In: Arthritis and allied conditions. 14th ed. Koopman WJ, editor. Baltimore: Lippincott, Williams and Wilkins; 2000. p. 83–104.
22. Sholter DE, Russell AS. Synovial fluid analysis and the diagnosis of septic arthritis. In: Rose B, Schur PH, editors. UpToDate. Waltham (MA): UpToDate; 2006.
23. Gabay C, Kushner I. Acute-phase proteins and other systemic responses to inflammation. N Engl J Med 1999;340:448–54.
24. Volanakis J. Acute phase proteins in rheumatic disease. In: Koopman WJ, editor. Arthritis and allied conditions. 14th ed. Baltimore: Lippincott, Williams and Wilkins; 2000. p. 505–14.
25. Miller A, Green M, Robinson D. Simple rule for calculating normal erythrocyte sedimentation rate. Br Med J (Clin Res Ed) 1983; 286:266.
26. Wener MH, Daum PR, McQuillan GM. The influence of age, sex, and race on the upper reference limit of serum C-reactive protein concentration. J Rheumatol 2000;27:2351–9.
27. Kushner I, Rzewnicki D, Samuels D. What does minor elevation of C-reactive protein signify? Am J Med 2006;119:166.e17–28.

Diagnostic Imaging

JOHN A. CARRINO, MD, MPH

Diagnostic medical imaging may reveal the presence of a previously unknown process, may aid in the characterization of a clinically suspected arthropathy, or may show an articular complication of a known disease process. When reviewing imaging of patients with suspected arthritis, it is useful to go through a checklist of findings (Table 1). Plain radiography remains the primary modality for evaluation of arthritis. However, other modalities, such as ultrasound (US), computed tomography (CT), and magnetic resonance imaging (MRI), play an increasingly important role in diagnosis and clinical management.

RADIOGRAPHY

Plain radiography using x-rays is dependent on differences in radiographic density. A radiograph is a 2-dimensional image of a 3-dimensional object. This is known as a projection imaging technique, in contrast to such cross-sectional modalities as CT, US, and MRI. One difficulty of image interpretation is superimposition of structures that may obscure pathology. Quality control is also very important, with patient positioning and radiographic exposure techniques optimized for visualization of subtle findings. Multiple views of an affected joint are often essential for detection of all relevant findings. In some areas of the body, "special" radiographic views in addition to or instead of "routine" views are helpful for identification of particular fractures, bone lesions, osteophytes, joint-space narrowing, erosions, or cysts.

COMPUTED TOMOGRAPHY (CT)

CT also utilizes x-rays to generate images, thus it maintains the strengths of projectional radiography in regard to exquisite bone and joint imaging and at the same time supersedes radiography with improved contrast and 3-dimensional imaging. The attenuation of tissues as the x-ray beam travels through it is measured from multiple angles and is related to the atomic number and density of the material being examined, as well as to the energy spectrum of the x-ray beam being emitted. CT can be useful in evaluation of the appendicular skeleton for fractures, subluxations, sclerotic and cystic bone lesions, and both pre- and postsurgical evaluation of hardware implantation. CT can also be used to assess bone mineral density. It can be useful in conjunction with arthrography. In all cases, one must weigh the increased patient exposure to radiation versus the potential benefit of an accurate diagnosis.

ULTRASOUND

Ultrasound imaging utilizes the interaction of sound waves with living tissue to produce an image of the tissue or, in Doppler-based modes, to determine the velocity of a moving tissue, primarily blood. Ultrasound is useful for evaluation of joint effusions, tenosynovitis, and ganglion cysts originating from joints and tendon sheaths. Erosions may be detected in rheumatoid arthritis. The addition of power Doppler offers

potential for evaluation of synovial vascularity, which may be related to disease activity in inflammatory arthropathies. Although ultrasound is user dependent and requires an experienced musculoskeletal sonographer to provide real-time assessments, this technology is increasingly utilized in rheumatology. Ultrasound can also be used to enhance the ability to identify accessible bursitis and tendinitis and improve the accuracy of injections. Many joints and structures, however, cannot be adequately assessed in all planes with ultrasound evaluation.

MAGNETIC RESONANCE IMAGING (MRI)

MRI is based on the absorption and emission of energy in the radiofrequency range of the electromagnetic spectrum. MRI produces images based on spatial variations in the phase and frequency of radiofrequency energy being absorbed and emitted by the imaged object. A variety of

Table 1.   Basic radiographic approach to arthritis

Soft tissues
  Effusion
  Pannus
  Calcification
  Masses
Mineralization
  Diffuse demineralization
  Periarticular demineralization
  Preservation of density
Joint space and subchondral bone
  Narrowing
  Subchondral white line
    Loss
    Sclerosis
  Subchondral lucencies or cysts
  Intraarticular bodies
  Ankylosis
Erosions
  Central (articular surface)
  Marginal (bare area)
  Periarticular
  Proliferative
  Mutilans
Proliferation
  Osteophytes or enthesophytes
  Periostitis
  Buttressing
Deformity
  Epiphyseal deformity
  Varus or valgus
  Flexion or extension
  Subluxation or dislocation
  Collapse or migration
  Disorganization
Distribution
  Monarticular
  Pauciarticular or polyarticular
    Symmetric
    Asymmetric
    Scattered

systems are used in medical imaging, ranging from open MRI units with magnetic field strength of 0.3T, extremity MRI systems with field strengths up to 1.0T, and whole-body scanners with field strengths up to 3.0T (in clinical use). Advantages of MRI over other imaging modalities include absence of ionizing radiation, superior soft-tissue contrast resolution, high-resolution imaging, and multiplanar imaging capabilities. The time to acquire an MRI scan has been a major weakness. MRI can be useful for identification of tenosynovitis, joint effusions, synovial proliferation, cysts, ganglia, erosions, cartilage loss, and reactive bone changes.

SCINTIGRAPHY

Nuclear scintigraphy provides both morphologic and physiologic information regarding the metabolic state of tissues. The most commonly used agent in musculoskeletal imaging is technetium-99m methylene diphosphanate (Tc-MDP). This agent affixes to bone surface by the process of chemisorption by attaching to hydroxyapatite crystals in bone and calcium crystals in mitochondria. Scintigraphy has a limited role in evaluation of arthritis. Three-phase "bone scan" using Tc-MDP can detect synovial hyperemia on the vascular (angiographic) and blood pool phases and periarticular uptake on the delayed phase in joints affected by inflammatory arthritis. Uptake is nonspecific, however, and is generally not used for narrowing the differential diagnosis in cases of suspected arthropathy. Bone scans can be useful, however, in identifying the number and distribution of joints involved and can help distinguish an articular from a nonarticular process. Because uptake of radiotracer is nonspecific, skeletal scintigraphy should be evaluated in conjunction with radiographs of areas with abnormal uptake.

IMAGING IN SPECIFIC ARTICULAR DISEASES

Osteoarthritis

Osteoarthritis (OA) may be present in primary or secondary forms. Imaging hallmarks of OA are joint-space narrowing, osteophytes,

and subchondral bone changes (marrow edema, sclerosis, and cysts) (Figure 1). Joint effusions are common. Erosions generally are absent unless OA is secondary to an underlying inflammatory arthropathy. Early osteophyte formation is seen as sharpening of the joint edges. Deformity results from more severe involvement. The distribution of primary OA is fairly characteristic. Weight-bearing joints or load-bearing compartments of joints are more susceptible. Other modifiers of disease distribution include prior trauma, infection, or other joint insult.

OA in the hand affects the proximal and distal interphalangeal (IP) joints and the scaphoid-trapezium-trapezoid or triscaphe joint. The thumb is frequently affected, involving the carpometacarpal and metacarpophalangeal (MCP) joint. In the shoulder girdle, acromioclavicular joint involvement is common. Rotator cuff arthropathy refers to glenohumeral OA related to rotator cuff degeneration and tearing with a resultant high-riding proximal humerus that may articulate with the undersurface of the acromion, causing reciprocating osseous changes. Degenerative arthritis of the spine is very common, and occurs at many different articulations, including facet (zygoapophyseal) joints and costovertebral joints. The intervertebral discs represent symphyses and thus do not undergo OA, per se. Degenerative disc disease is also called spondylosis deformans or often is referred to just as spondylosis. Scoliosis and accentuated lumbar lordosis add biomechanical stress and accelerate the degenerative process. The distribution of spondylosis is most common at the lower lumbar spine (L4–5, L5–S1) and at the lower cervical spine (C5–6). Spondylosis is commonly seen at multiple levels of the thoracic spine in older patients, but is not generally a source of pain, possibly due to relative lack of motion, which is limited by the semirigid thoracic cage. OA occurs in the facet, costovertebral, and synovial portions of the sacroiliac joints. In the hips, supracetabular subchondral cysts can enlarge and can be mistaken for a lytic neoplastic lesion. Buttressing stress reaction manifested as increased sclerosis is seen at the medial aspect of the femoral neck. Meniscal or cruciate ligament injuries, such as from contact sports and athletic injury, can lead to resultant knee OA typically limited to the injured side and more severe in the internal deranged compartment. Patellofemoral involvement is also commonly detected in lateral radiographs. Cartilage degeneration and subsequent OA can occur in younger individuals who have tracking abnormalities of the patella or instability of the extensor mechanism. In the ankle, tibiotalar OA is usually secondary to joint incongruity from prior trauma or ligamentous instability.

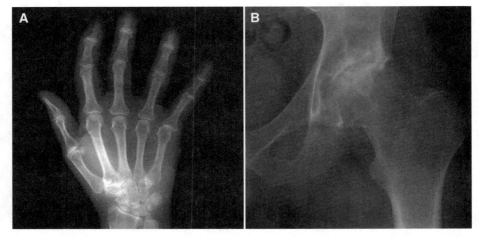

Figure 1. Osteoarthritis. **A,** Hand (distribution): Anteroposterior projection radiograph of the hand shows the classic distribution with involvement of the scapho-trapezium-trapezoid (STT or triscaphae) articulation, thumb carpometacarpal (CMC), thumb metacarpophalangeal (MCP), and interphalangeal (IP) joints of all the digits. **B,** Hip (superolateral migration): Anteroposterior projection radiograph shows acetabulofemoral joint narrowing that predominantly involves the superior load-bearing aspect of the articulation with associated subchondral sclerosis and cystic lesions. Also present is buttressing of the femoral neck with medial cortical thickening.

A developmentally square-shaped first metatarsal head can predispose to OA; large dorsal osteophytes develop with limitation of dorsiflexion, a condition called hallux rigidus or hallux limitus.

Erosive Osteoarthritis. Erosive OA, or inflammatory osteoarthritis, has a characteristic radiographic appearance typically affecting the IP joints of the hands. Separating this entity from conventional OA is the presence of central erosions creating an appearance likened to a seagull. Similar findings may also be seen in some cases of psoriatic arthritis. In later stages, this may progress to ankylosis.

Rheumatoid Arthritis

The distribution of joints affected in rheumatoid arthritis (RA) is different than that in OA. This disorder is characterized by synovial proliferation (pannus) and also includes bursitis and nodules (Figure 2). Bursitis can cause areas of ill-defined soft-tissue planes and prominances on radiographs, most evident in the retrocalcaneal and olecranon bursae. Rheumatoid nodules appear as focal soft-tissue masses, most commonly at areas undergoing chronic friction, especially at the olecranon (which can simulate bursitis) but also in the hands and feet. Tenosynovitis is evident radiographically as more diffuse soft-tissue swelling, seen most commonly at the wrist. Muscle atrophy can occur in later stages, related to disuse or part of an inflammatory myopathy. Extremity periarticular osteoporosis can be an early radiographic appearance (but is often technique related), although a generalized pattern of demineralization is often seen.

Marginal (bare area) erosions are characteristic of RA; a result of pannus eroding the bone at the apposition of the articular cartilage located at the margin of the joint capsule where redundant synovium exists. Persistent synovitis results in concentric uniform narrowing from diffuse cartilage loss. Osseous proliferation is generally absent in active RA; however, osteophyte formation can be seen in the setting of secondary OA. Subchondral cysts are seen and may grow to a large size.

The earliest radiographic manifestations are typically seen in the distal extremities (hands and feet); ulnar styloid soft-tissue swelling and erosion from tenosynovitis of the extensor carpi ulnaris is a common early finding as well.

Deformities are common, with subluxations at the MCP and metatarsophalangeal (MTP) joints, causing digits to deviate in an ulnar or lateral direction resulting in a windswept appearance. Carpus erosion causes ligamentous disruption and laxity with resultant instability. Erosion of the radiolunatotriquetral ligament causes the carpus to slip ulnarly

(ulnar translocation). RA involvement in the hands and feet is characteristically more proximal than distal, affecting the carpus, MCPs, and proximal interphalangeals but sparing the distal interphalangeals.

Involvement of the elbow causes displacement of the fat pads from pannus and, in the later stages, shows erosions. Acromioclavicular joint pannus often causes erosion of the distal clavicle. Synovial proliferation in the more capacious glenohumeral and knee joints may not cause erosions until later in the disease process. Shoulder pannus causes eventual tearing of the rotator cuff that results in instability and action of the dominant deltoid muscle, which then results in subluxation of the humeral head superiorly (i.e., high riding). The hips are commonly involved with concentric joint narrowing and axial migration, advancing to protrusio acetabulae.

In the ankle, characteristic erosions of the distal tibiofibular syndesmosis occur. The earliest radiographic manifestation in the foot is usually soft-tissue swelling and erosion at the fifth MTP joint. Erosions in the feet can precede radiographic changes in the hands in 10–15% of patients, which is why it is important to perform x-rays of both the hands and feet in the assessment of RA. Tendinopathies of the foot are common; posterior tibialis tendon dysfunction leads to pes planus and hindfoot valgus with forefoot abduction.

Involvement of the spine favors the cervical segments. Pannus of the synovial recesses around the C1 dens can cause erosion and laxity of the transverse ligament, leading to excessive atlantoaxial motion and instability; defined as widening of the inferior margin of the predental space >2.5 mm. The instability is best assessed with flexion and extension radiographs of the cervical spine. MRI is useful for determining the extent of pannus and degree of spinal canal compromise. Involvement of other intervertebral levels is common, appearing as minimal multilevel anterolistheses (step ladder subluxations). The sacroiliac joints are spared in RA.

Juvenile Chronic Arthritis

Some radiographic findings of juvenile chronic arthritis (JCA) mimic the adult form of RA (Figure 3). Unlike adult-onset RA, erosions are not a prominent feature. In systemic JCA, periostitis is often seen adjacent to affected joints. Deformity, rather than joint narrowing and erosion, is the main feature of systemic JCA, separating it from adult forms. This often results in secondary OA, despite remission of disease.

Active synovitis leads to hyperemia around the joint. When this occurs during periods of bony development, a relatively squared appearance of

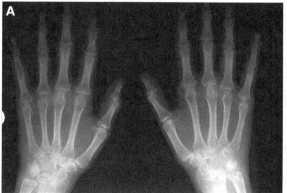
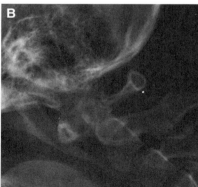
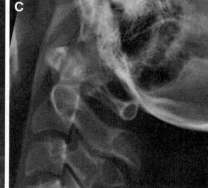

Figure 2. Rheumatoid arthritis. **A,** Hand (distribution): Anteroposterior projection radiograph of the hand shows the classic distribution with bilateral symmetric involvement of the metacarpophalangeal (MCP), proximal interphalangeal (PIP), and distal interphalangeal (DIP) joints of all the fingers. **B and C,** Atlantodental instability: Lateral projection cervical spine radiographs performed with flexion and extension show a widening of the atlantodental interval >3 mm between the arch of C1 and the odontoid process of C2, reflecting erosion of the transverse ligament related to pannus.

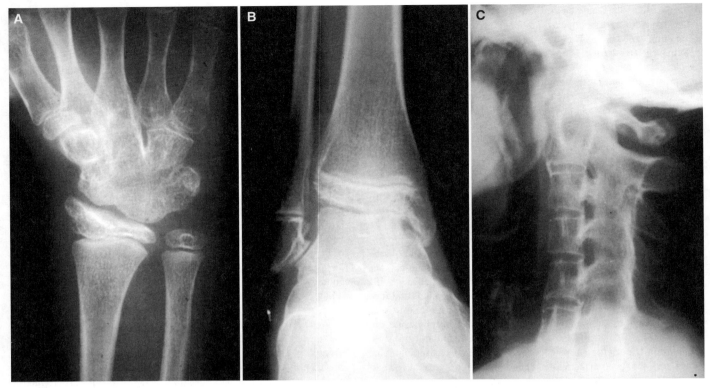

Figure 3. Juvenile rheumatoid arthritis. **A,** Hand: Anteroposterior radiograph shows fusion (ankylosis) of the carpal bones. **B,** Ankle: Oblique radiograph shows medial downward sloping of the talar dome (tibiotalar slant). **C,** Cervical spine: Lateral radiograph shows straightening with loss of the normal cervical lordosis, fusion (ankylosis) of the facet joints, and a small syndesmophyte-like calcification along the anterior margin of the C2-3 intervertebral disc.

the epiphyses is seen, with rapid transition to gracile (thin) diaphyses (overtubulated pattern). This early physeal fusion can cause growth disturbance, with bone shortening if the epiphysis fuses uniformly or with angular deformity of the epimetaphysis if only partial early fusion occurs. JCA causes ankylosis at a much higher frequency than in adult-onset RA and can affect any joint. In the cervical spine facet joint, anklyosis over numerous levels causes vertebral growth disturbance. Fusion of the carpal or tarsal bones is also relatively common.

Seronegative Spondyloarthropathies

Psoriatic and Reactive Arthritis. Radiographically, these disorders have a similar appearance that is characterized by erosions and bony proliferation; this contrasts with RA, in which new bone formation is not a characteristic finding (Figure 4). Differentiating psoriatic from reactive arthritis is distribution: psoriatic arthritis favors involvement of the hand, but reactive arthritis is more common in the foot. Both conditions tend to be asymmetric or occur in a "ray" distribution (involving multiple joints along a digit). Both can involve the axial skeleton, occurring at the upper lumbar spine or thoracolumbar junction; in contrast, ankylosing spondylitis (AS) generally starts at the lumbosacral junction and progresses superiorly. Soft-tissue findings in psoriatic and reactive arthritis consist of fusiform soft-tissue swelling around the joints of the digits. With more severe involvement, the whole digit can become swollen (dactylitis or sausage digit). Focal soft-tissue swelling can also be seen at the entheses, characterized by indistinct (fluffy) margins in comparison to mechanical traction-related spurs and erosions at attachment sites. Marignal erosions are often associated with adjacent bone proliferation showing a fluffy or whiskered quality and periostitis adjacent to an affected joint. Deformity is generally limited to the digits of the hands

and feet, with subluxations and angular deformity. Erosions can become quite severe, with pencilling of the end of the bone (appearing as if put through a pencil sharpener) and with the reciprocating articular surface becoming cupped (pencil-in-cup deformity). With severe involvement, shortening of the digit from telescoping of one bone into the other may occur or the articular surfaces can undergo complete destruction (arthritis mutilans). Erosions can also occur around the odontoid process, resulting in atlantoaxial instability; but this occurs less frequently than in RA. Sacroiliitis is common but tends to be asymmetric. Bony ankylosis can occur with chronic involvement at any affected joint, but is most commonly present at the IP, sacroiliac, and facet joints. Paravertebral ossification occurs in the spine, resulting in osseous bridging between 2 or more vertebral bodies. Typically, asymmetric ossification in psoriatic and reactive arthritis tends to be large, prominent, and protrude laterally, unlike the more uniform, smaller, and vertical syndesmophytes of AS. In comparison to spondylosis (degenerative disc disease and arthritis), the ossification in psoriatic and reactive arthritis emanates from the vertebral body (as opposed to the disc margin in spondylosis), and interverterbral disc height may be preserved.

Ankylosing Spondylitis. The imaging changes in AS characteristically begin at the sacroiliac joints and lumbosacral junction and progress cranially (Figure 5). Findings are sometimes initially recognized at the thoracolumbar junction.

The sacroiliac joints initially show poor definition of the subchondral white line and discrete erosions form subsequently, causing a widened appearance of the joint. Erosions occur early on the iliac side (which has thinner cartilage) at the anterior and inferior aspect, which is the synovial portion (the posterosuperior aspect is ligamentous). Reactive sclerosis at the joint margins ensues, with eventual fusion and decreased sclerosis.

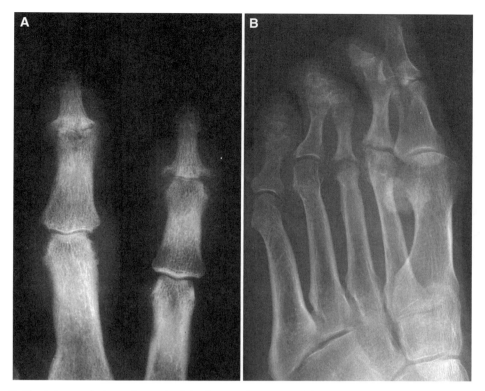

Figure 4. **A,** Psoriatic arthritis: Anteroposterior radiograph of the fingers shows synovial-type bare area erosions with adjacent bone proliferation (periostitis). **B,** Reactive arthritis: Oblique radiograph of the forefoot shows erosive arthropathy of the second and third metatarsophalangeal joint. The third digit demonstrates the pencil-in-cup deformity.

Early radiographic changes in the spine include squaring of the anterior vertebral body with loss of normal concavity. Enthesitis at the anulus fibrosis anterior endplate attachments causes erosion and irregularity (whiskering), with subsequent reactive sclerosis (shiny corners). Sharpey's fibers (outer anulus) progressively mineralize, leading to osseous bridging across the discs (syndesmophytes). Ossification also occurs along the interspinous ligaments. The margin of the ossification tends to be straight or slightly undulating (*bamboo spine*). The facet joints and costovertebral joints can also become involved and fuse.

The thoracic spine can become fixed, with a prominent kyphotic deformity. Stress from motion at the craniocervical junction with relative immobility of the cervical spine can lead to laxity of the transverse ligament of the dens and atlantoaxial instability. Minor trauma can result in spinal fractures with unusual patterns, and fracture healing is often poor, resulting in pseudarthrosis.

Outside the axial skeleton, the hips are the most commonly involved joints, showing concentric bilateral symmetric joint narrowing and axial migration with or without erosions. Shoulders, knees, acromioclavicular joints, sternal articulations, or distal extremities are affected less commonly (10–30%). Very advanced end-stage disease is characterized by ankylosis at affected joints.

Crystal-Associated Disorders

Gout (Monosodium Urate Monohydrate Arthropathy). The radiographic appearance of gout generally consists of erosions and masses, with a predilection for peripheral joints (Figure 6). The masses may appear dense either from the crystal itself or associated calcification. Gouty erosions are juxtaarticular from adjacent soft-tissue tophi or intraosseous crystal deposition. When intraosseous, they frequently

appear rounded and well circumscribed with a thin sclerotic margin. The stimulation of periosteal new bone formation can create a characteristic overhanging margin. Bone mineralization is normal in the early stages, and joint space is preserved until later stages, when secondary OA occurs. Deformity may occur early, initially related to soft-tissue masses and later related to enlarging masses, erosions, and arthritis. Common sites include the feet (first MTP, IP, and the tarsometatarsal [Lisfranc] articulations) and the hands (MCP, IP, and carpometacarpal articulations). The most characteristic and frequently (50%) involved area is the first MTP joint. Involvement of the wrist by gout may simulate RA (i.e., a spotty carpus). Olecranon and prepatellar bursitis occur and may calcify.

Calcium Pyrophosphate Dihydrate Deposition Disease (CPPD). In general, CPPD arthropathy manifests as OA in an atypical distribution with robust features (prominent osteophytosis). Soft-tissue calcification may be seen in the joint capsule, synovium, bursa, tendons, ligaments, and periarticular soft tissues. Chondrocalcinosis (cartilage calcification) is linear and regular for articular cartilage or coarse for fibrocartilage. Joints involved may or may not manifest chondrocalcinosis. Intraarticular bodies are frequent, but are typically fewer in number and larger in size than primary synovial chondromatosis. Although erosions are not present, subchondral cysts are a prominent feature. No periosteal reaction or new bone proliferation is seen, and bone mineralization is normal. Deformities occur secondary to accelerated OA.

The frequency for distribution of chondrocalcinois is in the following order: knee > symphysis pubis > wrist > elbow > hip. Hooked osteophytes are often identified with idiopathic or familial CPPD arthropathy. The radiocarpal articulation has severe degenerative changes with scapholunate ligament disruption, this is known as a scapholunate advanced collapse wrist. The wrist will frequently show ligamenous calcification involving the lunatotriquetral and scapholunate ligaments

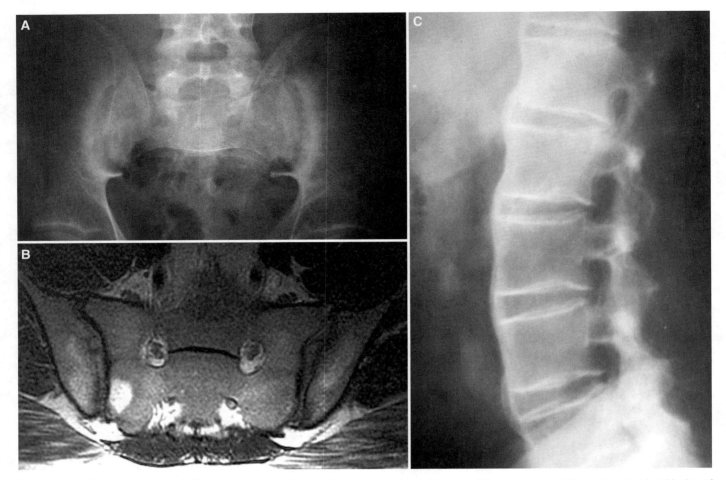

Figure 5. Ankylosing spondylitis. **A,** Sacroiliac joints (radiography): Anteroposterior radiograph of the pelvis shows bilateral symmetric widening of the sacroiliac joints reflecting erosions. Improved visualization of the sacroiliac joints, especially the synovial anteroinferior portion can be obtained with a modified "Ferguson view" (not shown). **B,** Sacroiliitis (magnetic resonance image): Axial oblique T1-weighted image through the mid-sacriliac joints shows erosions with joint-space widening and loss of the normal low-signal cortex on the iliac side of the joint. Subchondral bone reaction is also present. **C,** Lumbosacral spine: Lateral projection radiograph shows anterior intervetebral ossification reflecting syndesmophytes.

as well as chondrocalcinosis of the triangular fibrocartilage. The shoulder is a less commonly involved site but appears as glenohumeral OA with articular chondrocalcinosis. The spine typically manifests annulus fibrosis calcification. The pelvis commonly shows chondrocalcinosis of the pubic symphysis and the hip joints. The knee is commonly the initial site of clinical symptoms, and radiography characteristically shows disproportionate patellofemoral OA. Although the elbow, ankle, and foot articulations are not commonly involved, tendinous calcification related to CPPD may be encountered in the Achilles, triceps, or quadriceps tendons.

Hemochromatosis and Hepatolenticular Degeneration (Wilson Disease). Both conditions are associated with OA-like changes. The imaging findings are similar to CPPD arthropathy. Although the presence of hooklike osteophytes at the medial aspect of the second and third metacarpophalangeal joints (OA changes at non-OA joints) has been touted as characteristic, this finding is not truly specific for these disorders.

Hydroxyapatite Deposition Disease (Calcific Periarthritis). Basic calcium phosphate (BCP) deposition most commonly exists as hyrdoxyapatite. The clinically symptomatic disorders associated with BCP deposition have many synonyms, the more common being hydroxyapatite deposition disease (HADD), calcific periarthritis, and calcific tendinitis. The most common sites of deposition are the periarticular musculoskeletal-related structures, such as tendons, bursae, and ligaments. Periarticular calcifications are often detected on radiography

as incidental findings, especially at tendinous and ligamentous attachments not necessarily associated with symptoms. Hydroxyapatite (BCP) is frequently identified at periarticular or intraarticular locations, including intervertebral discs.

The radiographic appearance of BCP is a periarticular amorphous calcific opacity without features of ossification (i.e., trabecula). The size and shape typically have no relationship to the presence of symptoms. In an acute symptomatic presentation, crystals may migrate out of the tendon (burst out) into adjacent soft tissues, especially into a bursa—causing acute bursitis. Over time (several days), a well-defined homogeneous calcification in tendons may transform into a faint diffuse calcification in the bursa or may become ill defined, smaller, and disappear (dissolve).

Normal bone mineral density is exhibited. Enthesial erosions may be apparent at the pectoralis major tendon insertion and gluteus maximus tendon insertion, but are uncommon. In the periarticular form of HADD, there is no osseous proliferation and no joint deformity.

The shoulder is by far the most common joint involved, most often in the supraspinatus tendon, which may extend into the subacromial/subdeltoid bursa. The hand and wrist is a common area usually demonstrating a solitary focus of the extensor carpi ulnaris or flexor carpi ulnaris tendons or around the MCP or IP joints. Pelvic involvement is common around the hip, especially the greater trochanteric bursa. Hands and feet are also involved and usually show a solitary focus of

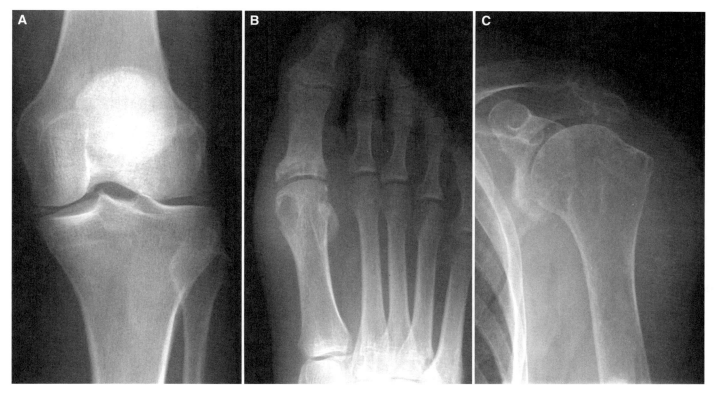

Figure 6. Crystal-associated arthropathies. **A,** Pyrophosphate arthropathy: Anteroposterior radiograph of the knee shows chondrocalcinosis present within the fibrocartilage of the menisci. There are small marginal osteophytes of the tibial spines. **B,** Gouty arthropathy: Anteroposterior radiograph of the forefoot shows juxtaarticular erosions with overhanging margins about the first metatarsophalangeal joint related to adjacent soft-tissue masses that are the gouty tophi. **C,** Hydroxyapatite deposition disease: Anteroposterior radiograph of the shoulder shows calcification in the rotator cuff (supraspinatus tendon) and in the subdeltoid bursa.

a periarticular soft-tissue calcific opacity in no particular area. The elbow and knee are not commonly involved.

The differential diagnosis for periarticular calcific opacities includes metastatic calcification, other crystal diseases, connective tissue diseases associated with soft-tissue calcifications, tumoral calcinosis, dystrophic calcifications (vascular, neuropathic, thermal, or traumatic), early heterotopic ossification (myositis ossificans), synovial cell sarcoma, juxtacortical chondroma, accessory ossicles (hands and feet), and infection (parasitic, leprosy).

Intraarticular Hydroxyapatite. Intraarticular BCP, typically composed of hyrdoxyapatite, probably represents a different phenomenon than periarticular deposition. This has been described in association with a rapidly destructive arthritis without osteophytosis or subchondral sclerosis. One of the original descriptions was in the shoulder and has been called Milwaukee shoulder syndrome or idiopathic destructive arthritis. Hydroxyapatite may also be found in joint aspirates of patients with primary OA.

Other Rheumatic Diseases

Scleroderma (Systemic Sclerosis). Radiography may show acrosteolysis secondary to pressure erosions from tight skin and soft-tissue calcifications. A true arthritis, which may or may not be erosive, occurs in 50%. CREST (calcinosis, Raynaud phenonmenon, esophageal dysmotility, sclerodactyly, and telangectasias) is a limited form of scleroderma with only facial and hand fibrosis, but radiography may demonstrate subcutaneous soft tissue calcification of the fingers.

Systemic Lupus Erythematosus (SLE). In SLE, the arthritis is nonerosive but deforming, characterized on radiography by

subluxations without erosions. The differential diagnosis is Jaccoud's arthropathy, which develops in about 4% of patients with rheumatic heart disease.

Mixed Connective Tissue Disease (MCTD) and Overlap Syndrome. MCTD favors a small-joint distribution. Soft-tissue swelling with sausage digits and associated calcinosis is common. Bone demineralization may be juxtaarticular or diffuse. Joint narrowing occurs as part of the inflammatory arthropathy. Erosions develop in 2 patterns: distal phalangeal tuft erosions (25–70%) and synovial marginal erosions. Osseous proliferation is not a feature. Flexion deformities and subluxations contribute to malalignment. Ankylosis is a late finding, typically occurring at the MCP and IP joints.

Differential Diagnosis

Several connective-tissue diseases share radiographic features, confounding the imaging differential diagnosis. The diagnosis of an overlap syndrome is facile when a constellation of classic findings of 2 different disorders exist in a single patient. However, since MCTD is not necessarily the full expression or complete combination of >1 disorder, atypical patterns predominate. Involvement by MCTD includes distal IP joints versus RA, where these articulations are uncommonly affected, and MCTD tends to be more asymmetric than RA. Synvoial-type erosions are uncommon in scleroderma and SLE. Scleroderma has frequent calcinosis, whereas uncomplicated SLE shows only occasional soft-tissue calcifications. The presence of both calcinosis and synovial-type marginal erosions should raise the possibility of an overlap syndrome, MCTD, or a rheumatic disorder complicated by end-stage renal disease (secondary hyperparathyroidism).

Recommended Reading

Allman RM, Brower AC, Kotlyarov EB. Neuropathic bone and joint disease. Radiol Clin North Am 1988;26:1373–81.

Bassett LW, Blocka KL, Furst DE, Clements PJ, Gold RH. Skeletal findings in progressive systemic scelrosis (scleroderma). AJR Am J Roentgenol 1981;136:1121–26.

Brower AC. Arthritis in black and white. Philadelphia: WB Saunders Co; 1988.

Cronin ME. Musculoskeletal manifestations of systemic lupus erythematosus. Rheum Dis Clin North Am 1988;14:99–116.

Espada G, Babini JC, Maldonado-Cocco JA, Garcia-Morteo O. Radiologic review: the cervical spine in juvenile rheumatoid arthritis. Semin Arthritis Rheum 1988;17:185–95.

Fernandez-Madrid F, Karvonen RL, Teitqe RA, Miller PR, Neqendank WG. MR features of osteoarthritis of the knee. Magn Reson Imaging 1994;12:703–9.

Hayes CW, Conway WF. Calcium hydroxyapatite deposition disease. Radiographics 1990;10:1031–48.

Kaye JJ. Radiologic assessment of osteoarthritis: new techniques. Rheum Dis Clin North Am 1993;19:659–72.

Rabinowitz JG, Twersky J, Guttadauria M. Similar bone manifestations of scleroderma and rheumatoid arthritis. Am J Roentgenol Radium Ther Nucl Med 1974;121:35–44.

Reed MH, Wilmot DM. The radiology of juvenile rheumatoid arthritis: a review of the English language literature. J Rheumatol Suppl 1991;31: 2–22.

Resnick D. Inflammatory disorders of the vertebral column: seronegative spondyloarthropathies, adult-onset rheumatoid arthritis, and juvenile chronic arthritis. Clin Imaging 1989;13:253–68.

Uri DS, Martel W. Radiologic manifestations of crystal-related arthropathies. Semin Roentgenol 1996;31:229–38.

Weissman B, editor. Imaging of arthropathies. Special issue. Radiol Clin North Am 1996;34(2):195–455.

Weissman BN. Imaging techniques in rheumatoid arthritis. J Rheumatol Suppl 1994;42:14–9.

Functional Ability, Health Status, and Quality of Life

DONNA J. HAWLEY, EdD, RN; as updated by KEVIN R. FONTAINE, PhD

Functional status, health status, health-related quality of life, and quality of life are terms used to summarize disease outcomes that go beyond the physiologic cost of disease. As outcomes, they describe to varying extents the physical, social, and emotional consequences of disease as perceived and reported by the individual. These outcomes are the result of a subjective judgment intended to represent what is important from the viewpoint of the patient.

DEFINITIONS

Moving along the continuum from functional status to quality of life, the terms become increasingly abstract and as such, more difficult to measure and quantify. *Functional status* is the ability to do such usual self-care activities of daily living as eating, dressing, grooming, and toileting.

Health status is broader than functional ability and encompasses total physical, mental, and social wellbeing (1). It includes important aspects of health, such as emotions and mood, symptoms (e.g., pain, fatigue), cognitive abilities, and social activities and roles.

Quality of life (QOL) is more comprehensive and abstract than either functional or health status. It is influenced by numerous factors unrelated to an individual's health or disease (e.g., safe water, adequate housing, crime, and educational opportunities). Furthermore, the perception of one's QOL has meanings, preferences, and priorities unique to the individual (2). As such, the totality of QOL is difficult to define and measure. For these reasons, evaluating the effect of disease on a person's quality of life has become more narrowly focused as health-related quality of life (HRQOL), which refers to a combination of functional ability, disease symptoms, social roles, and emotions. Thus, HRQOL represents a subjective judgment or perception of one's well-being. Although HRQOL is more comprehensive than health status, the terms are frequently used interchangeably. Both refer to the aggregate effects of disease on the individual's life as perceived and evaluated by the individual (1). In this chapter, the term "health status" will be used to refer to both HRQOL and health status. "Functional status" will refer to the ability to perform activities of daily living.

Note: A comprehensive Quality of Life Instruments Database was initiated by Mapi Research Institute to provide all those involved in health care evaluation a comprehensive and unique source of information on patient-reported outcomes and QOL measures. It was renamed PROQOLID, short for Patient-Reported Outcome and Quality of Life Instruments Database, in January 2005 and is available at http://www.proqolid.org/.

ASSESSING FUNCTIONAL ABILITY AND HEALTH STATUS

Assessment of functional ability and health status is typically a supplement to the information obtained through more traditional assessments of health history, physical examination, laboratory tests, and radiography.

Traditional assessments provide data about disease status and specific disease-related parameters, such as number of tender joints, current degree of inflammation, and number of erosions documented by physical examination, laboratory tests, x-rays, and the like. Health status assessments provide additional information about how the patient perceives his or her disease and its physical, social, and emotional consequences. Direct observation, physician estimation of functioning, and self-report questionnaires have been used to assess functional ability and health status.

Direct Observation

There are several standardized observational methods that may be used to evaluate one or more aspects of functional status. Hand function (button test), hand and arm strength (grip strength), lower extremity movement (walk time and timed-stands test), and range of motion (Keitel index) are described in Table 1. With the exception of the timed 50-foot walk test (3,4), these measures have been shown to be valid and sensitive to change in clinical studies. Each, however, relies on the motivation and cooperation of the patient. The amount of time needed to complete the Keitel index (>10 minutes) may limit its use in routine clinical practice. The specially designed equipment needed for the button test and the timed-stands test requires an initial expenditure. Grip strength can be assessed quickly in a busy clinic setting at minimal cost. It is a standard outcome measure for many clinical trials and is sensitive to improvement in inflammation as well as function for a person with rheumatoid arthritis (RA) (3).

Clinician Estimation

Two common methods for assessing function are physician global estimate of disease activity and the American College of Rheumatology (ACR) Revised Criteria for Classification of Functional Status in Rheumatoid Arthritis. Physician global assessment is based on the subjective interpretation of the patient's symptoms, apparent functioning, and laboratory tests (4). Assignment of scores from 0 (no disease activity) to 4 (very severe activity) is recommended by some authors (4). Although this measure has been shown to be sensitive to short-term change during clinical trials (3), similar findings have not been reported in practice situations (5,6). Physicians tend to overestimate physical limitations compared with patients' perceptions, especially at higher levels of impairment in persons with RA (5). If health care professionals plan to use professional judgment to evaluate functioning in routine clinical practice, validating one's judgment through discussion with the patient would be appropriate.

Functional status may be classified using the ACR Revised Criteria for Classification of Functional Status in Rheumatoid Arthritis. These criteria, as listed in Table 2, may be used for the "rapid, global assessment of functional status by health professionals" (7). They are helpful in classifying groups of RA patients at 1 specific point in time; however, using these criteria to monitor change over time for individual patients

Table 1. Examples of standardized measures for evaluating physical functioning in chronic rheumatic disorders using direct observation

Test	Purpose	Measurement method	Comments
Grip strength (4)	Measurement of hand, wrist, and forearm strength	Patient squeezes the cuff of a sphygmomanometer inflated to 30 mm Hg as hard as possible. The highest level on the mercury column of 3 attempts is recorded. May also be measured with Martin Virgorimeter (50).	Motivation, handedness, pain threshold, and muscle weakness will modify scores as well as involvement of any joint from the elbow to the hand. Grip strength has been shown to be sensitive to change in clinical trials (3).
Thumb to index strength	Measurement of hand and finger function	Measured with Martin Virgorimeter (55).	Same as grip strength measurement.
Time to walk 50 feet (4)	Measurement of lower extremity function	Individual walks 50 feet on a flat surface using any aids or assistive devices. Time is recorded to the nearest 0.1 second.	Motivation is influential. Low reliability, insensitive to changes in disease (3).
6-minute timed walk (35,56)	Field test of fitness	Measure of distance walked in 6 minutes.	Motivation is influential. Low correlation with standard laboratory tests of physical fitness. Sensitive to change in exercise clinical trial in fibromyalgia. Little information available for other disorders (35,56).
Jepson Hand Function Test, Grip Ability Test, Grip Function Test, Arthritis Hand Function Test	Various measures of hand function tested in persons with arthritis. Activities tested are based on activities of daily living	Specific tasks (e.g., picking up cards, pouring water from a jug, writing) are performed in presence of evaluator.	May be used in clinical trails of specific hand treatments, following hand surgery, and in long-term outcome studies. Some tests require special equipment (3,57,58).
Button test (3,59)	Measurement of hand function, can used in clinical practice	Standard board with 5 buttons. Patients are timed while they unbutton and button using both right and left hands separately. Two scores are averaged.	Motivation is an important factor. Useful in disorders with direct effect on hand function (e.g., rheumatoid arthritis).
Timed-stands test (3,60)	Measurement of lower extremity function	Number of seconds used in standing up and sitting down 10 times from a chair using only the lower extremities.	Motivation, age, and nonmusculoskeletal comorbid conditions may affect scores. Sensitivity to change has not been determined (3,60).
Keitel index (4,61)	Upper and lower extremity function with emphasis on range of motion.	Measures 24 standard tasks of peripheral and axial joint motion performed by patients. Evaluation is by trained observer. Completion time is 10–15 minutes (4).	Motivation may be a factor. Time and personnel to observe and score tasks are a factor in its use. Scale is sensitive to short-term change (3,62).

is not recommended (7,8). More detailed assessments are needed to determine important clinical change over time.

Self-Report Questionnaires

Numerous instruments and questionnaires have been developed to measure health status. These instruments vary in complexity from those measuring a single domain (such as ability to do activities of daily living or self-reported pain levels) to more comprehensive instruments

Table 2. American College of Rheumatology revised criteria for classification of functional status in rheumatoid arthritis*

Class	Description
Class I	Completely able to perform usual activities of daily living (self-care, vocational, and avocational)
Class II	Able to perform usual self-care and vocational activities, but limited in avocational activities
Class III	Able to perform usual self-care activities, but limited in vocational and avocational activities
Class IV	Limited ability to perform usual self-care, vocational, and avocational activities

* Usual self-care activities include dressing, feeding, bathing, grooming, and toileting. Avocational (recreational and/or leisure) and vocational (work, school, homemaking) activities are patient-desired, and age- and sex-specific. Reprinted with permission from reference 7.

having several subscales that measure different aspects of health status. In addition to functional status, the multidimensional instruments contain measures of pain, mood, and emotional wellbeing; symptoms such as sleep disturbance, fatigue (energy level), gastrointestinal distress, and morning stiffness; social activities and role; cognitive ability; and work and work disability. Patients' global perceptions of health and disease and their satisfaction with their overall health are included in some instruments. Less commonly evaluated are perceived priority areas for health, attribution of health problems, indirect and direct costs of disease, and drug side effects.

Instruments are classified as generic or disease specific. Generic instruments may be used to evaluate a variety of chronic conditions and provide a common measure so that comparisons can be made across different diseases. Comparison with the general population or with "healthy" groups is also possible (9). Disease-specific instruments are more sensitive to the particular set of problems or symptoms associated with a given disease (10). For example, pain is more important to evaluate in the rheumatic diseases than it is for patients with hypertension. Lower extremity function is especially important following hip or knee replacement for osteoarthritis (OA); however, limitations in activities related to hand functioning might be especially significant in early RA (11).

Disease-Specific Instruments

Health status instruments continue to be developed and validated for use across the rheumatic disorders, and more specific instruments are being developed for use in particular rheumatic diseases. The most widely used and general of these disease-specific instruments include the Health Assessment Questionnaire (HAQ) and its modifications, the Arthritis Impact Measurement Scales (AIMS) and its revision, and the McMaster Toronto Arthritis Patient Preference Disability Questionnaire (MACTAR). The Western Ontario and McMaster Universities Osteoarthritis Index (WOMAC), the Fibromyalgia Impact Questionnaire (FIQ), and the Bath Ankylosing Spondylitis Disease Activity Index (BASDAI) are examples of instruments for use with specific disorders. Each of these instruments is briefly described below; the domains included in each instrument are listed in Table 3.

Health Assessment Questionnaire. There are 2 versions of the original HAQ: the functional disability scale and the full HAQ, both developed in the early 1980s. The full HAQ is >20 pages long, changes periodically, and evaluates economic costs, medications and their side effects, use of health care services, comorbidity, functional disability, pain, and global disease severity. The second version, which is used extensively, is the short functional disability scale consisting of 24 questions. This instrument evaluates 8 activities of daily living,

including dressing, arising, eating, walking, hygiene, reach, grip, and general activities (e.g., running errands, getting in and out of a car) (12). HAQ scores range from 0 (able to perform all activities without difficulty) to 3 (unable to do activities even with help). Visual analog scales measuring severity of pain during the last week and global disease severity are frequently included as part of the HAQ. In contrast to the full questionnaire, this instrument may be completed and scored in <5 minutes and is suitable for use in both research and clinical practice settings. The HAQ functional disability scale has been translated into several languages and is used throughout the world (13,14). The instrument is sensitive to change in clinical trials and in long-term outcome studies, and it has been shown to predict mortality and future disabilities. It has been used in studies across the spectrum of rheumatic diseases and remains one of the most popular instruments. HAQ instruments are available at http://aramis.stanford.edu/HAQ.html.

Modified Health Assessment Questionnaire (M-HAQ). The M-HAQ includes a shortened version of the HAQ functional scale (8 items) plus items related to patient satisfaction with function and patient interpretation of his or her change in ability to perform routine activities (15).

Table 3. Domains of health status questionnaires, including major sections (X) and subsections (O)*

Domain	Disease-specific instruments										Generic instruments				
	F-HAQ	HAQ	CLIN-HAQ	M-HAQ	AIMS	AIMS2	WOMAC	FIQ	MACTAR	BASDAI	SF-36	SIP	FSS	FQ	MAF
Functional disability	X	X	X	X	X	X	X		X		X	X			
Eating												O			
Body care						O						O			
Mobility					O	O						O			
Dexterity					O	O									
ADL/self-care					O	O									
Arm function						O									
Physical function					O	O									
Pain	X	X	X	X	X	X	X	X		X	X				
Social activities and roles					X	X			X		X	X			
Social roles/function					O	O					O				
Home management												O			
Social activities					O	O					O				
Recreation/pastime												O			
Social interaction/isolation												O			
Social support						O									
Communication												O			
Work/work disability	X		X			X		X			X	X	X		
Symptoms															
Sleep/rest			X					X			X				
Stiffness				X			X	X		X					
Fatigue/energy			X	X				X			X		X	X	X
Gastrointestinal problems			X	X											
Alertness/cognition												X	X		
Adverse drug reactions	X		X												
Global measures															
Global disease severity	X	X	X	X											
Global health/wellbeing			X	X				X			X				
Satisfaction			X	X	X										
Emotions/mood			X	X	X	X		X	X		X	X			
Depression			O			O	O	O							
Anxiety			O			O	O	O							
Helplessness/attitude				O											
Financial aspects	X														
Indirect costs	O														
Direct costs	O														
Other areas															
Attribution of problems						X									
Priority areas: self-stated						X		X							

* F-HAQ = Full HAQ; HAQ = Health Assessment Questionnaire functional disability scale; CLINHAQ = clinical HAQ; M-HAQ = modified HAQ; AIMS = Arthritis Impact Measurement Scales; AIMS2 = Arthritis Impact Measurement Scales, version 2; WOMAC = Western Ontario and McMaster Universities Osteoarthritis Index; FIQ = Fibromyalgia Impact Questionnaire; MACTAR = McMaster Toronto Arthritis Preference Disability Questionnaire; BASDAI = The Bath Ankylosing Spondylitis Disease Activity Index; SF-36 = Medical Outcomes Study 36-Item Short Form Health Survey; SIP = Sickness Impact Profile; NHP = Nottingham Health Profile; FSS = Fatigue Severity Scale; FQ = Fatigue Questionnaire; MAF = Multidimensional Assessment of Fatigue Scale. Modified from reference 14, with permission.

The M-HAQ has been used extensively in clinical trials and long-term observational studies. Studies comparing the original HAQ functional ability scale to the M-HAQ have indicated that the M-HAQ does not describe the full range of disability (i.e., minimal impairment through inability to do the activities of daily living) as well as the HAQ, but nonetheless, has been recently shown to perform reasonably well when compared with longer versions of the HAQ (13,16).

Multi-Dimensional Modified HAQ (MD-HAQ). The MD-HAQ is most appropriate for routine clinic practice. It includes the M-HAQ plus items related to activity levels (walking, running, climbing stairs), pain, psychological distress, fatigue, global status, review of systems, and medications. It can be used to provide quantitative data for standard care of all patients with all rheumatic diseases (17).

CLIN-HAQ. The CLIN-HAQ is a derivative instrument that integrates several scales and subscales from established instruments as well as including new ones (14). It contains the HAQ functional disability scale, 5 visual analog scales (i.e., pain, global disease severity, sleep disturbance, gastrointestinal distress, and fatigue), a pain diagram, and the anxiety and depression subscales from the original AIMS instrument. This instrument has been used for numerous reports of long-term outcome in the rheumatic diseases as well as in ongoing clinical practice (14,18).

Arthritis Impact Measurement Scales. The AIMS, a comprehensive rheumatic disease health status instrument, has been published in 2 versions (19,20). Both instruments have been extensively validated and translated into several languages. The original AIMS examined the impact of arthritis in terms of both physical function (scales for mobility, physical activity, dexterity, and activities of daily living) and psychosocial aspects (subscales for social role, social activities, pain, depression, and anxiety). AIMS2, published in 1992, added new components that addressed issues of patient satisfaction, patient preference or priority areas for health status improvement, and attribution of symptoms/problems to arthritis. The length of both instruments (>20 minutes to complete) and the complexity of scoring have limited their use in routine clinical practice and clinical studies (21).

A shortened version of the AIMS2, the AIMS-SF, has been developed (22). The abbreviated instrument retains the original 5-component structure (physical functions, symptoms, affect, social interaction, and role) of the AIMS2 but reduces the number of items by 50%.

McMaster Toronto Arthritis Patient Preference Disability Questionnaire. The MACTAR, an interviewer-administered questionnaire, is designed to elicit patient priorities or preferences. Patients are asked to describe limitation in activities, including physical functioning (self-care); household, work, and leisure activities; social roles; and sexuality. They then are to rank the importance of doing those various activities without pain (23,24). The interviewer probes for answers using a detailed protocol. The instrument has been shown to be "valid and highly responsive" in clinical trials, but the cost of administration might limit its applicability for clinical practice and long-term outcome studies (24).

Western Ontario and McMaster Universities Osteoarthritis Index. The WOMAC is a self-administered instrument designed to measure dimensions particularly relevant to OA. It specifically measures pain, stiffness, and physical function associated with OA of the hip or knee (25). The instrument has been used extensively and is the most popular instrument for OA trials (26–31). The WOMAC correlates strongly with pain, fatigue, and psychological distress, demonstrating that the instrument has a global outlook (25). Its brevity (<10 minutes to administer) and responsiveness to change make it appropriate for use in clinical practice settings. The instrument has been translated into several languages and has been well validated.

Fibromyalgia Impact Questionnaire. The FIQ is a brief 20-item questionnaire designed to assess the effects of fibromyalgia on several domains. It includes items pertaining to physical function, work status, depression, anxiety, sleep, pain, stiffness, fatigue, and wellbeing (32). The physical function component assesses ability to do such common tasks as shopping, making beds, walking several blocks, laundry, vacuuming, and yard work. Participants have the option of not responding to items that are not relevant to them. The FIQ is the most widely used clinical and research instrument for measuring the effect of fibromyalgia, as well as change resulting from intervention (32–35).

The Bath Ankylosing Spondylitis Disease Activity Index. The BASDAI is a 6-item questionnaire designed to assess and evaluate disease activity in patients with ankylosing spondylitis (36). The BASDAI assesses spinal pain, fatigue, joint pain and swelling, areas of tenderness, and morning stiffness duration and severity on a 10-point scale, ranging from 1 (no problem) to 10 (the worse problem). The BASDAI is easy to administer and displays acceptable measurement properties and sensitivity to change.

Generic Health Status Measures

Generic health status measures assess the impact of a disease on important physical, social, and emotional domains of functioning. They are frequently used to assess health of the population; therefore, they may be used with both "healthy" subjects and those with illness and symptoms. These instruments are usually multidimensional and may include subscales that address different domains, such as pain, social isolation/interaction, and fulfillment of roles. They permit comparison across diseases and cultures, as well as comparisons with healthy populations (9). Table 3 lists common generic health status instruments.

Nottingham Health Profile (NHP). The NHP was developed in England and has been translated and tested in several languages. It includes 38 dichotomous questions that evaluate physical abilities, pain, sleep, social isolation, emotional reactions, and energy level from the patient's viewpoint (37). The simple format and short completion time (10 minutes) are advantages, although the yes/no response format does not allow the respondent to rate the extent to which a given item affects them. This makes it less sensitive to change over time (38).

Sickness Impact Profile (SIP). The SIP has been widely used in North America and Europe across numerous chronic diseases, including the rheumatic disorders. It contains 312 items within the dimensions of physical and psychosocial functioning. Specific sections include sleep and rest, eating, work, home management, recreation and pastimes, ambulating, mobility, body care and movement, social interaction, alertness behavior, emotional behavior, and communication (39). The SIP, and its modified variants, can be self-administered or administered by an interviewer and takes 20–30 minutes to complete. Although the SIP is one of the most comprehensive generic multidimensional health status questionnaires, its lack of a pain scale limits its value for people with rheumatic disorders (40).

The Medical Outcomes Study Short Form 36 (SF-36). The SF-36 is the most widely used generic instrument and is frequently paired with a disease-specific instrument in clinical drug trials, long-term observational studies, and other clinical investigations (9,41). It evaluates 8 domains of health status, including limitation in physical activities because of health problems, limitation in social activities because of health problems, limitation of social activities because of physical or emotional problems, limitation in usual role because of health problems, bodily pain, general mental health (psychological distress and wellbeing), vitality (energy and fatigue), and general health perceptions. The 8 domains can be scored individually, or physical component and mental component summary scores can be calculated. The instrument can be completed and scored quickly, and may be used in clinical practice, research, health policy, and population surveys. The

SF-36 has been extensively tested in large populations, and normative information is available for the US and several European countries. Moreover, the SF-36 has been used with a variety of chronic disease populations. The SF-36 is an important instrument due to its use as an outcome measure for US health policy research. Ongoing efforts to translate and validate the instrument in many countries further illustrate its significance. Shorter versions (i.e., SF-12, SF-8) of the SF-36 have also been developed to minimize patient burden.

Measures of Fatigue

Fatigue is increasingly recognized as a significant contributor to impaired functioning and HRQOL in rheumatic disease patients (42). Several measures have been developed to assess fatigue, including the **Fatigue Severity Scale** (FSS), the **Fatigue Questionnaire** (FQ), and the **Multidimensional Assessment of Fatigue Scale** (MAF). The FSS (43) is a 9-item questionnaire that assesses general fatigue. The FSS can be completed in 1–2 minutes and appears to offer a reliable and valid means of assessing fatigue associated with a given health condition. The FQ (44) is an 11-item questionnaire that assesses physical fatigue and mental fatigue with higher scores indicative of greater fatigue. Finally, the MAF (45) is a 16-item questionnaire that assesses 4 dimensions of fatigue (degree and severity, amount of distress it causes, its frequency, and the degree to which it interferes with activities of daily living).

HEALTH STATUS ASSESSMENT IN CHILDREN

Assessment of HRQOL and health status in children is complex. Developmental milestones, roles and tasks at different ages, discrepancies between parent and child, and normal variability in growth and behavior are just some of the issues that complicate the use of health status assessments with children. Nonetheless, health status instruments for children are being developed that complement the reliable and well-validated instruments for assessment of adults. Although functional classification systems, including the ACR Functional Class and the Chronic Activity Limitations Scale, have been used to describe functional limitations in children with rheumatic diseases, they have failed to describe adequately the physical limitations of these children. Use of these instruments, however, is suboptimal in that >85% of the disabilities of children with juvenile rheumatoid arthritis (JRA) have been categorized in classes indicating no or only minor disruptions in functional ability (46,47).

The **Childhood HAQ** (C-HAQ), the most commonly used instrument for children, is adapted from the functional status scale of the HAQ. It assesses functional ability, pain, and global severity. Each activity of daily living area from the adult HAQ (e.g., dressing, eating, and arising) has an age-appropriate assessment item. For example, able to remove socks was added to the dressing and grooming area because a healthy 1-year-old can perform this activity but could not accomplish the other listed activities. The instrument may be completed by the child or by parents as appropriate (48).

The **Juvenile Arthritis Quality of Life Questionnaire** (49) and the **Childhood Arthritis Health Profile** (50,51) are more comprehensive instruments than the C-HAQ. Each addresses the HRQOL domains beyond function, such as pain, psychosocial functioning, symptoms, and areas of family, friends, and school. Both instruments are beginning to be used in clinical practice.

Other instruments developed for use in children include the **Juvenile Arthritis Functional Assessment Scale** (JAFAS) and the **Juvenile Arthritis Functional Assessment Report** (JAFAR). The JAFAS includes 10 activities of daily living (e.g., buttoning a shirt or blouse, cutting food, walking, and bending) that are observed and evaluated by a health professional. In children 7 years and older, this instrument has been shown to discriminate between healthy children and children with JRA, and between different ability levels of chronically ill children (52). The JAFAS and JAFAR, an adaptation of the JAFAS, include 23 items and are designed as self-report instruments. Separate versions for proxy reports by parents or self-administration by the child are available (53).

USE OF HEALTH STATUS MEASURES IN CLINICAL PRACTICE

A variety of health status instruments have been developed and validated in clinical studies. They have been used as outcome measures in clinical trials evaluating medications, educational interventions, and joint replacement surgery. These measures are sometimes used to predict health care costs, length of stay in rehabilitation facilities, and even mortality. Although their usefulness in rheumatology outpatient care has been demonstrated (54), widespread integration of health status measures into routine clinical practice is difficult and time consuming, but remains an important goal.

In selecting an instrument for use in clinical care, the length of the instrument and appropriateness to the practice setting are the major concerns. For routine monitoring of outpatients in a rheumatology practice, the HAQ functional ability scale, the M-HAQ, and the CLIN-HAQ are widely used. They measure the important aspects of health status, such as functional ability, pain, psychological distress, fatigue, and satisfaction, yet responding to all items takes <5 minutes. Patients may complete the questionnaires while sitting in a waiting room so that disruption of clinical routine is minimal. Scoring can be done quickly; it is even possible for these assessments to be completed on a computer terminal so that important information (depression level, pain severity, and functional ability) is available immediately during the clinic visit (17). A standardized protocol to evaluate rheumatoid arthritis has been proposed by Pincus, and is available at http://www.clinexprheumatol.org/pdf/vol23/s39/s39_pdf/18pincus.pdf.

In rehabilitation settings and evaluations following orthopedic surgery, other instruments may be used to assess outcome of treatment. Perhaps the more comprehensive AIMS or AIMS2 would be helpful, especially if repeated administrations are not required. Time for completion is longer than for the HAQ, M-HAQ, or the CLIN-HAQ; however, more comprehensive information is obtained. If one is studying outcome in OA following orthopedic surgery, the WOMAC might provide the most meaningful information. The trade-off between cost of administration and comprehensive information remains the issue in selecting an appropriate instrument.

In primary care clinics, where a variety of chronic health problems are seen in addition to rheumatic diseases, the SF-36 (or its shorter versions) may be the best choice. The availability of both normative and disease-specific data in both the US and Europe make adoption of this instrument for a primary practice clinic appealing. As shown in Table 3, domains included in the SF-36 are similar to the AIMS and AIMS2 and to aspects of the HAQ, CLIN-HAQ, and M-HAQ. Like the disease-specific HAQ, CLIN-HAQ, and M-HAQ, patients can complete the SF-36 in a few minutes without assistance. Rapid scoring is feasible, providing the health professional with ready access to important information.

An RA-specific tool available on the internet that patients can use to monitor disease activity over time is the RA Activity Minder (http://www.hopkins-arthritis.som.jhmi.edu/arthritis_sa/home.cfm). Patients are able to track their weekly disease activity and print reports to take to their health care providers. The Activity Minder is free and patient data is stored on a secure server. No user-identifiable information is transmitted either during printing of reports or while data is stored on the database.

SUMMARY

Health status assessment has become integrated with traditional assessment tools of history taking, physical examination, laboratory tests, and radiography. Although physical functioning may be evaluated by direct observation, this approach is time consuming, expensive, and limited to the few tasks that are observable in the clinic. Reliable, well-validated self-report health status instruments have been developed for use in clinical research and practice. These instruments may be specific to the rheumatic diseases or may be multidimensional assessments of HRQOL. Some, such as the SF-36 or versions of the HAQ, are more appropriate for routine clinical care. Others, such as AIMS or SIP, are best used for clinical research or in comprehensive outcome studies. Regardless of instrument used, the assessment of health status is essential to the comprehensive understanding of how a disease affects someone's life; therefore, such assessment is also essential to providing comprehensive, high-quality patient care.

REFERENCES

1. Liang MH. The historical and conceptual framework for functional assessment in rheumatic disease. J Rheumatol 1987;14(Suppl 15):2–5.
2. Gill TM, Feinstein AR. A critical appraisal of the quality of quality-of-life measurements. JAMA 1994;272:619–26.
3. Anderson JJ, Felson DT, Meenan RF, Williams HJ. Which traditional measures should be used in rheumatoid arthritis clinical trials? Arthritis Rheum 1989;32:1093–9.
4. Decker JL, McShane DJ, Esdaile JM, Hathaway DE, Levinson JE, Liang MH, et al. Dictionary of the rheumatic diseases. Volume 1. Signs and symptoms. New York: Contact Associates International; 1982.
5. Kwoh CK, O'Connor GT, Regansmith MG, Olmstead EM, Brown LA, Burnett JB, et al. Concordance between clinician and patient assessment of physical and mental health status. J Rheumatol 1992;19:1031–7.
6. Kivela SL. Measuring disability–do self-ratings and service-provider ratings compare? J Chronic Dis 1984;37:115–23.
7. Hochberg MC, Chang RW, Dwosh I, Lindsey S, Pincus T, Wolfe F. The American College of Rheumatology 1991 revised criteria for the classification of global functional status in rheumatoid arthritis. Arthritis Rheum 1992;35:498–502.
8. Stucki G, Stoll T, Bruhlmann P, Michel BA. Construct validation of the ACR 1991 revised criteria for global functional status in rheumatoid arthritis. Clin Exp Rheumatol 1995;13:349–52.
9. Stewart AL, Greenfield S, Hays RD, Wells K, Rogers WH, Berry SD, et al. Functional status and well-being of patients with chronic conditions: results from the Medical Outcomes Study. JAMA 1989;262:907–13.
10. Fowler FJ, Cleary PD, Magaziner J, Patrick DL, Benjamin KL. Methodological issues in measuring patient-reported outcomes: the agenda of the work group on outcomes assessment. Med Care 1994;32:JS65–76.
11. Stewart AL, Painter PL. Issues in measuring physical functioning and disability in arthritis patients. Arthritis Care Res 1997;10:395–405.
12. Fries JF, Spitz P, Kraines RG, Holman HR. Measurement of patient outcome in arthritis. Arthritis Rheum 1980;23:137–45.
13. Wolfe F. Which HAQ is best? A comparison of the HAQ, MHAQ and RA-HAQ, a difficult 8-item HAQ (DHAQ), and a rescored 20-item HAQ (HAQ20): analyses on 2,491 rheumatoid arthritis patients following leflunomide initiation. J Rheumatol 2001;28:982–9.
14. Wolfe F. Health status questionnaires. Rheum Dis Clin North Am 1995;21:445–64.
15. Pincus T, Summey JA, Soraci SA Jr, Wallston KA, Hummon NP. Assessment of patient satisfaction in activities of daily living using a modified Stanford Health Assessment Questionnaire. Arthritis Rheum 1983;26:1346–53.
16. Uhlig T, Haavardsholm EA, Kvien TK. Comparison of the Health Assessment Questionnaire (HAQ) and the modified HAQ (MHAQ) in patients with rheumatoid arthritis. Rheumatology (Oxford) 2006;45:454–8.
17. Pincus T, Yazici Y, Bergman M. Development of the multi-dimensional health assessment questionnaire for the infrastructure of standard clinical care. Clin Exp Rheumatol 2005;23 (5 Suppl 39):S19–8.
18. Wolfe F, Skevington SM. Measuring the epidemiology of distress: the rheumatology distress index. J Rheumatol 2000;27:2000–9.
19. Meenan RF, Gertman PM, Mason JH. Measuring health status in arthritis: the Arthritis Impact Measurement Scales. Arthritis Rheum 1980;23:146–52.
20. Meenan RF, Mason JH, Anderson JJ, Guccione AA, Kazis LE. AIMS2: the content and properties of a revised and expanded Arthritis Impact Measurement Scales health status questionnaire. Arthritis Rheum 1992;35:1–10.
21. Haavardsholm EA, Kvien TK, Uhlig T, Smedstad LM, Guillemin F. Comparison of agreement and sensitivity to change between AIMS2 and a short form of AIMS2 (AIMS2-SF) in more than 1000 rheumatoid arthritis patients. J Rheumatol 2000;27:2810–6.
22. Guillemin F, Coste J, Pouchot J, Ghézail M, Bregeon C, Sany J, et al, The French Quality of Life in Rheumatology Group. The AIMS2-SF: a short form of the Arthritis Impact Measurement Scales 2. Arthritis Rheum 1997;40:1267–74.
23. Tugwell P, Bombardier C, Buchanan WW, Goldsmith CH, Grace E, Hanna B. The MACTAR patient preference disability questionnaire–an individualized functional priority approach for assessing improvement in physical disability in clinical trials in rheumatoid arthritis. J Rheumatol 1987;14:446–51.
24. Verhoeven AC, Boers M, van der Linden S. Validity of the MACTAR questionnaire as a functional index in a rheumatoid arthritis clinical trial. J Rheumatol 2000;27:2801–9.
25. Bellamy N, Buchanan WW, Goldsmith CH, Campbell J, Stitt LW. Validation study of WOMAC: a health status instrument for measuring clinically important patient relevant outcomes to antirheumatic drug therapy in patients with osteoarthritis of the hip or knee. J Rheumatol 1988;15:1833–40.
26. Bellamy N, Kean WF, Buchanan WW, Gerecz-Simon E, Campbell J. Double blind randomized controlled trial of sodium meclofenamate (Meclomen) and diclofenac sodium (Voltaren): post validation reapplication of the WOMAC Osteoarthritis Index. J Rheumatol 1992;19:153–9.
27. Grace D, Rogers J, Skeith K, Anderson K. Topical diclofenac versus placebo: a double blind, randomized clinical trial in patients with osteoarthritis of the knee. J Rheumatol 1999;26:2659–63.
28. Peloso PM, Bellamy N, Thomson GTD, Harsanyi Z, Babul N, et al. Double blind randomized placebo control trial of controlled release codeine in the treatment of osteoarthritis of the hip or knee. J Rheumatol 2000;27:764–71.
29. Klein G, Kullich W, Schnitker J, Schwann H. Efficacy and tolerance of an oral enzyme combination in painful osteoarthritis of the hip: A double-blind, randomized study comparing oral enzymes with non-steroidal anti-inflammatory drugs. Clin Exp Rheumatol 2006;24:25–30.
30. Brazier JE, Harper R, Munro J, Walters SJ, Snaith ML. Generic and condition-specific outcome measures for people with osteoarthritis of the knee. Rheumatology (Oxford) 1999;38:870–7.
31. Quintana JM, Escobar A, Arostegui I, Bilbao A, Azkaratej J, Geonaga JI, et al. Health-related quality of life and appropriateness of knee or hip joint replacement. Arch Intern Med 2006;166:220–6.
32. Burckhardt CS, Clark SR, Bennett RM. The fibromyalgia impact questionnaire: development and validation. J Rheumatol 1991;18:728–33.
33. Wolfe F, Hawley DJ, Goldenberg DL, Russell IJ, Buskila D, Neumann L. The assessment of functional impairment in fibromyalgia (FM): Rasch analyses of 5 functional scales and the development of the FM Health Assessment Questionnaire. J Rheumatol 2000;27:1989–99.
34. Richards SCM, Scott DL. Prescribed exercise in people with fibromyalgia: parallel group randomized trial. BMJ 2002;325:185–8.
35. Assis MR, Silva LE, Alves AM, Pessanha AP, Valim V, Feldman D, et al. A randomized controlled trial of deep water running: clinical effectiveness of aquatic exercise to treat fibromyalgia. Arthritis Rheum 2006;15:57–5.
36. Garrett S, Jenkinson T, Kennedy LG, Whitelock H, Gaisford P. Colin A. A new approach to defining disease status in ankylosing spondylitis: The Bath Ankylosing Spondylitis Disease Activity Index. J Rheumatol 1994;21:2286–91.
37. Hunt SM, McKenna SP, McEwen J, Backett EM, Williams J, Papp E. The Nottingham Health Profile: subjective health status and medical consultations. Soc Sci Med [A] 1981;15:221–9.
38. Fitzpatrick R, Ziebland S, Jenkinson C, Mowat A. A comparison of the sensitivity to change of several health status instruments in rheumatoid arthritis. J Rheumatol 1993;20:429–36.

39. Bergner M, Bobbitt RA, Carter WB. The Sickness Impact Profile: development and final revision of a health status measure. Med Care 1981;19:787–5.

40. Anderson RT, Aaronson NK, Wilkin D. Critical review of the international assessments of health-related quality of life. Qual Life Res 1993;2:369–95.

41. Ware JE, Sherbourne CD. The MOS 36-item short-form health survey (SF-36). 1. Conceptual framework and item selection. Med Care 1992;30:473–83.

42. Pollard L, Choy EH, Scott DL. The consequences of rheumatoid arthritis: quality of life measures Clin Exp Rheumatol 2005;23(5 Suppl 39):S43–52.

43. Krupp LB, LaRocca NG, Muir-Nash J, Sternberg AD. The fatigue severity scale: application to patients with multiple sclerosis and systemic lupus erythematosis. Arch Neurol 1989;46:1121–3.

44. Chalder T, Berelowitz G, Pawlikowska T, Watts L, Wessely S, Wright D, et al. Development of a fatigue scale. J Psychosomatic Res 1993;37:147–53.

45. Belza B. Comparison of self-reported fatigue in rheumatoid arthritis and controls. J Rheumatol 1995;22:639–43.

46. Feldman BM, Grundland B, McCullough L, Wright V. Distinction of quality of life, health related quality of life, and health status in children referred for rheumatologic care. J Rheumatol 2000;27:226–33.

47. Tucker LB. Whose life is it anyway? Understanding quality of life in children with rheumatic diseases. J Rheumatol 2000;27:8–11.

48. Burgos Vargas R. Assessment of quality of life in children with rheumatic diseases. J Rheumatol 1999;26:1432–5.

49. Singh G, Athreya BH, Fries JF, Goldsmith DP. Measurement of health status in children with juvenile rheumatoid arthritis. Arthritis Rheum 1994;37:1761–9.

50. Duffy CM, Arsenault L, Duffy KNW, Paquin JD, Strawczynski H. The juvenile arthritis quality of life questionnaire development of a new responsive index for juvenile rheumatoid arthritis and juvenile spondyloarthritides. J Rheumatol 1997;24:738–46.

51. Duffy CM, Tucker LB, Burgo-Vargas R. Update on functional assessment tools. J Rheumatol Suppl 2000;58:11–4.

52. Lovell DJ, Howe S, Shear E, Hartner S, McGirr G, Schulte M, et al. Development of a disability measurement tool for juvenile rheumatoid arthritis: the Juvenile Arthritis Functional Assessment Scale. Arthritis Rheum 1989;32:1390–5.

53. Howe S, Levinson J, Shear E, Hartner S, McGirr G, Schulte M, et al. Development of a disability measurement tool for juvenile rheumatoid arthritis: the Juvenile Arthritis Functional Assessment Report for children and their parents. Arthritis Rheum 1991;34:873–80.

54. Wolfe F, Pincus T. Data collection in the clinic. Rheum Dis Clin North Am 1995;21:321–58.

55. Jones E, Hanly JG, Mooney R, Rand LL, Spurway PM, Eastwood BJ, et al. Strength and function in the normal and rheumatoid hand. J Rheumatol 1991;18:1313–8.

56. Pankoff B, Overend T, Lucy D, White K. Validity and responsiveness of the 6 minute walk test for people with fibromyalgia. J Rheumatol 2000;27:2666–70.

57. Dellhag B, Bjelle A. A five-year followup of hand function and activities of daily living in rheumatoid arthritis patients. Arthritis Care Res 1999;12:33–41.

58. Dellhag B, Bjelle A. A grip ability test for use in rheumatology practice. J Rheumatol 1995;22:1559–65.

59. Pincus T, Callahan LF. Rheumatology function tests–grip strength, walking time, button test and questionnaires document and predict long term morbidity and mortality in rheumatoid arthritis. J Rheumatol 1992;19:1051–7.

60. Newcomer KL, Krug HE, Mahowald ML. Validity and reliability of the timed-stands test for patients with rheumatoid arthritis and other chronic diseases. J Rheumatol 1993;20:21–7.

61. Sullivan M, Ahlmen M, Bjelle A, Karlsson J. Health status assessment in rheumatoid arthritis. II. Evaluation of a modified Shorter Sickness Impact Profile. J Rheumatol 1993;20:1500–7.

62. Kalla AA, Smith PR, Brown GMM, Meyers OL, Chalton D. Responsiveness of Keitel functional index compared with laboratory measures of disease activity in rheumatoid arthritis. Br J Rheumatol 1995;34:141–9.

Additional Recommended Reading

McDowell I, Newell C. Measuring health: a guide to rating scales and questionnaires. 2nd ed. Oxford (UK): Oxford University Press; 1996.

Katz PP (Ed). Patient outcomes in rheumatology: a review of measures. Arthritis Rheum 2003;49 (5 Suppl):S1–235.

Streiner DL, Norman GR. Health measurement scales: a practical guide to their development and use, 2nd ed. New York: Oxford University Press; 2003.

Bibliography of Criteria, Guidelines, and Health Status Assessments Used in Rheumatology. Available at http://www.rheumatology.org/publications/abbreviations/r.asp.

Psychological Assessment

JERRY C. PARKER, PhD, and KAREN L. SMARR, PhD

Characterizing the psychological aspects of the rheumatic diseases is difficult due to the diversity of diagnostic categories. Arthritis almost always results in pain and restricted movement, but some acute conditions, such as gout and septic arthritis, respond quickly to treatment and have minimal long-term psychological impact. However, in chronic conditions such as rheumatoid arthritis (RA) and systemic lupus erythematosus (SLE), years of pain, functional losses, and deteriorated health are major challenges to the coping process. Many persons with chronic, debilitating arthritis manage to cope successfully. In some cases, however, either the disease-related stressors are too severe or the environmental resources are not sufficient to sustain a successful coping effort. Consequently, some persons with arthritis display psychological symptoms secondary to disease. In other cases, persons with arthritis present with pre-existing psychological problems.

PREVALENCE OF PSYCHOLOGICAL PROBLEMS

The prevalence of psychological distress is difficult to estimate across rheumatic conditions and socioeconomic settings. Useful data, though, can be obtained from the primary care literature, where the prevalence of psychological problems has been shown to be relatively high. One study found that 26% of patients met criteria for a psychiatric disorder using the Diagnostic and Statistical Manual of Mental Disorders, 3rd Edition, Revised (1,2). A survey of urban, low-income patients found that 18.9% screened positive for depression (3). Another study found that 15–40% of primary care patients met the criteria for a diagnosable mental disorder (4). There is little doubt that primary care settings are confronted with a high prevalence of mental, emotional, and behavioral problems.

In most rheumatology settings, psychological problems appear to be similarly prevalent. Estimates suggest that ~20% of persons with RA present with major depression (5). In a study of persons with SLE, 20.5% were found to have a concomitant psychiatric disorder (6). Approximately one-half of persons with either RA or osteoarthritis (OA) may experience losses in social relationships (7), which is a risk factor for depression. Although such psychological problems are far from universal, a substantial number of persons with arthritis will encounter psychological distress at some point in their lives. Those providing care to arthritis patients should be both vigilant regarding psychological problems and familiar with the process of psychological assessment.

IMPORTANCE OF PSYCHOLOGICAL PERSPECTIVE

Beyond recognizing the relatively high prevalence of psychological problems in medical settings, arthritis health professionals also need a keen appreciation of psychological concepts to provide optimal care for patients. Three broad psychological perspectives are important in the management of rheumatic disease: 1) the biopsychosocial model of illness; 2) the Institute of Medicine enablement model of disability; and 3) the empirical foundations for psychological interventions.

Biopsychosocial Model

For the past 400 years, the conceptualization of physical illness has been dominated by a biomedical framework. Illness has been viewed as a physiochemical abnormality requiring biologic management. The biomedical model is highly valid under many circumstances, and it has led to impressive therapeutic breakthroughs in such acute illnesses as infectious disease. Increasingly, though, the inadequacy of the biomedical model has been recognized, especially in such chronic diseases as arthritis. In these conditions, there is an intermingling of biologic, psychologic, and sociologic determinants with regard to the onset, course, and outcomes of illness. Engel (8) coined the term, *biopsychosocial model*, to convey the multiple determinants of physical illness. For optimal health care, the psychological and social aspects of rheumatic disease must be thoroughly assessed and treated.

Institute of Medicine Enablement Model of Disability

Another psychological concept derives from the Institute of Medicine "enabling-disabling process" model of disability (9). Traditionally, tissue abnormalities or physiologic imbalances have been viewed as the primary determinants of disability. However, many persons with abnormalities at the cellular level never develop failure of an entire organ system. Even persons who experience organ-system failure do not necessarily develop functional disability. The *enablement model* views the individual's environment as either enabling or disabling. Enabling factors, such as personal resilience (e.g., effective coping), access to appropriate care, and assistive devices, allow for independence and enhanced functioning. Disability can occur when barriers exist and these factors are lacking. Therefore, disability is not a purely biologic phenomenon but is also determined, to a great extent, by behavioral factors and the psychological processes of coping and adaptation. Consequently, from the disability perspective, the psychological status of people with arthritis should be carefully assessed.

Psychological Interventions

The effectiveness of psychological interventions also should be understood by health care professionals. In general, psychological treatments work reasonably well. A meta-analysis of the effectiveness of cognitive therapy for depression found that the average therapy patient did better than 98% of the control subjects (overall effect size = 0.99) (10,11). In comparison, the average effect size for drug treatment in arthritis ranges from only 0.45 to 0.77 (12). Even in severe psychiatric disorders, such as major depression, behavioral treatments are effective in ~55% of cases (13).

Cognitive-behavioral or self-management interventions for RA or OA are also associated with improvements in pain, depressive symptoms, coping abilities, self-efficacy, and other self-management behaviors (14). In addition, a stress management program for persons with RA has been shown to decrease helplessness, improve confidence in coping ability, and reduce pain, with benefits lasting up to 15 months (15). Evidence for the effectiveness of psychological interventions for persons with arthritis is impressive. Thus, psychological assessment can be viewed as an important prelude to identifying those who may benefit from psychological interventions.

APPROACHES TO PSYCHOLOGICAL ASSESSMENT

Psychological assessment is not a uniform procedure; it is a variety of approaches to the characterization of psychological and behavioral processes. There are 3 general approaches to psychological assessment: 1) diagnostic criteria; 2) unstructured clinical interviews; and 3) psychometric assessment. These approaches are not mutually exclusive. In fact, they often can be used in combination.

Diagnostic Criteria

A common approach to the assessment of psychological or psychiatric difficulties is the use of specific diagnostic criteria. In this approach, the symptoms characteristic of a given syndrome are systematically elaborated. The most common example is the Diagnostic and Statistical Manual-IV of the American Psychiatric Association (16), in which a classification of psychological and psychiatric states has been developed. The person conducting an assessment can search for the constellation of symptoms that characterize a particular diagnosis.

Diagnostic criteria have several advantages. The assessment process takes place in the context of a broad diagnostic classification system. Structured interviews guide the data-gathering process and minimize errors of omission. Also, when a psychological or psychiatric diagnosis is formulated, the associated clinical characteristics of the syndrome, such as natural history and prognosis, can usually be inferred. However, there are disadvantages to this approach. Many psychological manifestations do not conveniently fit into a structured diagnostic framework. Especially in the case of subclinical conditions, standard diagnostic frameworks simply may not apply. Diagnostic criteria are most useful in cases of moderate to severe conditions.

Clinical Interviews

Psychological assessment also can be approached through the use of unstructured clinical interviews. The examiner seeks to create a comfortable environment in which the examinee will feel free to discuss any psychological problems. The client-centered concepts of Carl Rogers provide the theoretical foundation for this approach (17). The interviewer asks open-ended questions and then listens in an accepting, nonjudgmental way. Subsequently, most examinees will articulate their individual, psychological concerns. The interviewer is thus able to gain an in-depth understanding of the patient's unique circumstances.

The unstructured interview provides an opportunity to access highly personal information that might otherwise be overlooked in a structured search for signs and symptoms. Another advantage is the rapport-building that usually occurs during a client-centered assessment; an excellent foundation may be established for future provider-patient interactions. The primary disadvantage of the client-centered approach is the lack of standardization of the data-gathering process. Determining the severity of a patient's psychological problems compared with other people may be difficult. Additionally, some patients are unable to articulate their personal problems because they do not fully recognize or understand them. Therefore, unstructured clinical interviews are most valuable when augmented by other structured approaches.

Psychometric Assessment

Psychometric assessment refers to the examination of psychological characteristics or related behaviors through the use of psychological tests. A psychological test is defined as an "objective and standardized measure of a sample of behavior," (18). The behavioral characteristic to be examined must be objective and must be observable by others. Collection of test data must be standardized so that the stimuli and demands of the test can be reproduced. A psychological test is typically restricted to a sample of behaviors because the full range of an examinee's responses is not accessible. In short, psychological testing is simply a rigorous way of observing behavior.

There are several advantages to this approach. The quantification inherent in psychological testing permits an assessment of how much of a specific psychological or behavioral characteristic exists. Thus, the establishment of norm groups is possible. A second advantage is that the error inherent in psychological tests can be estimated, which permits a confidence interval to be established for a test score. Third, the psychometric approach is rigorous in terms of statistical and quantitative methodology; however, only a narrow range of behaviors are sampled. Thus, a psychological test may not adequately focus on a person's primary psychological concerns. The effectiveness of psychological tests may vary across populations due to ceiling or floor effects (i.e., scores primarily at the top or bottom of the scale). In general, such tests are most useful when complemented by other types of clinical data.

DOMAINS OF PSYCHOMETRIC ASSESSMENT

There are literally hundreds of well-validated psychological tests that could be used in a rheumatology setting. However, the psychological domains most applicable for persons with arthritis include helplessness, depression, self-efficacy, coping and adaptation, social support, marital and family functioning, life stress, vocational preference, personality, and cognitive functioning. Each of these assessment domains warrants brief discussion. Specific psychological tests and instruments are referenced in more detail in Parker and Wright (19).

Helplessness

The domain of helplessness is particularly relevant to the care of persons with arthritis and is related to health outcomes (20). For many forms of arthritis, symptoms wax and wane; flares are generally unpredictable. Similarly, treatments for many forms of arthritis are only palliative. Therefore, persons with arthritis may perceive themselves as helpless and as having minimal control over their disease.

Depression

Although not universal, depression is a significant clinical problem for some persons with arthritis. Persons with chronic diseases have a higher probability of developing depression than do persons who are healthy (21). Social isolation and economic distress have been identified as factors that can contribute to depression (22).

Self-efficacy

Self-efficacy refers to a person's belief in his or her ability to accomplish a task or cope with a stressor (23). Self-efficacy for function, for pain, and for other symptoms have all been found to be related to important clinical outcomes, such as functional capacity and health status. In addition, self-efficacy is an important factor in the success of patient education interventions (24).

Life Stress

Stress is a common but potentially confusing term. Sometimes it can refer to environmental stimuli that are judged to be taxing by the individual. At other times, stress may refer to a person's biologic response to taxing stimuli. It can also refer to an interaction between a person and environment that is dependent on the person's perception of his or her situation, rather than on the situation itself. Despite this diversity of definitions, stress is a common problem for many people with arthritis. Disease-related problems such as chronic pain, functional losses, employment difficulties, and economic worries contribute to life stress.

Coping and Adaptation

In the face of numerous stressors, persons with arthritis must adapt to rapidly changing circumstances. The coping process usually involves a primary appraisal or judgment as to whether a stressor poses a risk of threat or harm. If a threat or harm is perceived, a secondary appraisal typically occurs as to whether sufficient resources exist to cope with the stressor. If persons perceive that they do not possess sufficient coping resources, then the stressfulness of the situation dramatically intensifies. Thus, assessment of the coping and adaptation process is important in the care of persons with arthritis.

Social Support

Social support refers to interpersonal relationships that are beneficial to a person's wellbeing. At best, social relationships offer support and understanding. At worst, they may offer criticism and blame. High levels of social support are generally associated with better adherence to medical regimens and more effective coping (25), although such findings are not universal (26).

Marital and Family Functioning

In chronic illness, marital and family functioning are often severely challenged. When health status changes for one family member, adaptation is often required by other family members as well. In arthritis, changes in work capacity or the ability to perform social roles can contribute to marital and family distress.

Vocational Assessments

One of the greatest challenges for persons with arthritis is maintaining gainful employment. Work-related difficulties and economic losses are common occurrences in the context of rheumatic diseases such as RA (27). Vocational assistance can lead to dramatically improved quality of life. Vocational assessments can elucidate aptitudes and functional work capacities.

Personality Testing

Personality testing refers to the examination of enduring psychological or behavioral traits of an individual. In rheumatology settings, personality testing is typically reserved for situations in which serious psychological problems appear to be developing or when mental health difficulties precede rheumatic disease.

Cognitive Functioning

Rheumatic diseases do not typically involve cognitive dysfunction. The most notable exception is SLE, in which cognitive functioning and psychiatric symptomatology may become prominent. Cognitive dysfunction also may occur in patients taking high-dose corticosteroids or certain other medications. In addition, arthritis patients may present with comorbidities that affect cognitive status, such as strokes, head injuries, or dementias. In these situations, neuropsychological testing can be helpful.

SCREENING FOR PSYCHOLOGICAL SIGNS AND SYMPTOMS

In rheumatology settings, sensitivity to the importance of screening for psychological signs and symptoms is required. Specifically, patients should be asked about their mood, sense of wellbeing, and general concerns; professional assessment of areas such as depression, anxiety, family discord, or life stress should be added as needed. Beyond verbal responses, some signs and symptoms of psychological distress also can be inferred from direct behavioral observation, if the examiner is vigilant and appropriately attuned to psychological issues.

INDICATIONS FOR CONSULTATION

Health care providers also need to know when and how to request psychological or mental health consultations. An initial step is to carefully explain the rationale for referral. Understandably, persons with arthritis view their health-related problems as primarily medical, so a psychological referral may seem inappropriate or unwarranted if not carefully explained. Conversely, many persons with arthritis recognize that their chronic disease constitutes a major challenge to their coping capacities. When psychological referral is presented as being secondary to their arthritis, patients often can more easily accept, or even welcome, the opportunity to receive help. There are 5 key areas for which psychological or mental health consultation may be helpful: 1) psychiatric diagnosis; 2) psychotropic medications; 3) chronic psychological distress; 4) acute adjustment reactions; and 5) psychoeducational treatments.

Psychiatric Diagnosis

In the management of rheumatic disease, a well-formulated psychiatric diagnosis is sometimes critical. For example, treatments for depression vary widely depending on the specific diagnosis. For major depression, pharmacologic treatment is usually indicated. Conversely, for adjustment reaction with depressed mood, supportive counseling is typically the treatment of choice. Cognitive dysfunction may be secondary to such diverse etiologies as adverse effects of medication, major depression, or dementia; treatment varies depending on the specific etiology. Therefore, psychological assessment should be obtained in situations where psychological or psychiatric diagnoses may effect treatment strategies. (Note: Psychologists and other licensed mental health professionals with advanced training are qualified to render psychiatric diagnoses.)

Psychotropic Medications

A related situation in which mental health assessment and consultation is indicated involves psychotropic medication. Many rheumatology health professionals do not possess extensive familiarity with either mental illness or psychotropic medications. A referral for psychological assessment or mental health consultation can result in more effective psychopharmacologic intervention for arthritis patients with concomitant psychiatric problems. If the rheumatologist elects to manage the psychotropic medication, referrals to other mental health professionals may still be indicated for various forms of supportive psychological care or therapy.

Chronic Psychological Distress

Patients may present with an extensive history of psychological distress, even though they do not show evidence of full-blown psychiatric disturbance. For some patients, the burden of living with a chronic disease eventually overpowers their coping capacities. Patients who show signs of chronic psychological distress should not be overlooked; referral for psychological assessment and subsequent intervention can lead to improved quality of life.

Acute Adjustment Reactions

Acute adjustment reactions sometimes occur in persons with rheumatic disease, just as they do in the physically healthy population. Acute marital conflicts or family disturbances may develop. Concerns regarding employment, finances, or social circumstances may arise. Although acute life stressors are unavoidable, they are often particularly severe in the context of a chronic disease. Careful psychological assessment can lead to effective interventions.

Psychoeducational Treatments

There are numerous reports regarding the effectiveness of psychoeducational interventions. For example, the Arthritis Self-Management Program has been shown to be beneficial for persons with arthritis (28), and rheumatology teams are increasingly using the services of psychologists, counselors, and educators. Psychological assessment can be helpful prior to implementing a psychoeducational intervention. For some arthritis patients, group treatments that enhance opportunities for socialization are indicated. For others, an individual treatment approach may be more viable. When there is uncertainty about the best psychoeducational strategy, psychological assessment should be considered.

CATEGORIES OF MENTAL HEALTH CONSULTANTS

Mental health consultants can be used from several disciplines, and there is considerable overlap in the range of services provided. A brief overview of mental health referral strategies follows.

Psychiatry

Referrals to psychiatrists are indicated when diagnosis of psychiatric conditions or medication management or consultation is needed. Psychiatrists are physicians, and many of them are well-trained to provide psychotherapeutic interventions.

Psychology

Referrals to psychologists are indicated for a full-range of mental health services, with the exception of medication management or other services that can be provided only by physicians or nurses. Psychologists are particularly well-trained in the areas of assessment and psychological interventions.

Social Work

Referrals to social workers are indicated for a wide-range of mental health services. Social workers typically are well trained in the provision of social and environmental support. Some social workers are also well prepared to provide supportive psychosocial interventions.

Nursing

Referrals to advanced-practice nurses with credentials in the mental health arena are indicated for a wide range of services, including medication management and psychotherapeutic care.

Counseling

Referrals to counselors are indicated for less severe forms of psychosocial distress, particularly for assistance managing adjustment reactions or situational life crises. Counselors are usually licensed, but credentials and training vary considerably across states. As a cautionary note, there is little restriction on the label "therapist" in many jurisdictions, so referrals in this category must be made carefully.

COLLABORATIVE CARE

There are 2 ways in which rheumatologists and mental health professionals can work together. First, psychologists and other mental health professionals can be treated as consultants; arthritis patients with concomitant psychological problems can simply be referred to mental health professionals working outside the arthritis team. The consultant model is easy to establish, but the mental health consultants may have little understanding of the unique needs of arthritis patients. In addition, some arthritis patients may not be comfortable receiving care in a mental health environment.

The second strategy for collaboration involves the direct participation of mental health professionals as members of the arthritis rehabilitation team. In this model, mental health professionals gain the opportunity to develop a deeper understanding of the needs of arthritis patients, and they can deliver their interventions within the overall context of the rheumatology setting.

REFERENCES

1. American Psychiatric Association. Diagnostic and statistical manual of mental disorders, 3rd ed, revised. Washington (DC): American Psychiatric Association; 1987.
2. Spitzer RL, Williams JBW, Kroenke K, Linzer M, deGruy FV, Hahn SR, et al. Utility of a new procedure for diagnosing mental disorders in primary care: The PRIME-MD 1000 study. JAMA 1994;272:1749–56.
3. Olfson M, Shea S, Feder A, Fuentes M, Nomura Y, Gameroff M, et al. Prevalence of anxiety, depression, and substance use disorders in an urban general medicine practice. Arch Fam Med 2000;9:876–83.
4. Jencks SF. Recognition of mental distress and diagnosis of mental disorders in primary care. JAMA 1985;253:1903–7.

5. Creed F, Ash G. Depression in rheumatoid arthritis: aetiology and treatment. Int Rev Psychiatry 1992;4:23–34.
6. Hay EM, Black D, Huddy A, Creed F, Tomenson B, Bernstein RM, et al. Psychiatric disorder and cognitive impairment in systemic lupus erythematosus. Arthritis Rheum 1992;35:411–6.
7. Wright GE, Parker JC, Schoenfeld-Smith K, Smarr KL, Buckelew SP, Slaughter JR, et al. Risk factors for depression in rheumatoid arthritis. Arthritis Care Res 1996;9:264–72.
8. Engel GL. The need for a new medical model: a challenge for biomedicine. Science 1977; 196:129–36.
9. Brandt EN Jr, Pope AM. Enabling America: assessing the role of rehabilitation science and engineering. Washington (DC): National Academy Press; 1997.
10. Dobson KS. A meta-analysis of the efficacy of cognitive therapy for depression. J Consult Clin Psychol 1989;57:414–9.
11. Gloaguen V, Cottraux J, Cucherat M, Blackburn IM. A meta-analysis of the effects of cognitive therapy in depressed patients. J Affect Disord 1998;49:59–72.
12. Felson DT, Anderson JJ, Meenan RF. The comparative efficacy and toxicity of second line drugs in rheumatoid arthritis. Arthritis Rheum 1990;33:1449–61.
13. Depression Guideline Panel. Depression in primary care: volume 2. Treatment of major depression. Clinical practice guideline, number 5. Rockville (MD): US Department of Health and Human Services; 1993.
14. Hawley DJ. Psycho-educational interventions in the treatment of arthritis. Baillière's Clin Rheumatol 1995;9:803–23.
15. Parker JC, Smarr KL, Buckelew SP, Stucky-Ropp RC, Hewett JE, Johnson JC, et al. Effects of stress-management on clinical outcomes in rheumatoid arthritis. Arthritis Rheum 1995;38:1807–18.
16. American Psychiatric Association. Diagnostic and statistical manual of mental disorders, 4th ed. Washington (DC): American Psychiatric Association; 1994.
17. Raskin NJ, Rogers CR. Person-centered therapy. In: Corsini RJ, Wedding DFE. Current psychotherapies. Itasca (IL): Peacock Publishers; 1989.
18. Anastasi A. Psychological Testing. New York: Macmillan Publishing Company, 1988.
19. Parker JC, Wright G. Psychologic assessment in rheumatology. Rheum Dis Clin North Am 1995;21:465–80.
20. Callahan LF, Brooks RH, Pincus T. Further analysis of learned helplessness in rheumatoid arthritis using a "Rheumatology Attitudes Index". J Rheumatol 1988;15:418–26.
21. Rodin G, Craven J, Littlefield C. Depression in the medically ill: an integrated approach. New York: Brunner/Mazel; 1991.
22. Hamilton M. Development of a rating scale for primary depressive illness. Br J Soc Clin Psychol 1967;6:278–96.
23. Bandura A. Self-efficacy: toward a unifying theory of behavioral change. Psychol Rev 1977;84:191–215.
24. Fetzer Institute. Multidimensional measurement of religiousness/spirituality for use in health research: a report of the Fetzer Institute/National Institute on Aging Working Group. Kalamazoo (MI): John E. Fetzer Institute; 1999.
25. Wallston BS, Alagna SW, DeVellis BM, DeVellis RF. Social support and physical health. Health Psychol 1983;2:367–91.
26. Spanier GB. Measuring dyadic adjustment: new scales for assessing the quality of marriage and similar dyads. J Marriage Family 1976;1:15–28.
27. Holland JL. Making vocational choices a theory of careers. New Jersey: Prentice-Hall; 1973.
28. Lorig K, Lubeck D, Kraines RG, Seleznick M, Holman HR. Outcomes of self-help education for patients with arthritis. Arthritis Rheum 1985;28:680–5.

Additional Recommended Reading

Blalock SJ, DeVellis RF, Brown GK, Wallston KA. Validity of the Center for Epidemiological Studies Depression Scale in arthritis populations. Arthritis Rheum 1989;32:991–7.

Parker JC, Bradley LA, DeVellis RM, Gerber LH, Holman HR, Keefe FJ, et al. Biopsychosocial contributions to the management of arthritis disability: blueprints from an NIDRR-sponsored conference. Arthritis Rheum 1993;36:885–9.

Pincus T, Callahan LF. Depression scales in rheumatoid arthritis: criterion contamination in interpretation of patient responses. Pat Educ Counsel 1993;20:133–43.

Pincus T, Callahan LF, Bradley LA, Vaughn WK, Wolfe F. Elevated MMPI scores for hypochondriasis, depression, and hysteria in patients with rheumatoid arthritis reflect disease rather than psychological status. Arthritis Rheum 1986;29:1456–66.

CHAPTER 12

Social and Cultural Assessment

LAURA ROBBINS, DSW, MSW

Clinicians today are challenged by the increasing number of patients from many cultures who speak different languages, have varying levels of acculturation, and come from varied socioeconomic backgrounds. These patients have unique ways of understanding illness and health, and they develop health care behaviors based on these beliefs. There has been a tendency to view patients of diverse cultures through the identification of specific, unifying characteristics that generalize cultural traits within groups (1). This unacceptable approach tends to stereotype patients. Instead, a patient-centered biopsychosocial approach that assesses culture as one aspect of the patient's experience is becoming more widely accepted (2–4, 5).

When living with a chronic illness, there are many emotional and physical challenges to everyday life activities and interpersonal relationships, often requiring a reevaluation of long-term goals. Moreover, rheumatic diseases are often unpredictable, resulting in the need for emotional and social support from family members, friends, and ultimately the health care team. Although social workers are trained to assess a patient's social and cultural background, it is not unusual for other health professionals to conduct similar assessments. Rheumatology health professionals should possess the basic knowledge, skill, and training to evaluate a patient's coping patterns and level of social adjustment, as well as how that patient's culture determines medical understanding of the disease and its etiology. Clinicians should also have the tools to assess how patients may decide to take action to address their disease.

This chapter addresses the components of a comprehensive social and cultural assessment. Understanding the patient in the appropriate social and cultural context can enable you to make referrals to appropriate education and support programs that have been demonstrated to influence health outcomes (6) and assist you in developing effective treatment plans.

ASSESSMENT METHOD

A comprehensive social and cultural assessment begins with evaluation of the patient's physical status, emotional state, and support systems. This approach focuses on the person, the situation, and the interaction between them (7). In the health care setting, the person is the patient, the situation may be medical crisis, and the interaction is the process that evolves between the patient and his or her support system in an attempt to cope with the medical condition. The emphasis is on the *process* by which people learn to function within their social network. The method also emphasizes communication skills and the patient's ability to articulate emotional, social, and physical needs to other people within their environment (8).

The patient is seen as an integral member of the medical team, bringing a unique history and understanding of the disease and participating actively in the treatment process. Effective emotional and social functioning is more likely to occur when patients become a part of the evaluation and contribute to developing the treatment plan. The goal of the assessment is to gain an understanding of the patient's emotional, social, and physical reactions to the medical situation to provide appropriate care. By working together, rheumatology health professionals and patients can assess the impact of the disease over time.

The first step is a comprehensive social and cultural assessment. This assessment may take from 1 to several sessions. Whenever possible, an evaluation that becomes part of the medical record should be written during each hospitalization and updated during routine office visits. Ongoing review is important because of disease flares.

THE SOCIAL ASSESSMENT

The Patient as Person

The goal of the social assessment is to evaluate the person's life history and the impact of the illness on current functioning. The patient is the best source of information, and scheduling an interview with the patient alone is optimal. If this is not possible, ask family members for some time alone during the interview with the patient. It is not unusual, for example, for an older person to have family members present who will answer questions addressed to the patient. When this occurs, patients should be encouraged to answer the questions themselves. Because disease is a family issue in some culturally diverse populations, it may be appropriate for the family to be present during the assessment. Assuring family members that their input is important can be useful and demonstrates that the family is vital to the patient as they learn to cope and adjust to the medical situation. It also allows assessment of the family's adjustment to the patient's illness.

Begin with the collection of demographic information (age, marital and parental status, education, sexual identity, work history, medical insurance, and religious affiliation). It is important to explore prior and current alcohol and drug use, as well as patient concerns related to housing arrangements, proximity to health care services, and available transportation. Ask questions that will elicit concrete responses (see Table 1). Responses can be used to evaluate the family constellation, support systems, belief systems, and the impact of arthritis on the patient's life.

Perhaps the most difficult part of the evaluation involves assessing physical and emotional changes the patient has experienced during interactions with people in their environment. Rapid, unplanned episodes of disease (such as flares, increased pain, or medication side effects) present unique challenges. Ask simple, direct questions that evaluate changes that have occurred with significant persons in the patient's immediate environment since the onset of symptoms (see Table 1). Similar questions should be asked about relationships in the patient's extended environment (work colleagues, school peers, religious congregations, and recreational contacts). Generally, these questions begin with "*What is different about …*" or "*How has your life changed since….*" Alterations in daily routines due to physical limitations can also shift social relationships and result in emotional distress. For example, the patient who has had to stop working due to rheumatoid arthritis may lose not only contact with colleagues but also the supportive listening of available friends.

Comparable questions about intimate personal relationships also need to be explored. Questions about role shifts in family responsibilities

Table 1. Social assessment sample questions

Social impact questions
Do you live close to the medical center?
Who lives in your household with you?
How do you get to and from the medical center?
Are you presently working?
What has changed about your current work schedule?
Do you go to school?
Who in your family is responsible for the cooking, shopping, child rearing, or the wellbeing of aging parents?

Emotional impact questions
How has the relationship with your children changed since you learned that you have arthritis?
How has your family reacted to the fact that you can no longer contribute to the household responsibilities?
How do your friends react to you since you told them about your arthritis?

Interpersonal impact questions
What did you and your partner enjoy that you can't enjoy now due to your arthritis?
What do you discuss with your husband about your osteoarthritis?
What are the kind of things that you and your husband routinely discuss?
How does your spouse feel about the changes in your relationship since you developed arthritis?
Have your sexual relationships changed since being diagnosed?

Nonverbal assessment questions
Does the patient ask questions during the interview?
Does the patient indicate that he or she is listening by a head nod as I am talking?
Does the patient appear distressed and perhaps too emotional to respond to questions?

---

between spouses and children are essential and should focus on the major daily responsibilities for the patient within the family system. Personal relationships and sexual relationships should also be explored (see Chapter 42), although it is important to be aware that not all cultures perceive sexual activity as something to be discussed outside of the relationship. It is always helpful to first develop trust before asking personal questions, and in some populations it may be essential. A direct approach to questions is most effective, particularly when the information required is personal and private. Knowledge about changes in sexual functioning will assist in making appropriate referral and in the treatment process.

Communication Skills

Good communication skills are fundamental in the patient—provider relationship. Learning how to enhance discussions and increase the exchange of information will facilitate the ability to ask questions that are personal and confidential. This includes not only spoken language but nonverbal interactions as well.

Specific tools can enhance communication between patients and providers. For example, through role modeling, you can demonstrate skills such as the ability to ask for help, how to verbalize questions and concerns, active listening, and asking for clarification and additional information. Questions that begin with "how," "what," and "why" are effective because they tend to elicit answers that require explanations, whereas questions that lead to "yes" and "no" answers tend to hinder information exchange. Direct questions might include "*What do you discuss with your husband about your osteoarthritis?*" or "*How does your spouse feel about the changes in your relationship since you developed arthritis?*"

Communication skills also can be evaluated through observation. You can observe whether someone is listening by asking yourself a series of questions (see Table 1). Awareness of how you, as the health professional, ask questions can greatly enhance the outcome of the assessment. Encourage patients to fully express their concerns about their medical

situation. Urge them to ask all their questions regardless of how relevant they seem.

The Social Environment

Patients with rheumatic diseases often experience changes in physical mobility, financial status, role function, and emotional health. The goal of social assessment is to evaluate the extent to which changes have occurred in relationships between the patient and the social factors that make up his or her social environment. These factors are inextricably linked to culture and affect the patient's self-worth and self-esteem (9).

When living with chronic illness, personal relationships also include doctors, nurses, hospital personnel, and health insurance companies. In some cultural groups, this can include whole communities. Through this expanding social network, the patient is confronted with many new and unique situations that can be perceived as opportunities as well as obstacles. The way in which people cope with chronic illness depends largely on previous experience. Availability of food, shelter, transportation, medical care, employment, education, and recreational activities are examples of some resources necessary for basic survival.

Patients also have psychosocial realities, such as role identity, self-esteem, and perceived self-worth, that are challenged when dealing with crisis (10). For example, when illness mandates that a woman change from a full-time professional, wife, and mother to full-time patient and part-time wife and mother, she may experience a direct assault on her identity and perceived self-worth. Family structure and family members' perceptions of the patient's roles also change. Psychosocial challenges are as important as the concrete realities of food and shelter, and can dramatically influence the patient's ability to cope effectively. Although the individual exercises some control by choosing friends for social support, most social relationships with parents, siblings, and extended family members are inherited. The quality of these relationships can have a potent effect and create pressures over which the individual has no control (11). With chronic illness, there is an increased need for intermittent dependency, which can make patients feel out of control and cause increased stress and anxiety.

THE CULTURAL ASSESSMENT

Health Beliefs and Behaviors

Culture has a significant impact on treatment outcomes. People acquire their own perceptions and beliefs about the origin of diseases and treatments that are learned in childhood, sanctioned within their culture, and expressed through behaviors. Through shared cultural beliefs we come to value what is worthwhile, desirable, and important for our wellbeing. However, our cultural identity may differ from those of people we encounter in our daily contacts. There is a tendency to view our own cultural orientation as the standard against which other cultures are judged (12). Therefore, assessment requires a culturally enlightened and sensitive approach.

Culture is a filter through which we interpret experiences. A patient has certain beliefs, concerns, and perceptions about the medical diagnosis as well as the encounter with the health professional (13). In Western societies, illness explanations are typically rooted in natural phenomena, such as infection with microorganisms, mechanical dysfunction, or more recently stress. However, many cultures attribute disease and illness to very different causes, such as folklore and pragmatic experiences that are passed on from one generation to the next (14). How a person defines and copes with chronic disease and the health care experience can greatly modify the treatment plan and delivery of services.

Table 2. Cultural self-assessment sample questions

Health professional self-assessment
- What is my cultural heritage?
- What was the culture of my parents and my grandparents?
- With what cultural group do I identify?
- What values, beliefs, opinions, and attitudes do I hold that are consistent with the dominant culture? Which are inconsistent? How did I learn these?
- What unique abilities, aspirations, expectations and limitations do I have that might influence my relations with culturally diverse individuals?
- How do I communicate with my patients?
- Do I change my communication styles to enhance discussion with my patients who come from different cultures than I do?

It is important to recognize how your own health beliefs and practices differ from those of other populations. Currently, most health professionals do not have specific training in cultural sensitivity. Although you may strive to be open minded about different cultural groups, even the most well-intentioned professionals bring ethnocentric biases to the assessment of a person with different cultural attitudes and beliefs. In the Anglo-American culture, values of mastery over nature, individualism, competition, and directness vary significantly from values of harmony with nature, group welfare, cooperation, and indirectness characteristic of some ethnocultural groups (15). Recognizing and understanding the differences in these values will lead to understanding of culture-specific behaviors that influence health behaviors.

Awareness of self is the first step to understanding others (16). A cultural assessment should begin with self-assessment. Recognizing one's own cultural identity and how it influences personal values, beliefs, and behaviors is a precursor to understanding and being able to assess a patient's cultural orientation. Self-assessment questions, such as those in Table 2, can help you recognize your own cultural identity and orientation and offer a general understanding of the influence of culture-specific beliefs and attitudes on health behaviors.

The cultural assessment must emphasize the patient's global beliefs, practices, and behaviors as well as health-specific ones. However, the goal is not only to understand beliefs, attitudes, and subsequent behaviors, but to identify how they are important to self-concept. Self-concept develops through socialization within the family unit, social networks, and community groups. We develop a perception of ourselves through interactions within our cultural group. Self-concept is formed by several factors, including language, sex, and behaviors. Questions about health care attitudes and beliefs can reveal information about health behaviors practiced by the patient (see Table 3). These questions can also provide insight into how patients within a cultural group define and treat diseases, as well as the patient's perception of how they cope and function.

For example, when assessing a Latina woman newly diagnosed with RA, it would not be unusual for the patient to consult with family members about what and how much to discuss with the physician. Latinos frequently consult with other family members before following a recommended medical treatment (17). When working with Latinos, cultural practices have to be recognized and respected to develop patient–provider trust. In addition, a Latina woman may not follow the prescribed treatment plan without consulting first her husband or family. Although she has her own concept of self-identity, it is determined in relation to family roles. In general, there are many cultures in which it is expected that the husband (or dominant male figure) be consulted about important decisions, particularly if decisions will affect the family unit (18).

The Importance of Language

Language shapes our world, defines our roles within society, and is the way in which we express our self-concept and identity (19, 20). It can be challenging to understanding the impact of chronic illness when language differences hinder communication.

Ask patients what language they primarily speak, read, write, and think in when at home or with friends and family. In the health care setting, patients who speak different languages often attempt to understand physician questions because their culture values respect for authority figures. Their marginal understanding of English can be conveyed by a nod of the head or by "yes" or "no" responses to questions, even though the patient usually does not fully understand the question. Whenever language may be a barrier, refrain from using questions that result in yes/no answers, and always ask the patient to repeat the information as an indicator of comprehension.

If there is any indication that the patient may not comprehend your questions, you should use a trained translator. However, there are important concerns and considerations about this approach. First, it is inappropriate to use family members to translate during an assessment. Commonly family members (especially young children) or close friends serve as translators during interviews. This can result in breach of patient confidentiality, inaccurate translation of questions and responses, and can cause emotional distress for family members who themselves are coping with the patient's medical condition (21). When family members are not present, staff may be asked to translate if they speak the same language. This practice is also inappropriate for many of the reasons outlined above. In addition, staff will often paraphrase the questions and provide their own interpretation of the patient's medical situation in an earnest attempt to assist the patient. Important information can be misinterpreted and stripped of its significance, contributing to poor treatment outcomes.

However, translators (especially those who are bilingual and bicultural) can be effective if utilized appropriately (17). Community agencies can provide professionally trained translators, and a growing number train translators to be available via phone. Another effective model is the use of bilingual, bicultural patient advocates who are trained as translators for other patients from the same cultural group. Although this model may appear to be labor intensive, the training and supervision of a cadre of patients is worth the initial investment to ensure the wellbeing of new patients. This also allows for assessment of the patient's level of language and communication skills, as well as a determination of cultural health beliefs and practices.

Specific cultures also have clearly defined health beliefs and practices that differ from those of Western medicine. It is unrealistic to

Table 3. Patient assessment*

Cultural identity
To what ethnic group do you belong?
What language do you speak most often with your family? With your friends?
What religious group do you belong to? Do you attend services regularly? In what ways do you practice your religion?

Health beliefs
How would you describe your arthritis symptoms?
What does having arthritis mean to you?
How do you believe that your arthritis can be treated?
What do you believe caused your arthritis?

Health behaviors
Who in the family makes the major decisions?
Who do you go to in your community for advice about medical problems or treatment?
When do you go for advice or treatment?
Do you go to a healer or any other person for advice about your health (Chinese herbalist, spiritualist, minister)? What advice do you follow?
What foods do you eat that you believe makes your arthritis better?
What foods do you eat that you believe makes your arthritis worse?
What other things do you do to deal with your arthritis?

* Adapted from reference 12.

expect health professionals be knowledgeable about the plethora of cultures they may encounter. Cultural sensitivity is a place to start. To ensure ongoing cultural understanding, it may be necessary to engage a community leader as a key informant about the patient's culture to assist you in obtaining information (22). Community leaders often are identified within cultural groups as the informant for group-specific norms, beliefs, and attitudes. There are large community health agencies serving Asian, Latino, African American, and Native American groups. Enlisting a cultural informant greatly enhances communication and can help break down barriers that lead to the mistrust, fear, and intimidation that some cultural groups feel toward Anglo-American institutions (23). A cultural informant does not replace the patient; rather, the informant collaboratively serves as a verbal translator and advocate for the patient. The patient's consent and permission must always be obtained prior to engaging a third party in the assessment process.

Acculturation

Culturally determined health beliefs and practices may vary within cultural groups due to the length of time the patient has lived in the United States. Acculturation occurs as people learn new behaviors when they are exposed to new cultures. If a patient from Russia has lived in the US for 15 years, the patient may be relatively familiar with Anglo-American health beliefs and behaviors. It should be standard practice during an assessment to ask a brief question such as *"How long have you lived in …."* The patient's response can then guide you when conducting the full cultural assessment.

THERAPEUTIC INTERVENTIONS

Once a social and cultural assessment is completed, it may be necessary to refer the patient for psychosocial treatment. Many therapeutic interventions are available; however, the type of referral depends upon the assessment. Licensed social workers use counseling to assist the patient in making emotional adjustments to chronic illness. Social workers can help the patient with concrete needs, such as financial evaluations and referrals for assistance. They also assist with problems relating to housing, medical insurance, disability, and transportation. Additionally, if it is determined that the patient is experiencing significant psychological difficulties (e.g., depression, anxiety disorder, personality problems), referral to a psychologist or psychiatrist may be appropriate.

When there are difficulties among family members, family therapy may be needed. Referrals should be made to family social workers or licensed marital and family counselors who can work effectively with the entire family. Consulting with a key informant, such as a clergy member, can be beneficial with some cultural groups to determine an appropriate referral.

For many who are experiencing mild difficulty with the common adjustments of living with a chronic illness (mild depression, anger, or sadness) self-management or support groups can be extremely beneficial. The Arthritis Foundation (www.arthritis.org) provides a list of such programs offered through its local chapters. Over time, participants in self-management programs report a decrease in depression, an increase in self-confidence, and an increase in self-management skills (24). Programs like these are excellent vehicles for empowering patients by providing educational information and social support.

Finally, traditional therapeutic interventions may not be relevant to some cultural groups. For many people, support and empathy originate from systems within the cultural group. For African Americans, religious affiliations often provide spiritual support and are a source of comfort during medical crises. In some Latino cultures, herbs and botanicals are obtained from within the community and are used to take control of the medical illness. And in some Asian cultures patients in emotional distress will keep their concerns within the family rather than seek outside assistance. When working with culturally diverse patients, the goal is to understand the client's emotional and social supports.

A social and cultural assessment is a key component of comprehensive evaluation of patients with rheumatic diseases. Sociocultural assessments are important contributors to the overall medical diagnosis, management, and treatment of the person who is challenged by a chronic disease.

REFERENCES

1. Carrillo JE, Green A, Betancourt J. Cross-cultural primary care: a patient-based approach. Ann Intern Med 1999;130:829–34.
2. Berlin EA, Fowkes WC Jr. A teaching framework for cross-cultural health-care: application in family practice. West J Med 1983;139:934–8.
3. Scott CJ. Enhancing patient outcomes through an understanding of inter-cultural medicine: guidelines for the practitioner. Md Med J 1997;46: 175–80.
4. Goldstein E, Bobo L, Womeodu R, Kaufman L, Nathan M, Palmer D, et al. Intercultural medicine. In: Jensen NM, van Kirk JA, editors. A curriculum for internal medicine residency: the University of Wisconsin program. Philadelphia: American College of Physicians; 1996.
5. Betancourt J, Green A, Carrillo JE. Cultural competencies in health care: emerging frameworks and practical approaches. The Commonwealth Fund, Field Report, October, 2002. Accessed June 16, 2006. URL: http://www.cmwf.org/publications/publications_show.htm?doc_id=221320.
6. Robbins L. Patient education. In: Paget SA, Beary JF III, Gibofsky A, editors. Hospital for Special Surgery manual of rheumatology and outpatient orthopedic disorders: diagnosis and therapy. 5th ed. Philadelphia: Lippincott Williams & Wilkins; 2005.
7. Hollis F. Casework: a psychosocial therapy. 2nd ed. New York: Random House; 1972.
8. Turner F, editor. Social work treatment: interlocking theoretical approaches. New York: Free Press; 1979.
9. Helman CG. Culture, health and illness: an introduction for health professionals. 3rd ed. Boston: Butterworth-Heinemann, 1994.
10. Perlman H. Social casework: a problem solving process. Chicago: University of Chicago Press; 1957.
11. Billingsley A. Black families in white America. Englewood Cliffs (NJ): Prentice-Hall; 1968.
12. Locke D. Increasing multicultural understanding: a comprehensive model. Newbury Park (CA): Sage; 1992.
13. Eisenberg L. Disease and illness: distinctions between professional and popular ideas of sickness. Cult Med Psychiatry 1977;1:9–23.
14. Allegrante JP, Sleet D, editors. Derryberry's educating for health: a foundation for contemporary health education practice. San Francisco: Jossey-Bass; 2004.
15. Sigelman L, Welch S. Black Americans' views of racial inequity: the dream deferred. New York: Cambridge University Press; 1991.
16. Lum CK, Koreman SG. Cultural-sensitivity training in U. S. medical schools. Acad Med 1994;69:239–41.
17. A primer for cultural proficiency: towards quality health services for Hispanics. Washington (DC): The National Alliance for Hispanic Health, Estrella Press; 2001.
18. Locke DC. Cross-cultural counseling issues. In: Pakmo AJ, Weikel WJ, editors. Foundations of mental health counseling. Springfield (IL): Charles C Thomas; 1986. p. 23–30.
19. Sotomayor M. Language, culture and ethnicity in developing self-concept. Soc Casework 1977;41:195–203.
20. Quillte J. Barriers to effective communication. In: Lipkin M Jr, Putnam SM, Lazare A, editors. The medical interview: clinical care, education and research. New York: Springer-Verlag; 1995. p. 110–21.
21. Putsch RW. Cross-cultural communication: the special case of interpreters in health care. JAMA 1985;254:3344–8.
22. Breckon D, Harvey J, Lancaster R. Community health education: settings, roles, and skills for the 21st century. Gaithersburg (MD): Aspen; 1994.
23. Robbins L, Allegrante JP, Paget S. Adapting the Systemic Lupus Erythematosus Self-Help (SLESH) course for Latino SLE patients. Arthritis Care Res 1993;6:97–103.

24. Robbins L. Patient education. In: Klippel J, Weyland C, Wortman R, editors. Primer on the rheumatic diseases. 12th ed. Atlanta: Arthritis Foundation; 2001.

Additional Recommended Reading

Braithwaite R, Taylor S, editors. Health issues in the black community. San Francisco: Jossey-Bass; 1992.

Journal of Multicultural Social Work. New York: The Haworth Press.

Carlson V. Social work and general systems theory. Berkeley: University of California, School of Social Welfare; 1957.

Molina C, Molina-Aguirre M, editors. Latino health in the US: a growing challenge. Washington (DC): American Public Health Association; 1994.

National Alliance for Hispanic Health. A primer for cultural proficiency: towards quality health services for Hispanics. Washington (DC): Estrella Press; 2001.

Ponterotto J, Casas J, Suzuki L, Alexander C, editors. Handbook of multicultural counseling. Thousand Oaks (CA): Sage; 1995.

Rogler L. Implementing cultural sensitivity in mental health research: convergence and new directions (3-part series). Psychline Inter-Transdisciplinary Journal of Mental Health 1999;3(1–3).

International Classification of Functioning, Disability and Health (ICF): A Basis for Multidisciplinary Clinical Practice

ALARCOS CIEZA, PhD, MPH, and GEROLD STUCKI, MD, MS

A patient's diagnosis alone provides limited information. It tells little about what patients can do, what their prognosis is, what they need, etc. Because functioning is a central dimension in working with patients with rheumatic diseases, concepts, classifications, and measurements of functioning and health are important to clinical practice, research, and teaching in this field (1). The approval of the International Classification of Functioning, Disability and Health (ICF) by the World Health Assembly in May 2001 can be considered a landmark event in establishing a new era of patient-oriented clinical practice, research, and teaching (2,3).

The ICF offers information about how people live with their health conditions. It is based on an integrative biopsychosocial model of functioning, disability, and health developed by the World Health Organization (WHO) (2). Rehabilitative medicine also places an emphasis on functioning and disability. It targets functioning, the environment, and modifiable personal factors because functioning is seen as being in close interaction with the environment and the person's characteristics (4). Moreover, functioning represents not only an outcome, but also the starting point of the clinical assessment, development of a treatment plan, and evaluation and quality assessment of the plan.

The ICF has the potential to enhance the care of patients by providing a universal language of functioning and disability. It provides a framework to guide treatment and coordinate care among the health care team. The ICF can be applied regardless of the culture or health condition, and is applicable to all health professionals. Use of the ICF in clinical settings has the potential to significantly increase the quality of care by providing a common language and understanding of functioning and disability. Although there has been a general description of the principals and benefits of applying the ICF to facilitate interdisciplinary communication, little has been written about how to integrate the ICF into clinical practice. The objective of this chapter is to describe in practical terms how the ICF can be applied in clinical practice in the context of a multidisciplinary rheumatology team. The example of a patient with rheumatoid arthritis (RA) is used as an illustration. First, we begin with a review of ICF terms.

ICF TERMINOLOGY

In the ICF model, disability and functioning are viewed as outcomes of interactions between *health conditions* (diseases, disorders, and injuries) and *contextual factors* (2) (see Figure 1).

Health condition describes the disease, disorder, injury, or trauma. The health condition may also include other factors (e.g., aging, stress, congenital anomaly, or genetic predisposition) or information about pathogeneses or etiology. Potential interactions may occur between the health condition and all components of functioning (body functions and structures, activity, and participation).

Body functions are defined as the physiologic functions of body systems (including psychological functioning). *Body structures* are the anatomic parts of the body (e.g., organs, limbs, and their components). Abnormalities of function or structure are referred to as impairments, which are defined as a significant deviation or loss (e.g., deformity) of structures (e.g., joints) and/or function (e.g., reduced range of motion, muscle weakness, pain, and fatigue).

Activity is the execution of a task or action by an individual and represents the individual perspective of functioning. Difficulties are referred to as *activity limitations* (e.g., limitations in mobility, such as walking, climbing steps, grasping, or carrying).

Participation refers to the involvement in life situations and reflects the societal perspective. Participation restrictions are problems the patient experiences in these areas (e.g., limitations in community life, recreation, and leisure). Note that limitations in walking may also be considered as a *participation restriction* if problems with walking limits participation in desired activities.

Contextual factors represent the entire background of an individual's life and living situation. Within the contextual factors, *environmental factors* make up the physical, social, and attitudinal environment in which people live and conduct their lives. These factors are external to individuals and can have a positive or negative influence, i.e., they can represent a facilitator or a barrier for the individual. *Personal factors* are the particular background of an individual's life and living situation and include features that are not part of a health condition (e.g., sex, age, race, fitness, lifestyle, habits, and social background). They can be referred to as those factors that define the person as a unique individual. Personal factors cannot be impaired, limited, or restricted. They can, however, have a positive or negative impact on disability and functioning.

THE ICF CLASSIFICATION SYSTEM

The biopsychosocial view guided the development of the ICF. Therefore, the components of the model correspond to the components of the classification. Each component contains an exhaustive list of ICF

Functioning and Disability

Functioning denotes the positive aspects and **disability**, the negative aspects of the interaction between an individual with a health condition and his or her contextual factors (environmental and personal factors). **Disability** is an umbrella term for impairments, limitations in activities, and restrictions in participation. This distinction can help when reading the medical literature. Disability is usually the preferred term. However, from the biopsychosocial perspective presented here, functioning is implicitly addressed when disability is studied, and vice versa (15).

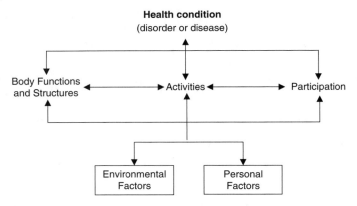

Health condition
(disorder or disease)

Body Functions and Structures ↔ Activities ↔ Participation

Environmental Factors   Personal Factors

Figure 1. A model of disability that is the basis for the International Classification of Functioning, Disability and Health. Reprinted from reference 2.

categories, which are the units of the classification. The ICF categories are hierarchically organized and are denoted by unique alphanumeric codes (see Figure 2). The categories are arranged in a stem/branch/leaf scheme within each component.

Each component consists of chapters (first level). Each chapter consists of second-level categories that, in turn, are composed of categories at the third level, which include fourth-level categories. The structure of the ICF is similar to that of a textbook in which the information is organized in chapters with subheadings that help the reader locate the information sought. An example from the component *body functions* is presented below:

b2	Sensory functions and pain	(first/chapter level)
b280	Sensation of pain	(second level)
b2801	Pain in body part	(third level)
b28013	Pain in back	(fourth level)

Qualifiers are used to denote the level of functioning and health or the severity of the problem. The WHO proposes that all categories in the classification be quantified using the same generic scale.

0 – NO problem (none, absent, negligible, ...)	0–4%
1 – MILD problem (slight, low, ...)	5–24%
2 – MODERATE problem (medium, fair, ...)	25–49%
3 – SEVERE problem (high, extreme, ...)	50–95%
4 – COMPLETE problem (total, ...)	96–100%
8 – not specified	
9 – not applicable	

Additional qualifiers specific to the different components are also used (see Table 1). For example, the second and third qualifiers of the component *body structures* are used to indicate the nature of a determined change and its location, respectively.

The ICF contains more than 1,400 categories, making it a highly comprehensive classification system. (A checklist of major categories of the ICF is available at http://www3.who.int/icf/checklist/icf-checklist.pdf.) This comprehensiveness is a major advantage and strength of the ICF. It is, however, also the major challenge to its practicality and use in clinical practice.

ICF CORE SETS

To enhance the applicability and usefulness of the ICF to clinicians and researchers working with people with specific disorders, *ICF Core Sets* were developed. ICF Core Sets were identified to select a subset of categories that can serve as minimal standards for the assessment and documentation of functioning and health in clinical studies, clinical encounters, and multiprofessional comprehensive assessment.

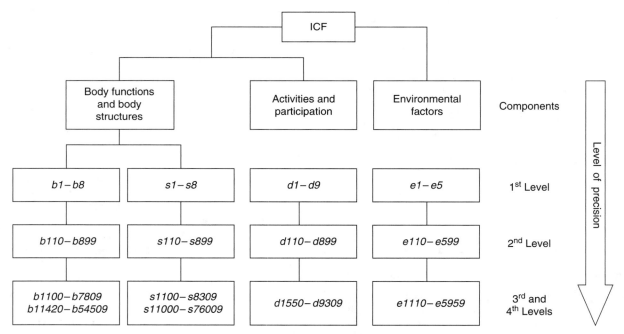

Figure 2. The different levels of the ICF. The ICF uses an alphanumeric system in which letters *b, s, d,* and *e* are used to denote *body functions, body structures, activities and participation*, and *environmental factors*, respectively. These letters are followed by a numeric code that starts with a chapter number (1 digit), followed by a second level (2 digits), and third and forth levels (1 digit for each). Source: International Classification of Functioning, Disability and Health (ICF). Genevar: World Health Organization, 2001.

Table 1. The ICF qualifiers used to quantify the level of functioning or the severity of the problem*

Components	First qualifier	Second qualifier
Body functions (b)	Generic qualifier with the negative scale used to indicate the extent or magnitude of an impairment	None
	Example: b167.3 to indicate a severe impairment in specific mental functions of language	
Body structures (s)	Generic qualifier with the negative scale used to indicate the extent or magnitude of an impairment	Used to indicate the nature of the change in the respective body structure:
	Example: s730.3 to indicate a severe impairment of the upper extremity	0 No change in structure 1 Total absence 2 Partial absence 3 Additional part 4 Aberrant dimensions 5 Discontinuity 6 Deviating position 7 Qualitative changes in structure, including accumulation of fluid 8 Not specified 9 Not applicable
		Example: s730.32 to indicate the partial absence of the upper extremity
Activities and participation (d)	Performance	Capacity
	Generic qualifier	Generic qualifier
	Problem in the person's current environment	Limitation without assistance
	Example: d5101.1 − to indicate mild difficulty with bathing the whole body with the use of assistive devices that are available to the person in his or her current environment	Example: d5101.−2 to indicate moderate difficulty with bathing the whole body; implies that there is moderate difficulty without the use of assistive devices or personal help
Environmental factors (e)	Generic qualifier, with negative and positive scale, to denote extent of barriers and facilitators, respectively	None
	Example: e130.2 to indicate that products for education are a moderate barrier. Conversely, e130+2 would indicate that products for education are a moderate facilitator	

*ICF = International Classification of Functioning, Disability and Health. Reprinted from reference 2.

The conceptual approach of the ICF Core Sets derives from 2 different perspectives: that of people experiencing an acute episode and that of people suffering from a chronic condition. The *acute* and *post-acute ICF Core Sets* apply to people experiencing an acute episode in the hospital setting and post-acute rehabilitation. From this perspective, the organ-system approach, rather than the condition-specific approach, reflects the reality of health care in most countries and seemed most practical (5–7).

ICF Core Sets for chronic conditions can be applied in any health care setting (8,9). Currently, ICF Core Sets are available for 12 chronic conditions. The Core Sets for rehabilitation research and practice were developed in collaboration with the ICF Research Branch of WHO ICF and the Department of Physical Medicine and Rehabilitation of the Ludwig-Maximilian University in Munich (http:\\www.icf-research-branch.org).

For each chronic health condition, both a *comprehensive* and a *brief ICF Core Set* have been established. The comprehensive ICF Core Set is a list that describes the typical spectrum of problems in functioning of patients with a specific condition and can be used to guide multidisciplinary assessments. The b*rief ICF Core Set* can be utilized in clinical or epidemiologic studies and is meant to serve as a *minimum data set to be documented in every clinical study* to comparably describe the burden of disease across studies. The brief ICF Core Sets include as few categories as possible to be practical, but as many as necessary to sufficiently describe the typical spectrum of problems in functioning of patients with a specific condition.

Examples of the comprehensive ICF Core Sets for rheumatoid arthritis are presented in Tables 2–4. Elements of the brief ICF Core Set are indicated in bold text.

USING THE ICF IN CLINICAL PRACTICE

ICF Core Sets can be useful for treatment planning and evaluation. Optimal treatment of rheumatic diseases often requires longitudinal, coordinated multidisciplinary care potentially involving specialists from such areas as physical medicine, rheumatology, orthopedics, nursing, physical therapy, occupational therapy, social work, podiatry, vocational counselling, and clinical psychology. The ICF Core Sets allow the rheumatology health care team to describe the impairments, limitations in activities, restrictions in participation, and the contextual factors of patient with rheumatic diseases. This result is the development of functional profile of each patient. This baseline profile can, in turn, serve as reference for followup assessments.

Table 2. Body functions/Body structures categories from the comprehensive International Classification of Functioning, Disability and Health (ICF) Core Set for rheumatoid arthritis*

ICF code	ICF category title
Body functions	
b130	Energy and drive functions
b134	**Sleep functions**
b152	Emotional functions
b180	Experience of self and time functions
b1801	Body image
b280	**Sensation of pain**
b2800	Generalized pain
b2801	Pain in body part
b28010	Pain in head and neck
b28013	Pain in back
b28014	Pain in upper limb
b28015	Pain in lower limb
b28016	Pain in joints
b430	Hematological system functions
b455	**Exercise tolerance functions**
b510	Ingestion functions
b640	Sexual functions
b710	**Mobility of joint functions**
b7102	Mobility of joints generalized
b715	Stability of joint functions
b730	**Muscle power functions**
b740	**Muscle endurance functions**
b770	**Gait pattern functions**
b780	**Sensations related to muscles and movement functions**
b7800	Sensation of muscle stiffness
Body structures	
s299	Eye, ear and related structures, unspecified
s710	**Structure of head and neck region**
s720	**Structure of shoulder region**
s730	**Structure of upper extremity**
s73001	Elbow joint
s73011	Wrist joint
s7302	Structure of hand
s73021	Joints of hand and fingers
s73022	Muscles of hand
s750	**Structure of lower extremity**
s75001	Hip joint
s75011	Knee joint
s7502	Structure of ankle and foot
s760	Structure of trunk
s7600	Structure of vertebral column
s76000	Cervical vertebral column
s770	Additional musculoskeletal structures related to movement
s810	Structure of areas of skin

*Categories included in the brief ICF Core Set are indicated in bold text.

We present an example of the use of the ICF for a hypothetical patient with rheumatoid arthritis (Mrs. Baker). Clinical characteristics of this RA patient are presented in Figure 3.

ICF AND THE REHAB CYCLE

The rehabilitation cycle (rehab cycle) is a structured approach to rehabilitation management with 4 key elements: assessment of the problems, assignment of intervention targets to health professionals and to intervention principles, implementation of the intervention plan using specific intervention techniques, and finally, the evaluation of goal achievement (see Figure 4)(10). (Note: Principles of the rehab cycle are applicable to both ambulatory and in-patient settings.)

Assessment of Problems

The assessment phase consists of the following 3 steps:
1. Identifying the problems and needs of the patient;
2. Determining the long-term, intervention-program, and cycle goals; and
3. Identifying intervention targets related to the cycle goals.

Step 1: Identifying the problems and needs of the patient. Initially, all members of the patient's health care team work together to comprehensively assess the patient's problems. On the ICF sheet (Figure 5), the patient-perspective section (upper part) provides a practical way to document the patient's problems entirely from his or her perspective using the patients' own words. From the patient history and information provided by proxies, personal factors and contextual factors relevant to the current problems can also be recorded with a + or a − sign, indicating whether they represent a barrier or a facilitator.

The health professional section (lower part) of the ICF sheet documents the findings from the medical history, the clinical examination, technical investigations (e.g., laboratory, imaging, and electrophysiologic examinations), and the ICD diagnosis.

The information collected from the medical history, the clinical examination, and technical investigations can be documented nonsystematically or systematically with the appropriate ICF Core Set. A systematic approach (alone or in combination with a nonsystematic approach) assures that all potentially relevant problems identified in the ICF Core Set development have been considered.

Responsibility for certain aspects of the assessment can be assigned to specific team members with the requisite expertise. Structured interviews or standardized tests (ranging from a simple observation to complex test batteries) can be used to collect data. For example, it may be decided that the physiotherapist will measure muscle strength and sensory-motor testing will be evaluated by the physician. Assignment of responsibilities optimizes efficiency and minimizes burden on the patient by avoiding duplication of effort.

Some aspects of completing the ICF sheet may require additional annotation in clinical practice. First, there is a single list of domains in the classification for both the *activities and participation* components. Therefore, the same ICF category can be seen either as an *activity* or *participation*, and the same ICF category can be noted under *activity* if it refers to a limitation in task and under *participation* if it refers to a restriction in life involvement. To complicate matters further, the same ICF category can also be rated as *performance* or as *capacity*. Performance describes what an individual does in his or her current environment. Because the current environment brings in a societal context, performance can be understood as "involvement in a life situation" or "the lived experience" of people in the actual context in which they live. Capacity describes an individual's ability to execute a task or an action. It indicates the highest probable level of functioning, i.e., the full ability of the individual. The assessment of *capacity*, therefore, requires observing a patient executing a specific task using standardized equipment or in a standardized environment. Typical examples are the six-minute walk test (11) and the Sequential Occupational Dexterity Assessment (SODA) (12). Other test situations may be constructed in a structured interview, like asking the patient about his capacity in a defined environment. Note that most self-administered patient questionnaires are typically pure performance measures. They ask what a person does in her or his environment and not what a person could do in a standardized or facilitating environment. An example of this would be the item "climbing one flight of stairs" in the Short-Form 36 (13).

Because the upper part of ICF sheet reflects the patients' perspective, it refers to *performance*. The lower part, containing the health

Table 3. Activities and participation categories from the comprehensive International Classification of Functioning, Disability and Health (ICF) Core Set for rheumatoid arthritis*

ICF code	ICF category title
d170	Writing
d230	**Carrying out daily routine**
d360	Using communication devices and techniques
d410	**Changing basic body position**
d415	Maintaining a body position
d430	**Lifting and carrying objects**
d440	**Fine hand use**
d445	**Hand and arm use**
d449	Carrying, moving, and handling objects, other specified and unspecified
d450	**Walking**
d455	Moving around
d460	Moving around in different locations
d465	Moving around using equipment
d470	**Using transportation**
d475	Driving
d510	**Washing oneself**
d520	Caring for body parts
d530	Toileting
d540	**Dressing**
d550	**Eating**
d560	Drinking
d570	Looking after one's health
d620	Acquisition of goods and services
d630	Preparing meals
d640	Doing housework
d660	Assisting others
d760	Family relationships
d770	**Intimate relationships**
d850	**Remunerative employment**
d859	**Work and employment, other specified and unspecified**
d910	Community life
d920	**Recreation and leisure**

*Categories included in the brief ICF Core Set are indicated in bold text.

Table 4. Environmental factors from the comprehensive International Classification of Functioning, Disability and Health (ICF) Core Set for rheumatoid arthritis*

ICF code	ICF category title
e110	Products or substances for personal consumption
e115	**Products and technology for personal use in daily living**
e120	Products and technology for personal indoor and outdoor mobility and transportation
e125	Products and technology for communication
e135	Products and technology for employment
e150	Design, construction and building products and technology of buildings for public use
e155	Design, construction and building products and technology of buildings for private use
e225	Climate
e310	**Immediate family**
e320	Friends
e340	Personal care providers and personal assistants
e355	**Health professionals**
e360	Other professionals
e410	Individual attitudes of immediate family members
e420	Individual attitudes of friends
e425	Individual attitudes of acquaintances, peers, colleagues, neighbours and community members
e450	Individual attitudes of health professionals
e460	Societal attitudes
e540	Transportation services, systems and policies
e570	**Social security services, systems and policies**
e580	**Health services, systems and policies**

*Categories included in the brief ICF Core Set are indicated in bold text.

professional perspective, refers to *capacity*. *Participation* issues are generally rated with respect to performance and are listed in the upper part of the ICF sheet, which also documents activities the patient experiences as a limitation. Hence, the upper section of a typical ICF sheet often contains many ICF categories belonging to the *participation* component and few belonging to the *activity* component. Most of the ICF categories of the *activities* component are listed in the lower section.

With respect to body functions and structures, it is important to emphasize that only problems perceived by the patient should be recorded in the upper section. These include symptoms such as pain, stiffness, perceived weakness, muscle tone, depression, or emotional problems. All potentially relevant impairments in functions and structures are examined and recorded by the professional team. Therefore, the ICF sheet typically contains many items referring to the *body function* and *structure* component in the lower section, and only a few items in the upper section.

Using the example of Mrs. Baker, one would systematically go through all the ICF categories of the comprehensive ICF Core Set for RA after having collected the information from her medical history, the clinical examination, and technical investigations (see Figure 5). The ICF categories that are impaired, limited or restricted and the relevant environmental factors would then be marked. The ICF categories that are relevant to Mrs. Baker's current situation are then transferred to the health professional part of the ICF sheet. Published methods for linkage (14) can be used to guide which pieces of information from the medical history, clinical examination, and technical investigations correspond to the various ICF categories.

Step 2: Determining the long-term, intervention-program, and cycle goals. The next step in the assessment phase is to define the long-term, intervention-program, and cycle goals. This step should involve the entire team when possible. The physician's responsibility is not only to coordinate the team in defining the goals, but also to attend to the patients' medical and physical safety needs, including an assessment of the amount of stress the patient can comfortably tolerate.

Although long-term and intervention-program goals are typically defined on the level of *participation*, cycle goals are typically selected from the *activity* component. Cycle goals reflect the next goal to be achieved within the following days or weeks. Because patient resources are limited, it is best to limit this to no more than 2 or 3 goals at the same time.

Patients and their families can be very helpful when formulating long-term and program goals. These goals are generally expressed as *can do* or *can not do*. Typical long-term and program goals include "can live independently at home," "can go out independently for shopping," "can move safely inside the house," "can safely perform transfer and get dressed," and "can resume working," etc.

The cycle goals are typically marked in the patient perspective part of the ICF sheet, reflecting the importance of the patient's perspective in the process.

In the example of Mrs. Baker, the long-term goal is to foster her independence in self-care and housework. Although she had to give up her job at this time, she does not want to remain unemployed the rest of her life. Hence, the long-term goal is vocational retraining. The initial cycle goals set by the team at the beginning of therapy may be reduction of the pain in her hands and fingers and difficulties in self-care.

Step 3: Identification of potential intervention targets related to cycle goals. Once cycle goals have been established, intervention targets can be identified. Intervention targets should be directly related to cycle goals and must be potentially modifiable. Familiarity with the literature about the factors influencing a certain cycle goal (e.g., pain) is important. The team may review the literature for the most relevant

Personal Information:
Born: 01.02.62, Munich, Germany
Years of formal education (school + professional): 15 years
Diagnosis of rheumatoid arthritis: 10 years ago in August.
10 months ago: Hospitalization due to rheumatoid arthritis.

X-ray of both hands:
Subluxation of metacarpophalangeal joints 2 and 3 right, beginning ulnar
drift right; degenerative changes in proximal and distal interphalangeal joints right hand,
2nd and 3rd fingers

s73011 Wrist joint
s73021 Joints of hand and fingers

Laboratory parameters:
• Rheumatoid factor seropositive
• Anti-cyclic citrullinated peptide antibody positive
• Erythrocyte sedimentation rate 25 mm/hour
• C-reactive protein 3 mg/dl
• Hemoglobin 10 g/dl

b430 Haematological system functions
b435 Immunological system functions

Pharmacotherapy:
• Methotrexate: 10 mg 1× /week orally
• Etanercept: 50 mg 1× /week subcutaneous
• Folic acid 1 mg 1× /day orally

e110 Products and substances for personal consumption

Activities of daily life:
Household:
• Cleaning: complete impairment in making beds, cleaning the windows, carrying full buckets.
• Laundry: complete impairment in wringing out and hanging up clothes.
• Kitchen: complete limitations in opening cans, bottles, screw caps, using a pair of scissors

d640 Doing housework
d430 Lifting and carrying objects
d445 Hand and arm use
d445 Hand and arm use
d550 Eating
d560 Drinking
d630 Preparing meals
d440 Fine hand use

Clinical examination:
Rheumatoid nodule, right elbow

s770 Additional musculoskeletal structure related to movement

6-minute walk
220 meters; while walking latent pain in the knee, severe increasing pain in both feet,
and feeling of instability in the knee.

d450 Walking
d28016 Pain in joints
d28015 Pain in lower limb
b715 Stability of joints functions

Gait pattern
Duchenne's sign on the left side

b770 Gait pattern functions

Transfer
Seat – stand
Dorsal position – face-down position } No pathologic findings
Dorsal position – seat

d410 Changing basic body position

Physical examination
Hands: Right hand:
                     ulnar drift
                     swan-neck deformity of 5th finger
                     boutonnière deformity of 2nd finger
                     fingers and wrist joints swollen
Feet: both ankle joints swollen
                     bunion in hallux valgus position, right > left
Knees: right one swollen
Trunk: no pathological findings

s7302 Structure of hand
s73011 Wrist joint
s73021 Joints of hand and fingers
b715 Stability of joint functions
s7502 Structure of ankle and foot
s75011 Knee joint
s760 Structure of trunk

Assessment of muscle power
Dynamometer for grip strength

b730 Muscle power functions

	right	21.4 pounds		
	left	47.3 pounds		
Elbow				
flexion	right	5/5	left	5/5
extension	right	5/5	left	5/5
Knee				
flexion	right	3-4/5	left	5/5
extension	right	4/5	left	5/5

Figure 3. Clinical findings of Mrs. Baker.

(Continued)

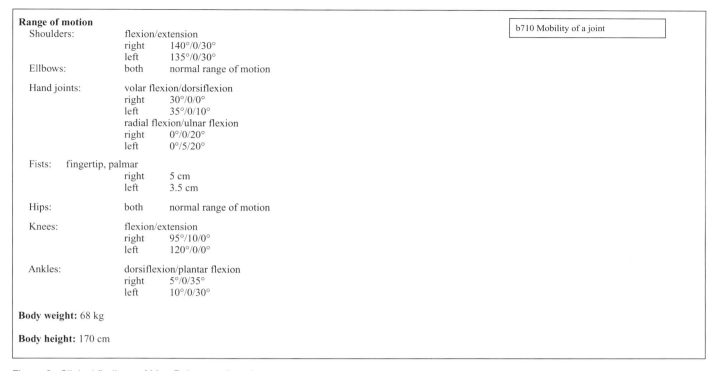

Range of motion

Shoulders:	flexion/extension	
	right	140°/0/30°
	left	135°/0/30°
Ellbows:	both	normal range of motion
Hand joints:	volar flexion/dorsiflexion	
	right	30°/0/0°
	left	35°/0/10°
	radial flexion/ulnar flexion	
	right	0°/0/20°
	left	0°/5/20°
Fists:	fingertip, palmar	
	right	5 cm
	left	3.5 cm
Hips:	both	normal range of motion
Knees:	flexion/extension	
	right	95°/10/0°
	left	120°/0/0°
Ankles:	dorsiflexion/plantar flexion	
	right	5°/0/35°
	left	10°/0/30°

b710 Mobility of a joint

Body weight: 68 kg

Body height: 170 cm

Figure 3. Clinical findings of Mrs. Baker, continued.

intervention targets for the cycle goal. For more information see the review by Cieza and Stucki (15).

Intervention targets usually are derived from the component directly to the left of the cycle goal. For example, when pursuing a cycle goal in the *participation* component, the targets are typically at the level of the *activity* component. When selecting a cycle goal for *activity*, the intervention targets are derived from *body functions and structures*. Personal factors and environmental factors also have to be considered as intervention targets. For example, motivation, lack of family support, and current living conditions (e.g., living on the 4th floor in a building with no elevator) are important, potentially negative factors that may be modified through team intervention.

Most of the intervention targets for the cycle goal "pain in hands and fingers" are derived from *body functions and structures*. Medication (an *environmental* factor) may also be a relevant target related to pain. Intervention targets for the second cycle goal referring to self-care are derived from the *body functions and structures*, *environmental* factors, and *activity* components.

In the case of Mrs. Baker, the intervention targets selected by the team in relation to the cycle goals ("pain in hand and fingers" and "difficulties in getting dressed and problems in brushing teeth and combing hair") are circled. All intervention targets are listed in the lower half of the ICF sheet. Note that a connecting line has been drawn between both cycle goals, indicating a strong relationship between them. Improvement in pain is likely to have a positive effect on self-care activities.

Assignment of Targets

The next step is to match interventions to relevant health professionals or intervention principles. More than one or even all team members may be assigned to many intervention targets. Assignment also includes identifying the intervention principle (e.g., manual therapy, thermotherapy, hydrotherapy) and specific team member. Team members are thereby aware of all relevant intervention principles that will be used to achieve the identified goals.

In the case of Mrs. Baker, the intervention targets "mobility and stability of joints," "muscle power," and "degenerative changes in fingers" would be assigned to physical therapists who may use manual therapy as the intervention principle. The occupational therapist could also be assigned to the intervention target "mobility and stability of joints" as well as "fine hand use" and "hand and arm use." In addition to providing appropriate assistive devices, they may apply movement training and compensation strategies as intervention principles. The "swelling in finger and wrist" might be assigned to the massage therapist who would use thermotherapy and hydrotherapy. The physician would be responsible for monitoring and controlling inflammation and pain through medications. Hence, each of the intervention targets would be assigned to the different team members and to the corresponding intervention principles.

Implementation of Intervention

The next steps are to have each team member
- define her or his intervention technique in relation to the intervention principle;
- identify a measure to follow the progress made; and
- define a goal (measured value) to be achieved and timeframe to achieve the goal.

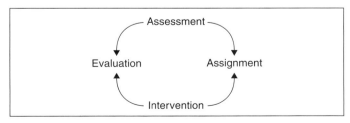

Figure 4. The rehabilitation cycle.

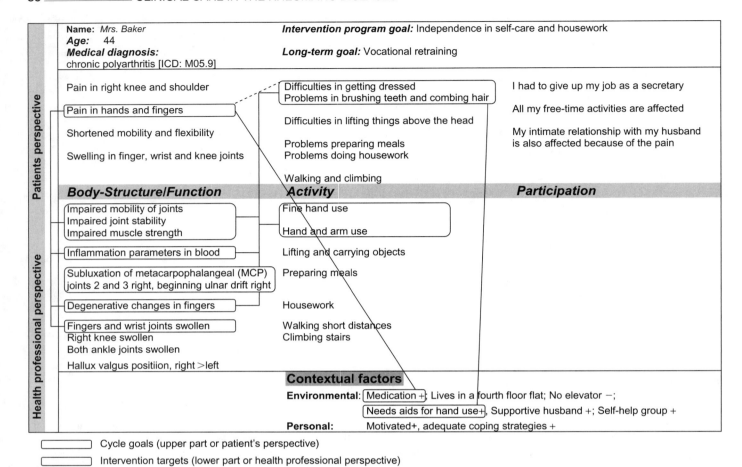

Figure 5. The International Classification of Functioning, Disability and Health sheet including the intervention-program, the long-term goals, and the cycle goals.

For example, if the intervention principle is manual therapy, isometric muscle strengthening might be the technique used. In this case, the ICF qualifier scale can be used to monitor progress. However, more precise measures that take into account the patient's age, general health status, comorbidities, or settings may also be used.

Evaluation

The regular evaluation of progress toward achieving cycle goals and intervention targets is essential. This evaluation is the basis for deciding whether to add intervention targets or to change the intervention principle. At predetermined intervals (or when cycle goals have been achieved), the team should reassess areas outlined in the appropriate brief ICF Core Set. New cycle goals and intervention targets may be proposed, or a decision may be made to continue with the existing treatment plan.

CONCLUSION

In summary, the endorsement of the ICF by the Word Health Assembly in May 2001 marks an important milestone in health services provision and research. The ICF and the model of functioning, disability and health upon which it is based are increasingly integrated into practice by health care providers, researchers, health authorities, and insurers.

The WHO model of functioning, disability and health provides a useful framework to structure the process of multidisciplinary care of rheumatology patients. In this chapter, we have used the comprehensive ICF Core Set for RA to show how the model can be applied to the assessment, creating a comprehensive treatment plan and monitoring outcomes. Use of the ICF Core Set sheet helps clinicians to address the complexity of the different possible interactions among the wide range of factors that influence a patient's level of functioning and disability. ICF Core Sets can also be used to ensure that treatments provided to rheumatic patients address their specific needs and optimize long-term care and health outcomes.

The authors want to thank Alexandra Rauch and the whole team of the ICF Research Branch for their valuable contribution to this chapter.

REFERENCES

1. Stucki G, Ewert T, Cieza A. Value and application of the ICF in rehabilitation medicine. Disabil Rehabil 2003;25:628–34.
2. World Health Organization. International classification of functioning, disability and health: ICF. Geneva: World Health Organization; 2001.
3. Cieza A, Stucki G. New approaches to understanding the impact of musculoskeletal conditions. Best Pract Res Clin Rheumatol 2004;18: 141–54.
4. Enabling America: assessing the role of rehabilitation science and engineering. Washington DC: National Academy Press; 1997.
5. Stucki G, Ustun TB, Melvin J. Applying the ICF for the acute hospital and early post-acute rehabilitation facilities. Disabil Rehabil 2005;27: 349–52.

6. Stucki G, Stier-Jarmer M, Grill E, Melvin J. Rationale and principles of early rehabilitation care after an acute injury or illness. Disabil Rehabil 2005;27:353–9.

7. Grill E, Ewert T, Chatterji S, Kostanjsek N, Stucki G. ICF core sets development for the acute hospital and early post-acute rehabilitation facilities. Disabil Rehabil 2005;27:361–6.

8. Stucki G, Grimby G. Applying the ICF in medicine: foreword. J Rehabil Med 2004;36:5–6.

9. Cieza A, Ewert T, Ustun TB, Chatterji S, Kostanjsek N, Stucki G. Development of ICF core sets for patients with chronic conditions. J Rehabil Med 2004;44(Suppl):9–11.

10. Stucki G, Sangha O. Clinical quality management: putting the pieces together. Arthritis Care Res 1996;9:405–12.

11. Enright PL. The six-minute walk test. Respir Care 2003;48:783–5.

12. van Lankveld W, van't Pad BP, Bakker J, Terwindt S, Franssen M, van Riel P. Sequential occupational dexterity assessment (SODA): a new test to measure hand disability. J Hand Ther 1996;9:27–32.

13. Ware JE Jr, Sherbourne CD. The MOS 36-item Short-Form Health Survey (SF36). 1. Conceptual framework and item selection. Med Care 1992;30:473–81.

14. Cieza A, Geyh S, Chatterji S, Kostanjsek N, Ustun B, Stucki G. ICF linking rules: an update based on lessons learned. J Rehabil Med 2005;37:212–8.

15. Cieza A, Stucki G. Understanding functioning, disability, and health in rheumatoid arthritis: the basis for rehabilitation care. Curr Opin Rheumatol 2005;17:183–9.

The Patient's Experience

KATHLEEN S. LEWIS, RN, CMP, LPC

I arrived at the Atlanta Visiting Nurse Association early to get some things done before a staff meeting. As I rushed about, I began having chest pains. They were like the pains I experienced 3 months earlier. I'd thrown a clot to my lung, spending a week in the hospital and a month out of work.

I called my supervisor to one side. She checked me out and had me call my doctor. It was arranged that another nurse would drive me to the doctor's office after the staff meeting. I left work never to return again.

THE DIAGNOSIS

A perfusion lung scan showed a clot in my left lung exactly at the spot of the previous clot, even though I was taking coumadin. I felt scared. The next few days were filled with tests. The end result was that the doctors made a diagnosis of exertional asthma.

That diagnosis didn't explain what was happening in my body— chest pain, shortness of breath, fatigue, fever, joint pain, hair loss, and other symptoms that had been evolving over the past 8 years. A month later, in preparing to go on a trip to Hawaii with my husband, I got a sun lamp to begin a suntan. A rash developed on my chest. I headed back to the doctor.

My doctor ran more tests. My life was changing rapidly. I had only enough energy to be up for short periods of time. It was difficult to carry out my activities of daily living, and roles as mother and wife. I was getting more anxious. At the same time, we were getting ready for our trip.

Later that week, 2 days before we were to leave for Hawaii, I called my doctor to get my lab results. "Kathleen, it looks like you have systemic lupus erythematosus. You need to see a rheumatologist. Be sure you wear sunscreen when you are in the sun." His voice came across the phone like a cannon exploding in my ears and kept ringing in my ears as I drove to pick up my sons at soccer practice. At age 34 with 2 boys (8 and 10 years old), a husband, and a career, life would never be the same.

That day I left the office, I went instantaneously from being employed to being disabled. It took one and a half soul-wrenching years to go through the disability process. People handle retirement best when it's their choice, their health is good, and they have adequate financial resources. I had none of those when going on disability.

As a visiting nurse, I saw acutely and terminally ill patients. I had no idea what it was like to live with a chronic illness, such as a rheumatic disease. Only after living with many chronic diseases have I learned what it is like to live with illness daily. In working and living with chronic illness for 28 years, I have become aware that there are different challenges in living with acute, terminal, and chronic illness.

Acute illness rapidly reaches crisis and resolution, resulting in death or cure. Terminal illness is considered fatal, with a limited lifespan. I was only familiar with illness where you get sick, get better, and are well or illness where you get sick, get worse, and die. With chronic illness, I'd neither die nor get well, but would live with ongoing fluctuating illness for a lifetime.

It seemed people around me thought I was a failure, a malingerer, neurotic, different, or weird. I began to recognize the stigma associated with illness and disability. The implication seemed to be that maybe I wasn't doing something right, was being punished, or just didn't have

enough faith. It is hard to believe that with modern medicine there isn't a cure for every ache or pain. Television commercials make it seem there is a pill to treat any ailment—from hair loss to impotence.

CHALLENGES OF LIVING WITH CHRONIC ILLNESS

Victor Frankl says living with a chronic illness is like being a prisoner of war: "Where there's an end of certainty … there's uncertainty of an end," (1). With acute and terminal illness, time is short. An end is in sight. Chronic illness lasts a lifetime. It is open-ended and ongoing, with unpredictable fluctuations.

Additional health problems arose secondary to aging, rheumatic disease, and side effects of medications. I developed antibiotic-resistant infections in my sphenoid and ethmoid sinuses, reactions to most antibiotics, and kidney failure secondary to medications and rheumatic disease. All this has been a bit much for others to comprehend, leaving me feeling alone.

Significant support people (health care professionals, family, friends, work associates) have come and gone. I have experienced a shifting of whole support systems. When meeting people, it is difficult to know what, when, and how to tell them about my health and limitations. It takes a lot of emotional energy to try to "pass" as "normal." I can only be comfortable with others when I am comfortable with myself.

The Physician–Patient Relationship

The long-term physician–patient relationship becomes like a marriage (2). It has been one of the most important bonds for me—with give and take, agreements and disagreements. It is a relationship best maintained with honesty, concern, and respect. A balanced working relationship is essential. Normal emotions are played out. For me, anger, anxiety, and frustration are a part of the relationship. Sometimes a power struggle develops to determine who is in control. The physician and I might displace our feelings on each other.

Some patients tend to "doctor shop" to find a magic cure. If a treatment doesn't work they move to another physician without letting the original physician know anything about it. They complicate their illness, diagnosis, and treatment by not working on being honest with their doctor or letting them know when treatments do or don't work.

My physician's opinions and judgments reach into many areas of my life. I have been frightened and at my lowest, both physically and emotionally, when initiating and maintaining these relationships. I have had as many as 8 doctors at one time. It can be maddening to try to relate to so many doctors. They may not agree with or even talk to one another.

At times, my physicians have seemed God-like and like my lifeline. I've realized that no physician can keep me in good health. The physician can only tell me what I need to do, learn to listen to my body, and try to interpret what it is saying. Understanding this point has taken a lot of time and patience for me.

A physician's training is focused on relieving pain and suffering— not helping patients learn how to live with them. When treatments don't work, some physicians seem to feel they have failed. My chronic distress has presented my physicians with personal distress (4). They have had to admit they just did not know what to do. Physicians and patients each have their special needs. How these needs blend and collide has a bearing on the quality of health care (5).

In the extremely expensive and constantly changing managed care setting, I have been forced to give up trusted, familiar health care professionals as insurance plans merged, changed, and physicians jumped from one plan to another. In the 28 years that I have lived with rheumatic diseases, I have had to create completely new health care teams several times while juggling serious health problems. Managed care can dictate who you see as well as what tests, treatments, or procedures are done and how often. Medicare has only recently begun offering prescription benefits; but those benefits are limited, at best.

It has been frightening, difficult, and sometimes devastating to have to start all over with a new health care professional. Physicians need patients, just as patients need physicians. They are both involved differently with illness (5). I cannot replicate my medical history in spoken or written words to fully convey what a previous clinician has seen me through. It can take a year or more to create the open, trusting relationship needed for good medical care.

Education about my illness and test results has been essential to relate my medical history and condition as clearly as possible when I go to another physician. Getting copies of all of my lab results, summary letters, and diagnostic test results over the years has proved invaluable. I learned that lesson after 12 years of my medical records were lost.

Support Network

Chronic illness presents challenges to your entire support community. Significant others have tired, worn out, and become impatient over the years. Research has shown that spouses of patients experiencing chronic pain have higher levels of depression than the general population (6). The patient may live but the family may die.

Significant support people, like my husband, had their own needs but often lacked adequate resources to have them met. There were times when he needed a break and doubted his ability to go the distance. He seemed to become numb to my constant health needs and lose the ability to tell what was and wasn't important. After living with my health problems for 6 years, as well as other family and life stresses, he left and filed for divorce.

We needed a broad base of support to balance the demands of my illness and life. This base might have included health care professionals, support groups, chat rooms, counselors, church affiliates, nuclear and extended family, friends, and neighbors. With a network of support, the burden could have been spread around so that everybody had a better chance of being able to go the distance.

When I was finally diagnosed with lupus, my response was that I would rather die than live for a lifetime like I was feeling. My husband felt we could handle anything as long as I did not die. He wanted to go for lunch to celebrate. We switched stances over the years.

We got caught up in the fear of what might happen in the days and years ahead, while we waited and longed for remission. Both flares and remissions present challenges. It can be quite depressing to feel better for awhile only to feel worse again. These fluctuations can confuse and irritate all concerned.

Credibility Gap

Many times I look great and my lab work appears normal, but I feel horrible. Other times I feel great but my labs are abnormal. I begin to feel crazy when my external and internal reality don't jibe. This dynamic sets up a credibility gap between me and my support network. Doubt, uncertainty, and confusion exist over what is real.

At times I feel isolated, alone, and convinced that no one understands. I have been defensive, argumentative, and combative trying to prove my complaints. At other times, I smile in denial and say everything is fine, only to crash later. There'd also be periods when I would withdraw and become bitter, angry, and confused.

Strangely, when you are ill, people seem compelled to tell you how good you look. When I became ill, you'd have thought I'd entered a beauty contest. I felt caught in a dilemma of whether to dress to cover my illness or to display my illness to appear credible. I found I became emotionally healthy when the illness became only a part of me. I began to dress to accentuate all of who I was.

I learned how to dress up a neck brace with scarves and turtlenecks. People didn't even realize I was wearing a brace. Wearing skirts and pants with pleats and belts helped conceal a lumbar support. I found colorful wrist splints, and attractive silver ring splints to support finger joints.

Hats, sunscreens, and opaque makeup protected me from UV rays. Hats also covered my scant hair, and eventually became my trademark. I found it healthy to do these things, if my adaptive efforts were to be an expression of all of me—style and illness. Trying to forget something is the best way to remember it.

I am asked by patients to "make" their support people understand what they are experiencing. I cannot make anyone understand my situation or me, theirs. I get caught in a power/control struggle when I try. When I can accept my situation and establish realistic expectations for myself, others, and life, I am more at ease with myself and others. I can then identify key significant people who can support me, and let go of those who cannot. I understand that it may have more to do with them than me.

Health care professionals need to accept patients as individuals and listen. Patients need to be educated as to which complaints can be realistically treated and which ones cannot be treated—all without diminishing the reality of their complaints or their credibility. It has taken a long time to learn what my individual disease flare patterns are and to understand that not everything can be treated. Even though there may be no additional treatment, and laboratory tests may not validate how I feel, I can accept myself and feel credible.

Rheumatic diseases don't have the recognition factor or credibility of cancer. Patients who have had both cancer and rheumatic disease say that rheumatic disease was harder to live with. I had a cancer scare right before my ex-husband left. He told me that if I'd had cancer, he'd have stayed and said nothing.

Keeping a Record

Learning to keep a record of my health fluctuations helps me to see my disease patterns and report them to my health professionals in an organized fashion. With documentation, I possibly appear more credible and help the doctor see what is happening. A monthly calendar with symptoms and schedules jotted down can help to keep up with my disease activity and schedule. There are health journals available to keep records.

I used to become frustrated with physician visits because there would be so much to discuss in a limited time. I discovered that compiling an update of everything that has gone on since the last visit, including personal and financial factors, helped me make the best use of time and set an agenda for a very important business meeting. My update is as brief and succinct as possible. I keep a copy and give one to my physician.

Some clinicians fear that keeping records will cause patients to focus on their symptoms and illness. I have found keeping records helps me become more scientifically objective about my illness to see what correlates to what—especially when starting or stopping a treatment. By writing symptoms down I can forget about them and leave them on paper. I can see times when I feel better and keep everything from becoming blurred together. Health care professionals can also help the patient focus on what is important and needs to be kept updated, thus allowing the patient more of a role in medical care (7).

Pacing

Acute and terminal illness come with sprints of frantic activity, rush orders, heroic efforts, heightened attention, and vigilance. Living with a chronic illness like rheumatic disease is more like running a marathon; it requires pacing, endurance, commitment, and flexibility.

I rarely experience rush orders or empathy. It may take several months to find out the results of tests unless I ask the doctor to send me copies. Only my symptoms are treated, not the illness itself. I must endure the illness, side effects of medications, and treatments—without a lot of frantic activity, empathy, or support. For me, illness-related activities need to simply become a way of life.

Expensive tests need to be done and medications need to be taken on an ongoing basis, without getting back to "normal." Sometimes I become impatient, frustrated, or discouraged with how slowly things move. Patient education has helped me understand the need for ongoing lab results, what they mean, and how medications are geared to balance gains against the risk of side effects. It has taken months, even years, of trial-and-error to find the medication combination that works best for me, only to possibly lose it years later due to side effects.

Interspersed with the slow pace of the chronic illness can be acute and potentially life-threatening episodes. The tempo speeds up, tests are done quickly, and I receive a lot of attention and empathy. When my kidneys initially began to fail, there was much concern and activity surrounding the biopsy and outcome. However, once the disease activity leveled off, everyone switched gears back to the marathon methodical pace. I am still in kidney failure, but it has become a part of who I am, my normal abnormal.

Switching back and forth from a marathon to sprints can be difficult. The sprints break up the rhythm of my life and drain my energy. After an acute episode, I may not be able to return to my usual level of activity. All those concerned for me can become sick and tired of my being sick and tired.

It takes time, flexibility, patience, and communication for all involved to find a new routine and way of living with so many changes. I found it was important to keep as much structure and schedule in my life as possible. I needed to deal with my illness one day at a time; to not get stuck in the past or the future.

In a marathon, runners say that the 21st mile can feel like a wall. They don't think they can make it, and want to give up. Their lungs burn. Their legs feel like lead. Those involved with chronic illness may hit a similar emotional wall from time to time as the years stretch out. Patients may think of suicide when they hit a wall.

The chronically ill are at a greater risk of committing suicide than the terminally ill (8). Health care professionals need to be acutely aware of this fact during times of increased stress, a sudden flare after a time of feeling better, a failed treatment, or long periods of no improvement. I have considered suicide at times, but have fought my way through to a better place.

In some illnesses, it can be healthy to fight the disease, push beyond your limits, and not listen to your pain and fatigue. A hero mentality—take the bullet and keep on going—gets rewarded. With rheumatic disease, you need to learn how to live alongside your illness, not fight it or run away.

With rheumatic disease, you can turn on, turn up, and prolong your disease activity if you don't incorporate the 4 P's into your life: pace, prioritize, problem solve, and plan. You need to balance rest and activity. Sometimes you don't know you are pushing too hard, until after the fact. You may feel the price is worth what you're able to do. To me, successful living with chronic illness is to live to the edge of my limitations, which may fluctuate day to day or hour to hour, without going over.

Stress

With acute and terminal illness, stress is intense and short-lived. Long-term stress associated with chronic illness requires long-term coping skills. My thoughts can be one of my greatest stressors. My body responds to every thought, creating a mind–body feedback loop that changes my hormone release, heart and respiration rates, muscle tension, immune functions, and more. McWilliams (9) states that "positive thoughts (joy, happiness, fulfillment, achievement, worthiness) have positive results (enthusiasm, calm, well-being, ease, energy, love). Negative thoughts (judgment, unworthiness, mistrust, resentment, fear) produce negative results (fear, anxiety, alienation, anger, fatigue)."

To be healthy, I try to balance my positive and negative thoughts—maybe 2 positive thoughts for each negative one. I need negative thoughts as a part of my wisdom. Heath professionals can help patients balance their thoughts with realistic expectations through patient education, listening, and not discounting their fears and concerns.

Family members may experience the greatest stress when the patient reaches a plateau and all involved realize that this is as good as it gets. I distinctly remember the day my ex-husband realized that my limited ability to engage in activity was not going to change. The dream of complete remission and "normal" was vanquished. That was probably a major turning point in our marriage.

My family and I needed help to become familiar and comfortable with my illness. Discussing the illness and associated thoughts and feelings with my doctors or in support groups provided a type of systematic desensitization that helped reduce the fear of symptoms and encouraged learning about my disease patterns. Instead of feeling phobic about chest pain, slowly we learned to tell the differences of pain caused by pleurisy, pericarditis, costochondritis, and pulmonary emboli.

Stress comes not only from a chronic illness, but also from associated daily events. The major life event of a diagnosis may translate into myriad daily life hassles, such as a poor night's sleep, remembering when and what medications to take, side effects of medications, fatigue, pain, dealing with the health care system, changing roles in the family, and loss of substantial gainful employment, etc. Richard Lazarus at the University of California, Berkeley suggests that you can balance stress effects of every perceived hassle experienced if you have 2 perceived uplifting experiences, ranging from a pleasant time with your family to getting enough sleep (10).

Dealing with the health care system can be a major hassle or stress for me, starting with the receptionist and continuing through the entire experience to the rescheduling clerk and the ever-present reimbursement battle. Every person in the physician's office can present as either a hassle or an uplift. No matter how good the physician may be, the rest of the staff can neutralize the beneficial effects of an office visit. I desperately need my encounters with physicians and their staffs to be as uplifting and supportive as possible.

When perceived demands are equal to perceived resources, you are balanced. When perceived resources do not equal perceived demands, you are in distress (11). When I perceive my health care professionals as resources rather than demands, it makes a great difference.

Since my diagnosis, perceived demands have increased and perceived resources have decreased. I've worked to increase my resources by attending support groups and self-help classes, engaging in exercise at my level of fitness, practicing meditation and relaxation techniques, educating myself about my illness and treatments, pacing to balance rest and activities, getting counseling, learning how to ask for what I need, leaving a physician when he or she is not working for me, balancing 1 negative thought with 2 positive ones, praying, and journaling. These resources have helped me balance the load to make it through one challenge, day, and event at a time. For me, working on a mind–body–spirit level is essential for maintaining as much health as possible. The resources I have fostered through these activities include self-disclosure, self-directness (assertiveness), confidence, acceptance, social support, financial freedom, physical health, physical fitness, stress monitoring, tension control, structuring, problem solving, cognitive restructuring, functional beliefs, and social ease (12).

THE GRIEF PROCESS

Being diagnosed with a chronic illness may initiate a lifelong grief process for patients and their loved ones. This process is different from that associated with acute or terminal illness.

I grieved present losses and losses yet to come, including my former good health, a good night's sleep, independence, privacy, body image, sense of control, relationships as they had been, established roles inside and outside the family, former social status, the ability to find health or life insurance, a sense of self-confidence, dreams and plans for the future, gainful employment and financial security, familiar daily routines, hobbies, getting suntanned in a bikini, modes of expressing sexuality. The list could go on and on.

Grieving losses resulting from chronic illness presents special difficulties. The grieved object is present for all to see and reminds everyone of what was lost. I needed to do my own grieving while experiencing the grief of others. Every person grieves in his or her own manner and timeframe.

Experts say it takes 2–4 years to grieve a significant loss (13). Almost everything about me had changed or was affected to some degree. Flares and the promise of remission made it difficult to determine which losses were permanent and which temporary. It took years to assess my fluctuating limitations and losses due to the illness.

Important tasks and maintaining family roles interrupted and delayed my personal grieving process. Seeing others grieve and not being able to continue many of my old familiar roles made me feel guilty. I felt compelled to keep up the morale of others. I found that my delayed grief could manifest itself as an immediate reaction of coldness, inability to express feelings that burst forth uncontrollably at a later time, or illness that didn't respond to treatment (14).

Grieving a chronic illness involves losses that may also be resources that are ongoing and open-ended, complicating and extending the time needed to grieve. I have found the emotional reaction to a chronic illness can be more crippling and enduring than the physical aspects of the illness (15). As Simonton (16) pointed out, "Harmony—balance among the physical, mental, and spiritual aspects of being—is central to health."

The all-absorbing identity of an illness and disability threatened my sexual identity, and my ability to relate to others that usually penetrated the fabric of my being. I became lupus and disability. When I introduced myself, the most important thing for people to know was that I had lupus. The perceived loss of sexual identity along with the loss of a secure way of relating to others initiated more grief. The grief process

itself caused more difficulty in relating to others. Significant attachments were threatened by this breakdown, creating yet another loss. Purtilo (17) stated that of the things that might be lost with chronic illness, privacy, body image, and relationships are the most important. It took years to shrink lupus and disability down to size so that they became only a part of who I am and not all of me.

Remissions, or feeling somewhat better, can reinforce denial. Depression kicks back up with a flare or feeling worse again. Patients and their significant others can bounce back and forth between denial and depression, and never make it to acceptance. When a patient gets stuck in any of the stages of the grief process and is not able to move back and forth on his or her own, a counseling referral may be necessary.

Without grieving my losses, I ran the risk of developing dysfunctional behaviors such as severe reactions to separation, unexplained somatic responses, specific medical diseases, and altered relationships with others (18). When I did not grieve my losses, I couldn't make the lifestyle changes needed to accommodate my illness and treatment. The illness continued to control my life at an unconscious level.

As grieving is worked through, "one can get the past in perspective and find meaning in the present" (19). As I grieved my losses, I began to accept my limitations and see new potentials. I then began to wade back into life and find new creative ways to carry out my life, be productive, express my sexuality, and relate to those around me. Through mind–body–spirit work, I was able to recapture some of my losses and count them once again as resources.

Labeling what I was feeling as grief was very helpful to me and gave me permission to grieve, let go, and continue with my life. Grief can be reawakened by a failed treatment, intercurrent illness, significant family transitions, increased loss of function, a disease flare, changes in the health care team, etc. (7). When health care professionals are aware of the grief process, they may help patients anticipate and understand emotional challenges. I have come to believe that dying is the easy part. Living, not just suffering with a chronic illness, is where the real challenge lies.

SICK ROLE OR HEALTHY ROLE

The sick role in medical sociology requires the patient to be dependent, submissive, passive, unhappy, nondirective, childlike, clingy, depressed, and *look sick*. The sick role sanctions and grants temporary relief from personal, social, and vocational responsibility. The sick role is permitted for a limited amount of time only, and the person is expected to function to the optimum degree his or her condition will allow (20).

When I claim to be ill without acting out the sick role, many people will insist that I am not really ill because I *look* so good. The chronically ill learn not to exhibit pain or fatigue behaviors. I try to live with illness without claiming the sick role all the time. Living in the sick role all the time can be demeaning, limiting, and crippling. I need to listen to my body as a guide to activity, but not let my body be my god and determine my mood or attitude.

I haven't found many healthy role models for how to manage illness. Some patients may become dependent and clingy from fear of their illness, a sense of vulnerability, or because they are living out the expected sick role. Other patients may choose fierce, rigid independence, 1) because it is lauded and encouraged by our society's hero mentality, 2) out of fear of rejection, inferiority, embarrassment, or always being on the receiving end, or 3) they may be afraid of being labeled a complainer, a hypochondriac, or lazy. Too much dependence or independence can create codependency. Interdependence seems to be the healthier choice.

I try to accept my limitations and identify my need for assistance. Being able to ask for what I need and set boundaries in an assertive, kind, firm, clear, specific, and direct manner can help greatly. In this way, I learn to bargain my limitations in a matter-of-fact, business-like way without whining, complaining, or demanding. This type of communication can happen as I accept myself, develop realistic expectations, and transact the business of communicating my needs. However, it has taken counseling, study, and failure for me to reach this point.

My two sons and I started family counseling as my ex-husband and I were separating. We tried to negotiate realistic expectations for each other. Once we visited our counselor before I had surgery. We discussed which people they preferred to bring food. We set boundaries on their behavior with the house sitter during my hospital stay. What could have been a nightmare turned out to be as pleasant as possible under the circumstances. I continue to see the same counselor for assistance and guidance when I lose my way or perspective.

Many times patients are seen as noncompliant, resistant, and problematic when they are independent, think for themselves, want to be active participants in their health care, and look good. Patients today tend to be educated consumers about their illness and its treatment. Although it may take more time, energy, and effort, health professionals need to educate patients, or refer them to good sources of information that will allow them to make informed decisions about their lives and illness. Patients may become advocates for themselves and others experiencing similar conditions. See Cheryl Koehn's chapter on "finding normal again" (chapter 47) for more insight.

With rheumatic disease treatment options, I try to be active in weighing risks and benefits of treatment. Being able to participate in these choices often makes a difference in my adhering to the treatment. A patient's power is decreased and the clinician's power is increased when there is uncertainty in the course of an illness, outcome of treatment, or future actions of the clinician. In my experience, the situation is improved when clinicians allow patients to be equal partners, to take an active role in their treatment, and to assume responsibility for themselves (5).

NEW HOPE AND GOALS

In the first 2 years after my diagnosis, I shifted from the couch to the bed and to the hospital. I realized that I needed realistic hopes and goals for the future. I began writing poems and articles to occupy my time. I even wrote an article on systemic lupus erythematosus that was published in *Nurse Practitioner*. Eventually, I wrote a book and articles on living with chronic illness. My writing gave me something to fill my time, a sense of purpose, recognition by winning some literary contests, and much-needed structure. I now speak around the country to patient and professional groups.

I learned that grief accompanies any big transition in life. I started doing grief support with friends facing significant transitions. After the first 2 years, I attended a chaplaincy program. It was very difficult to keep the 2-morning-per-week schedule. I ended up in a 3-month flare and in the hospital for a week. I made it back to the program and finished.

From that experience, I investigated what training I needed for counseling the chronically ill. I found a Master's degree program in rehabilitation counseling that would let me specialize in chronic illness and accommodate my limitations. It took me 5 years to complete a year and a half of coursework.

During that time, I had 7 surgeries, went through a divorce, placed my mother in a nursing home, became the single mother of 2 teenage sons, had my first book published, began a counseling ministry out of my home, led SLE support groups, worked with the Arthritis Foundation developing the SLE Self–Help course, and lived with chronic illness on a daily basis. In trying to fill my time and provide structure for my life, I found a whole new involvement in life and talents I didn't know I had. Recently, I've needed to adjust my life by living with one of my sons and his family.

CONCLUSION

I must emphasize the importance of my time with my health care professionals. Although any appointment is only a moment in the time in the battles of living with chronic illness, it may be a "holy moment." Often I have waited a long time for the visit, and will play and replay the meeting in my mind. My anxiety levels may be elevated. Later I may not remember or comprehend what was said. Many questions may come to mind the minute I walk out the office door.

Having my health provider reinforce what is discussed is a lifesaver for me. Checklists, pamphlets, or written information in any form is helpful for me and my family. A sense that my physician hears me and takes me seriously is invaluable. I can leave the office feeling I have a partner and an advocate rather than an adversary.

Having gone through my grief process over and over, I feel better prepared to live my life successfully with rheumatic disease. I've learned a great deal about my disease and how to cope better in working partnerships with my doctors, my family, my friends, and the world. I hope my future holds better treatment and management options and that my confidence in dealing with the stresses and challenges put to me will continue to grow.

My family has changed, my activities have changed, and my life has changed—with negative as well as positive consequences. Although I would prefer *not* to have experienced some of the changes, my involvement and focus on communication makes the challenge of living with a chronic rheumatic disease a part of my life to learn and grow.

If you, too, are a patient, take heart. In all likelihood, you will be able to grow, develop, and stretch from the challenges presented to you. If you are a health care professional, please communicate and work with your patients and their families. Education and communication are key components to making your patients' disease less burdensome. If you are a researcher, remember that we are hoping for a cure, but are willing to accept medications with fewer side effects. If you are a family member or simply a concerned reader, please recognize that many rheumatic diseases are multifaceted and have tremendous positive as well as negative impacts on our lives.

REFERENCES

1. Frankl EV. Man's search for meaning. Boston: Beacon Press; 1962.
2. Lewis KS. Successful living with chronic illness. Celebrating the joys of life. Dubuque, IA: Kendall/Hunt; 1994.
3. Chyatte SB. On borrowed time. Living with hemodialysis. Oradell, NJ: Medical Economics; 1979.
4. Lewis KS. Celebrate life: new attitudes for living with chronic illness. Atlanta: Arthritis Foundation; 1999.
5. Benet G. Physicians and their patients. London: Ballaire Tindale; 1979.
6. Lewis KS. Chronic illness and marriage: endings and beginnings. Humane Medicine 1989;5:54–7.
7. Lewis KS. Emotional adjustment to chronic illness. Prim Care Practice 1998;2:38–51.
8. Ford RD. Health assessment handbook. Springhouse, PA: Springhouse Corporation; 1987.
9. McWilliams R. You can't afford the luxury of a negative thought. Los Angeles: Prelude Press; 1995.
10. Lazarus RS: Little hassles can be hazardous to your health. Psychology Today 1981; pp. 58–62.
11. Matheny KB. Stress coping: a qualitative and quantitative synthesis with implications for treatment. Counsel Psychol 1986;14:499–549.

12. Matheny K. The coping resources inventory for stress: a measure of perceived resourcefulness. Clin Psychol 1993;49:815–30.

13. Werner-Beland JA. Grief responses to long-term illness and disability. Reston, VA: Reston Publishing; 1980.

14. Mezer RR. Dynamic psychiatry. New York: Springer Publishing Company; 1976.

15. LeMaistre J. Beyond rage: the emotional impact of a chronic physical illness. Oak Park, IL: Alpine Guild; 1985.

16. Simonton OC. The healing journey. New York: Bantam Books; 1992.

17. Purtilo R. Similarities in patient response to chronic and terminal illness. Phys Ther 1976;56:279–84

18. Lindeman. Symptomology and management in grief. In: Crisis intervention: selected readings. New York: Family Service Assoc of Am; 1965.

19. Cox-Gedmark J. Coping with physical disabilty. Philadelphia: The Westminister Press; 1980.

20. Shontz CS. The psychological aspects of physical illness and disability. Reston, VA: Reston Publishing; 1975.

SECTION B: COMMON RHEUMATIC DISEASES

CHAPTER

15

Acute Inflammatory Arthritis and Gout

ARYEH M. ABELES, MD, PAMELA B. ROSENTHAL, MD,
and MICHAEL H. PILLINGER, MD

Acute inflammatory arthritis constitutes painful swelling of 1 or more joints, with onset in minutes to days. Rapid joint capsule distension often results in an exquisitely painful condition, even when the problem is benign. Although some acute inflammatory arthritides presage potential damage if not properly diagnosed and treated, the prognosis for most is excellent if quickly recognized and managed.

DIAGNOSTIC APPROACH

The differential diagnosis of acute inflammatory arthritis includes infections (bacterial, mycobacterial, fungal, viral, and postinfectious), crystal arthropathies (gout, pseudogout), trauma, and autoimmune-mediated inflammatory arthritis (rheumatoid arthritis, psoriatic arthritis, etc.). Although other forms of arthritis may present acutely, they are more commonly chronic.

A thorough history and physical exam are crucial to establish appropriate diagnosis and treatment (Table 1). Serum and blood testing, although helpful, are rarely diagnostic in acute arthritis. Laboratory tests can indicate the level of systemic inflammation (erythrocyte sedimentation rate [ESR], C-reactive protein [CRP]), the likelihood of infection (white blood cell count), and risk factors for particular kinds of arthritis (e.g., elevated serum urate in gout). Specific laboratory tests (antibodies to microorganisms, blood cultures, etc.) occasionally permit identification of systemic diseases that present with acute arthritis. Because the acute process itself does not result in immediate bony destruction, plain radiography is rarely diagnostic, but can identify previously unrecognized chronic arthropathy. Unequivocally, the most important test in evaluating any acute inflammatory arthritis is aspiration (arthrocentesis) and examination of synovial fluid from the involved joint(s). To the patients' disadvantage, however, arthrocentesis is often deferred or even eschewed prior to treatment initiation, potentially leading to unclear diagnoses or inappropriate therapy.

ACUTE INFECTIOUS ARTHRITIS

Bacterial Infection

Bacterial joint infection is a medical emergency because failure to address the problem for even a few days may result in irremediable joint destruction. Accordingly, in the setting of any acute arthritis, ruling out bacterial infection should assume the highest priority. A recent skin break in the area of the affected joint should always be sought because it may have provided a port of entry for bacteria. Alternatively, bacterial joint infection may occur via hematogenous spread from another source; evidence of local infection elsewhere in the body or bacteremia should also be considered. Individuals with a history of intravenous drug use are at particular risk for introducing infection directly into the bloodstream, and can simultaneously have bacterial endocarditis and infectious arthritis. Individuals at high risk for general infection—for example, patients taking immunosuppressive therapy or with immunocompromised conditions—should also be considered at particular risk. The timing of symptom onset should be taken into consideration; most cases of septic arthritis develop over 1–2 days because part of the disease pathogenesis involves local elaboration of the causative organism, whereas gouty attacks typically peak in just a few hours from onset.

A prior history of chronic or episodic arthritis does not rule out superimposed infection. Indeed, the presence of preexisting joint damage, with or without chronic effusion, provides a hospitable environment for bacterial infection. Thus, individuals with chronic arthritides are at higher risk for infection. Patients with prosthetic joints are particularly susceptible to infections; an acute arthritis in a prosthetic joint should be presumed to be infected until proven otherwise. Individuals with tophaceous gout may also be susceptible to developing infection within a tophus, a particularly difficult problem to treat because tophi are avascular and poorly penetrated by antibiotics.

Although virtually any joint may become infected, the pattern of involvement can be helpful in suggesting infection. Most helpful is the distinction between monarticular and polyarticular arthritis. For reasons that may relate to local bacterial penetration, most acute infectious arthritis is monarticular. When more than 1 joint is involved, the index of suspicion for infection may be lower; nonetheless, a lack of infection should still be proven rather than presumed. The likelihood that an acute polyarthritis represents infection rises dramatically in patients with generalized sepsis or compromised immunity.

The specific joints involved may also provide diagnostic clues. Although acute arthritis of the acromioclavicular joint is rare, it is a common site of infection in intravenous drug users. The arthritis of disseminated gonococcemia most typically occurs in the wrists, elbows, and ankles (1), whereas most other cases of septic arthritis present in larger, weight-bearing joints.

Virtually any organism can infect a joint, but by far the 2 most common bacteria infecting joints are *Staphylococcus aureus* and *Neisserria gonorrheae*. Infection with non-group A, beta-hemolytic streptococci is also common. Staphylococcal infection may occur in any age group; affected individuals frequently, but not universally, offer histories of local skin breaks. In contrast to staphylococci infections, septic arthritis caused by

Table 1. Evaluation of a patient with acute arthritis*

History

General
- Age
- Sex
- Prior history of arthritis
- Prior hyperuricemia
- Hypertension or renal insufficiency
- Medications
- Immunocompromise (HIV, diabetes)
- Prior joint replacement surgery
- Recent infections
- Exposure to pathogens through household contacts and/or behaviors

Current Disease
- Monoarticular or polyarticular
- Site of involvement
- Duration of current problem (hours, days)
- Degree of inflammation
- Associated fevers

Physical exam
- Joint(s) involved
- Painful or tender
- Degree of swelling
- Joint involvement versus periarticular (bursa, tendon) problem
- Erythema (possible cellulites)
- Rash (punctuate, plaque-like, plantar, genital, other)
- Cardiac murmur
- Pharyngitis

Laboratory exams

Joint fluid
- Gram stain and culture
- Cell count
- Microscopic exam for crystals (polarizing microscope)
- Special stains and culture, when indicated (mycobacterial, fungal)
- PCR when indicated

Blood work
- Complete blood count
- Serum electrolytes (including calcium, phosphate)
- BUN/creatinine
- ESR
- CRP
- Serum uric acid level
- Blood cultures when indicated
- Serologies (ASO, RF, Lyme titers, etc.) when indicated

* HIV = human immunodeficiency virus; PCR = polymerase chain reaction; BUN = blood urea nitrogen; ESR = erythrocyte sedimentation rate; CRP = C-reactive protein; ASO = antistreptolysin O; RF = rheumatoid factor.

N. gonorrheae preferentially affects a younger population, with gonococcal arthritis the most common joint infection among young, sexually active men and women (1). It is transferred to the joint by hematogenous spread after sexual transmission and typically is accompanied by venereal disease, which may not be clinically apparent. Gonococcal arthritis is often accompanied by tenosynovitis and small, subtle, nonpainful pustules. Intravenous drug users and immunocompromised patients are also prone to infection with pseudomonas and gram-negative organisms. Additionally, virtually any microorganism that causes bacteremia can be hematogenously spread to joints.

Mycobacterial and Fungal Infection

In addition to traditional bacterial infections, other infections should be considered in the setting of acute-onset arthritis. Mycobacterial and fungal articular infections are uncommon and, when present, tend to present as a chronic rather than acute arthritis (2). Nonetheless, these infections can have a rapid onset, particularly in the immunocompromised. Tuberculous articular infection is not necessarily preceded by obvious pulmonary involvement. Although infection with the spirochete *Borrelia burgdorferi* can cause acute polyarthralgia, classic Lyme arthritis tends to be monarticular or oligoarticular, most commonly affecting the knee. Lyme arthritis also tends to be less inflammatory than most infectious arthritides, frequently causing large effusions in the absence of severe pain (3).

Viral Infection

Viral infections most typically cause a migratory or additive polyarthritis, probably from immune complex formation within the joints, and may be accompanied by a rash (4). Recent infection with hepatitis B can cause polyarthritis, often before other clinical symptoms or the onset of liver function abnormalities. Parvovirus B19, which in children results in a slapped-cheek appearance of the face, can present in adults as polyarthritis without the characteristic rash, often accompanied by flu-like symptoms (5). Most typically, viral arthritides are nondestructive and resolve with resolution of the viral illness.

Postinfectious Arthritides

Several infections may not cause infectious arthritis, but instead result in a postinfectious autoimmune reaction to joint components. One such condition is reactive arthritis, which occurs weeks to months after either dysentery or urethral infection with *Chlamydia* (which may occur with gonoccocal infection) (6). Individuals who are HLA–B27-positive are most susceptible to developing reactive arthritis, the clinical picture of which is characterized by a subacute to acute large-joint monarticular or oligoarticular arthritis, primarily of the lower extremities. *Reactive arthritis* is frequently accompanied by inflammation of tendons and entheses. It may also be accompanied by sterile inflammation of the eyes and urethra; when the complete triad is present, the designation *Reiter's syndrome* is sometimes applied. Skin findings typical of reactive arthritis include keratoderma blennhoragicum (a psoriasiform-like rash of the palms and soles) and circinate balanitis (a serpiginous ulcerative lesion of the glans penis). See also Chapter 27, Spondyloarthropathies.

Individuals with group A beta-hemolytic streptococcal throat infections may also develop postinfectious arthritis, typically in a migratory polyarticular pattern (7). Individuals exhibiting a wider range of clinical features after a group A streptococcal infection (most particularly carditis) can be said to have the complete syndrome of acute rheumatic fever (8).

Diagnosis of Infectious Arthritis

Examination of a septic joint will typically show the cardinal signs of inflammation (heat, swelling, redness, and pain). A full examination of other joints, as well as any other complaints of the patient, is critical to define the pattern and extent of the process (Table 2). Fever (with or without chills) is consistent with infection, but can be seen with virtually any type of acute inflammatory arthritis, particularly gout. Care should be taken to examine for possible skin breaks and to delineate the extent of the swelling. It is essential to distinguish between true joint involvement and involvement of related structures.

Although laboratory evaluation for a possibly infected joint tends to be relatively simple, blood tests will typically not distinguish between infection and inflammation from other causes. ESR or CRP can be elevated in any systemic inflammatory process. A peripheral white blood cell count, if elevated (and particularly if the neutrophil count is

Table 2. Characteristics of infectious arthritis

Infectious arthritis	Pathogen	Clinical setting	Most typical joint involvement	Diagnosis/culture
Bacterial	*Staphylococcus aureus*; non-group A, beta-hemolytic strep	Idiopathic or immunocompromised host	Large weight bearing	Joint fluid culture / blood culture
	S aureus, pseudomonas	Intravenous drug users	Acromioclavicular	Joint fluid/ blood culture
	Gram-negative organisms	Immunocompromised		Joint fluid/ blood culture
	Neisseria gonorrheae	Sexually active hosts	Wrists, elbows, ankles	Joint fluid culture <50% sensitive; must culture, throat, rectum, and urethra for *Neisseria*
Spirochete	*Borrelia burgdorferi* (Lyme disease)	Endemic zone host + tick exposure; arthritis is probably postinfectious	Knee (can be oligoarticular)	Serologies
Viral	Hepatitis B; Parvovirus B-19		Polyarticular	Serologies
Postinfectious	*Salmonella, Shigella, Yersenia, Enterobacter, Chlamydia*	Most commonly, HLA–B27-positive patient	Monarticular or oligoarticular; syndrome associated with sterile eye and uretheral inflammation + rash	Active infection likely in the past; stool or urethral cultures often negative

elevated), is highly consistent with infection, though other inflammatory arthritides may cause an elevated white blood count. Blood should be cultured, particularly in the presence of fever or other infection. When appropriate, cultures of the throat, rectum, and urethra should be obtained to rule out gonoccocal infection, because their yield may be higher than joint fluid. If pustules are present, these should also be cultured. If suspicion is high, viral serologies, Lyme titers, stool or urethral cultures (reactive arthritis), throat cultures, and antistreptolysin O titers (poststreptococcal arthritis) should be considered. Serum chemistries and liver function tests may be helpful in defining the context in which the event is occurring (i.e., diabetes, renal failure, hepatic disease). Other laboratory studies may indicate alternative diagnoses, such as serum uric acid level for gout.

Radiography of the affected joint (and the contralateral joint for comparison) is important for baseline analysis but is unlikely to provide definitive information, because x-rays taken early in the disease are unlikely to show joint destruction. Nevertheless, they should always be obtained in patients with a trauma history, and may identify underlying chronic arthritis (9). Moreover, if bacterial arthritis has been allowed to go untreated for a number of days, early joint destruction may be evident.

Without question, the most important diagnostic procedure for evaluating potential joint infections is the joint aspiration. Aspiration should be done in virtually every case of an acutely swollen joint. In experienced hands, joint aspiration is rapid, safe, minimally invasive, and provides the most reliable data in the workup for acute arthritis. Care should be taken to sterilize the skin thoroughly prior to arthrocentesis, and to avoid passing the needle through any cutaneous or subcutaneous infections (i.e., cellulitis), which could introduce bacteria into what may still be a sterile joint. Although joint aspiration techniques are beyond the scope of this chapter, the operator should ensure that the needle is of sufficient gauge to permit easy fluid flow, and a reasonable attempt should be made to drain the maximum amount of fluid possible for both diagnostic and therapeutic purposes. If more than 1 joint is swollen, the practitioner may need to decide whether to aspirate 1, several, or all swollen joints. The appearance and viscosity of the fluid should be noted. Inflammatory joint fluids are most typically cloudy and nonviscous (owing to the presence of neutrophils and the enzymatic destruction of hyaluronic acid). Once collected, the joint fluid should be sent for Gram stain, culture, cell count with differential, and examination for the presence of crystals under polarized microscopy. Where the index of suspicion warrants, the practitioner should also consider ordering special cultures (e.g., gonococcus, mycobacteria, fungi) or bacterial polymerase chain reaction (Lyme disease). A common error among nonspecialists is to initiate empiric antibiotic

therapy prior to joint aspiration; such an approach should be avoided aggressively, because it may dramatically reduce the diagnostic yield and impair the evaluation. Synovial fluid levels of protein, glucose, and lactate dehydrogenase are not diagnostically useful.

A joint fluid white blood cell count of >100,000 cells/mm^3, although not definitive for infection, should generally be considered infectious until proven otherwise. However, bacterial infections not uncommonly induce joint fluid leukocytosis to a lesser degree (2,000–100,000 range, most commonly >50,000), and so a lower joint fluid count should not be presumed to definitively exclude infection (10). This is particularly true in the case of gonococcal and Lyme arthritis, which tend to produce a less robust inflammatory response. Typically, a bacterially driven leukocyte count will consist predominantly of polymorphonuclear leukocytes; the presence of a monocytosis should lead to the consideration of fungal or mycobacterial infection. Gram stains offer the opportunity for rapid confirmation of infection and identification of the offending organism. However, Gram stain analysis is, to some extent, operator-dependent and some organisms may be more difficult to identify than others. Consequently, a negative Gram stain does not rule out infection, and if suspicion remains high, the clinician should consider empiric antibiotic therapy pending final culture results. Depending on the offending organism, even culture results may not be definitive, as cultured fluid from gonococcus-infected joints yield a sensitivity of ~50%. Complicating the analysis of infectious arthritis is the fact that the presence of another disease (e.g., identification of crystals in the joint fluid) does not rule out the possibility of coinfection.

Therapy for Infectious Arthritis

Therapy for a bacterial joint infection should consist of early and aggressive antibiosis accompanied by thorough drainage. The selection of antibiotic should be empiric at first, guided where possible by the results of the Gram stain. The clinical setting (unique patient characteristics and local knowledge about infectious organisms in the community) may guide the decision for empiric therapy. Consultation with an infectious disease specialist may be desirable. Coverage of staphylococcal infection is typically the most pressing consideration (11). Subsequently, the outcome of joint fluid culture may permit the selection of a more specifically active agent. To prevent joint damage, the removal of all joint fluid is considered critical. Where the fluid is readily accessible, the joint may be needle aspirated to remove the fluid; aspirations must be performed regularly until fluid ceases to reaccumulate (11). When the joint fluid is not adequately drained by aspiration or if the synovial white count does not improve rapidly, the joint should be drained arthroscopically. Early consultation with the orthopedic service (usually on the day of admission) is mandatory, and will assist in the decision about approach to drainage. Antibiotic therapy should typically be continued for a total of 4 weeks (usually divided evenly between intravenous and oral therapy).

Therapies for viral-related arthritides should be directed at the underlying viral infection; no direct joint intervention is typically necessary. Therapy for postinfectious arthritis should first consist of confirming that the triggering infection is no longer present and therefore does not require antibiotics. Subsequent therapy is then based on the use of antiinflammatory drugs, and in some instances steroids and immunosuppressants, to control the inflammatory response.

GOUT

Particularly among men, gout is among the most common of acute inflammatory arthritides. In gout, an acute inflammatory response to crystals of uric acid in the joint, either newly precipitated or released from preestablished pools in the soft tissue, results in symptoms. Gout is distinctly uncommon among premenopausal women because they are typically protected from hyperuricemia by mechanisms not entirely understood, but apparently relating to estrogen-dependent alterations in renal urate handling. Therefore, a diagnosis of gout should be considered with skepticism in premenopausal women, unless a particularly compelling risk factor can be identified (aggressive diuretic use, renal insufficiency, documented hyperuricemia).

It is important to obtain a detailed history of the current attack, as well as of the presence of chronic risk factors for gout. History of previously diagnosed gout, or to a lesser extent hyperuricemia, is one of the strongest risk factors for a current episode. The health care provider should define the nature of prior attacks, including which joints were affected. The frequency of past attacks (particularly the recent past) provides information as to disease severity and as to how likely it is that the patient is suffering another attack at presentation. A diagnosis of gout is assigned frequently, and sometimes incorrectly, by caregivers who have not definitively established the diagnosis via joint aspiration and crystal identification. For instance, bursitis of the hallux valgus can mimic podagra (gouty arthritis of the first metatarsophalangeal [MTP] joint) and is often mislabeled and mistreated as gout, especially in young women (12). It is therefore necessary to confirm a prior gout diagnosis by establishing whether an aspiration has been performed, and determining the qualifications of the caregiver who made the diagnosis.

Because gout is a consequence of elevated serum uric acid, establishing risk factors for hyperuricemia is also helpful in determining one's level of suspicion for the diagnosis (13). Common risks include renal insufficiency and a high purine diet. Although obesity is also associated with hyperuricemia, the extent to which this reflects diet is not well established. Regular alcohol consumption, particularly in the form of beer or ales, which not only contain alcohol but are rich in purines, is a well-established risk. Of the various forms of alcohol consumed, wine seems to have the least effect on serum urate, possibly because of a uricosuric effect. A number of drugs may also result in hyperuricemia. Drugs such as diuretics may induce prerenal azotemia; others (nonsteroidal antiinflammatory drugs [NSAIDs], angiotensin-converting enzyme inhibitors) may reduce glomerular filtration. Drugs that are weak acids may directly compete with urate in the kidney; aspirin and salicylates at low doses act in this manner to decrease urate excretion, but at high doses (4–6 gm/day) have a uricosuric effect. The chronic or recent use of any of these agents may predispose a patient to hyperuricemia and gout. Finally, the recent use of agents that lower urate can paradoxically increase the risk of gout by releasing occult pools of uric acid stored in extravascular tissues. Thus, a patient with previously diagnosed gout is at increased risk for attacks in the immediate period following initiation of a urate-lowering agent.

Clinical Picture and Evaluation

The onset of acute gout is typically extremely rapid, occurring over hours. The classic presentation is of a man with hyperuricemia who, after a heavy meal accompanied by significant alchohol, goes to bed to awaken hours later with an extremely painful arthritis. The affected joint is typically red, warm, swollen, and exquisitely painful, which

Table 3. Features of infectious arthritis versus gout*

	Infectious Arthritis	Gout
Joint exam: red, hot, swollen, painful	+++	+++
Monarticular	+++	+++
Polyarticular	+	++
Joint fluid: WBC (neutrophils)	50,000 typical; >100,000 nearly pathognomonic	2,000–100,000; occasionally higher
Joint fluid: microscopy	Pathogenic organism (occasionally missed)	Negatively birefringent, needle-shaped uric acid crystals
Fever	+++	++
Elevated systemic inflammatory markers (ESR, CRP)	+++	+++
Serum uric acid level	Not informative	+++ (during acute attack level can occasionally be normal)
Onset of inflammation	Typically 1–2 days	Typically hours
Risk factors	Skin break in proximity of joint; immunocompromise; prosthetic joint; IVDU; underlying joint pathology including tophaceous gout	Renal insufficiency; hypertension; obesity; antihypertensive medication; history of prior gout
Therapy	Antimicrobial therapy (intravenous followed by oral); typically 4 weeks; aggressive joint drainage and lavage	Antiinflammatory therapy (colchicine, NSAID, or glucocorticoid) for days until resolution of symptoms

* WBC = white blood cells (per mm³); ESR = erythrocyte sedimentation rate; CRP = C-reactive protein; IVDU = intravenous drug use; NSAID = nonsteroidal anti-inflammatory drug.

cannot be distinguished on physical examination from a septic joint (Table 3). The most commonly affected joint in acute gout is the first MTP of either foot; ~90% of first gout attacks occur in this location. Most, but not all, first attacks of gout are monarticular (14). Subsequently, gouty attacks can occur in almost any joint in the body (knees and ankles being next most common) and can be polyarticular; the presence of acute polyarticular inflammation in an otherwise well individual may sway the differential diagnosis toward gout or another crystal disease and away from sepsis.

The evaluation of acute gout typically involves a series of laboratory studies. An elevated ESR or CRP confirms inflammation, but does not distinguish between gout and infection; gouty attacks can cause the ESR to be ≥100 mm/hour. Similarly, an elevated white blood cell count may be seen in both infection and acute gout. Routine serum chemistries are useful to assess renal function. An elevated serum uric acid level establishes hyperuricemia and is supportive of, but not pathognomonic for, acute gouty arthritis. Indeed, a normal or even low serum urate level can sometimes be seen in acute gout as a consequence of the uricosuric effects of cytokines on the renal tubule. A 24-hour urine collection for uric acid should not be ordered during the acute attack, since the results obtained are neither reliable during the acute period nor useful for treating the attack.

Radiographs of the affected joint are not helpful in diagnosing an acute gouty episode. Nevertheless, in certain situations (e.g., in a patient with years of recurrent podagra), radiography may identify characteristic changes of chronic gout, including subcortical lucencies with overhanging edges of bone near the bone—cartilage margin (15). Such findings indicate tophaceous erosions and point toward a history of longstanding gout.

The most useful—indeed, the only—way to definitively diagnose an acute attack of gout is to aspirate the affected joint and examine the fluid for the presence of urate crystals and white blood cells (16). Uric acid crystals are slender, needle-shaped, and negatively birefringent; they are best appreciated under polarized microscopy but may be visible under regular light microscopy. Urate crystals may be plentiful or rare; an experienced observer may need to examine the specimen for an extended period of time before reaching a conclusion.

Confusingly, the presence of uric acid crystals makes the diagnosis of acute gout likely, but not definite, because old crystals from prior attacks may be retained without causing inflammation, for reasons that are not entirely clear. Accordingly, the diagnosis of gout also requires the presence of an inflammatory response in the joint, defined as a synovial fluid white blood cell count of ≥2,000 cells/mm³. Most attacks of acute gout, however, will cause much higher white cell counts, occasionally >100,000. The definitive diagnosis of an acute gouty attack actually rests on the presence of uric acid crystals within the cytoplasm of neutrophils, indicating that the inflammatory response is directed toward the crystals. Even when uric acid crystals are seen, the joint fluid should also be examined for the simultaneous presence of other crystals, especially calcium pyrophosphate crystals, and should undergo Gram stain and culture to rule out coinfection.

Treatment of Acute Gout

Treatment of acute gout is always directed at the inflammatory response, and not the presence of crystals, per se. Three general approaches are available: colchicine, cyclooxygenase inhibitors, and glucocorticoids (17).

Colchicine is one of the oldest drugs known to man, and generally acts to inhibit neutrophil function by disruption of cellular microtubules. In the acute setting, colchicine is administered orally, 0.5 or 0.6 mg per hour, until one of the following targets is achieved: 1) the

---

Rehabilitation Considerations in Acute Inflammatory Arthritis

- Patients presenting with acute inflammatory arthritis should be referred directly to a rheumatologist for evaluation and treatment.
- Range-of-motion exercises are necessary following acute phase to ensure maintenance of joint mobility.
- Joint pain arising from Lyme disease generally presents as large effusions in the absence of severe pain. Frequently, a bull's eye rash may be evident on inspection. Referral to a rheumatologist for antibiotics is necessary to prevent joint and other complications from the disease.

---

patient begins to note symptom relief; 2) the patient begins to experience gastrointestinal (GI) intolerance (usually diarrhea); or 3) a predetermined total maximum dose is reached, in the range of 4–6 mg. Because of the frequency of causing severe diarrhea in a patient with difficulty ambulating, many practitioners will use colchicine as adjunctive therapy only at low dose (0.5–0.6 mg once or twice per day) to avoid this very unpleasant side effect. Patients receiving colchicine for acute gout should not receive additional colchicine (either acutely or for daily prophylaxis) for several weeks because the half-life of the drug is quite long. Toxicities of colchicine at high doses are numerous and, in addition to GI intolerance, include bone marrow and renal failure and neuromyopathies; these toxicities are more common in patients with renal failure, and high doses of colchicine should be avoided in such patients.

Colchicine is most effective early in an acute attack (i.e., within the first hours of symptom onset), when only a few doses may be required. However in a well-established attack (hours to days), higher more toxic doses tend to be required and still may not be efficacious. Other therapeutic options should therefore be considered. Intravenous colchicine (1–2 mg every 12 hours for 1 or 2 doses) causes little GI intolerance, but poses significant risk: fatalities have been reported, particularly in individuals with renal disease. It should be used rarely, if ever, and only by physicians with expertise in the drug (17).

Cyclooxygenase inhibitors (NSAIDs, COX-2 inhibitors) can be quite effective in reversing acute gout, and have the added benefit of providing analgesia (17). Maximal doses are typically required to control inflammation. Although all NSAIDs are probably effective, indomethacin has been best studied. A typical regimen of indomethacin for gout would be 50 mg orally 3 or 4 times daily, with a taper over 3–7 days as the condition improves. Indomethacin however has significant central nervous system (CNS) and GI toxicities; its use should be considered carefully, especially in the elderly. Since some patients treated with NSAIDs may rebound with a new flare during the taper (particularly those with very high serum urate levels), practitioners may wish to consider simultaneous prophylaxis with low-dose daily colchicine (0.6 mg once or twice daily, depending on renal function) for several weeks to prevent recurrence. A decision to initiate an NSAID for gout is determined largely on the patient's risks for toxicity, particularly renal failure, GI ulcers or bleeding, and hypertension; individuals at risk for these problems may warrant consideration of another therapy, although the GI risk of NSAIDs may be reduced by concurrent administration of a proton-pump inhibitor. COX-2–selective inhibitors may also be effective.

Glucocorticoids are extremely potent antiinflammatory agents and have excellent efficacy in gout. The mechanism of action of these agents is extremely complex but involves their ability to bind to and activate cellular glucocorticoid receptors, which regulate nuclear transcription. Glucocorticoids may be administered orally; a typical dosage of prednisone is 40–60 mg daily for several days, followed by a taper over

Nursing Considerations in Acute Inflammatory Arthritis

- Advise patient to discontinue colchicine when pain is relieved or vomiting and/or diarrhea begins.
- Encourage adequate fluid intake.

1–2 weeks once relief begins. For individuals with liver problems, hypertension, or congestive heart failure, methylprednisolone (16–24 mg/day to start) may be more appropriate because it does not require liver metabolism and has less mineralocorticoid acitivity than prednisone. In the acute hospitalized setting, methylprednisolone may be administered intravenously, followed by changeover to the oral equivalent. The potential side effects of glucocorticoids are well known, and include hyperglycemia, hypertension, fluid retention, adrenal suppression, and CNS side effects. Accordingly, care should be taken in using glucocorticoids in individuals at risk for these problems. Another approach to administration of glucocorticoids is to inject it directly into the affected joint. Local steroid injection is safe, well-tolerated, and greatly diminishes the systemic side effects of the agent. Particularly in monarticular gout, it is both effective and practical. The major consideration limiting the use of intraarticular steroid is the care that one must take to avoid introducing the drug into an infected joint. Accordingly, joint fluid must first be aspirated and examined, including expert appraisal of the Gram stain to rule out likely infection, before returning to the patient for injection. Many patients are reluctant to undergo a second procedure. Patients who experience soft-tissue or polyarticular gouty attacks, but have relative contraindications to systemic steroid therapy, often respond to an intramuscular depo steroid injection. Finally, intramuscular injection of a depo formulation of adrenocorticotropic hormone is highly effective in inducing glucocorticoid production by the adrenals, and thus treating gout without causing adrenal suppression; once a favored therapy, this approach is currently used less often due to a lack of availability of the longer-acting formulation (18).

Under no circumstances should a clinician attempt to address the patient's hyperuricemia during an acute attack, such as by instituting allopurinol or discontinuing urate-lowering therapies. Such strategies may impede the patient's recovery, because either lowering or raising the serum urate often results in worsening or renewed attacks (18). Consequently, changes in urate-lowering strategies should not be started until weeks after the acute attack.

After an acute attack has resolved, the practitioner must consider what, and whether, chronic management is warranted. Virtually all patients with gout should be encouraged to limit their purine intake, in the form of alcohol reduction and minimizing intake of high-purine foods, such as organ meats and shellfish. The practitioner should also examine whether the patient takes any medications that promote hyperuricemia (e.g., diuretics), and if so, whether effective substitutes may be initiated. If such alterations succeed in lowering the serum urate, ideally below 7.0 mg/dl, no further management may be needed.

Patients who experience acute attacks only on a rare or occasional basis do not necessarily require chronic treatment, although this decision must be determined on a case-by-case basis. Individuals manifesting their first attack also should generally not be committed to long-term prophylaxis, as subsequent attacks often do not occur for quite some time. However, for individuals whose acute attacks come frequently (at least 3 times annually), pharmacologic prophylaxis is warranted. Initial prophylaxis may be accomplished by preventing inflammation, reducing serum urate, or both. In contrast to high-dose colchicine in the acute setting, the use of colchicine (0.6 mg twice daily; adjusted for renal function) for long-term prophylaxis is generally well tolerated, frequently

effective, and may be simpler than managing the serum urate. However, for patients who continue to have attacks, have tophi on exam, demonstrate gouty erosions on radiography, or whose uric acid is exceptionally high (>9.5 mg/dl), lowering uric acid is necessary.

Serum uric acid may be lowered by 1 of 2 approaches: either reducing urate production or increasing urate excretion by the kidney. Increasing urate excretion is accomplished through the use of probenecid, an agent that acts to block urate resorption in the proximal tubule. Probenecid is a generally safe and effective drug. However, it is only effective in patients with a normal creatinine clearance for whom the cause of hyperuricemia is uric acid underexcretion; underexcretion can be determined by measuring the uric acid in a 24-hour urine collection. Typically, underexcretion is defined by a 24-hour excretion of <800 mg/dl, although the specific value may vary with the individual lab. Despite its utility and safety, the use of probenecid is relatively unpopular among physicians and patients. Probenecid must be taken three times daily. Because it induces urate excretion, probenecid increases the risk of urate nephrolithiasis, necessitating generous water consumption and, in some instances, alkalinization of the urine to avoid stone formation. Individuals with a history of uric acid stones should therefore avoid probenecid.

The currently available alternative, allopurinol, lowers serum urate by inhibiting xanthine oxidase and consequently blocking urate synthesis. Allopurinol is generally dosed once daily, and is efficacious for both overproducers and underexcreters of urate. For individuals with renal stones or tophaceous gout, allopurinol is the first choice for therapy. However, allopurinol should not be prescribed cavalierly. Although allopurinol toxicity is rare (~1%), it is also potentially severe and can result in Stevens-Johnson Syndrome, liver and marrow failure, and death. Accordingly, patients started on allopurinol should be instructed to discontinue the drug in the presence of rash or other adverse effects. Since allopurinol is metabolized by the liver and excreted by the kidney, it should be used carefully in patients with hepatic or renal dysfunction. Allopurinol should initially be started at 100 mg daily and gradually titrated up to achieve a serum urate <7.0 mg/dl. In the case of patients with tophi, lower serum urate levels (<5.0 mg/dl) should be targeted to induce dissolution of tophi. For most individuals, the dosage will not exceed 300 mg/day, although some patients may require as much as 600 mg/day (in divided doses) to achieve the urate target.

Several agents are currently in development that may represent alternative ways to lower serum urate. Febuxostat is a nonpurine analog of uric acid that, like allopurinol, inhibits urate synthesis. Because it is not renally excreted, it may be easier to use in individuals with renal insufficiency. It may also offer an alternative for patients intolerant of allopurinol. Rasburicase is a recombinant form of uricase, an enzyme that humans lack but that has the capacity to rapidly lower serum urate levels. Under what circumstances these agents may be useful and cost-effective remains to be determined.

CALCIUM CRYSTAL DISEASES

Uric acid crystals are not unique in their ability to induce inflammation; other crystals, most notably crystals containing calcium, can have similar effects. Although several kinds of calcium crystals have been identified, calcium pyrophosphate dihydrate (CPPD) crystals are most common and cause an entity known as pseudogout (19).

Pseudogout

The clinical presentation of pseudogout (CPPD deposition disease) is similar to acute gout; attacks are highly inflammatory, come on rapidly,

Table 4. Conditions associated with calcium pyrophosphate dihydrate deposition disease

Metabolic derangements, including abnormalities of calcium/phosphate levels	Direct cartilage disruption
Hyperparathyroidism	Osteoarthritis
Familial hypocalciuric hypercalcemia	Hemochromatosis
Hypophosphatasia	Gout
Hypomagnesemia	Amyloidosis
Hypothyroidism	Trauma
	Neuropathic joints
	Aging

and may be monarticular or polyarticular. In contrast to gout, attacks are most often seen in the knee, followed by the wrist (20). The results of laboratory studies are often similar to gout and infection, with elevated ESR, CRP, and white count. In contrast to gout, which is a disease of elevated systemic urate levels, pseudogout is only rarely associated with hypercalcemia, and in fact, recent studies suggest that pseudogout may relate instead to local production of calcium pyrophosphate in the joint (21). Hypothyroidism has also been associated with pseudogout, but many of the conditions associated with pseudogout—including aging, osteoarthritis, hemochromatosis, and gout—may be linked more by a predisposition to disrupt normal cartilage architecture than by any systemic effect (Table 4). Radiographs of an affected joint may demonstrate chondrocalcinosis: the characteristic pattern of CPPD deposition, appearing as a thin white line that runs parallel to and just beneath the surface cartilage. Chondrocalcinosis only confirms a risk factor because pseudogout may occur without radiographic chondrocalcinosis, and chondrocalcinosis can exist in the absence of pseudogout. Aspiration of the joint fluid in pseudogout reveals positively birefringent, rectangular or rhomboid calcium pyrophosphate crystals, both extraarticular and within the cytoplasm of neutrophils. These are smaller, paler and more difficult to appreciate than urate crystals, and are easily missed. Gout and infection must also be ruled out, as these conditions may coexist with acute pseudogout.

Therapy for acute pseudogout is directed at the inflammatory response rather than the crystal component. NSAIDs, glucocorticoids, and colchicine may all be considered (20), although colchicine may be less effective in acute management than the other therapies. Long-term treatment of pseudogout can be difficult, because no known therapies are available to regulate the deposition of calcium pyrophosphate crystals (21). Low-dose colchicine (0.6 mg once or twice daily, depending on renal function) may be used to prevent attacks. NSAIDs may also be sufficient to provide pseudogout prophylaxis in patients with coexistent osteoarthritis.

Other Calcium Crystal Diseases

A number of other calcium-based crystals can produce acute musculoskeletal inflammation. Most common are hydroxyapatite crystals, which typically deposit in tendons, periarticular soft tissue, and synovia. Risk factors include renal failure and chronic dialysis with hyperphosphatemia, local deposition following corticosteroid injection, connective tissue diseases, milk-alkali syndrome, and CNS insults. Hydroxyapatite deposition may be asymptomatic and picked up on x-ray only, where it often appears as calcification of periarticular soft tissue. In contrast, it may produce severe acute inflammatory disease,

which can affect both periarticular and articular structures and occasionally lead to significant joint destruction (16). Involvement of the shoulder is sometimes called Milwaukee shoulder, but virtually any joint may be affected. Diagnosis depends on history and radiography because crystal identification requires electron microscopy. Treatments for acute attacks include NSAIDs, colchicine, and local steroid injections. Identifying and correcting an underlying cause of hypophosphatemia or hypercalcemia may reduce the risk of future attacks.

Calcium oxalate may also cause acute arthritis; its identification in joint fluid requires special staining with alizarin red dye.

OTHER CAUSES OF ACUTE JOINT INFLAMMATION

Other potential causes of acute joint inflammation include osteoarthritis, rheumatoid arthritis, or other chronic arthritides presenting acutely; trauma, including multiple repetitive or minor; and bursitis.

REFERENCES

1. Cucurull E, Espinoza LR. Gonococcal arthritis. Rheum Dis Clin North Am 1998;24:305–22.
2. Messner RP. Arthritis due to tuberculosis, fungal infections, and parasites. Curr Opin Rheumatol 1991;3:617–20.
3. Massarotti EM. Lyme arthritis. Med Clin North Am 2002;86:297–309.
4. Smith JW. Infectious arthritis. Infect Dis Clin North Am 1990;4:523–38.
5. Calabrese LH, Naides SJ. Viral arthritis. Infect Dis Clin North Am. 2005;19:963–80, x.
6. Amor B. Reiter's syndrome: diagnosis and clinical features. Rheum Dis Clin North Am 1998;24:677–95, vii.
7. Mackie SL, Keat A. Poststreptococcal reactive arthritis: what is it and how do we know? Rheumatology (Oxford) 2004;43:949–54.
8. Carapetis JR, McDonald M, Wilson NJ. Acute rheumatic fever. Lancet 2005;366:155–68.
9. Siva C, Velazquez C, Mody A, Brasington R. Diagnosing acute monoarthritis in adults: a practical approach for the family physician. Am Fam Physician 2003;68:83–90.
10. Pascual E, Jovani V. Synovial fluid analysis. Best Pract Res Clin Rheumatol 2005;19:371–86.
11. Goldenberg DL. Septic arthritis. Lancet 1998;351:197–202.
12. Cooper SM. Pseudopodagra in young women. Arthritis Rheum 1990;33:607–8.
13. Agudelo CA, Wise CM. Gout and hyperuricemia. Curr Opin Rheumatol 1991;3:684–91.
14. Reginato AJ, Schumacher HR Jr. Crystal-associated arthropathies. Clin Geriatr Med 1988;4:295–322.
15. Uri DS, Dalinka MK. Imaging of arthropathies: crystal disease. Radiol Clin North Am 1996;34:359–74, xi.
16. Schumacher HR. Crystal-induced arthritis: an overview. Am J Med 1996;100(Suppl 2A):46S–52S.
17. Abramson SB. Treatment of gout and crystal arthropathies and uses and mechanisms of action of nonsteroidal anti-inflammatory drugs. Curr Opin Rheumatol 1992;4:295–300.
18. Terkeltaub RA. Clinical practice: gout. N Engl J Med 2003;349:1647–55.
19. Weinstein A, Urman JD, Abeles M, Lowenstein M. The chondrocalcinosis—pseudogout syndrome (calcium pyrophosphate dihydrate deposition disease). Conn Med 1977;41:693–5.
20. Kerr LD. Inflammatory arthritis in the elderly. Mt Sinai J Med 2003;70:23–6.
21. Ea HK, Liote F. Calcium pyrophosphate dihydrate and basic calcium phosphate crystal-induced arthropathies: update on pathogenesis, clinical features, and therapy. Curr Rheumatol Rep 2004;6:221–7.
22. Zimmermann B 3rd, Mikolich DJ, Ho G Jr. Septic bursitis. Semin Arthritis Rheum 1995;24:391–410.

Fibromyalgia

RAYMOND M. PERTUSI, DO, RAHUL K. PATEL, MD, and BERNARD R. RUBIN, DO, MPH

Fibromyalgia is a syndrome characterized by chronic diffuse pain and sleep disturbances that are often accompanied by a variety of non-specific complaints. Patients typically exhibit exquisite tenderness to palpation of specific points on the body. There are no significant laboratory or pathologic findings that aid in the diagnosis (1). The management team includes physicians, nurses, mental health professionals, and rehabilitation providers.

The syndrome's cause is uncertain, but patients may report a prior traumatic experience—either physical or emotional (2). The pathophysiology of fibromyalgia is poorly understood. The sleep disturbance reflects an inability to achieve restful sleep. Arousals (awakening) occur before the patient can achieve rapid eye movement (dream) sleep. Other potential etiologies for the development or persistence of fibromyalgia may involve genetic predisposition to disordered epinephrine/norepinephrine, dopamine, serotonin, 5-hydroxytryptophan, cytokines, substance P, and N-methyl-D-aspartate receptor mechanisms (1).

Limited understanding of the causes and mechanisms underlying fibromyalgia has resulted in management based upon anecdote, experience, and trial and error. At this time, there are no pharmaceuticals approved for fibromyalgia, but a few agents are currently under consideration by the Food and Drug Administration. The lack of understanding of the condition and its treatment is reflected in the poor response to treatment often observed, despite the best efforts of the management team (3).

The difficulty in treating fibromyalgia may create a culture of avoidance or even disdain toward these patients from their caregivers. Practitioners must recognize and address their own issues as they relate to caring for such patients (4). Patients with fibromyalgia should be given the opportunity to improve their condition. However, both patients and their providers must establish realistic goals and expectations—acknowledging the likelihood that cure or even significant improvement is low in many cases.

PREVALENCE

Fibromyalgia has been diagnosed in both sexes, with women between the ages of 30 and 50 being disproportionately affected (5). Prevalence estimates range from 2% to 8% (6). Patients may have experienced a traumatic episode that they often relate to the development of fibromyalgia (2). Before being diagnosed, these patients have frequently visited multiple practitioners over years and have had many tests, the results of which have been normal or unhelpful. Patients are often frustrated as a result of their experience with practitioners.

Major depression occurs in 30% of fibromyalgia patients (7). The relationship between pain and depression in fibromyalgia is unclear. Pain processing in the central nervous system (CNS) may not differ between fibromyalgia patients and controls, however, reaction to the same painful stimulus may vary considerably. Depressed fibromyalgia patients react to pain differently than control fibromyalgia patients (8). Fibromyalgia patients who catastrophize about their pain appear to have unique functional magnetic resonance images (9).

The exaggerated response to pain upon tender point palpation may be partially explained by such phenomena.

DIAGNOSIS

Fibromyalgia syndrome comprises a variety of signs and symptoms. There are no diagnostic criteria, however agreement among researchers have resulted in classification criteria that are useful as a diagnostic guideline (see Table 1) (10). These include pain in all 4 quadrants of the body and tender points at specific sites on the body that are elicited during physical examination.

Tender points are tender in most healthy individuals. However, fibromyalgia patients appear to exhibit an exaggerated response. They may complain or withdraw from the examiner. The location of the tender points is shown in Figure 1. Enough pressure to blanch the examiners fingernail is adequate. The patients face and body posture should be observed while applying the pressure. It's best not to solicit a response by asking whether it hurts; but it is better to observe the patient's reaction to the applied pressure (11).

A variety of nonspecific complaints may accompany the syndrome (1). Musculoskeletal complaints in addition to pain include subjective swelling of muscles and joints. Tempromandibular joint complaints are common.

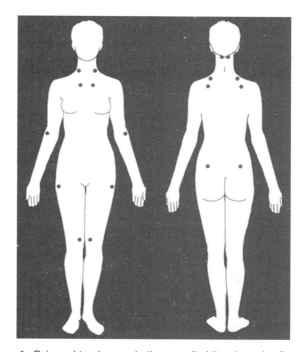

Figure 1. Pain and tenderness in the so-called "tender points" are the defining characteristics of fibromyalgia, so medical care providers focus on the features of the pain to distinguish it from other rheumatic disorders. Reprinted from the ACR Slide Collection on the Rheumatic Diseases, with permission from the American College of Rheumatology.

Rehabilitation Considerations in Fibromyalgia

- Active versus passive interventions are encouraged with this patient population to promote self-management.
- Fatigue, pain, and sleep disturbances impact function. It is important to teach techniques to adjust physical activity to accommodate these factors.
- Fine motor weakness may be present. Careful examination of fine motor activities should be conducted.
- Combine cognitive behavioral with exercise interventions to promote adherence and enhance outcomes of care.
- Aerobic exercise up to 30 minutes, 3 times per week is recommended to prevent deconditioning and enhance functional independence.

Fatigue is almost always present and may be reported as the most limiting feature of the patient's condition. Patients frequently complain of *cognitive dysfunction* characterized by forgetfulness and difficulty focusing. Studies, however, have failed to demonstrate an objective loss in cognitive function (12). Other nervous system complaints may include *paresthesias* in patterns that are neither dermatomal nor physiologically understandable. These paresthesias may be fleeting or constant. *Headaches* are common. Subjective *fine motor weakness* is frequently expressed as the inability to hold objects without dropping them. Restless leg syndrome may contribute to sleep disturbance.

Patients may complain of *chest pain* with or without respiration, but pleurisy is rarely identified. The pain is usually reproducible with palpation. Shortness of breath may relate to deconditioning because no clear cardiopulmonary pathology has been identified, with the possible exception of sleep apnea (13). *Raynaud's phenomena* occurs in ~20% of fibromyalgia patients, although criteria for an underlying connective tissue disease are usually absent.

Gastrointestinal complaints include dysphagia, which usually occurs in the pharyngeal or upper esophageal area. It is usually intermittent and nonprogressive, which distinguishes it from most organic causes. Alternating diarrhea and constipation typical of *irritable bowel syndrome* are common complaints. *Irritable bladder syndrome* has also been reported. Some patients have been identified as having interstitial cystitis (14), but a clear relationship does not exist.

Exclusion of other conditions that may produce similar complaints is important, but the approach should be rational. Therefore, unless a complete history and physical exam or initial laboratory tests point toward an explanation other than fibromyalgia, expensive scanning procedures should be avoided.

Laboratory Studies

Agreement on initial laboratory tests is not complete among experts. A complete blood count, extended chemistry panel, an inflammatory marker (such as erythrocyte sedimentation rate or C-reactive protein) and a thyroid stimulating hormone level are probably adequate. A creatine kinase level is often performed to rule out any primary or iatrogenic muscle disease (usually caused by statins). Antinuclear antibodies and rheumatoid factors may be positive in fibromyalgia patients in the absence of any underlying autoimmune disease. They should not be ordered unless clinically indicated by the existence of signs and symptoms associated with lupus, rheumatoid arthritis, or other autoimmune disorders. The most common differential diagnoses for fibromyalgia are listed in Table 2.

Sleep History

A careful sleep history is needed to identify an underlying organic sleep disorder, seen particularly in men (13). When possible, family members should be queried about the patient's sleep. Emphasis should be placed upon whether the patient snores loudly, startles frequently during sleep, and has had observed apneic episodes. The presence of apneic episodes, in particular, warrants further investigation for obstructive sleep apnea given its high association with cardiovascular disease, hypertension, and sudden death (14). It is helpful to demonstrate to family members and the patient's bed partner what apneic episodes may look like. Identification of these features should generate referral to a pulmonologist or sleep specialist.

Typically, patients have seen multiple specialists and have had many tests before the diagnosis of fibromyalgia is established. After the diagnosis is established there may be a period of time where utilization of services declines (15).

Table 1. Criteria for the classification of fibromyalgia*

1. History of widespread pain.
Definition. Pain is considered widespread when all of the following are present: pain in the left side of the body, pain in the right side of the body, pain above the waist, and pain below the waist. In addition, axial skeletal pain (cervical spine or anterior chest or thoracic spine or low back) must be present. In this definition, shoulder and buttock pain is considered as pain for each involved side. "Low back" pain is considered lower segment pain.

2. Pain in 11 of 18 tender point sites on digital palpation.
Definition. Pain, on digital palpation, must be present in at least 11 of the following 18 sites:
Occiput: Bilateral, at the suboccipital muscle insertions.
Low cervical: bilateral, at the anterior aspects of the intertransverse spaces at C5–C7.
Trapezius: bilateral, at the midpoint of the upper border.
Supraspinatus: bilateral, at origins, above the scapula spine near the medial border.
Second rib: bilateral, at the second costochondral junctions, just lateral to the junctions on upper surfaces.
Lateral epicondyle: bilateral, 2 cm distal to the epicondyles.
Gluteal: bilateral, in upper outer quadrants of buttocks in anterior fold of muscle.
Greater trochanter: bilateral, posterior to the trochanteric prominence.
Knee: bilateral, at the medial fat pad proximal to the joint line.

Digital palpation should be performed with an approximate force of 4 kg.
For a tender point to be considered "positive" the subject must state that the palpation was painful. "Tender" is not to be considered "painful."

For classification purposes, patients will be said to have fibromyalgia if both criteria are satisfied. Widespread pain must have been present for at least 3 months. The presence of a second clinical disorder does not exclude the diagnosis of fibromyalgia.

* Reprinted with permission from reference 10.

Table 2. Conditions that may mimic fibromyalgia

Drug-induced myopathy
Thyroid disorders (hypo, hyper)
Hyperparathyroidism
Polymyalgia rheumatica
Rheumatoid arthritis
System lupus erythematosus
Depression

MANAGEMENT

A rheumatologist may affirm the diagnosis, however, many rheumatologists will refer the patient back to the primary care provider with recommendations for management. Whether rheumatologists should treat fibromyalgia patients is controversial. There is no clear line of evidence showing that fibromyalgia patients have better outcomes in the hands of specialists (16).

Patient education is important for alleviating fear and improving outcomes (17). Patients are often relieved because they erroneously expect to become deformed, disfigured, and disabled. The Arthritis Foundation (AF) provides informative pamphlets and material on their Web site (www.arthritis.org) that is suitable for patients. Alternatively, the patient can be referred to the local AF chapter to learn about local resources including support groups. (Additional sources of credible information, including the American College of Rheumatology, can be found in Chapter 48). Patients should be reminded that many Web sites are not run by professional associations and others are purely for profit. These should be approached with caution.

As a chronic complex pain syndrome, fibromyalgia is managed using a *multidisciplinary approach* addressing sleep restoration, pain management, psychosocial treatment, and an exercise program (18). Compartmentalizing the approach into these distinct categories is often a matter of convenience rather than practicality. The effects of many interventions impact 2 or more categories.

Pain syndromes like fibromyalgia are sometimes depicted as having reciprocal interactions. In this model, pain, sleep disturbance, deconditioning, and mood disturbance are all affected by one other. Occasionally a single treatment may result in improvement in all areas. More often, all 4 areas need to be addressed simultaneously to achieve a reasonable degree of improvement in the patient's condition. Medications commonly used to treat fibromyalgia are listed in Table 3.

Sleep

Sleep hygiene is an obvious but often overlooked topic of discussion with the patient. Patients should be reminded to establish a sleep routine that includes regular hours, comfortable temperatures, and limited noise. Stimulants, alcohol, and exercise should be avoided in the hours prior to sleep. They should be reminded that the bed should be used for only 2 things and 1 of them is sleep (they may laugh when you say this). Food, pets, hobbies, and television should be kept out of the bedroom.

Sleep may be improved with a tricyclic antidepressant, such as amitriptyline, taken about an hour before bedtime (19). The usual starting dose is 10–25 mg. The dose can be titrated upward according to effect. Patients may experience daytime drowsiness as a side effect. Taking the medication a little earlier and allowing enough time for a full 8 hours of sleep may help.

Patients with fibromyalgia may have such significant sleep disturbance that they never dream. The recurrence of dreaming is a good sign, but patients may experience extraordinarily vivid dreams or even nightmares while under therapy with amitriptyline. They may be reluctant to increase the dosage, which may be required to promote a deeper level of sleep such that they are not awakening during their dreams.

Alternatively, cyclobenzaprine in doses of 10–20 mg an hour before bedtime may be used (20). If refractory to amitriptyline and cyclobenzaprine, alprazolam, trazadone, or hypnotics (zolpidem or eszopiclone) can be tried, but referral to a sleep specialist may be needed to exclude an underlying organic sleep disturbance that is preventing the treatment from restoring restful sleep (13).

Pain

Amitriptyline has also been shown to relieve pain (19), however this effect is often delayed. Patients should not expect the more immediate analgesia that is seen with opioids. Opioids are effective at relieving fibromyalgia pain (21), but tolerance may occur if they are used chronically, and dose escalation should be expected. The dependence that may develop is contrary to most principles of chronic benign pain management, which focuses on restoration of function (22). As a result, opioids should be avoided. One exception may be tramadol. This unique agent has both opiod-like and tricyclic antidepressant-like features. Dependence and abuse are rare, such that it is not scheduled as other opioids and narcotics according to the Food and Drug Administration (23).

A newer agent, duloxetine, is indicated for depression and diabetic peripheral neuropathy, but has been studied in fibromyalgia and appears to be an effective pain reliever (24). Pramipexole has been approved for Parkinson's disease and has been used off label for restless leg syndrome, which may be seen in fibromyalgia patients. Pramipexole has been shown to relieve pain and promote sleep in fibromyalgia patients through its effect on dopamine receptors in the CNS (25). Side effects may be limiting at the dosages used in the study.

Two other medications indicated for neuropathy have been reported to help fibromyalgia pain. Gabapentin and pregabalin may modulate or partially block neuronal calcium channels, resulting in a reduction in the release of pain-mediating neurotransmitters (26).

Nonsteroidal antiinflammatory agents are commonly used despite a paucity of evidence demonstrating any significant efficacy (27). Considering the gastrointestinal and cardiovascular side effects, the risk–benefit ratio weighs against their use. If used, their efficacy should be determined within 1 or 2 weeks of initiating therapy, and they should be immediately discontinued if they are not clearly effective. Glucocorticoids are not effective in fibromyalgia (27). Sometimes they can be helpful if there is the suggestion of a concomitant inflammatory condition. If lack of response after a brief trial suggests otherwise, they should be discontinued.

Table 3. Medications commonly used in the treatment of fibromyalgia

Drug(s)	Dosage (mg)
Amitriptyline	10–50 at bedtime
Cyclobenzaprine	10–20 at bedtime
Fluoxetine	20–80 each morning
Tramadol	50–100 four times per day (titrated)
Tramadol/ER	100–300 per day (titrated)
Venlafaxine	37.5 twice per day
Duloxetine	60 twice per day
Gabapentin	up to 1800 per day (divided)
Pregabalin	up to 450 per day (divided)
Pramipexole	0.25–4.5 each bedtime (titrated)
Zolpidem	5–10 each bedtime

Mood

Mood and pain are often addressed together using single or combination approaches. Tricyclic antidepressants, which have been around for ≥50 years, such as amitriptyline and cyclobenzaprine, have proven useful for addressing both mood disturbance and pain. The combination of using a serotonin-specific reuptake inhibitor (e.g., fluoxetine, sertraline) in the morning and amitriptyline in the evening also is effective (28). Newer mixed reuptake inhibitors, such as venlafaxine, which have combined effects on serotonin and norepinephrine, also may be helpful (29). Duloxetine has antidepressant effects and may have a greater impact on mood over pain in fibromyalgia patients (24).

Most patients should be referred to a psychologist or psychiatrist for thorough evaluation and possibly comanagement of significantly depressed mood. Depression may need to be managed aggressively if severe, because suicide is a potential risk. Psychologists also help patients to develop pain coping skills through biofeedback, visualization techniques, and counseling (see chapter 33 on cognitive-behavioral therapy). The *Arthritis Foundation Self-Help Program* is a group-education program that gives fibromyalgia patients an opportunity to learn and practice self-management skills. Trained volunteers, many of whom have arthritis or fibromyalgia, teach these courses. Some patients consider support groups helpful (30), but some caution is warranted because support groups may not be run by mental health or arthritis professionals and can have highly variable methods and goals.

In many practice settings, most of the coaching and counseling is provided by nursing providers. These front-line caregivers are the first to learn when a treatment isn't working or the patient has experienced a setback.

Physical Activity and Exercise

Exercise has been shown to reduce pain and fatigue as well as improve sleep and mood (31,32). It may be the most empowering thing a patient can do to manage their condition.

If cleared from a cardiopulmonary standpoint, all patients should be encouraged to participate in a regularly scheduled, graded, low-impact aerobic exercise program. Walking in a warm water pool may be an excellent starting point for severely affected patients. The warmth may be therapeutic and the water's buoyancy reduces the effect of gravity on the muscles and joints. The *Arthritis Foundation Aquatic Program* is offered in many community pools and YMCAs throughout the United States. The resistance from walking in water allows the heart rate to rise with less effort. If successful, patients can progress to land-based exercises. For less affected patients, a stationary bicycle or treadmill may be a reasonable starting point.

Regardless of the exercise chosen, the goals and rules are the same. The patient should eventually perform continuous aerobic activity for 30 minutes at least 3 times a week. The greatest obstacle to exercise is the pain it generates. Instruct patients to start at a level they know they can handle and to gradually increase the time they exercise each session, until they reach 30 minutes of sustained aerobic activity. They

should then begin to increase the speed or vigor of their activity until they are exercising at a moderate intensity. This can be determined using a standard aerobic exercise heart rate chart (Figure 2).

At times, patients may need to reduce the duration or intensity of their exercise if they feel they have advanced too quickly with resulting pain. The biggest mistake patients make is to do too much too soon, such that they never want to exercise again. Encouraging a go-slow approach should prevent this from occurring and will reduce the likelihood of them quitting the exercise program. This approach may require months for the patient to be reconditioned, but remind them that the effort is worth it.

Physical therapists and certified exercise specialists may also assist in the development of an exercise program by teaching the patients how to avoid injury through ergonomics and by stretching and strengthening related muscle groups. Passive techniques such as massage, heat, cold, and ultrasound may provide pain relief, but should be primarily used to maintain function rather than relieve pain. Over reliance on these techniques for the purpose of pain relief fosters dependence that is contrary to the main goal of pain management. Patients can be taught to perform some of the passive techniques on themselves. Passive and active techniques used in combination with a graded aerobic exercise program can enable patients to achieve their conditioning goals.

Rehabilitation specialists have played a central role in both multimode and multidisciplinary rehabilitation programs. The latter may not be as effective as the former (18,33).

OUTCOMES

It is unreasonable to expect a cure. However, most patients are eager to get any relief from their pain and fatigue. Outcomes frequently depend more on what the patient does than what the caregivers do to them. Encouragement to continue their prescribed management program, particularly the exercise component, may be the most important thing we offer the patient. A good support group may also assume this function. Support group dynamics are variable and therefore group therapy may not always serve the desired purpose. Certain Arthritis Foundation chapters sponsor local support groups that may be monitored by an employee of the chapter to assure that the group functions appropriately.

Up to 30% of fibromyalgia patients may apply for disability from a private insurer or through the Social Security Administration (34). Patients should be encouraged and supported in their efforts to remain functional and employed as long as possible. Disability insurers and examiners are beginning to recognize fibromyalgia as a potentially disabling condition. Regardless, the lack of objective laboratory and

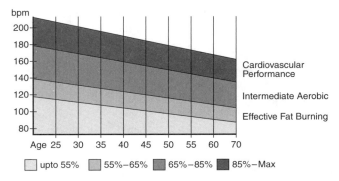

Figure 2. Standard heart rate chart.

radiographic findings, along with the limited physical features associated with the condition, make it difficult for patients to get a disability settlement (35).

CONCLUSION

Fibromyalgia is difficult to manage. Health care providers may do more harm than good by prescribing inappropriate medications or performing unnecessary procedures (36). These behaviors may result from the sense of impotence and frustration that providers feel when they assume total responsibility for healing the patient. This can be avoided by assuring that the provider and the patient have a realistic understanding of the nature of the condition, the management approach, and the likelihood for improvement.

REFERENCES

1. Mease P. Fibromyalgia syndrome. Review of clinical presentation, pathogenesis, outcome measures and treatment. J Rheumatol. 2005;32:6–21.
2. Greenfied S, Fitzcharles MA, Esdail JM. Reactive fibromyalgia syndrome. Arthritis Rheum 1992;35:678–81.
3. Baumgartner E, Finskh A, Cedraschi C, Vischer TL. A six year prospective study of a cohort of patients with fibromyalgia. Ann Rheum Dis 2002;61:644–5.
4. Asbring P, Navanen AL. Ideal versus reality: physician's perspective on patients with chromic fatigue syndrome and fibromyalgia. Soc Sci Med 2003;57:711–20.
5. Wolf F, Ross K, Anderson J. The prevalence and characteristics of fibromyalgia in the general population. Arthritis Rheum 1995;38:19–28.
6. Lawrence RC, Helmick CG, Arnett FC, Deyo RA, Felson DT, Giannini EH, et al. Estimates of the prevalence of arthritis and selected musculoskeletal disorders in the United States. Arthritis Rheum 1998;41:778–99.
7. Burckardt CS, O'Reilly CA, Wien AN. Assessing depression in fibromyalgia patients. Arthritis Care Res 1994;1:35–9.
8. Gieseke T, Gracely RH, Williams DA. The relationship between depression, clinical pain and experiential pain in a chronic pain cohort. Arthritis Rheum 2005;52:1577–84.
9. Gracely RH, Geisser ME, Giesecke T, Grant MA, Petzke F, Williams DA, et al. Pain catastrophizing and neural responses to pain among persons with fibromyalgia. Brain 2004;127:835–43.
10. Wolfe F, Smythe HA, Yunus MB, Bennett RM, Bonbardier C, Goldenberg DL, et al. The American College of Rheumatology 1990 criteria for the classification of fibromyalgia: report of the multicenter criteria committee. Arthritis Rheum 1990;33:160–72.
11. Okifuji A, Turk DC, Sinclair SD. A standardized manual tender point survey. J Rheumatol 1997;24:377–83.
12. Hirshberg L, Jaffer AM, Reid RT, et al. Absence of demonstrable cognitive abnormalities in fibromyalgia patients. American College of Rheumatology Annual Meeting. October 2003, abstract # 528.
13. May KP, West SG, Baker MR, Everett DW. Sleep apnea in male patients with the fibromyalgia syndrome. Am J Med 1993;94:505–8.
14. Shivalkar B, Van De Heyning C, Kerremans M, Rinkevich D, Verbraecken J, De Backer W, et al. Obstructive sleep apnea syndrome: more insights on structural and functional cardiac alterations, and the effects of treatment with continuous positive airway pressure. J Am Coll Cardiol 2006;47:1433–9.
15. Hughes G, Martinez C, Myon E, Taïeb C, Wessely S. The impact of a diagnosis of fibromyalgia on health care resource use by primary care patients in the UK. Arthritis Rheum 2006;54:177–83.
16. Schachana L, Littlejohn G. Primary care and specialist management optional. Bailliers Res I Pract Res Clin Rheumatol 1993;13:469–77.
17. Burckhardt CS, Bejelle A. Education programmes for fibromyalgia patients; description and evaluation. Baillieres Clin Rheumatol 1994;8:935–55.
18. Pfeiffer A, Thompson JM, Nelson A, Tucker S, Luedtke C, Finnie, et al. Effects of a 1.5-day multidisciplinary outpatient treatment program for fibromyalgia: a pilot study. Am J Phys Med Rehabil 2003;82:186–91.
19. O'Malley PG, Balden E, Tomkins G, Santoro J, Kroenke K, Jackson JL, et al. Treatment of fibromyalgia with antidepressants : a meta-analysis. J Gen Intern Med 2000;15:659–66.
20. Tofferi JK, Jackson JL, O'Malley PG. Treatment of fibromyalgia with cyclobenzaprine: a meta-analysis. Arthritis Rheum 2004;51:9–13.
21. Bengtsson M, Bengtsson A, Jorfeldt L. Diagnostic epidural opioid blockade in primary fibromyalgia at rest and during exercise. Pain 1989;39:171–80.
22. Jane C, editor. The Massachusetts General Hospital handbook of pain management. Philadelphia: Ballantyne Lippincott Williams & Wilkins. 3rd ed. 2006. p. 628.
23. Bennett RM, Kamin M, Karim R, Rosenthal N. Tramadol and acetaminophen combination tablets in the treatment of fibromyalgia pain: a double-blind, randomized, placebo-controlled study. Am J Med 2003;114:537–45.
24. Arnold LM, Rosen A, Pritchett YL. A randomized, double blind, placebo-controlled trial of duloxetine in the treatment of women with fibromyalgia with or without major depressive disorder. Pain 2005;119:5–15.
25. Holman AJ, Myers RR. A randomized, double-blind, placebo-controlled trial of pramipexole, a dopamine agonist, in patients with fibromyalgia receiving concomitant medications. Arthritis Rheum 2005;52:2495–505.
26. Crofford LJ, Rowbotham MC, Mease PJ, Russell IJ, Dworkin RH, Corbin AE, et al. Pregabalin for the treatment of fibromyalgia syndrome: results of a randomized, double-blind, placebo-controlled trial. Arthritis Rheum 2005;52:1264–73.
27. Goldenberg DL, Burckhardt C, Crofford L. Management of fibromyalgia syndrome. JAMA 2004;92:2388–95.
28. Goldenberg DL, Mayskly M, Mossey CJ, Ruthazer R, Schmid C. A randomized, double-blind crossover trial of fluoxetine and amitriptyline in the treatment of fibromyalgia. Arthritis Rheum 1996;39:1852–9.
29. Sayar K, Aksu G, AK I, Tosun M. Venlafaxine treatment of fibromyalgia. Ann Pharmacother 2003;37:1561–5.
30. Williams DA. Psychological and behavioral therapies in fibromyalgia and related syndromes. Rest Pract Res Clin Rheumatol 2003;17:649–65.
31. Richards SCM, Scott DL. Prescribed exercise in people with fibromyalgia: parallel group randomized trial. Br Med J 2002;325:185–8.
32. Gowans SE, deHueck A, Voss S, Silaj A, Abbey SE. Six-month and one-year follow-up of 23 weeks of aerobic exercise for individuals with fibromyalgia. Arthritis Rheum 2004;51:890–8.
33. Bennett RM, Burckhardt CS, Clark SR, O'Reilly CA, Wiens AN, Campbell SM. Group treatment of fibromyalgia: a 6 month out patient program. J Rheumatol 1996;23:521–8.
34. White KP, Speechley M, Harth M, Ostbye T. Comparing self-reported function and work disability in 100 community cases of fibromyalgia syndrome versus controls in London, Ontario. Arthritis Rheum 1999;42:76–83.
35. Bennett RM. Fibromyalgia and the disability dilemma: a new era in understanding a complex multi-dimensioned pain syndrome. Arthritis Rheum 1996;39:1627–34.
36. Kinder AJ, Dawes PT, Clement D, Hollows C. Do patients with fibromyalgia undergo unnecessary operations? Rheumatology 2004;43(Suppl 2):ii72.

CHAPTER 17

Knee Pain

BRIDGET T. WALSH, DO, and MICHAEL J. MARICIC, MD

Knee pain is one of the most common musculoskeletal complaints presenting to the primary care, rheumatology, and orthopedic clinics (1). This chapter will focus on the most common conditions presenting with knee symptoms and will review the most cost-effective evaluation and treatment options available.

ANATOMY

Having a basic understanding of the knee's anatomy is helpful to sort out possible underlying etiologies of knee pain. The knee is comprised of 3 compartments: the medial tibiofemoral, the lateral tibiofemoral, and the patellofemoral. There is just 1 synovial cavity encompassing 3 knee compartments. Additionally, the popliteal fossa is located posteriorly and is a common source of pain, stiffness, and limited motion when fluid has collected in it. In ~40% of the population, there is a small connection between the synovial cavity of the knee and the popliteal fossa. The fluid, however, can only go from anterior to the posterior fossa area due to a one-way valve-like process; so when fluid is under pressure anteriorly, it can collect posteriorly.

There are several bursa surrounding the knee that can become inflamed and cause pain. The most common of these include the prepatellar bursa just distal to the patella, the anserine bursa located ~4–6 cm below the medial tibial plateau and medial to the tibial tuberosity, and a medial collateral ligament bursa that lies adjacent to the medial collateral ligament.

EXAMINATION

Inspection

It is first necessary to inspect the knee for alignment, swelling, and redness. Observing the knee in a standing position will allow the clinician to determine whether there is a valgus alignment (the ankle being more lateral in relation to the knee, giving a knock-knee appearance) or varus alignment (the ankle being more medial in relation to the knee, giving a bowlegged appearance). Additionally, the clinician should make note of any flexion contracture or hyperextension. It is important to also make note of the overall posture and alignment of the hips. Flexion contractures and of the hips can contribute to flexion contractures at the knee (e.g., as seen in ankylosing spondylitis). By observing the knees posteriorly, one can appreciate if there is swelling in the popliteal fossa suggestive of a Baker's cyst.

Assessment of Motion

Because the knee is a hinged joint, the only motion the knee should have is flexion and extension. When assessing flexion and extension, one needs to evaluate for adequate flexion of ~140–160° and adequate extension (180°); <180° suggests a flexion contracture and >180° suggests a hypermobility syndrome. Obese individuals, those with an underlying chronic arthritic condition, or those with a popliteal cyst (Baker's cyst) may have decreased motion. The medial and lateral collateral ligaments on the side and the anterior and posterior cruciate ligaments internally keep the knee stable. If there is a derangement or tear in any of these ligaments, the knee may have motion in other planes besides just flexion and extension.

Assessment for Stability

A valgus stress test to assess medial collateral ligament instability is performed with one hand stabilizing the lateral thigh and the other hand placing outward pressure on the medial calf. A varus stress test to assess lateral collateral ligament instability is performed with one hand stabilizing the medial thigh and the other hand placing inward pressure on the medial calf. Pain or excessive opening of the knee compared with the other side suggests an injury to the respective ligament being tested. The anterior drawer sign to assess anterior cruciate stability is performed with the patient's knee flexed 90° and the foot held down firmly. The proximal tibia is pulled forward with both hands, noting any pain or excessive motion compared with the opposite knee. The posterior drawer sign to assess posterior cruciate stability is performed in a similar manner, except that the proximal tibia is pushed backward. The patient's muscles must be relaxed during testing, as quadriceps contraction may mask signs of instability.

The menisci cover the medial and lateral tibial plateaus, serve as a cushion during ambulation, and are a frequent cause of knee pain when torn. Assessing for meniscal tears is performed by palpating the medial and lateral joint lines for tenderness. Another test for meniscal pathology is McMurray's test, performed by passively flexing the knee, applying the thumb and index finger over the lateral and medial joint lines, respectively, and then medially rotating the knee to test the lateral meniscus and laterally rotating the knee to test the medial meniscus, all the time applying torque through the foot. These tests are more sensitive for posterior meniscal tears than anterior ones, and a negative test does not exclude meniscal pathology. Magnetic resonance imagery (MRI) may have to be performed if there is no easily explainable reason for the patient's pain based on physical examination (2,3).

Assessment for an Effusion

Inspection is performed first looking at the patellar contours. If there is a loss of the sharpness of the patellar outline, there may be an effusion present. This may be very difficult to see in an obese individual. Assessing for patellar ballottement is performed by taking the left hand and coming from the superior aspect of the knee and forcing fluid from the suprapatellar pouch into the knee. With the right hand index finger firmly pressing the patella down against the femoral condyles, one checks to see if the patella seems to bob up and down or give way, suggestive of an effusion. Next, by pressing medially along and just below the patellar border, the clinician forces any fluid laterally. Then by gently pressing laterally, one can see if the fluid returns medially; this is called a fluid wave.

The Noisy Knee

Creaking, snapping, grinding, and clicking are common noises the patient will hear with underlying osteoarthritis (OA) of the knee or patellofemoral syndrome. Some patients will describe a snapping sound laterally that may signify iliotibial band syndrome.

ANTERIOR KNEE PAIN

Patients presenting with anterior knee pain will often present with one of the following conditions: prepatellar bursitis, patellofemoral syndrome (chondromalacia patella), or patellar tendinitis.

Prepatellar Bursitis

The prepatellar bursa is located between the patella and overlying skin on the lower half of the patella, extending to the superior portion of the infrapatellar ligament. Prepatellar bursitis is most commonly caused by trauma, especially repetitive kneeling, which causes friction of the bursa ("housemaid's knee"), but can also be due to an infection or crystalline process, such as gout (Figure 1).

Patients with prepatellar bursitis can present with significant and abrupt swelling, redness, and pain made worse by bending, walking stairs, and kneeling.

There typically is swelling or bogginess in the anterior patellar region, warmth, erythema, and tenderness. The pain will be worse

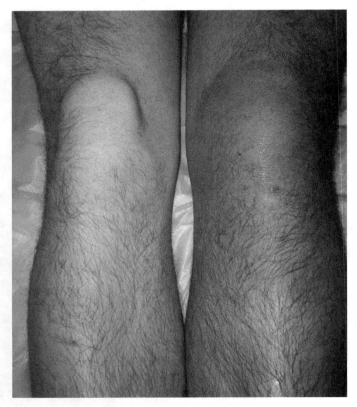

Figure 1. Septic prepatellar bursitis with an extensive cellulitic reaction of the surrounding soft tissue. Maximum tenderness overlies the bursa. There is neither suprapatellar nor popliteal fullness or tenderness. Aspiration of the bursa yielded purulent fluid. Reprinted with permission from the ACR Slide Collection on the Rheumatic Diseases.

on palpation and flexion of the knee. Although there is typically no effusion in the joint itself, it sometimes is difficult to assess for effusion because of the tenderness while attempting to ballot the patella. Assessing for an effusion by pressing medially along the joint line and then again laterally to assess for fluid wave should be negative. Passive range of motion of the knee is typically normal, except that flexion will aggravate the pain and may be limited due to the inflammation and swelling. A septic prepatellar bursitis may simulate or be accompanied by adjacent cellulitis.

The history and physical should confirm this diagnosis. If infection is suspected, the prepatellar bursa should be aspirated and the fluid sent for culture. Radiographic studies are typically not needed, as this should be a clinical diagnosis. If, however, there is a concern for possible knee effusion, radiographic or ultrasound evaluation may be beneficial. If there is a concern for septic prepatellar bursitis and very little fluid is obtained on aspiration, antibiotics may need to be instituted empirically.

Nonsteroidal antiinflammatory drugs (NSAIDs) or topical therapy may be tried, or a cortisone injection can be given as long as no infection is suspected. Antibiotics should be instituted if there is suspicion of a septic prepatellar bursitis. Unlike a septic joint, a patient with a septic prepatellar bursitis does not typically need to be admitted to the hospital or the bursa drained repeatedly. Treatment can be done on an outpatient basis with oral antibiotics to cover for gram-positive organisms.

Patellofemoral pain syndrome

This is a common cause of knee pain in young women and had been called chondromalacia patella in the past, although patellofemoral pain syndrome is the preferred term (4). Patients will complain of pain and stiffness in the anterior knee, especially after going from periods of rest to activity. Pain is worse with flexion, stair climbing, and prolonged walking.

The knee usually looks normal at inspection. Flexion and extension of the knee may elicit crepitation. Compressing the patella against the femoral condyles with lateral motion will elicit pain; this is the one of the most sensitive ways to make the diagnosis. Joint effusions are uncommon. Patellar malalignment is usually the underlying etiology.

The diagnosis may be made clinically and supported by radiographic tangential or sunrise views of the knee (Figure 2). Quadriceps strengthening exercises, hamstring stretching, and other conservative therapies may be beneficial.

Infrapatellar Tendinitis

This condition is common among individuals doing a lot of jumping, and is seen predominantly in athletes. Pain is described along the infrapatellar tendon and its insertion to the tibial tuberosity. Pain will be elicited on palpation of the area and during full knee extension.

In general, the knee will look normal with no evidence of an effusion. There will be focal tenderness to palpation of the infrapatellar tendon and pain will be worse when forcing extension against resistance.

The diagnosis is made by the history and physical exam. Conservative therapy is generally all that is needed. NSAIDs can be used along with ice and rest.

Osgood-Schlatter Disease

Another cause of anterior knee pain in actively growing adolescents is Osgood-Schlatter disease. This is an inflammation of the epiphysis (the

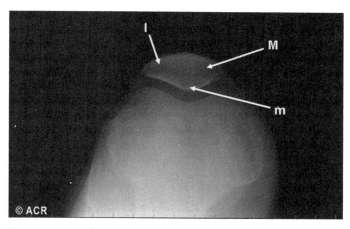

Figure 2. Normal knee (radiograph, tangential patellar view). The tangential patellar view may be obtained in a number of ways. When analysis of patellar subluxation is specifically sought, minimal knee flexion and a relaxed quadriceps allow mild degrees of subluxation to be detected. The normally longer lateral patellar facet (l), the median ridge (m), and the medial facet (M) are visible. Reprinted with permission from the ACR Slide Collection on the Rheumatic Diseases.

insertion of the patellar tendon to the tibia) that results in focal anterior knee pain at the tibial tubercle. Radiographs are not indicated unless the patient has atypical complaints, fever, or pain not directly over the tibial tubercle. Treatment is conservative and includes stretching and strengthening of the quadriceps muscles. The disorder gradually improves with time.

MEDIAL KNEE PAIN

Pain in the medial aspect of the knee is a common presenting complaint. Conditions that will elicit medial knee pain include anserine bursitis, medial meniscal tear, and medial knee osteoarthritis.

Anserine Bursitis

The anserine bursa is located ~4–6 cm below the medial tibial plateau. It is a common cause of pain for overweight middle-aged or elderly individuals, predominantly women with OA of the knee. Pain is worse with walking, bending, and stair climbing.

On examination, there will be a focal tenderness 4–6 cm below the medial tibial plateau. There should be no knee effusion or laxity unless other conditions are associated with the bursitis.

Typically the history and physical are all that are needed to make the diagnosis. In the elderly person or the individual that has been taking corticosteroids for a long time, consideration of tibial osteonecrosis should be considered and a radiograph or MRI might be necessary. Often, just injecting the anserine bursa with lidocaine followed by prompt resolution of symptoms can aid the clinical diagnosis.

Treatment for anserine bursitis includes rest, ice, topical analgesics, or corticosteroid injection into the bursa using ~20 mg of triamcinolone or equivalent corticosteroid along with 1% lidocaine without epinephrine.

Medial Collateral Ligament Injury

This should be considered in the young athlete or in those with a history of trauma. Patients may report discomfort on weight bearing, walking, and climbing or descending stairs. There is often an associated history of trauma.

Results of the knee exam may vary depending on the extent of the injury. If there is no evidence of ligamentous laxity but discomfort on palpation of the tendon, then one may be dealing with a first-degree strain. Should the ligament be partially torn, there will be increased pain and temporary opening of the knee joint on medial stress indicative of a second-degree separation. A complete tear of the ligament will elicit persistent pain and significant instability on medially applied stress.

An MRI is probably the best way to make the diagnosis, to assess the degree of the medial collateral ligamentous injury, and to differentiate from a meniscal tear or other pathology. Treatment will depend on the severity of the damage.

POSTERIOR KNEE PAIN

The most common problem in the posterior knee is a Baker's cyst (popliteal cyst). Patients will typically report fullness in the back of the knee that is worse with flexion. Oftentimes they will report that flexion is limited. Baker's cysts may rupture into the posterior calf muscle, and this can result in fairly severe swelling and pain in the calf (pseudothrombophlebitis syndrome). Any condition resulting in a knee effusion can produce a popliteal cyst. There is a naturally occurring communication between the synovial complex anteriorly and the semimembranosus-gastrocnemial bursa in ~40% of the population. This bursa is located beneath the medial head of the gastrocnemius muscle. A one-way valve-like mechanism may develop between the anterior synovial chamber and the bursa, resulting in fluid being forced posteriorly when there is increased pressure from the synovial effusion of the anterior knee.

The best way to check for a popliteal cyst is to evaluate the popliteal fossa from the rear with the patient standing. With the patient supine, the clinician may palpate the fullness posteriorly. There will often be an effusion in the anterior chamber of the knee. Cyst rupture may result in significant pain and swelling in the calf and evidence of bleeding above the ankle at the medial malleolus (the crescent sign) (Figure 3). This crescent sign may help distinguish the calf swelling from thrombophlebitis.

The diagnosis can most often be made on physical examination along with a suggestive history. If the cyst has ruptured and there is a concern of pseudothrombophlebitis, then ultrasound may be required. An MRI may also be helpful.

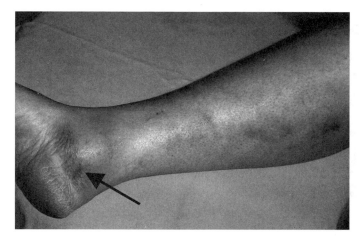

Figure 3. A 48-year-old woman with rheumatoid arthritis developed a ruptured popliteal cyst, which resulted in swelling and ecchymosis of the lower extremity. Pooling of blood at the ankle and foot produces the classic "crescent sign." Reprinted with permission from the ACR Slide Collection on the Rheumatic Diseases.

An injection of corticosteroids into the anterior compartment (never inject into the knee posteriorly due to the danger of hitting the popliteal artery) will help decrease the swelling. NSAIDs may also be used if the condition is not as urgent.

LATERAL KNEE PAIN

Lateral compartment OA, trauma to the lateral collateral ligament, and lateral meniscal tears may lead to lateral knee pain. Physical examination and radiographs or an MRI will help differentiate these conditions. In the young athlete, the most common reason for lateral knee pain is a condition called iliotibial band syndrome.

Iliotibial Band Syndrome

The iliotibial band extends from the ileum down to the lateral tibial plateau. It courses over the femoral condyles laterally, and this is the area where pain is typically generated. This condition is common in runners, especially those doing long-distance running and running on uneven surfaces. The problem is caused by repetitive flexion and extension of the hip as the tensor fascia lata pulls the iliotibial band forward when the hip is flexed and the gluteus maximus pulls it posteriorly when the hip is extended (5).

Patients may describe a snapping sound in the lateral femoral condylar area. Patients report pain, aching, and sometimes burning along the band that is worse in the lateral femoral condylar area. As time goes on, the area becomes focally tender to palpation.

Examination will typically reveal normal alignment, the lack of an effusion, and no laxity. There will be focal knee pain over the lateral femoral condyle. Pain may be accentuated by standing with the knees slightly flexed. There may be a mild varus alignment of the knee. A tight iliotibial band may be appreciated with the patient lying on the unaffected side, taking the hip and knee in flexion with the hip abducted. Then extend the hip and knee and adduct the hip; the iliotibial band will get stuck on the femoral condyle. This maneuver is called Ober's test.

Diagnosis is made by the history and physical exam. Tenderness and clicking over the lateral femoral condyles with the remainder of the knee exam being normal is very suggestive of iliotibial band syndrome. Conservative therapy is typically all that is needed. The patient should be told to decrease the amount of running, especially on uneven surfaces. NSAIDs and ice may be helpful.

OSTEOARTHRITIS

Osteoarthritis of the knee is one of the most common conditions of the elderly (6). Patients may be asymptomatic despite the fact that radiographs show joint-space narrowing, sclerosis, and osteophytes, or they may have severe symptoms with minimal changes radiographically (7).

Patients may have mild stiffness in the morning but it usually lasts <30 minutes. The pain will be worse at the end of the day or after prolonged weight bearing and walking. Differentiating intraarticular pain of OA from periarticular pain from anserine bursitis, medial collateral ligament bursitis, or other conditions needs to be assessed.

Inspection will frequently reveal mild bony enlargement and possibly a valgus or varus knee alignment. The knee will typically feel cool, although an OA flare may have a mild inflammatory component and the knee may feel a little warm. There may be a small to moderate effusion. Patients with OA frequently have quadriceps atrophy and may have mild medial or lateral ligamentous laxity.

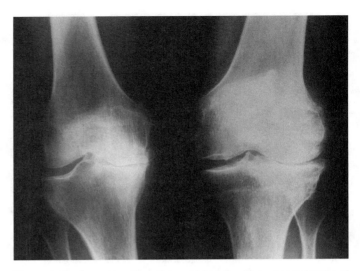

Figure 4. Radiographs of medial and lateral cartilage degeneration of knee joint. **Left,** the anteroposterior projection of the knee shows marked narrowing of the medial compartment and moderate sclerosis of adjacent bony margins. Involvement of the medial aspect of the knee joint is much more common than of the lateral compartment. **Right,** the anteroposterior projection of the knee shows narrowing of the lateral compartment and sclerosis of adjacent bony margins. The intercondylar tibial tubercles are elongated, and there is flattening of the medial femoral condyle. Unicompartmental joint-space loss and reactive new bone formation help differentiate degenerative from inflammatory arthritis. Reprinted with permission from the ACR Slide Collection on the Rheumatic Diseases.

Osteoarthritis in the strict sense is diagnosed radiographically. The medial compartment is most commonly involved, but the lateral and patellofemoral compartments may be involved as well. Joint-space narrowing, sclerosis, and osteophyte formation are the radiographic hallmarks of OA (Figure 4). It is typically not needed to do an MRI to make the diagnosis of OA. However, a meniscal tear, ligamentous, or other internal pathology is suspected, then an MRI will need to be performed. If there is an effusion present it should be aspirated and fluid sent for cell count and crystal investigation. The typical white blood cell count of OA fluid will be <1,000 cells/mm^3.

The treatment options for OA range from conservative therapy to joint replacement surgery. Because there is no definitive therapy to slow the progression of osteoarthritis, symptomatic treatment is the mainstay. Physical therapy, particularly quadriceps-strengthening exercise, is helpful and has been shown to decrease pain and the need for NSAIDs. If there is instability noted on examination, bracing may be necessary. Many patients find that topical remedies help relieve their pain. Capsaicin has been studied in a randomized controlled trial and was comparable in its pain-relieving affects to NSAIDs. The American College of Rheumatology recommends starting with acetaminophen at doses up to 4 grams per day before proceeding to NSAIDs. Lower doses should be utilized in the elderly, those with preexisting renal or hepatic dysfunction, or those taking other medications that could affect the liver. Monitoring liver enzymes will be essential in these patients. Many patients with OA find that acetaminophen is not helpful, and trying different NSAIDs is usually the next alternative. In the elderly patient for whom NSAIDs are contraindicated, opioid analgesics may be necessary.

THE ACUTE PAINFUL KNEE

There are several considerations that need to be made when the patient presents with an acutely painful knee. First, the clinician must determine if this is a monarticular inflammatory process or one involving several

Rehabilitation Considerations in Persons with Knee Disorders

- Comprehensive examination and history are necessary to design appropriate interventions for the various forms of knee disorders
- Management of anterior knee pain resulting from conditions such as patellofemoral pain syndrome and infrapatellar tendinitis can be managed with ice (10–20 minutes), reduction of physical activity that causes excessive pounding on the legs (e.g., running), low-impact activity, and quadriceps strengthening.
- An magnetic resonance image is probably the best way to make the diagnosis and degree of the medial collateral ligamentous injury, and to differentiate from a meniscal tear or other pathology. Rehabilitation intervention will depend on the severity of the damage.
- Patients presenting with the abrupt onset of a painful, red, swollen, warm knee should be evaluated on an urgent basis and referred to their physician.
- Patients with osteoarthritis commonly present with mild stiffness in the morning but it usually lasts <30 minutes, and pain that is worse at the end of the day or after prolonged weight bearing and walking.
- Patients with osteoarthritis should be encouraged to remain physically active and engage in regular exercise to maintain range of motion, prevent deconditioning, and maximize function.

joints, or if it is an exacerbation of a chronic condition or an acute traumatic injury. A traumatic injury should be self-evident from the history, and will not be discussed further, except to say that if there is an effusion associated with trauma it is best to aspirate the fluid assessing for blood (hemarthrosis) and fat globules indicative of a fracture (8).

Patients presenting with the abrupt onset of a painful, red, swollen, warm knee should be evaluated on an urgent basis (9). A monarticular inflammatory knee process may be a septic joint that requires hospitalization, intravenous antibiotics, and repeated aspirations. Differentiating between an acute crystalline arthritis (gout or pseudogout) and a septic joint requires aspiration of the fluid for analysis and polarized microscopy (10). See Chapter 15, Acute Inflammatory Arthritis and Gout, for a complete discussion.

REFERENCES

1. Jackson JL. O'Malley PG. Kroenke K. Evaluation of acute knee pain in primary care. Ann Intern Med 2003;139:575–88.
2. Solomon DH, Simel DL, Bates DW, Katz JN, Schaffer JL. The rational clinical examination. Does this patient have a torn meniscus or ligament of the knee? Value of the physical examination. JAMA 2001;286:1610–20.
3. Terry GC, Tagert BE, Young MJ. Reliability of the clinical assessment in predicting the cause of internal derangements of the knee. Arthroscopy 1995;11:586–76.
4. Yates C, Grana WA. Patellofemoral pain: a prospective study. Orthopedics 1986;9:663–7.
5. Messier SP, Edwards DG, Martin DF, Lowery RB, Cannon DW, James MK, et al. Etiology of iliotibial band friction syndrome in distance runners. Med Sci Sports Exerc 1995;27:951–60.
6. Altman R, Asch E, Bloch D, Bole G, Borenstein D, Brandt K, et al., Diagnostic and Therapeutic Criteria Committee of the American Rheumatism Association. Development of criteria for the classification and reporting of osteoarthritis: classification of osteoarthritis of the knee. Arthritis Rheum 1986;29:1039–49.
7. Claessens AA, Schouten JS, van den Ouweland FA, Valkenburg HA. Do clinical findings associate with radiographic osteoarthritis of the knee? Ann Rheum Dis 1990;49:771–4.
8. Hardaker WT Jr, Garrett WE Jr, Bassett FH 3rd. Evaluation of acute traumatic hemarthrosis of the knee joint. South Med J 1990;83:640–4.
9. Cibere J. Rheumatology: 4. Acute monoarthritis. CMAJ 2000;162: 1577–83.
10. Felson DT, Anderson JJ, Naimark A, Kannel W, Meenan RF. The prevalence of chondrocalcinosis in the elderly and its association with knee osteoarthritis: the Framingham Study. J Rheumatol 1989;16:1241–5.

Low Back and Neck Pain

DAVID BORENSTEIN, MD

Low back and neck pain are among the most common symptoms evaluated and treated by primary care providers. The common cold is the only medical illness associated with more lost days from work than spine disorders (1). In any 12-month period in the United States, 15–20% of the population has an episode of lumbosacral pain.

Low back and neck pain are symptoms associated with more than 70 disorders, including both mechanical and medical illnesses (2). Mechanical disorders of the spine cause more than 90% of all episodes of back and neck pain. Mechanical spine pain may be defined as pain secondary to overuse of a normal anatomic structure (i.e., muscle strain) or pain secondary to trauma or deformity of an anatomic structure (spinal stenosis). These disorders are characterized by exacerbation (e.g., during sustained spinal extension) and alleviation (e.g., while in supine position) of pain in direct correlation with particular physical activities. The most common mechanical disorders of the spine include muscle strain, herniated intervertebral discs, and spondylosis.

Medical illnesses of the spine may include infections, neoplasms, spondyloarthropathies, and metabolic disorders. These systemic illnesses are treated specifically for the associated medical disorder; for example, antibiotics are prescribed for vertebral osteomyelitis and parathyroidectomy for hyperparathyroidism.

A wide range of therapies, including limiting rest, medications, physical modalities, behavior modification, and surgery, are available to treat mechanical spine pain. The abundance of interventions has resulted in confusion for primary care providers concerning the choice of effective therapy for specific forms of mechanical spine pain. This absence of consensus was documented in a study of 2,897 physicians who responded to a questionnaire concerning the prescribing of therapy for patients with acute muscle strain, sciatica, and chronic low back pain (3). Treatment recommendations chosen by the respondents followed a pattern consistent with the specialty of the physician—that is, surgery was chosen by orthopedic surgeons, rehabilitation by physiatrists, and so on. These choices often conflicted with published guideline recommendations for diagnosis and management of low back pain (4).

The practicing physician must be able to determine a cost-effective method of diagnosing and treating spinal pain. Except in the rare circumstance of individuals with a surgical emergency, such as cauda equina syndrome, ruptured abdominal aneurysm, or cervical myelopathy with cord compression, nonsurgical treatment is effective for the majority of patients with acute spine pain. However, only a minority of patients are totally pain-free at 12 months after the onset of their event (5). Also, relapses will occur in up to 75% of individuals with a new episode of back pain within the next 12 months (6). Acute spine pain is defined by a duration of <12 weeks, whereas chronic spine pain has a duration of ≥12 weeks.

MECHANICAL DISORDERS OF THE AXIAL SKELETON

Common mechanical disorders of the lumbar and cervical spine include muscle strain, whiplash, intervertebral disc herniation, spondylosis, and spinal stenosis. The clinical characteristics of these disorders are listed in Table 1. The *Primer on the Rheumatic Diseases*, 12th edition, contains descriptions of the clinical symptoms, signs, and diagnostic methods to identify these mechanical disorders.

Muscle strain is preceded by a physical event, such as lifting a weight greater than the forces that can be supported by the muscular and ligamentous structures of the spine. Back or neck pain associated with muscle injury radiates up and across the paraspinous muscles, with radiation limited to the buttocks or the shoulders, respectively.

Whiplash, or cervical hyperextension injuries of the neck, are associated with rear-collision motor vehicle accidents (7). Impact from the rear causes acceleration–deceleration injury to the soft tissue structures in the neck. The symptoms of stiffness and pain with neck motion are first noticed 12–24 hours after the accident. Headache is commonly reported. Patients may have difficulty swallowing or chewing and may have paresthesias in the arms.

Intervertebral disc herniation occurs with a sudden physical event, such as lifting a heavy object or sneezing. Herniation of the disc causes nerve impingement and inflammation resulting in radiating pain in the leg (sciatica) or arm (brachialgia). Back or neck pain may be present, but it is not universally noted by individuals with a disc herniation.

Spondylosis, or osteoarthritis (OA) of the spinal zygapophyseal joints, may cause localized low back or neck pain. As the intervertebral disc degenerates, intersegmental instability and approximation of the vertebral bodies shift the compressive forces across the zygapophyseal joints. The transition of these facet joints from non–weight-bearing to weight-bearing joints leads to zygapophyseal OA. As a result, patients develop lumbar or cervical pain that increases at the end of the day and radiates across the low back or shoulders.

Spinal stenosis/myelopathy occurs as a consequence of spinal cord compression by osteophytes, ligamentum flavum, or intervertebral disc. Cervical spondylotic myelopathy is the most common cause of spinal cord dysfunction in individuals older than 55 years of age (8). With disc degeneration, osteophytes develop posteriorly and project into the spinal canal, compressing the spinal cord and its vascular supply. Clinical symptoms include a history of peculiar sensations in the hands, associated with weakness and lack of coordination. Neck pain is mentioned by only one-third of patients with myelopathy. In the lower extremities, this disorder can cause gait disturbances, spasticity, leg weakness, and spontaneous leg movements. Older patients may describe leg stiffness, foot shuffling, and a fear of falling. Incontinence is a late manifestation.

Lumbar spinal stenosis causes chronic low back pain, frequently lasting >12 weeks. Progression of the disorder causes increased narrowing of the spinal canal, resulting in stenosis and compression of neural elements. The clinical manifestation of spinal stenosis is neurogenic claudication. Narrowing of the spinal canal, which may occur at single or multiple levels, causes radiating lower extremity pain when walking or standing.

DIAGNOSTIC EVALUATION

History and physical examination are the cornerstones of the diagnostic evaluation for these spinal pain patients (9). Most individuals with systemic causes of spinal pain are identified with these

Table 1. Mechanical disorders of the axial skeleton

	Muscle strain	Herniated nucleus pulposus	Spinal stenosis	Whiplash	Spondylosis	Myelopathy
Typical age at onset, years	20–40	30–50	>60	30–40	>50	>60
Pain pattern						
Location	Back/neck	Back/leg	Neck/arm/leg	Neck	Back/neck	Arm/leg
Onset	Acute	Acute	Insidious	Acute	Insidious	Insidious
Extension	Increase	Decrease	Increase	Increase	Decrease	Increase
Flexion	Decrease	Increase	Decrease	Decrease	Increase	Decrease
Straight leg raising	−	+	+ with stress	−	−	+ with stress
Plain x-ray	−	−	+	−	+	+
Computed tomography	−	Disc herniation	Canal narrowing	−	Joint arthritis	Canal narrowing
Magnetic resonance	−	Disc herniation	Canal narrowing	−	Joint arthritis	Canal narrowing

methods. Patients with systemic disorders have fever or weight loss, severe nocturnal pain, prolonged morning stiffness, pain associated with fracture, or viscerogenic pain from the cardiovascular, gastrointestinal, or genitourinary systems. Additional radiographic and laboratory tests confirm the suspicions generated during the general examination. Radiographic examination for mechanical spinal pain reveals nonspecific findings that may be unassociated with pain generation. Individuals who are asymptomatic may have abnormal findings on magnetic resonance (MR) imaging (10). In addition, MR scans are unable to predict who is at risk of developing spinal pain over time (11). The majority of individuals with spinal pain can be treated with nonsurgical management without the need for diagnostic testing that involves invasive procedures.

THERAPEUTIC INTERVENTIONS

Treatment of acute spinal pain differs from treatment of chronic spinal pain. Therapies that are appropriate for individuals with chronic pain may not be indicated for patients with acute symptoms. A reasonable goal for therapy of acute spine pain is 100% pain relief and return to normal function, whereas the goal for therapy of chronic spine pain is maximizing function. Total relief of pain may not be achieved when pain has been present for an extended period of time. Many therapies have been proposed for spinal pain without clinical investigation to determine their efficacy. Scientifically proven therapies for acute or chronic spinal pain are few compared with other common medical disorders.

Treatment Guidelines for Spinal Pain

In December 1994, the Agency for Health Care Policy and Research (AHCPR) published a 160-page *Clinical Practice Guideline* booklet on the diagnosis and management of acute low back pain, based on recommendations of a multidisciplinary panel of practitioners that reviewed 3,918 published scientific articles (12). The panel made recommendations concerning initial assessment, clinical care, and special studies and diagnostic considerations, including surgery. The articles for diagnosis and therapy were rated from A (studies with strong research-based evidence) to D (those with published articles that did not meet inclusion criteria for study design). Greatest support was given to randomized, controlled trials. In the absence of such trials, evidence was described as weak or indirect. In these circumstances, the potential benefit of an intervention had to outweigh its potential risks to be considered cost effective.

Therapeutic interventions recommended by the panel are listed in Table 2. Most recommendations are based on a small number of articles, although thousands were reviewed. In addition, certain therapies

were not recommended because of the absence of scientific studies demonstrating efficacy, not because of the absence of possible benefit. For example, muscle relaxants were not recommended. Additional studies, however, have been added to the medical literature that support the use of muscle relaxants (13). Study design may also limit the potential to demonstrate efficacy. For example, investigations of epidural corticosteroid injections that measure benefit at 1 week and at 6 months will miss the beneficial effects of the therapy that occur in the 2nd to 12th weeks (14). The relationship between specific disorders and treatment recommendations is lacking. It is also important to remember that the guidelines do not apply to disorders associated with chronic low back pain.

Other diagnostic and treatment plans have been developed based upon evidence-based guidelines and best-practice principles (15). Thoughtful therapeutic plans are available that describe the relative benefits of physical, pharmacologic, and cognitive-behavioral therapies for acute, subacute, and chronic spinal pain (16). The problem is not the existence of guidelines, but their application in the clinical setting.

Therapy for Acute Mechanical Spine Pain

The therapy of acute mechanical low back and neck pain should incorporate some of the AHCPR guidelines along with practical recommendations that patients can follow. Many of the recommendations for treatment of mechanical disorders of the low back are also applicable to the neck.

Muscle Strain. Therapy for acute muscle strain of the spine includes controlled physical activity, nonsteroidal antiinflammatory drugs (NSAIDs), muscle relaxants, and physical therapy. Muscle strains improve with gradually increased physical activity. However, there are upper limits on the extent of exercises early in the course of a spinal pain episode. Individuals who believe that an early return to usual exercise programs is appropriate are at risk of reinjury. Patients should be encouraged to remain in bed only for limited periods of time. A period as short as 2 days has been shown to be effective at relieving acute back and neck pain (17). Limiting physical activity initially allows the injured tissues to rest, permitting a greater opportunity for healing without reinjury; however, prolonged bed rest results in deconditioning that is detrimental to muscle function. As soon as acute pain diminishes, encourage patients to increase physical activity. This might include walking for increasing periods of time each day. Increasing evidence supports resumption of normal activity early in the course of muscle strain to maximize the return to full function. Research in Finland showed the efficacy of bed rest for 2 days, back-mobilizing exercises, or ordinary activity as tolerated for low back pain therapy (18). Better recovery, improved function, and fewer missed work days were associated with ordinary physical activity.

Table 2. Agency for Health Care Policy and Research (AHCPR) guidelines for management of acute low back pain

I. Patient education

Patients with acute low back problems should be given accurate information about the following (strength of evidence = B):
- A. Expectations for both rapid recovery and recurrence of symptoms based on natural history of low back symptoms.
- B. Safe and effective methods of symptom control.
- C. Safe and reasonable activity modifications.
- D. Best means of limiting recurrent low back problems.
- E. The lack of need for special investigations unless red flags are present.
- F. Effectiveness and risks of commonly available diagnostic and further treatment measures to be considered should symptoms persist.

II. Medications

Acetaminophen and nonsteroidal antiinflammatory drugs (NSAIDs)
- A. Acetaminophen is reasonably safe and is acceptable for treating patients with acute low back problems (strength of evidence = C).
- B. NSAIDs, including aspirin, are acceptable for treating patients with acute low back problems (strength of evidence = B).
- C. NSAIDs have a number of potential side effects. The most frequent complication is gastrointestinal irritation. The decision to use these medications can be guided by comorbidity, side effects, cost, and patient and provider preference (strength of evidence = C).

III. Physical treatments

Spinal manipulation
- A. Manipulation can be helpful for patients with acute low back problems without radiculopathy when used within the first month of symptoms (strength of evidence = B).
- B. A trial of manipulation in patients without radiculopathy with symptoms longer than 1 month is probably safe, but efficacy is unproven (strength of evidence = C).

IV. Activity modification

Activity recommendations for bed rest and exercise
- A. A gradual return to normal activities is more effective than prolonged bed rest for treating acute low back problems (strength of evidence = B).
- B. Prolonged bed rest for more than 4 days may lead to debilitation and is not recommended for acute low back problems (strength of evidence = B).
- C. Low-stress aerobic exercise can prevent debilitation due to inactivity during the first month of symptoms and thereafter may help to return patients to the highest level of functioning appropriate to their circumstances (strength of evidence = C).

Non-narcotic analgesics, such as NSAIDs, relieve pain and allow patients to be more mobile. Nonsteroidal drugs with a rapid onset of action and analgesic properties are most helpful in patients with acute pain (19). Muscle relaxants may be helpful for patients who have palpable, paraspinous muscular spasm on physical examination or difficulty sleeping at night because of muscle pain. The muscle relaxant may be given 2–3 hours before sleep to limit somnolence the following morning. Cyclobenzaprine is effective as a muscle relaxant without causing somnolence (13). The combination of an NSAID with a muscle relaxant is better than an NSAID alone at improving pain relief in acute low back pain patients with muscle spasm (20). Physical modalities, in the form of ice massage initially or warm baths subsequently, may also decrease pain and diminish spasm.

Local areas of muscle spasm in the lumbar or cervical spine may be resistant to oral medications. On physical exam, the areas of spasm are identified to be firm to palpation, with radiation of pain to surrounding muscles. This "trigger point" may be injected with a combination of a local anesthetic and semisoluble corticosteroid preparation. These injections are effective in breaking the pain–spasm cycle that results in muscle tightness. If injections are contraindicated (for example, in patients with sensitivity to local anesthetics), acupressure over the trigger point may also offer symptomatic relief.

Many health care professionals play important roles in the recovery of patients with low back or neck pain. Physical therapists offer pain-relieving modalities early in the course of back or neck strain. Subsequently, range-of-motion and strengthening exercises restore function to baseline levels as pain lessens. Manipulation by a chiropractor may be helpful early in the course of back pain that is unassociated with leg pain. Massage therapy improves the range of motion of contracted muscles. Although these therapeutic modalities are frequently prescribed, the clinical evidence that proves the efficacy of these interventions is limited (21).

Whiplash. Treatment of whiplash with active cervical rotation is better than standard care, which includes initial rest, soft cervical collar, and gradual self-mobilization (22). A cervical collar increases muscle stiffness and slows recovery; therefore, whiplash patients are encouraged to discontinue the use of a cervical collar within a few days of the injury. Mild analgesics, NSAIDs, and muscle relaxants are prescribed

to encourage motion of the neck. Most patients improve after about 4 weeks of therapy. Patients with symptoms that persist longer than 6 months rarely experience significant improvement. The mechanism of chronic pain in whiplash patients remains to be determined. Prolonged disability from a whiplash injury is associated with litigation (23).

Acute Herniated Nucleus Pulposus. The treatment for most patients with a herniated disc is nonoperative; 80% will respond to conservative medical therapy. Patient education is essential for a successful outcome, as the patient must understand the natural history of resolution of disc herniation. The initial component of therapy is controlled physical activity with the patient in a semi-Fowler's position in bed. Once back and leg pain lessen, encourage the patient to walk. Bed rest does not hasten improvement compared with activity as tolerated, and it causes muscle deconditioning (24).

Drug therapy in the form of NSAIDs, analgesics, and muscle relaxants decreases pain and inflammation. NSAIDs are important for the control of leg and arm pain, because inflammation of the nerve root is the source of sciatica and brachialgia in disc herniation patients. NSAIDs with prolonged action may be better able to control symptoms. Analgesic medications, including narcotics, may be used for severe pain; however, other analgesics should be substituted for narcotics as soon as pain diminishes. Epidural corticosteroid injections are indicated for patients whose continued sciatica does not respond to 2–4 weeks of conservative therapy. Epidural injections are helpful in decreasing pain early in the course of sciatica (25).

Surgical intervention is reserved for patients in whom all forms of conservative therapy fail. Patients with sciatica, abnormal physical findings, and confirmatory radiographic tests are candidates for discectomy. The success rate for lumbar discectomy ranges from 70% to 95% depending upon the duration of followup (26,27). Surgical intervention for cervical disc herniation is also reported to be successful in a majority of patients with brachialgia and corresponding anatomic abnormalities. For cervical disc herniations, opinion is divided on the need for cervical fusion in addition to discectomy (28). Fusion requires a bone graft harvested from another surgical site (iliac bone), which may become an additional area of pain. However, patients with cervical fusions have a return to function and more rapid pain relief.

Rehabilitation Considerations for Spine

- Provide local application of heat or cold dependent on acuity and presentation of symptoms.
- Conduct ergonomic assessment to address ergonomic factors.
- Prescribe exercises that are specific to the condition and clinical presentation.
- Restore flexibility of associated muscle groups.
- Assess posture and store neutral posture.
- Patient education in self-management skills is important to avoid future injuries or to prevent exacerbation of symptoms.

Therapy for Chronic Mechanical Spine Pain

Myelopathy. Nonsurgical therapy should be attempted for cervical myelopathy patients without severe neurologic compromise or for those who are poor surgical risks. Conservative therapy includes immobilization with a firm cervical orthosis, NSAIDs, epidural corticosteroid injections, and cervical traction. However, in general, myelopathy is a surgical disease for individuals with associated neurologic abnormalities. The goal of surgery is to decompress the spinal cord to prevent further spinal cord compression and vascular compromise. Surgical intervention has the best opportunity to yield improvement before irreversible damage is sustained by the cervical spinal cord. Compared with medically treated patients, surgically treated patients have better early outcomes with greater functional recovery (29). However, the benefit may wane as individuals are tested at longer followup evaluations at 1 year or longer (30). This may be related to progression of the underlying arthritis.

Spinal Stenosis. Patients with lumbar spinal stenosis have pain that progresses over an extended period of time. The majority of individuals with spinal stenosis can be treated nonsurgically. Education about appropriate spinal biomechanics used in activities of daily living and those positions of the spine that exacerbate back and leg pain is a key component. Inflammation of the soft tissues in the spinal canal and neural foramina result in compression of neural elements.

NSAIDs are useful in decreasing inflammation, soft tissue swelling, and neural compression, and they may be used for an extended period of time while improvement of function continues. Due to the increased age in many patients with spinal stenosis, increased sensitivity to NSAID toxicities—particularly those of the gastrointestinal tract—must be considered. The utility of epidural corticosteroid injections for spinal stenosis is questionable, because they tend to be more effective for radicular pain associated with herniated intervertebral discs than for spinal stenosis. If used, I may prescribe the following course: order 1 lumbar epidural injection and observe the clinical response; then order another injection as soon as 8 weeks after the initial injection if leg symptoms return; a total of 3 injections may be given over 6 months; the series of 3 injections may be repeated every 6 months.

Surgical decompression should be considered for patients with neurogenic claudication that severely limits function. These patients are unable to walk one block or have radicular pain when standing. The first operation has the greatest opportunity for relief of symptoms. In a study of 251 patients with spinal stenosis who underwent decompression surgery, 67% had an excellent or good outcome (31). Good operative outcome was reduced to only 46% of 66 patients with repeat decompressive operations.

Chronic Pain Therapy

A small but significant proportion of spine patients do not respond to acute therapy and require prolonged nonsurgical management. In chronic pain management, the patient must be convinced that the goal of therapy is to maximize physical function. A combination of therapies is necessary to reach this goal. Exercise programs that improve aerobic conditioning and range of motion are helpful. Patients may benefit from increased NSAID dosages or switching to a different chemical class of NSAID. Tricyclic antidepressants offer additional pain relief mediated through the central nervous system. The use of narcotic analgesics is generally discouraged, but they may be used at a specific dosage to facilitate function. A study of patients with chronic low back pain receiving narcotic pain relievers demonstrated improvement of spinal pain without episodes of toxicity, addiction, or dose escalation (32). Long-acting narcotics may decrease pain to allow a return to work without the waxing and waning effect of short-acting agents. Once a regular work schedule is established, a gradual decrease of dosage is attempted while function is maintained. Some individuals are unable to reduce their narcotic requirement without a deterioration in physical function and require constant levels of narcotic medications for extended periods. The benefits and detriments of this form of therapy must be constantly reviewed by the physician and patient.

Return to employment or other productive pursuits is an important goal of therapy. Movement of the back or neck improves function and counters the inactivity that can exacerbate pain. The appearance of new symptoms or marked exacerbation of preexisting problems is an indication for reevaluation.

REFERENCES

1. Deyo RA, Weinstein JN. Low back pain. N Engl J Med 2001;344:363–70.
2. Borenstein DG, Wiesel SW, Boden SD. Low back and neck pain: comprehensive diagnosis and management. 3rd ed. Philadelphia: WB Saunders; 2004.
3. Cherkin DC, Deyo RA, Wheeler K, Ciol MA. Physician views about treating low back pain. The results of a national survey. Spine 1995;20:1–20.
4. Koes BW, van Tulder MW, Ostelo R, Kim Burton AK, Waddell G. Clinical guidelines for the management of low back pain in primary care: an international comparison. Spine 2001;26:2504–14.
5. Croft PR, Macfarlane GJ, Papageorgiou AC, Thomas E, Silman AJ. Outcome of low back pain in general practice: a prospective study. BMJ 1998;316:1356–9.
6. van den Hoogen HJ, Koes BW, Deville W, van Eijk JT, Bouter LM. The prognosis of low back pain in general practice. Spine 1997;22:1515–21.
7. Spitzer WO, Skovron ML, Salmi LR, Cassidy JD, Duranceau J, Suissa S. Scientific monograph of the Quebec Task Force on Whiplash-Associated Disorders: redefining "whiplash" and its management. Spine 1995; 20(8 Suppl):1S–73S.
8. Bernhardt M, Hynes RA, Blume HW, White AA 3rd. Cervical spondylotic myelopathy. J Bone Joint Surg Am 1993;75:119–28.
9. Carragee EJ. Clinical practice. Persistent low back pain. N Engl J Med 2005;352:1891–8.
10. Boos N, Semmer N, Elfering A, Schade V, Gal I, Zanetti M. Natural history of individuals with asymptomatic disc abnormalities in magnetic resonance imaging: predictors of low back pain-related medical consultation and work incapacity. Spine 2000;25:1484–92.
11. Borenstein DG, O'Mara JW Jr, Boden SD, Lauerman WC, Jacobson A, Platenberg C. The value of magnetic resonance imaging of the lumbar spine to predict low-back pain in asymptomatic subjects: a seven-year follow-up study. J Bone Joint Surg Am 2001;83A;1306–11.
12. Bigos S, Bowyer O, Braen G, Brown KC, Deyo RA, Haldeman S. Acute low back problems in adults. Rockville (MD): Agency for Health Care Policy and Research, Public Health Service, U.S. Department of Health and Human Services. December 1994. Clinical Practice Guideline No. 14. AHCPR Publication No.95-0642.
13. Borenstein DG, Korn S. Efficacy of a low-dose regimen of cyclobenzaprine hydrochloride in acute skeletal muscle spasm: results of two placebo-controlled trials. Clin Ther 2003;25:1056–73.
14. Spaccarelli KC. Lumbar and caudal epidural corticosteroid injections. Mayo Clin Proc 1996;71:169–78.
15. Weiser S, Rossignol M. Triage for nonspecific lower-back pain. Clin Orthop Relat Res 2006;443:147–55.
16. Nordin M, Balague F, Cedraschi C. Nonspecific lower-back pain: surgical versus nonsurgical treatment. Clin Orthop Relat Res 2006;443:156–67.

17. Deyo RA, Diehl AK, Rosenthal M. How many days of bed rest for acute low back pain? A randomized clinical trial. N Engl J Med 1986;315:1064–70.

18. Malmivaara A, Hakkinen U, Aro T, Heinrichs M, Koskenniemi L, Kuosma E. The treatment of acute low back pain—bed rest, exercises, or ordinary activity? N Engl J Med 1995;332:351–5.

19. van Tulder MW, Scholten RJ, Koes BW, Deyo RA. Nonsteroidal anti-inflammatory drugs for low back pain: a systematic review within the framework of the Cochrane Collaboration Back Review Group. Spine 2000;25:2501–13.

20. Cherkin DC, Wheeler KJ, Barlow W, Deyo RA. Medication use for low back pain in primary care. Spine 1998;23:607–14.

21. Cherkin DC, Sherman KJ, Deyo RA, Shekelle PG. A review of the evidence for the effectiveness, safety, and cost of acupuncture, massage therapy, and spinal manipulation for back pain. Ann Intern Med 2003;138:898–906.

22. Rosenfeld M, Seferiadis A, Carlsson J, Gunnarsson R. Active intervention in patients with whiplash-associated disorders improves long-term prognosis: a randomized controlled clinical trial. Spine 2003;28:2491–8.

23. Gun RT, Osti OL, O'Riordan A, Mpelasoka F, Eckerwall CG, Smyth JF. Risk factors for prolonged disability after whiplash injury: a prospective study. Spine 2005;30:386–91.

24. Vroomen PC, de Krom MC, Wilmink JT, Kester AD, Knottnerus JA. Lack of effectiveness of bed rest for sciatica. N Engl J Med 1999;340:418–23.

25. Buchner M, Zeifang F, Brocai DR, Schiltenwolf M. Epidural corticosteroid injection in the conservative management of sciatica. Clin Orthop Relat Res 2000;375:149–56.

26. McCullogh JA. Focus issue on lumbar disc herniation: macro- and micro-discectomy. Spine 1996;21(24 Suppl):45S–56S.

27. Awad JN, Moskovich R. Lumbar disc herniations: surgical versus nonsurgical treatment. Clin Orthop Relat Res 2006;443:183–97.

28. Irwin ZN, Hilibrand A, Gustavel M, McLain R, Shaffer W, Myers M. Variation in surgical decision making for degenerative spinal disorders. Part II: cervical spine. Spine 2005;30:2214–9.

29. Sampath P, Bendebba M, Davis JD, Ducker TB. Outcome of patients treated for cervical myelopathy. A prospective, multicenter study with independent clinical review. Spine 2000;25:670–6.

30. Fouyas IP, Statham PF, Sandercock PA. Cochrane review on the role of surgery in cervical spondylitic radiculomyelopathy. Spine 2002;27:736–47.

31. Herno A, Airaksinen O, Saari T, Silhoven T. Surgical results of lumbar spinal stenosis. A comparison of patients with or without previous back surgery. Spine 1995;20:964–9.

32. Mahowald ML, Singh JA, Majeski P. Opioid use by patients in an orthopedics spine clinic. Arthritis Rheum 2005;52:312–21.

Additional Recommended Reading

Borenstein DG. Disorders of the low back and neck. In: Klippel JH, editor. Primer on the rheumatic diseases. 12th ed. Atlanta: Arthritis Foundation; 2001. p. 165–73.

Borenstein DG. Back in control! A conventional and complementary prescription for eliminating back pain. New York: M Evans and Company; 2001.

Liebson C, editor. Rehabilitation of the spine: a practitioner's manual. 2nd ed. Philadelphia: Lippincott, Williams & Wilkins; 2007.

Myopathies

LISA CHRISTOPHER-STINE, MD, MPH

Idiopathic inflammatory myopathies (IIM) encompass 3 more common diseases—polymyositis (PM), dermatomyositis (DM), and inclusion body myositis (IBM)—and a number of rarer entities. The clinical, laboratory, and pathologic diagnostic criteria proposed by Bohan and Peter are the most familiar and accepted definitions of PM and DM and have been used in the majority of clinical trials (1,2). Additional useful classification criteria have been suggested by Tanimoto et al and by Targoff et al (Table 1) (3,4). IBM was not part of the original classification scheme but is now commonly included. Although other classification criteria systems for IBM have been devised (Table 2), characteristic muscle biopsy features remain the defining element (5).

ETIOLOGY AND EPIDEMIOLOGY

The inflammatory myopathies are rare conditions, and the etiology remains unknown. The incidence of PM is estimated to be between 2.18 and 7.7 cases per million per year. Medsger et al and Oddis et al (6,7) found an increasing incidence in 2 separate studies performed 20 years apart, although this may represent improved diagnostic accuracy rather than an actual increase. Incidence increases with age, with the highest rates being seen in the 35–44 and 55–64-year age groups. There are few epidemiologic studies that address incidence among nonwhite racial groups. Oddis et al found a 4-fold increase in incidence in black men compared with white men and a nearly threefold increase in black women compared with white women (6,7). Overall, there is a female:male ratio of ~2:1 in PM and DM. One study was undertaken to determine whether climactic and geographic factors influence the distribution of DM, PM, and associated autoantibodies. Of the variables evaluated in univariate and multivariate analyses, surface ultraviolet radiation intensity most strongly contributed to DM and was strongly related to anti–Mi-2 autoantibodies (8). This study suggested that ultraviolet radiation may modify the clinical and histopathologic expression of autoimmune muscle disease in various populations.

IBM, in contrast, is more common in men. IBM has only recently been recognized as a distinct entity from PM and is treated differently as well; thus, epidemiologic information about IBM is more limited. Several investigative groups have observed that IBM may be the most common inflammatory myopathy in individuals older than 50 years of age. The argument has been made, however, that IBM should not be included among the inflammatory myopathies because inflammation is often sparse with only a secondary role, and the response to antiinflammatory therapy is minimal (9).

In an international collaborative effort, the International Myositis Assessment and Clinical Studies Group is working to standardize diagnostic and classification criteria, particularly for clinical trials. It is anticipated that this working group will facilitate the development of future prospective multicenter interdisciplinary studies incorporating clinical, laboratory, and pathologic information using standardized and validated measures and methods (10).

PATHOGENESIS

The pathogenesis and mechanism of cell injury of autoimmune inflammatory myopathies remain unclear. Although there are cases of myositis in which frank inflammation is absent on muscle biopsy, it is generally accepted that inflammation, driven by autoimmunity, is the major cause of muscle damage. Accumulating data suggest that autoantigens are critical in driving the concomitant autoimmune response. Furthermore, unique changes in antigen expression may play a role in antigen selection and ongoing damage, as may conformational changes in both the immunizing tumor and target tissue when malignancy is present (11).

Autoantibodies—albeit not necessarily directed at muscle-specific antigens—are found in the majority of cases of PM and DM, but not commonly in IBM. In many cases these antibodies are unique to myositis. It remains unclear, however, whether the autoantibodies themselves play a pathogenetic role or whether they are epiphenomena. Many have observed that skeletal muscle fibers do not constitutively express major histocompatibility complex (MHC) class I molecules, yet the muscle fibers of patients with myositis demonstrate high levels of MHC class I expression. The logical assumption is that the MHC-expressing muscle cells present important self antigens to T cells residing in the inflamed muscle tissue, but this scenario is not verified and remains speculative. Because of the paucity of traditional costimulatory cells in muscle, the ability of muscle cells to function as professional antigen-presenting cells remains uncertain (12).

Significant advances have been made in better characterizing disease mechanisms in myositis. DM and PM have been most often distinguished clinically by the presence or absence of characteristic rashes; however, it is increasingly appreciated that muscle biopsy features, although overlapping, are also disparate (13). Some persuasive observations support a primary role for endomysial invasion by CD8+ T cells in PM, and a vasculopathy with a humoral immune basis in DM. Although certain immunopathologic features, which reflect different pathologic mechanisms, have been incorporated in the development of a new classification scheme (14), that effort may be premature because the proposed histologic findings are not generally available outside of academic settings. Furthermore, this scheme ignores other well-studied features without offering evidence that the prognosis and response to therapy—the true concerns of patients and physicians—are better represented.

Although apoptosis has not been recognized histologically in myositis, it is thought that granzyme B and perforin have roles, especially in PM (15,16). Casciola-Rosen and colleagues have determined that the development of some myositis-specific antibodies, as well as other autoantibodies, may involve the unique susceptibility of targeted antigens to granzyme B cleavage (17). The role of local cytokines has not been established, but some of the autoantigens—most notably Jo-1—have chemokine-like properties and may therefore recruit inflammatory cells to sites of muscle cell injury (18).

In earlier studies, careful investigation for candidate viruses showed negative results, but several other viral etiologies (including human immunodeficiency virus, human T-lymphotropic virus, hepatitis C,

Table 1. Current idiopathic inflammatory myopathy diagnostic criteria*

Bohan and Peter Criteria (1,2)	Targoff proposed criteria (3)	Tanimoto proposed criteria (4)
1. Symmetrical proximal muscle weakness	1. Symmetrical proximal muscle weakness	1. Symmetrical proximal muscle weakness
2. Skeletal muscle enzyme elevation	2. Skeletal muscle enzyme elevation	2. Skeletal muscle enzyme elevation
3. Abnormal EMG[†]	3. Abnormal EMG[†]	3. Abnormal EMG[†]
4. Muscle biopsy abnormalities[‡]	4. Muscle biopsy abnormalities[‡]	4. Muscle biopsy abnormalities[‡]
5. Typical skin rash of DM[§]	5. Typical skin rash of dermatomyositis[§]	5. Typical skin rash of dermatomyositis[§]
	6. **One of the myositis-specific antibodies**	6. **Muscle pain**
	7. **MRI may substitute for criterion 1 or 2**	7. **Positive anti-Jo-1 antibody**
		8. **Nondestructive arthritis/arthralgia**
		9. **Systemic inflammatory signs[#]**

* For the Bohan and Peter criteria: Possible PM = any 2 of the first 4 criteria; possible DM = criterion 5 (rash) plus any 2 criteria; probable PM = any 3 of the first 4 criteria; probable DM = criterion 5 (rash) plus any 3 criteria; definite PM = all 4 of the first 4 criteria; definite DM = criterion 5 (rash) plus all 4 other criteria. For the Targoff criteria: Possible IIM = any 2 criteria; probable IIM = any 3 criteria; definite IIM = any 4 criteria; MRI results consistent with inflammation may be substituted for criterion 1 or 2. For the Tanimoto criteria: Rash plus at least 4 of the other 8 items = DM; 4 of the items excluding rash = PM (no definite, probable, or possible categories). EMG = electromyography; DM = dermatomyositis; PM = polymyositis; IIM = idiopathic inflammatory myopathy; MRI = magnetic resonance imaging.
† Abnormal EMG may include polyphasic, short, small motor-unit potentials; fibrillation, positive sharp waves, insertional irritability; bizarre, high-frequency, repetitive discharges
‡ Muscle biopsy abnormalities may include degeneration/regeneration, perifascicular atrophy, necrosis, phagocytosis, fiber size variation, and mononuclear inflammatory infiltrate.
§ Skin rash would include Gottron's sign, heliotrope rash.
# Systemic signs may include temperature >37° C, elevated C-reactive protein, erythrocyte sedimentation rate >20 mm by Westergren method.

and parvovirus B-19) have been postulated, although not proven, in the etiology of some cases of inflammatory myopathy (19).

Proposed pathogenic mechanisms for IBM include increased transcription and accumulation of beta-amyloid precursor protein and its proteolytic fragment; abnormal accumulations of the components of lipid metabolism, and oxidative stress (20). These characteristics, in concert with misfolded or unfolded proteins in the context of a cellular aging environment, appear to contribute to the pathogenesis of IBM. Recently, mutations in the UDP-*N*-acetylglucosamine 2-epimerase/ *N*-acetylmannosamine kinase gene have been recognized in some cases of IBM (21).

CLINICAL PRESENTATION AND EXAMINATION

Muscular Manifestations

The clinical hallmark of PM and DM is the gradual onset over weeks to months of symmetrical proximal muscle weakness. Weakness is most often found in deltoids and hip flexors. Patients may complain of being unable to rise from a low-seated chair or to comb their hair. Although myalgiais are sometimes present at disease onset or during therapy, as muscle strength rebounds, it is *weakness* and not pain that is the defining muscle-related complaint. Dermatomyositis has, in addition, characteristic skin findings, including a heliotrope rash, Gottron's sign, and the shawl and V signs. Although patients with rashes typical of dermatomyositis but unaccompanied by muscle disease have been described, the appearance of diagnostic DM rashes is typically followed by myositis within 1 or 2 years in the majority of such cases. Some patients, however, remain free of muscle disease, and have so-called "amyopathic dermatomyositis" or "dermatomyositis sine myositis" (22).

IBM differs in its clinical presentation, as its hallmark is usually atrophy and weakness of the quadriceps and the wrist and finger flexors, producing both proximal (early) and distal (late) weakness. A "scooped out" forearm appearance is a specific phenotypic element that may alert the examiner as well. A history of frequent falls is common. In addition, polyneuropathy and facial weakness are occasional IBM-associated features seen only rarely in PM and DM. Extramuscular manifestations are not appreciated in IBM.

Extramuscular Manifestations of PM and DM

Organ systems affected in addition to muscle and skin include the heart (arrythmias, congestive heart failure, and myocarditis), lung (fibrosing alveolitis, aspiration, and most notably, interstitial lung disease), gastrointestinal tract (dysphagia and, in rare instances, intestinal vasculitis), and joints (arthralgia and nondeforming symmetric arthritis). As described below, autoantibody status may help to predict the extramuscular clinical phenotype.

Pulmonary Involvement. Several recent studies have helped to clarify pulmonary involvement in myositis. A survey of 70 people with clinical and radiographic evidence of pulmonary fibrosis or interstitial pneumonia was gathered from 973 patients evaluated at the Mayo Clinic. Surgical lung biopsies were carried out on 22. Of these, 18 had nonspecific interstitial pneumonia (NSIP), of whom 11 had fibrosis. Two had diffuse alveolar damage, and 1 each had usual interstitial pneumonia and bronchiolitis obliterans organizing pneumonia (23). In a series of 156 patients in France, 36 demonstrated pulmonary involvement. A high morbidity rate, including 5 deaths, was noted. In this series, a substantial proportion of patients (19.2%) improved or even showed a resolution of their lung disease (24). In a series from Japan, an unusually high incidence of interstitial lung disease was found; most patients had NSIP or usual interstitial pneumonia. Diffusion capacity and high-resolution computed tomography (CT) were especially sensitive in detecting this disease. An elevation in the serum level of KL-6, a pulmonary glycoprotein, acted as a marker of clinically active lung disease (25). A recent retrospective review of CT findings of 14 patients with NSIP associated with PM and DM over an average followup duration of 27.6 months (range 3–61 months) concluded that, with treatment, serial CT scans showed an improvement in ground-glass and/or reticular opacities with limited radiographic

Table 2.   Inclusion body myositis (IBM) diagnostic criteria

I.   **Diagnostic classification**
  A.   *Definite* IBM
     Patients must exhibit all muscle biopsy features.* None of the other clinical or laboratory features are mandatory if muscle biopsy features are diagnostic.
  B.   *Probable* IBM
     If the muscle biopsy shows inflammation and vacuolated fibers without other pathologic features of IBM, then a diagnosis of probable IBM can be given if the patient exhibits the characteristic clinical (II.A. 1,2,3) and laboratory (II.B. 1) features.

II.   **Characteristic features**
A.   Clinical features
  1.   Duration of illness >6 months
  2.   Age of onset >30 years
  3.   Muscle weakness
  Must affect proximal and distal muscles of arms and legs and patient must exhibit at least one of the following:
    a.   Finger flexor weakness
    b.   Wrist flexor > wrist extensor weakness
    c.   Quadriceps muscle weakness

B.   Laboratory features
  1.   Serum CPK <12 times the upper limit of normal†
  2.   Muscle biopsy
    a.   Inflammatory myopathy characterized by mononuclear cell invasion of necrotic muscle fibers
    b.   Vacuolated muscle fibers
    c.   Either
      Intracellular amyloid deposits or 15–18-nm tubulofilaments by electron microscopy
  3.   Electromyography must be consistent with features of an inflammatory myopathy

* Invasion of nonnecrotic fibers by mononuclear cells, vacuolated muscle fibers, and intracellular (within muscle fibers) amyloid deposits of 15–18 nm.
† CPK = creatine phosphokinase.

progression of the fibrosis (26). Patients with anti–aminoacyl–transfer RNA synthetase autoantibodies, such as anti–Jo-1 and related autoantibodies, are more likely to have interstitial lung disease. Patients with amyopathic DM may develop potentially fatal interstitial lung disease and need appropriate screening and imaging (27).

Cardiac Involvement. Clinically significant heart disease—heart failure as a result of myocarditis or significant cardiac arrhythmias—is uncommon in myositis. There is a reported association between anti–signal recognition particle (anti-SRP) antibodies and cardiac involvement, largely based on 2 studies including a total of 20 patients (28,29). Of these subjects, only 1 was diagnosed with a true cardiomyopathy. Most patients had associated cardiac palpitations without additional documentation. More recent evidence suggests that anti-SRP antibodies may not contribute to cardiac involvement to the degree that was once suspected (30).

Myositis and Malignancy. The association between inflammatory myopathy and malignancy is well known, and several recent articles have enhanced our understanding of the relationship, although not the basic underlying mechanism. Almost all studies have demonstrated a higher association of malignancy with DM than with PM (31–33). However, malignancy may be associated with PM with a higher prevalence than previously thought because of the better classification of inflammatory myopathies (33). A large population-based study found an increased risk of cancer with both PM and DM (34). In these large studies and in a combined analysis of 3 large Scandinavian studies, the increased incidence declined over the years following the diagnosis but was still measurable as long as 5 years later in DM patients (35).

Several investigators have evaluated risk factors associated with malignancy in patients with inflammatory myopathy. DM appears to confer more risk than PM, although estimates of the difference between these 2 subgroups are quite variable. Increasing age, capillary damage on biopsy, cutaneous necrosis, cutaneous leukocytoclastic vasculitis, and cutaneous mucinosis appear to be positive risk factors for myositis-associated malignancy (34,36–38). Many associated malignancies have been reported and are generally commensurate with the incidence in the general population. Notable exceptions are an increase in cancers of the ovary, breast, lung, stomach, colon, nasopharynx, pancreas, and bladder, and for non-Hodgkin's lymphoma (34–42).

The ideal cancer-screening regimen necessary for patients with a new diagnosis of myositis, as well as the interval needed between such screenings, is under debate (32,42,43). Most agree that an age- and

sex-specific evaluation should be performed, as well as routine laboratory investigations, including a complete blood count, erythrocyte sedimentation rate, comprehensive metabolic profile, urinalysis, and chest radiograph. In women, obtaining a Pap smear, mammogram, uterine ultrasound, and serum CA-125 level are warranted. It is generally accepted that a digital rectal prostate examination should be performed and a serum prostate-specific antigen measurement ascertained in male patients older than 50 years of age. Upper and lower gastrointestinal endoscopy are generally recommended, but the exact screening age is unclear. Patients in high-risk categories, such as those with a family history of colon or breast cancer, or smokers, should undergo a more thorough evaluation. Total body CT or magnetic resonance image (MRI) "pan-scans" are not routinely recommended.

There are insufficient data upon which to recommend when, after a negative workup for malignancy, the evaluation should be repeated. Heightened vigilance, including careful physical examinations and routine laboratory tests, for several years following a diagnosis of PM or DM is encouraged. There are published reports of ovarian carcinoma occurring as late as 5 years after the diagnosis of DM, suggesting that an annual CA-125 serum assay with an annual pelvic examination and transvaginal ultrasound are warranted (44).

DIAGNOSIS AND LABORATORY TESTING

Although there are established criteria for the diagnosis of myositis (Table 1), the definitive diagnosis of an inflammatory myopathy in adults requires a muscle biopsy. To confirm the diagnosis and rule out conditions that may clinically resemble myositis (Table 3), a biopsy

Table 3.   Differential diagnosis of idiopathic inflammatory myopathies

- Limb girdle muscular dystrophies
- Metabolic myopathies
- Mitochondrial myopathies
- Neurologic diseases: motor neuron disease, Parkinson's disease, spinal muscular atrophy, myasthenia gravis, channelopathies
- Endocrine/immunologic disease: myxedema, stiff man syndrome, thyroxicosis
- Toxic myopathy (drug-associated): corticosteroids, statins, azathioprine, chloroquine, colchicine

Call the Doctor and Red Flags

- Symptoms of weakness during or after exercise or fasting are uncommon in idiopathic inflammatory myopathies (IIM) and may indicate a metabolic myopathy.
- Myalgia exceeding weakness or asymmetrical painful limbs lead against the diagnosis of IIM and suggest alternative diagnoses, including pyomyositis.
- Patients with IIM who are treated with corticosteroids and continue to be weak or become weak again after initial therapy may have a steroid myopathy. A normal creatine phosphokinase (CPK) despite increasing weakness suggests this diagnosis. Gradual reduction in corticosteroid dosage often restores muscle strength.
- When diagnosing inflammatory myopathies, there are several clues that lead one away from that diagnosis. Unlike many other rheumatic diseases, inflammatory myopathies are not generally heritable. In general, a _family history of a similar illness_ is a red flag for other disease states, most notably limb girdle muscular dystrophies and metabolic myopathies.
- Phenotypic features, such as calf pseudohypertrophy, winging scapulae, or early muscle atrophy, suggest a muscular dystrophy.
- CPK elevations >100-fold often signify a metabolic myopathy or toxic myopathy with rhabdomyolysis. Patients with a history of rhabomyolysis are at risk for additional episodes and should be counseled to stay well hydrated and seek medical attention if they note wine-colored or dark urine.
- Treatment-resistant polymyositis is often either improperly diagnosed (i.e., limb-girdle muscular dystrophy) or associated with a tumor.
- Patients with myopathies secondary to a known drug exposure, such as statin cholesterol-lowering medications, generally improve over weeks to months. Continual muscle-related symptoms or elevated muscle enzymes should prompt another diagnosis and warrants further evaluation by a specialist. A muscle biopsy may be indicated.

should be performed on every patient in whom the diagnosis of an inflammatory myopathy is considered. Furthermore, biopsy provides a histologic sample for comparison should a repeat biopsy be warranted if disease course worsens despite treatment.

Overall, biopsy results have a false-negative rate of 10–25% due to the unevenness of distribution of the tissue pathology. Not only are some entire muscles neighboring inflamed muscles often spared, but the inflammation is also not uniformly distributed within a muscle or even within a fascicle. MRI guidance can reduce the false-negative rate by increasing sensitivity and enhancing the negative predictive value (45,46). Occasionally, a muscle biopsy may not demonstrate a mononuclear cell infiltrate if therapy has been started, but other pathologic changes may persist. Similarly, in some cases of subacute necrotizing myopathy, an inflammatory infiltrate may be absent, but this should not delay therapy because this entity may be steroid responsive (45–47).

In addition to a careful history, family history, and laboratory tests, both electromyography and imaging studies (particularly MRI) may serve as useful adjuncts to diagnosis. MRI can also be helpful in selecting a site for biopsy.

Muscle enzyme levels, including creatine kinase (CK) and aldolase, are almost universally elevated. Usually, aspartate aminotransferase and sometimes alanine aminotransferase or alkaline phosphatase (all of which may come from muscle as well as liver) may also be elevated, and they are often erroneously mistaken as indications of liver disease.

In a small number of cases (<5%), muscle enzyme measurements are not elevated even on repeated testing. Extreme elevations (>100-fold higher than the upper limit of normal) in CK are very rare in myositis and prompt a careful search for another diagnosis.

Electromyographic testing may demonstrate evidence of an "irritable myopathy" (polyphasic, short, small motor-unit potentials; fibrillation,

positive sharp waves, insertional irritability; bizarre, high-frequency, repetitive discharges).

Antinuclear antibody level is nonspecifically elevated in many PM and DM patients, but its absence should not preclude the disease. Other associated autoantibodies include anti-Ro and antisynthetase autoantibodies (including anti–Jo-1, which is the only commercially available myositis-specific antibody available).

TREATMENT AND MANAGEMENT PRINCIPLES

There is high morbidity and substantial mortality associated with IIM; therefore, prompt recognition and therapy is essential. A retrospective series determined the overall mortality rate to be as high as 22%, largely from cancer and pulmonary complications (48). To date, DM has proved the most treatable inflammatory myopathy, responding to steroids, intravenous immunoglobulin (IVIG), or immunosuppressants. PM is usually also responsive to immunosuppressant therapy, but the response may vary depending on autoantibody association and the clinical phenotype (49). IBM is the most treatment-resistant subset of myositis.

Corticosteroids

Corticosteroids remain the initial agents of choice in the treatment of all inflammatory myopathies. Corticosteroids improve clinical weakness and reduce serum muscle enzyme elevations. Corticosteroids appear to be most helpful for the improvement of DM and PM. There is clearly a much less robust and sustained response in IBM patients. Although no controlled trial supports the use of corticosteroids, many experts give an initial pulse dose of 1 gram of methylprednisolone intravenously daily for 1–3 days in an attempt to shorten disease course and to enhance the possibility of a clinical remission. The exact duration and dosage of subsequent corticosteroid oral therapy has not been studied systematically, and current dosing regimens are largely based on empirical data and anecdotal evidence. Steroid-sparing agents are required in a substantial number of patients to decrease long-term steroid side effects and to attain a satisfactory antiinflammatory response. In many clinics, supplemental immunosuppressive therapy is now started very early.

Steroid-Sparing Agents

Dermatomyositis and Polymyositis. Additional immunosuppressive agents currently used in the treatment of autoimmune inflammatory myopathies include azathioprine (50,51), methotrexate (51), IVIG, mycophenolate mofetil (52,53), intravenous gammaglobulin (54,55), tacrolimus (56), and cyclosporin A (57). Few randomized clinical trials have been conducted with these agents, and the impetus for their use arises from either small case series or the accumulated clinical experience gathered in large clinics (58). Several reports support the use of combinations of these immunosuppressive therapies. Tacrolimus, a calcineurin inhibitor used to prevent rejection in transplant patients, is a promising, effective, well-tolerated therapy for managing refractory interstitial lung disease and myositis as part of the antisynthetase syndrome (59).

Inclusion Body Myositis. IBM typically has a much slower course of response to therapy. A positive treatment benefit may only be realized after several years of treatment, but many clinical trial endpoints occur after a few months (60). A randomized, double-blind, parallel-group

Rehabilitation Considerations in Myositis

- The 3 more common diseases are polymyositis (PM), dermatomyositis (DM), and inclusion body myositis (IBM).
- There is high morbidity and mortality associated with these conditions.
- With PM and DM, gradual onset of symmetrical proximal muscle weakness (deltoids and hip flexors) over weeks to months is commonly seen. It is weakness not muscle pain that is the defining muscle-related complaint.
- Skin manifestations will also been seen with DM.
- The clinical presentation of IBM differs and is typically atrophy and weakness of the quadriceps and the wrist and finger flexors, producing both proximal (early) and distal (late) weakness. A "scooped out" forearm appearance is a specific phenotypic element, and a history of frequent falls is common.
- Exercise should not begin until medications have taken effect, and medication effects should be considered in the design of exercise programs and monitoring of patients during exercise (e.g., impact of steroids on blood pressure at baseline and during exercise).
- Pulmonary involvement is a common extramuscular manifestation of PM and DM and should be considered in designing exercise interventions.
- Exercise is not contraindicated except during periods of severe disease flare.
- Pain levels should be monitored and activity adjusted accordingly.
- Symptoms of weakness during or after exercise or fasting are uncommon in the inflammatory myopathies and may indicate a metabolic myopathy. Contact the physician immediately.

comparison of methotrexate versus placebo for IBM demonstrated no statistically significant change in improvement in muscle strength; serum CK activity was, however, decreased (61). Neither IVIG nor a testosterone analog, oxandrolone, proved significantly beneficial (55,62). A pilot study to assess the safety of a home exercise program on muscle function and histopathology found no change in the histopathology or serum creatinine kinase level;[AQ:3] however, there was a significant decrease in the areas that were stained for the endothelial cell marker EN-4 in the muscle biopsies after training (63). The authors concluded that the home exercise program was not harmful and did not appear to cause inflammation; thus, exercise may prevent further loss of muscle strength in patients with IBM. The use of interferon beta was studied in a pilot trial. Interferon beta was well tolerated in IBM; however, no differences in muscle strength or mass were observed between the placebo and interferon beta-1a groups at 6 months (64).

Other Therapeutic Options

A variety of experimental therapies have been reported, most often in single case reports. These therapies have been largely reserved for patients resistant to traditional therapies or those patients with severe disease manifestations. Therapies have, to date, included anti-tumor necrosis factor α (anti-TNFα) agents, interferon gamma (Avonex), hemopoietic stem cell transplantation, total body irradiation, and extracorporeal photochemotherapy (56). A randomized clinical trial to assess the efficacy of infliximab in the treatment of patients with inflammatory myopathies is currently ongoing at the National Institutes of Health. This is the first large-scale clinical trial of its kind and will help to clarify whether anti-TNFα therapies will be useful additional agents for myositis patients. A small pilot study of the anti–B-cell agent rituximab in refractory dermatomyositis showed promise and demonstrated sufficiently encouraging results to justify a more formal evaluation of this approach in the treatment of DM (65); thus,

a cooperative multicenter controlled trial of rituximab is currently underway.

Physical therapy is recommended to enhance muscle strength and endurance. Although most patients are not limited by pain, individuals who experience pain during physical therapy sessions should work with their therapist to find exercises that minimize discomfort. Overall, exercise is not contraindicated except during periods of severe disease flare.

There are no specific dietary restrictions for patients with IIM. No studies have shown benefit or harm of any specific dietary intake patterns. Patients should watch their caloric intake while taking corticosteroids, because this therapy is associated with an increase in appetite and often concomitant weight gain.

REFERENCES

1. Bohan A, Peter JB. Polymyositis and dermatomyositis (first of two parts). N Engl J Med 1975;292:344–7.
2. Bohan A, Peter JB. Polymyositis and dermatomyositis (second of two parts). N Engl J Med 1975;292:403–7.
3. Tanimoto K, Nakano K, Kano S, Mori S, Ueki H, Nishitani H, et al. Classification criteria for polymyositis and dermatomyositis. J Rheumatol 1995;22:668–74.
4. Targoff IN, Miller FW, Medsger TA Jr, Oddis CV. Classification criteria for the idiopathic inflammatory myopathies. Curr Opin Rheumatol 1997;9:527–35.
5. Griggs RC, Askanas V, DiMauro S, Engel A, Karpati G, Mendell JR, et al. Inclusion body myositis and myopathies. Ann Neurol 1995;38:705–13.
6. Medsger TA Jr, Dawson WN Jr, Masi AT. The epidemiology of polymyositis. Am J Med 1970;48:715–23.
7. Oddis CV, Conte CG, Steen VD, Medsger TA Jr. Incidence of polymyositis-dermatomyositis: a 20-year study of hospital diagnosed cases in Allegheny County, PA 1963–1982. J Rheumatol 1990;17:1329–34.
8. Okada S, Weatherhead E, Targoff IN, Wesley R, Miller FW. Global surface ultraviolet radiation intensity may modulate the clinical and immunologic expression of autoimmune muscle disease. Arthritis Rheum 2003;48:2285–93.
9. Plotz PH, Miller F, Hoffman E, Casciola-Rosen L, Rosen A. Workshop on inflammatory myopathy; Bethesda, 5–6 April 2000. Neuromuscul Disord 2001;11:93–5.
10. Rider LG, Giannini EH, Harris-Love M, Joe G, Isenberg D, Pilkington C, et al. Defining clinical improvement in adult and juvenile myositis. J Rheumatol 2003;30:603–17.
11. Duan-Porter WD, Casciola-Rosen L, Rosen A. Autoantigens: the critical partner in initiating and propagating systemic autoimmunity. Ann N Y Acad Sci 2005;1062:127–36.
12. Nagaraju K. Update on immunopathogenesis in inflammatory myopathies. Curr Opin Rheumatol 2001;13:461–8.
13. Engel AG, Arahata K, Emslie-Smith A. Immune effector mechanisms in inflammatory myopathies. Res Publ Assoc Res Nerv Ment Dis 1990;68:141–57.
14. van der Meulen MF, Bronner IM, Hoogendijk JE, Burger H, van Venrooij WJ, Voskuyl AE, et al. Polymyositis: an overdiagnosed entity. Neurology 2003;61:316–21.
15. Goebels N, Michaelis D, Engelhardt M, Huber S, Bender A, Pongratz D, et al. Differential expression of perforin in muscle-infiltrating T cells in polymyositis and dermatomyositis. J Clin Invest 1996;97:2905–10.
16. Hohlfeld R, Goebels N, Engel AG. Cellular mechanisms in inflammatory myopathies. Baillieres Clin Neurol 1993; 2:617–35.
17. Casciola-Rosen L, Andrade F, Ulanet D, Wong WB, Rosen A. Cleavage by granzyme B is strongly predictive of autoantigen status: implications for initiation of autoimmunity. J Exp Med 1999;190:815–26.
18. Howard OM, Dong HF, Yang D, Raben N, Nagaraju K, Rosen A, et al. Histidyl-tRNA synthetase and asparaginyl-tRNA synthetase, autoantigens in myositis, activate chemokine receptors on T lymphocytes and immature dendritic cells. J Exp Med 2002;196:781–91.
19. Leff RL, Love LA, Miller FW, Greenberg SJ, Klein EA, Dalakas MC, et al. Viruses in idiopathic inflammatory myopathies: absence of candidate viral genomes in muscle. Lancet 1992;339:1192–5.
20. Askanas V, Engel WK, McFerrin J, Vattemi G. Transthyretin Val122Ile, accumulated Abeta, and inclusion-body myositis aspects in cultured muscle. Neurology 2003;61:257–60.

21. Eisenberg I, Avidan N, Potikha T, Hochner H, Chen M, Olender T, et al. The UDP-N-acetylglucosamine 2-epimerase/N-acetylmannosamine kinase gene is mutated in recessive hereditary inclusion body myopathy. Nat Genet 2001;29:83–7.
22. Sontheimer RD. Cutaneous features of classic dermatomyositis and amyopathic dermatomyositis. Curr Opin Rheumatol 1999;11:475–82.
23. Douglas WW, Tazelaar HD, Hartman TE, Hartman RP, Decker PA, Schroeder DR, et al. Polymyositis-dermatomyositis-associated interstitial lung disease. Am J Respir Crit Care Med 2001;164:1182–5.
24. Marie I, Hachulla E, Cherin P, Dominique S, Hatron PY, Hellot MF, et al. Interstitial lung disease in polymyositis and dermatomyositis. Arthritis Rheum 2002;47:614–22.
25. Hirakata M, Nagai S. Interstitial lung disease in polymyositis and dermatomyositis. Curr Opin Rheumatol 2000;12:501–8.
26. Arakawa H, Yamada H, Kurihara Y, Nakajima Y, Takeda A, Fukushima Y, et al. Nonspecific interstitial pneumonia associated with polymyositis and dermatomyositis: serial high-resolution CT findings and functional correlation. Chest 2003;123:1096–103.
27. Sontheimer RD, Miyagawa S. Potentially fatal interstitial lung disease can occur in clinically amyopathic dermatomyositis. J Am Acad Dermatol 2003;48:797–8.
28. Love LA, Leff RL, Fraser DD, Targoff IN, Dalakas M, Plotz PH, et al. A new approach to the classification of idiopathic inflammatory myopathy: myositis-specific autoantibodies define useful homogeneous patient groups. Medicine (Baltimore) 1991;70:360–74.
29. Targoff IN, Johnson AE, Miller FW. Antibody to signal recognition particle in polymyositis. Arthritis Rheum 1990;33:1361–70.
30. Hengstman GJ, van Engelen BG, Vree Egberts WT, van Venrooij WJ. Myositis-specific autoantibodies: overview and recent developments. Curr Opin Rheumatol 2001;13:476–82.
31. Callen JP. Relationship of cancer to inflammatory muscle diseases. Dermatomyositis, polymyositis, and inclusion body myositis. Rheum Dis Clin North Am 1994;20:943–53.
32. Zantos D, Zhang Y, Felson D. The overall and temporal association of cancer with polymyositis and dermatomyositis. J Rheumatol 1994;21:1855–9.
33. Buchbinder R, Hill CL. Malignancy in patients with inflammatory myopathy. Curr Rheumatol Rep 2002;4:415–26.
34. Sigurgeirsson B, Lindelof B, Edhag O, Allander E. Risk of cancer in patients with dermatomyositis or polymyositis: a population-based study. N Engl J Med 1992;326:363–7.
35. Hill CL, Zhang Y, Sigurgeirsson B, Pukkala E, Mellemkjaer L, Airio A, et al. Frequency of specific cancer types in dermatomyositis and polymyositis: a population-based study. Lancet 2001;357:96–100.
36. Marie I, Hatron PY, Levesque H, Hachulla E, Hellot MF, Michon-Pasturel U, et al. Influence of age on characteristics of polymyositis and dermatomyositis in adults. Medicine (Baltimore) 1999;78:139–47.
37. Hunger RE, Durr C, Brand CU. Cutaneous leukocytoclastic vasculitis in dermatomyositis suggests malignancy. Dermatology 2001;202:123–6.
38. Tan E, Tan SH, Ng SK. Cutaneous mucinosis in dermatomyositis associated with a malignant tumor. J Am Acad Dermatol 2003;48:S41–2.
39. Higuchi I, Hashimoto K, Kashio N, Izumo S, Inose M, Izumi K, et al. Detection of HTLV-I provirus by in situ polymerase chain reaction in mononuclear inflammatory cells in skeletal muscle of viral carriers with polymyositis. Muscle Nerve 1995;18:854–8.
40. Barnes BE, Mawr B. Dermatomyositis and malignancy: a review of the literature. Ann Intern Med 1976;84:68–76.
41. Stockton D, Doherty VR, Brewster DH. Risk of cancer in patients with dermatomyositis or polymyositis, and follow-up implications: a Scottish population-based cohort study. Br J Cancer 2001;85:41–5.
42. Maoz CR, Langevitz P, Livneh A, Blumstein Z, Sadeh M, Bank I, et al. High incidence of malignancies in patients with dermatomyositis and polymyositis: an 11-year analysis. Semin Arthritis Rheum 1998;27:319–24.
43. Wakata N, Kurihara T, Saito E, Kinoshita M. Polymyositis and dermatomyositis associated with malignancy: a 30-year retrospective study. Int J Dermatol 2002;41:729–34.
44. Whitmore SE, Anhalt GJ, Provost TT, Zacur HA, Hamper UM, Helzlsouer KJ, et al. Serum CA-125 screening for ovarian cancer in patients with dermatomyositis. Gynecol Oncol 1997;65:241–4.
45. Adams EM, Chow CK, Premkumar A, Plotz PH. The idiopathic inflammatory myopathies: spectrum of MR imaging findings. Radiographics 1995;15:563–74.
46. Schweitzer ME, Fort J. Cost-effectiveness of MR imaging in evaluating polymyositis. AJR Am J Roentgenol 1995;165:1469–71.
47. Bronner IM, Hoogendijk JE, Wintzen AR, van der Meulen MF, Linssen WH, Wokke JH, et al. Necrotising myopathy, an unusual presentation of a steroid-responsive myopathy. J Neurol 2003;250:480–5.
48. Marie I, Hachulla E, Hatron PY, Hellot MF, Levesque H, Devulder B, et al. Polymyositis and dermatomyositis: short term and long term outcome, and predictive factors of prognosis. J Rheumatol 2001;28:2230–7.
49. Joffe MM, Love LA, Leff RL, Fraser DD, Targoff IN, Hicks JE, et al. Drug therapy of the idiopathic inflammatory myopathies: predictors of response to prednisone, azathioprine, and methotrexate and a comparison of their efficacy. Am J Med 1993;94:379–87.
50. Bunch TW. Prednisone and azathioprine for polymyositis: long-term followup. Arthritis Rheum 1981;24:45–8.
51. Villalba L, Hicks JE, Adams EM, Sherman JB, Gourley MF, Leff RL, et al. Treatment of refractory myositis: a randomized crossover study of two new cytotoxic regimens. Arthritis Rheum 1998;41:392–9.
52. Gelber AC, Nousari HC, Wigley FM. Mycophenolate mofetil in the treatment of severe skin manifestations of dermatomyositis: a series of 4 cases. J Rheumatol 2000;27:1542–5.
53. Mowzoon N, Sussman A, Bradley WG. Mycophenolate (CellCept) treatment of myasthenia gravis, chronic inflammatory polyneuropathy and inclusion body myositis. J Neurol Sci 2001;185:119–22.
54. Cherin P, Pelletier S, Teixeira A, Laforet P, Genereau T, Simon A, et al. Results and long-term followup of intravenous immunoglobulin infusions in chronic, refractory polymyositis: an open study with thirty-five adult patients. Arthritis Rheum 2002;46:467–74.
55. Dalakas MC, Sonies B, Dambrosia J, Sekul E, Cupler E, Sivakumar K. Treatment of inclusion-body myositis with IVIg: a double-blind, placebo-controlled study. Neurology 1997;48:712–6.
56. Oddis CV. Current approach to the treatment of polymyositis and dermatomyositis. Curr Opin Rheumatol 2000;12:492–7.
57. Vencovsky J, Jarosova K, Machacek S, Studynkova J, Kafkova J, Bartunkova J, et al. Cyclosporine A versus methotrexate in the treatment of polymyositis and dermatomyositis. Scand J Rheumatol 2000;29:95–102.
58. Mastaglia FL, Garlepp MJ, Phillips BA, Zilko PJ. Inflammatory myopathies: clinical, diagnostic and therapeutic aspects. Muscle Nerve 2003;27:407–25.
59. Wilkes MR, Sereika SM, Fertig N, Lucas MR, Oddis CV. Treatment of antisynthetase-associated interstitial lung disease with tacrolimus. Arthritis Rheum 2005;52:2439–46.
60. Rose MR, McDermott MP, Thornton CA, Palenski C, Martens WB, Griggs RC. A prospective natural history study of inclusion body myositis: implications for clinical trials. Neurology 2001;57:548–50.
61. Badrising UA, Maat-Schieman ML, Ferrari MD, Zwinderman AH, Wessels JA, Breedveld FC, et al. Comparison of weakness progression in inclusion body myositis during treatment with methotrexate or placebo. Ann Neurol 2002;51:369–72.
62. Rutkove SB, Parker RA, Nardin RA, Connolly CE, Felice KJ, Raynor EM. A pilot randomized trial of oxandrolone in inclusion body myositis. Neurology 2002;58:1081–7.
63. Arnardottir S, Alexanderson H, Lundberg IE, Borg K. Sporadic inclusion body myositis: pilot study on the effects of a home exercise program on muscle function, histopathology and inflammatory reaction. J Rehabil Med 2003;35:31–5.
64. Muscle Study Group. Randomized pilot trial of high-dose betaINF-1a in patients with inclusion body myositis. Neurology 2004;63:718–20.
65. Levine TD. Rituximab in the treatment of dermatomyositis: an open-label pilot study. Arthritis Rheum 2005;52:601–7.

Osteoarthritis

SHARI M. LING, MD, and KATHERINE RUDOLPH, PhD, PT

Osteoarthritis (OA) is the most common disease of the joints, affecting >20 million individuals in the United States alone (1). This translates into a significant cost to society that exceeds that of rheumatoid arthritis when both direct (physician visits, medications, surgery) and indirect costs (disability, time lost from work, inability to perform self care) are considered (2). Given the projected increase in the number and proportion of older adults in the US, the societal cost of this disease is anticipated to increase further over the coming decades. Osteoarthritis is an increasingly important and costly health problem in the United States.

PATHOLOGY AND PATHOGENESIS

Osteoarthritis develops insidiously and progresses slowly over years. Cartilage degeneration is the hallmark of this disease. Cartilage fibrillation and ulceration that begins superficially eventually extends into deeper layers. Subchondral bone can be involved along with cartilage defects. Eventually, bony spurs (osteophytes) develop. Focal synovial membrane inflammation can also be observed. Matrix metalloproteinases (MMPs) and proinflammatory cytokines (e.g., interleukin 1) secreted by synovial cells and chondrocytes appear to be important mediators of cartilage destruction. A number of growth factors and inhibitors of MMPs and cytokines are secreted in an unsuccessful attempt to counteract these degradative forces.

CLINICAL PRESENTATION AND DIAGNOSIS

Symptoms

Patients with OA complain of joint pain and sometimes stiffness. Stiffness of the joint after sleep or prolonged inactivity (gel phenomenon) is usually brief (5–30 minutes) and quickly abates with movement, unlike the morning stiffness associated with inflammatory joint diseases, which can persist for hours. Although joint stiffness may be the earliest symptom with OA, pain is the most common symptom that leads a patient with OA to seek a medical evaluation. Initially, pain usually occurs during activity and subsides with rest. However as the disease progresses, pain can persist despite rest and can deprive patients of restful sleep at night. Among the many possible etiologies of pain in OA are stretching of the joint capsule, increased vascular pressure in subchondral bone, surrounding muscle spasm, and the inflammatory irritation of innervated tissues surrounding the joint (bursitis) or within the joint (synovitis). It is certain that pain in OA does not arise from the cartilage because cartilage lacks nerve endings.

Physical Abnormalities

The joints most commonly involved in OA are summarized in Table 1. Bony enlargement of the medial and dorsolateral aspects of the distal interphalangeal (DIP) or proximal interphalangeal (PIP) joints (Heberden's and Bouchard's nodes, respectively) is a defining characteristic of OA.

These nodes usually develop slowly over time, and are occasionally preceded by more rapidly enlarging gelatinous cysts or chondrophytes that are radiographically silent. Erythema and warmth are usually absent or minimal. Movement and palpation of the joint can be painful and limited in its range. *Crepitus* (a grating sensation upon joint motion) can be elicited in accessible joints such as the thumb base and knee.

Laboratory and Radiographic Findings

There are no laboratory tests that can be used to reliably diagnose OA. Acute phase reactants, such as erythrocyte sedimentation rate, are not elevated, and synovial fluid analysis usually indicates a white cell count of $<2,000/mm^3$. Laboratory studies are more helpful to exclude alternative diagnoses, such as infectious arthritis, Lyme disease, or crystalline diseases (gout, calcium pyrophosphate dehydrate deposition).

The classic radiographic findings of OA are bony spurs at the joint margins, called osteophytes. Other findings include asymmetric narrowing of the joint space, subchondral sclerosis, and subchondral cyst formation. Radiographic severity of OA correlates with the clinical severity of disease in less than half of patients. Given the high prevalence of these radiographic abnormalities in older adults, it remains necessary for the evaluating clinician to ascertain whether the presenting symptoms are attributable to OA or if OA is an incidental finding.

Differential Diagnosis

The diagnosis of OA is based on symptoms, physical findings, and radiographic characteristics (3,4). Because effective treatment is highly dependent upon the correct diagnosis, exclusion of other conditions is exceedingly important. A history of systemic symptoms, such as unintentional weight loss, excessive fatigue, and prolonged morning stiffness, warn clinicians of an inflammatory condition such as polymyalgia rheumatica or rheumatoid arthritis, particularly when accompanied by an abnormal sedimentation rate, high C-reactive protein level, or inflammatory joint fluid. Signs of intense inflammation on physical examination (redness, significant warmth) are highly suggestive of either crystalline disease (gout or pseudogout) or infection of the joint or bone, and may warrant further evaluation including arthrocentesis if the symptomatic joint is accessible. Spondyloarthropathies (such as Reiter's syndrome, ankylosing spondylitis, or psoriatic

Table 1. Common sites of involvement in osteoarthritis

Cervical spine
First carpometacarpal joint
Distal interphalangeal joints
Proximal interphalangeal joints
Lumbar spine
Hips
Knees
First metatarsophalangeal joint

arthritis) with sacroiliac and lumbosacral spine involvement may be accompanied by painful and swollen fingers or toes (sausage digits) that are not restricted to the joint and can be differentiated by clinical and radiographic characteristics. Additionally, if painful symptoms and fatigue are due to such conditions as fibromyalgia or vitamin D deficiency superimposed upon OA, treatment with analgesics or anti-inflammatory agents will be ineffective. In addition, musculoskeletal pain can develop secondary to metabolic disturbances that affect bone (hyperparathyroidism), congenital abnormalities of the ligaments (hypermobility syndromes), and genetic defects of the connective tissue (Marfan, Ehlers-Danlos). Finally, pain that is elicited on active but not passive motion is highly suggestive of a periarticular problem (tendinitis, bursitis). Pain due to tendinitis and bursitis can usually be reproduced on direct palpation of the periarticular structure. In contrast, arthritis pain can be reproduced on palpation of the joint line and is painful during both passive and active movement.

Disease Subsets

Hand. The hand is the location in which the typical OA features can be easily appreciated on physical examination. The most commonly affected joints in the hand are the first carpometacarpal joint (at the thumb base), DIP joint, and PIP joints. Erosive OA of the hand is a variant in which there is prominent DIP and PIP involvement. Inflammatory flares result in joint erosion, deformity, and subsequent ankylosis.

Knee. Knee OA is often accompanied by a palpable effusion, crepitus, and periarticular muscle atrophy. Symptoms of locking and give-way weakness should be sought and if present further evaluated with maneuvers to evaluate the competence of the supporting ligaments and meniscus. In contrast, teenagers and young adults (particularly women) may present with anterior compartment or patellar pain due to *chondromalacia patellae*. This mostly self-limited condition, also referred to as patellofemoral syndrome, is most symptomatic when sitting in a movie theater, walking uphill, or walking up stairs. Although it is often grouped with OA, it can result from a variety of problems, including abnormal quadriceps angle and trauma. Knee pain that is aggravated by prolonged periods of kneeling and is accompanied by significant suprapatellar effusion is suggestive of prepatellar bursitis.

Hip. Symptoms are usually insidious in onset, but eventually result in pain most commonly localized to the groin, and less often to the lateral hip, buttocks, or knee. Painful and limited motion on internal rotation of the hip is characteristic. Occasionally, pain may arise from impingement of the lateral femoral cutaneous nerve (meralgia paresthetics). This can be reproduced by tapping over the site of impingement. Pain with tenderness on the lateral aspect of the upper thigh suggests trochanteric bursitis that can be superimposed upon hip OA.

Neck. OA of the neck can cause pain and limited movement. The movement can limit the patient's ability to look upward and side-to-side—a movement necessary for a full field of view when changing lanes and reversing while driving. Occasionally, patients can experience nerve impingement with referred pain to the shoulder or down to the hand. Osteophytes can enlarge to the point that patients can develop painful or difficult swallowing.

Spine. OA of the lower back can also result in pain that is worse with prolonged standing. Occasionally, OA of the facet joints of the lumbar spine can result in spinal stenosis. Symptoms of spinal stenosis include pain and pseudo-intermittent claudication—that is pain in the calf and leg that occurs with walking and is relieved by sitting down. Patients with spinal stenosis often adopt a stooped posture with loss of the normal lordotic curvature of the spine.

PREVENTION

Since OA is likely a heterogeneous disease, it is not possible to identify one single factor that, if modified, would reduce risk of all forms of OA. However, OA of weight-bearing joints has been strongly associated with excess weight (5–8). More recently, modest weight loss in OA has been accompanied by a decrease in symptoms (9), and reduced joint loads (10) suggest hope for reducing disease progression.

Severe joint injuries increase risk of OA development, and therefore suggest a need for programs to minimize risk of cruciate ligament (11,12) and joint injury (13,14), and also facilitate repair and recovery for young adults at risk. In contrast, the role of repetitive, relatively minor, trauma in development of OA is not clear. However, occupations involving considerable bending and lifting seem to be related to OA of the knees. Preventive measures may be indicated, including changes in certain repetitive motions, reduced significant trauma, and reduced bending.

MANAGEMENT

Guidelines for OA management have been developed by the American College of Rheumatology (15–18), the European League Against Rheumatism (19–21), and summarized in reviews by Felson (22,23). The treatments included in these guidelines should be tailored to each individual patient, carefully weighing adverse event risks relative to potential benefits. Pain relief and restoration of function remain the primary treatment objectives, and are best achieved medicinally together with a well-coordinated, individualized therapeutic program. This can be achieved efficiently by a multidisciplinary team (e.g., rheumatologist, physiatrist, orthopedist, physical therapist, occupational therapist, psychologist, psychiatrist, nurse/nurse coordinator, dietician, and social worker) who can provide patient education, physical measures, psychosocial interventions, medicinal and surgical interventions, and reinforced by followup contact either in person or by telephone.

Patient Education

Patient education provides the foundation for effective management of OA. Misconceptions often exist about this disease at both extremes. Older patients with OA may mistakenly attribute their symptoms and loss of function to growing older. Alternatively, patients with OA may be overly concerned about rapid progression to disability. Any of these scenarios can result in under-reporting of symptoms, nonadherence to recommended treatments, and misuse of both prescribed and nonprescription preparations. Patient education directed at lifestyle changes, such as exercise and weight control, might be helpful in altering the natural history of the disease. Patient adherence to recommendations is important for the effectiveness of medications and exercise; it also improves self-efficacy (24–27). Furthermore, use of over-the-counter preparations or alternative therapies should be discussed. Educational pamphlets, such as those available through the Arthritis Foundation, are a useful and practical source of information.

Pharmacologic Therapy

Alleviation of painful symptoms constitutes the primary focus of prescribed and over-the-counter medicinal management of OA. In general, treatments should utilize the least toxic and least expensive medications first. Furthermore, since there is no single best medication for any given patient, selection of specific agents should be based upon each patient's symptom severity and weighed against potential adverse events. Finally, it is important to recognize the complexity of treating painful symptoms in older patients who are more likely to endure comorbid medical conditions and multiple medications (28).

Topical Agents. Topical agents have a role in the treatment of OA (29). Capsaicin, derived from capsicum, the common pepper plant, is known to be effective in management of OA of the hands when applied 2–4 times daily. Its use results in a sensation of heat or burning for several days, until the nerve endings are depleted of substance P (a neurotransmitter). Care should be taken to avoid the inadvertent application of capsaicin in the eyes and other mucous membranes. Topical nonsteroidal antiinflammatory drugs (NSAIDs) may provide short-term relief of knee OA pain (30). Although generally well tolerated, use of other topical analgesic agents (e.g., nonprescription formulations of menthol and salicylate-based preparations) have not been proven more effective than placebo.

Simple analgesics. Acetaminophen remains the first-line drug of choice for OA management (31), although it may be less effective than NSAIDs or cyclooxygenase 2 (COX-2) inhibitors for patients with more severe pain (32). Acetaminophen should be used at a dosage not to exceed 1 gram 4-times daily (maximum US daily dose of 4 grams) and is well tolerated. However, acetaminophen can result in hepatotoxicity when ingested at high doses and thus should be used cautiously in patients with impaired liver function and should not be taken with alcohol. Despite some evidence of exacerbated renal insufficiency, it is a safer drug than NSAIDs for patients with renal impairment (32).

Tramadol is a mild inhibitor of the opioid receptor and also inhibits uptake of norepinephrine and serotonin. Tramadol is an effective analgesic in management of OA symptoms, and also has NSAID-sparing effects (33). A starting dosage of 25 mg/day for 3 days can be escalated slowly to a maximum dosage thereafter to achieve the desired analgesia. Potential adverse effects include nausea and drowsiness. Seizures and allergic reactions have also been reported at higher doses. Although tramadol is not a controlled substance, it can be abused in opioid-dependent patients.

Narcotic Analgesics. Narcotic analgesics can be effectively prescribed in management of OA pain. Long-acting preparations of oxycodone can be considered for patients with persistent, moderate-to-severe pain (34,35). Agents, such as codeine and propoxyphene, that have minimal addiction potential would be preferable if narcotic analgesics are required. It is anticipated that narcotic analgesic use may become more common in light of concerns of cardiovascular complications implicated with COX-2 inhibitors and possibly other NSAIDs (28).

Nonsteroidal Antiinflammatory Drugs. NSAIDs are the most commonly prescribed agents for treatment of both pain and inflammation in OA, and appear to be more effective in relieving moderate-to-severe pain than acetaminophen (36). Although NSAIDs all inhibit COX enzymes, patient responses to specific agents may vary considerably. Patients vary in their benefit and adverse reactions to various NSAIDs. Difference in half-lives of the NSAIDs may influence patient adherence and dosing. Despite their efficacy, NSAIDs should be prescribed with caution. Analgesia can often be achieved at low doses. Thus, treatment should begin with the lowest dosage and increased incrementally to identify the lowest effective dosage for each patient. Additionally, NSAIDs can be used intermittently and in combination with other analgesics.

Patients using NSAIDs should be monitored for gastrointestinal (GI) symptoms of dyspepsia, peptic ulcer disease, gastritis, and gastrointestinal bleeding; however, GI bleeding may occur in the absence of prior symptoms. In patients at risk of GI events, prophylaxis is highly recommended using 1 of 3 strategies (37–39). Once-daily proton-pump inhibitor (PPI) therapy decreases dyspepsia and also effectively decreases the development of NSAID-associated ulcers and recurrent NSAID-related ulcer complications. Prophylaxis is also indicated for high-risk patients taking low-dose aspirin. This includes patients taking nonselective NSAIDs with low dose aspirin, and patients on aspirin therapy who also have *Helicobacter pylori* infection. A second strategy to reduce GI events is cotreatment with misoprostol. Although misoprostol also decreases NSAID-induced ulcers and GI complications (40), its effectiveness depends upon frequent dosing that in itself can cause diarrhea and dyspepsia. H_2 blockers and sucralfate may reduce GI symptoms, but do not reduce the risk of ulcers or serious GI complications (38).

COX-2 Inhibitors. COX-2 inhibitors represent the third strategy for reducing NSAID-related GI complications. COX-2 inhibitors can provide effective pain relief from OA (37,41). Several studies of rofecoxib (42,43), including the Vioxx Gastrointestinal Outcomes Research (VIGOR) study (44), and celecoxib (42,43), including the Celecoxib Long-Term Arthritis Safety Assessment Study (CLASS) (45), have demonstrated a significant reduction in GI symptoms and serious GI adverse events, when compared with nonselective NSAIDs. However, the potential benefits of COX-2 use should be weighed against the potential risks (28,46). First, data showing an increased risk of acute cardiovascular events in association with the use of selective COX-2 inhibitors (45,47) has resulted in the removal of 2 of the 3 approved agents from the market (rofecoxib and valdecoxib), and a considerably more cautious approach to the use of the remaining agent (celecoxib). Although cotreatment with aspirin may be considered (48,49), concurrent use of low-dose aspirin may compromise the protective advantage of COX-2 selectivity. The efficacy of COX-2–selective inhibitors compared with NSAIDs in combination with other prophylactic strategies have not been well studied for primary prevention. Finally, COX-2–selective agents are as likely as nonselective NSAIDs to reduce kidney function, particularly in older adults with renal compromise (50–52). Because they do not have an effect on platelet function, COX-2 inhibitors are sometimes used in patients taking anticoagulants or with underlying bleeding diathesis; however, coagulation parameters should be carefully monitored in patients who add any medication to their anticoagulants because of potential drug–drug interactions. Thus the risks and benefits of COX-2–selective antagonists must be carefully considered in each patient.

Nutriceuticals. Patients with OA have used numerous nutriceuticals, with only limited well-controlled studies to indicate their efficacy. Oral glucosamine and chondroitin sulfate are available in the United States and have been used in the treatment of OA. Studies of glucosamine have been met with mixed reviews, some of which have shown symptom-relieving benefits (53), whereas others have failed to demonstrate effectiveness over placebo (54–57). This includes a recently conducted National Institutes of Health-sponsored study of >1,500 patients to assess the efficacy of glucosamine and chondroitin sulfate, alone or in combination, compared with placebo and a celecoxib comparator (the GAIT study). The study failed to demonstrate an effect of the supplements on the primary symptomatic outcomes in contrast to celecoxib (54). Recent studies demonstrating slower rates of joint-space narrowing in subjects treated with glucosamine or chondroitin sulfate over 2–3 years compared with placebo has been met with optimism for structure-modifying drugs in the near future; however, the particular methodology used for the structural outcome has been criticized (58). Interestingly, some studies demonstrating structure modification do not show concomitant symptom improvement. The GAIT study will have additional analysis reported to determine the possible structure-modifying benefits over 2 years. Fortunately, glucosamine and chondroitin sulfate are relatively well tolerated. Earlier concerns of hyperglycemia, exacerbated diabetes, and possible effects of chondroitin on coagulation parameters have not been seen in recent studies (54).

There is limited evidence supporting use of either S-adenosylme-thionine or methylsulfonylmethane. Although touted as natural products, these are manufactured chemicals that have limited proven value. Still other agents such as cat's claw and shark cartilage remain commercially available and are highly sought after despite the absence of scientific support for their use in the treatment of painful OA.

Intraarticular Agents. Intraarticular depot corticosteroids may be considered in management of accessible peripheral joints, and are proven to achieve short-term pain relief (59). However the previously held belief of greater efficacy in patients with a demonstrable effusion has not been supported in the literature. Although repeated and recurrent administration are well tolerated (60), the need for repeated intraarticular injections should lead to consideration of definitive surgical intervention. Complications, such as septic arthritis, are rare if proper aseptic technique is employed.

The intraarticular delivery of synthetic and naturally occurring hyaluronan derivatives have gained popularity in management of mild-to-moderate OA of the knee (61–62) and hip given their effectiveness in alleviating painful symptoms. Although effective, the mechanism of action of this therapy has not been delineated. Furthermore, additional studies are needed to evaluate the long-term effects of these agents (63). Several injections are required for the different compounds and some patients may experience a flare of symptoms after injection. The ideal population or stage of OA most amenable to these agents has not been well defined. Nonetheless these agents are an additional option in the management of OA pain, especially in those who may have contraindications to NSAIDs or are unable to tolerate other analgesics.

Future Disease-Modifying Agents. The progress made toward delineating the pathophysiology and development of methods for earlier diagnosis provides the basis for the development of effective disease-modifying therapies in the near future. Although definitive, structure- and disease-modifying therapies are not yet available for OA, several promising studies have been conducted that provide hope that such therapy is within reach. Diacerein has been proposed as a slow-acting, symptom-modifying and perhaps disease structure-modifying drug for OA (64). Doxycycline is of interest for its metalloproteinase-inhibiting activity, and has been shown capable of limiting joint-space narrowing in obese women, but does not appear to prevent disease development nor improve symptomatic outcomes (65). Risedronate, a bisphosphonate indicated for treatment of osteoporosis, has been recently shown to reduce markers of cartilage degradation and bone resorption (66). Other compounds with collagenase-inhibiting properties are being developed and investigated as structure- or disease-modifying agents for OA. Other agents of interest as potential OA structure modifiers include antagonists of interleukin 1 (67) and inhibitors of MMPs, inducible nitric oxide synthetase, intracellular signaling pathways such as P38, MEK-1/2, and peroxisome-proliferator activated receptors.

Physical Measures

Many physical modalities have been proven effective in reducing pain and stiffness and improving function. They comprise an integral part of OA management.

Exercise: Patients with OA should be encouraged to exercise—the myth that any exercise worsens arthritis should be dispelled. In patients with knee OA, exercise programs have been linked to pain reduction and improvements in knee function (68). In theory, improved muscle support of the joint may retard the progression of OA. (See also Chapter 32, Exercise and Physical Activity.)

Exercise is the most commonly employed physical measure in the treatment of patients with OA (69). Exercise is beneficial on several levels. On a systemic level, exercise can improve aerobic capacity, reduce the risk of cardiovascular disease, and combat obesity. Exercise can maintain joint motion and flexibility, which are important for cartilage nutrition and can reduce the accumulation of fluid in the knee (23). Fluid accumulation in any joint is particularly important because studies have shown that capsular distension contributes to reflex muscle inhibition (70). Reflex inhibition can contribute to quadriceps muscle weakness in people with knee OA (71) and may make volitional strength training ineffective (72,73). Studies have shown that neuromuscular electrical stimulation to induce high-force muscle contractions may produce greater strength gains in patients with reflex inhibition (74).

Exercise can also improve quadriceps femoris strength, which has been linked not only to higher function in patients with knee OA but may help prevent or slow progression of the disease. Some studies have shown that quadriceps weakness precedes the development of symptomatic knee OA (75,76) and leads to faster progression of knee OA; so, quadriceps strength training is often recommended (22). However, Brandt et al (75) found that quadriceps strength was not related to disease progression in women with knee OA. In fact, studies have shown that excessive knee laxity and knee malalignment, both common characteristics of people with knee OA, reduce the influence of quadriceps strength on improving knee function (77) and reducing OA progression (78). These findings suggest that factors other than quadriceps weakness are likely involved with progression of the disease and should be investigated (79).

Recently, self-reported knee instability, defined as the sensation of shifting, buckling, and giving way in the knee, has been shown in the majority of people with knee OA (80,81). Fitzgerald et al (82) found that self-reported instability influences knee function over and above other impairments, such as knee pain, reduced range of motion, and quadriceps strength, and suggested that effective rehabilitation may require interventions that address knee instability in addition to muscle strength. There is some evidence that neuromuscular training that reduces knee instability will also improve function in a patient with knee OA (83), however further research is needed to clarify the mechanisms underlying self-reported knee instability and its effect on OA progression.

Although recent evidence raises questions about the effect of strong quadriceps on disease progression, quadriceps strengthening is still the treatment of choice (22) because of its beneficial effect on patient function. Other exercise programs, such as a supervised fitness walking program, with patient education improve functional status without worsening OA of the knee (84). Care should be taken to choose exercises that maximize muscle strengthening and minimize stress on the affected joints (85). Aquatic therapy is particularly effective because it involves multiple muscle groups without placing undue stress on joints. Involvement in particular sports or activities may actually worsen symptoms and may need to be curtailed or modified. For example, chondromalacia patella may be worsened by activities involving high-force muscle contractions with the knee flexed, such as bicycling; lumbar facet OA may worsen with activities that involve hyperextension of the spine, such as occurs in swimming. A gradual progression of exercise intensity is vital because regimens that are advanced too quickly can worsen symptoms. Patients should always be advised that worsening pain during exercise is a warning sign that exercise tolerance has been reached and rest is needed.

Orthotic Devices. Orthotic devices (86), such as corsets, collars, knee braces, and foot orthotics can decrease pain by unloading joints or improving joint biomechanics, which may also reduce further injury. For example, a heel and/or sole lift can reduce the effect of a leg-length discrepancy that leads to functional scoliosis and excessive stress on the lumbar spine. Proper footwear, including orthotic shoes, is often of great value. Athletic shoes with good mediolateral support, good medial arch, and calcaneal cushion can reduce pain and provide support.

Foot orthotic devices or orthotic shoe inserts may help the patient with subluxed metatarsophalangeal joints (86). Wedged foot orthoses to reduce pain and increase function in people with knee OA have shown some promise (87). Studies have shown that laterally wedged insoles reduce the adduction moment at the knee, thereby reducing load on the medial compartment (88). Knee braces are also used to unload the knee typically on the medial side. Unloading braces are successful in reducing pain and improving function (89,90), but it is unclear what affect they have on disease progression.

Supports and orthotic devices are intended to allow patients to increase activity and retain functional independence; however, it is important to monitor their use. For example, initial use of a cervical collar for neck disease should be intermittent, and it should be checked for proper sizing and orientation. Devices that limit motion should be used with care because of the importance of motion and flexibility in cartilage nutrition and reducing fluid accumulation.

Assistive Devices. Canes, crutches, and walkers, when properly used, can increase the base of support, decrease loading, and reduce demands on the lower limb and its joints (91). A cane can unload an affected hip by as much as 60%. The total length of a properly measured cane should be equal to the distance between the upper border of the greater trochanter of the femur and the bottom of the heel of the shoe, resulting in elbow flexion of about 20 degrees. Patient education on proper cane use is important. The cane should be held in the hand contralateral to, and moved together with, the affected limb (92). The healthier limb should precede the affected limb when climbing up stairs. However, when descending stairs, the cane and the affected limb should advance first. Use of assistive devices should be monitored to ensure proper use and condition of the devices. For example, cane and crutch tips should be changed when worn to avoid slipping on smooth or wet surfaces.

Activity Modification. Altering activities of daily living may decrease symptoms of OA. For example, raising the level of a chair or toilet seat can be helpful because the hip and knee are subjected to the highest pressures during the initial phase of rising from the seated position. There is other evidence in the literature in support of modifying activities to reduce OA progression. Chang et al (93) found that patients with medial tibiofemoral OA who used a larger internal hip abduction moment had less likelihood of OA progression. They suggested that a large internal hip abduction moment can result from strong hip abductors that could reduce the tensile load on the lateral knee joint structures, thereby reducing load on the medial compartment. Whether hip abductor strengthening can or will affect hip abductor moments during walking is unknown. It is possible that strengthening along with appropriate gait training methods could increase hip abductor moments, thereby reducing the progression of knee OA. High knee adduction moments are common in people with medial knee OA and are linked to OA progression (94,95). Reduced walking speed has also been suggested as a means to reduce high knee adduction moments in people with more severe knee OA (96). However, slow walking requires higher energy cost and walking slowly may not be practical for all people.

Modalities. Thermal modalities can be particularly effective. The use of heat, cold, or alternating heat and cold are based on patient preference and not on any scientific superiority. Traditionally, the more acute the process, the more likely cold applications will be of benefit (reduction in blood flow and pain). Cold is mostly used in the form of cold packs or vapor-coolant sprays to relieve muscle spasm, decrease swelling in acute trauma, and relieve pain from inflammation. The use of heat can be subdivided into superficial and deep, with no proven advantage of one over the other. Hot packs, paraffin baths, hydrotherapy, and radiant heat are vehicles for providing superficial heat.

Nursing Considerations in Osteoarthritis

- Inform patients it may take up to 2 weeks to get full benefit of pain relief from nonsteroidal antiinflammatory drugs.
- Encourage lifestyle changes, such as weight loss and exercise.

Ultrasound can provide deep heat, usually for larger joints, such as hips. The therapeutic value of applying heat includes decreasing joint stiffness, alleviating pain, relieving muscle spasm, and preventing contractures. The use of heat is contraindicated over tissues with inadequate vascular supply, bleeding, or cancer. Heat should also be avoided in areas close to the testicles or near developing fetuses. The range of temperatures used is 40–45°C (104–113°F) for 3–30 minutes (97). Transcutaneous neural stimulation (98) has also shown some efficacy in reducing pain in patients with knee OA.

Several other physical modalities, with as yet unproven or limited value, include massage, yoga therapy, acupressure, acupuncture, magnets, pulsed electromagnetic fields, and spa therapy. (See also Chapter 38, Thermal and Electrical Agents Used to Manage Arthritis Symptoms and Chapter 36, Therapies from Complementary and Alternative Medicine.)

Psychosocial Measures

Psychological, social, and educational factors are relevant for patients with OA and may be amenable to intervention (99,100). Perception and reporting of pain and other symptoms (101,102) are highly influenced by psychosocial factors, and may represent a manifestation of depression or anxiety (103). Reassurance, counseling, and education may minimize the interference of psychosocial factors. Patients who participate in their care and understand their disease are more likely to accept and adapt to the challenges of living with OA. Beyond supportive care, depression and anxiety are amenable to psychosocial and pharmacologic intervention.

Psychosocial factors, such as self-efficacy, also influence medical decision making (104) and adherence with medical and lifestyle recommendations (25). This includes implementation of lifestyle changes to achieve weight loss for overweight and obese patients with OA (105,106). Additional evidence illustrates the importance of participation and adherence in exercise intervention and training (26,106–108). Finally, increasing physical activity has been proven beneficial for sedentary adults regardless of age (109), and is achievable using interventions to boost motivation (84).

Finally, psychosocial factors also influence the perception and reporting of physical function and functional limitations (110). The ability to perform valued life activities, the wide range of activities that individuals find meaningful or pleasurable above and beyond activities that are necessary for survival or self-sufficiency, has strong links to psychological wellbeing—in some cases, stronger links than functional limitations and disability in basic activities of daily living.

Surgical Intervention

Surgical intervention should be considered for patients with pain that has persisted despite maximal medicinal, physical, and rehabilitative therapies.

Arthroscopy, Tidal Irrigation, and Debridement. Arthroscopy is a surgical technique that utilizes a large-bore needle and fiber-optic viewing to allow visualization of the internal structures of the knee. The utility of this procedure as a means to alleviate painful symptoms has recently been challenged by a randomized, controlled study in which arthroscopy with tidal irrigation of the knee was no more effective in relieving pain or improving function than sham irrigation (111). However, arthroscopy with debridement remains useful in patients with meniscal injury and loose bodies that result in knee locking and give-way weakness. Synovectomy has not been proven effective for established OA.

Osteotomy. Surgical realignment to improve the biomechanics of an OA-affected joint is achieved by removing a segment of the tibia or hip as an alternative to arthroplasty in younger, overweight patients and in those with unicompartmental disease of the knee. High tibial osteotomy may be undertaken in patients with painful knee OA who have varus (bow legged) malalignment due to severe cartilage loss in the medial compartment (112). However, only 50% of patients with knee osteotomies have satisfactory results at 10 years. Hip osteotomy achieves less favorable results and thus is utilized less often.

Arthroplasty. Arthroplasty remains the procedure of choice for patients with severe, deforming OA whose symptoms and disability are unresponsive to maximal nonsurgical therapeutic interventions. Patellofemoral (total knee) arthroplasties achieve good-to-excellent long-term results. Unicompartment arthroplast, also referred to as minimally invasive arthroplasty, has been used since the 1970s. Although less frequently used, this procedure usually results in good outcomes (113). However, which of these prostheses should be used for any given patient is highly variable (114). Finally, hip resurfacing may be an option for patients with disabling OA of the hip (115). Even with these advances, however, the initial consideration should be whether the patient will be able to withstand the physiologic stressors of surgery (116). Second, comorbid medical conditions should be evaluated to ascertain whether competing impairments might limit functional recovery following joint replacement. Third, with severe bilateral osteoarthritis of the knee or hip, simultaneous replacement of both joints should be contemplated. However, the rate of perioperative complications may be slightly higher with simultaneous bilateral arthroplasties than with staged arthroplasty (117,118). Finally, it should be recognized that joint replacement surgery is elective, and should be considered after all more conservative therapies have been tried but before the patient develops generalized or cardiovascular deconditioning (115). As such, it may be worth reconsidering the utility and effectiveness of preoperative exercise and physical training (119).

Other surgical techniques. Techniques have been developed to rejuvenate failing cartilage by penetrating or fracturing the surface, or by transplanting cartilage or cartilage together with bone.

REFERENCES

1. Lawrence RC, Helmick CG, Arnett FC, Deyo RA, Felson DT, Giannini EH, et al. Estimates of the prevalence of arthritis and selected musculoskeletal disorders in the United States. Arthritis Rheum 1998;41:778–99.
2. Kramer JS, Yelin EH, Epstein WV. Social and economic impacts of four musculoskeletal conditions: a study using national community-based data. Arthritis Rheum 1983;26:901–7.
3. Kellgren JH, Lawrence JS. Radiological assessment of osteo-arthrosis. Ann Rheum Dis 1957;16:494–502.
4. Altman RD. The classification of osteoarthritis. J Rheumatol Suppl 1995;43:42–3.
5. Felson DT, Anderson JJ, Naimark A, Walker AM, Meenan RF. Obesity and knee osteoarthritis: the Framingham Study. Ann Intern Med 1988;109:18–24.
6. Felson DT, Goggins J, Niu J, Zhang Y, Hunter DJ. The effect of body weight on progression of knee osteoarthritis is dependent on alignment. Arthritis Rheum 2004;50:3904–9.
7. Hochberg MC, Lethbridge-Cejku M, Scott WW Jr, Reichle R, Plato CC, Tobin JD. The association of body weight, body fatness and body fat distribution with osteoarthritis of the knee: data from the Baltimore Longitudinal Study of Aging. J Rheumatol 1995;22:488–93.
8. Karlson EW, Mandl LA, Aweh GN, Sangha O, Liang MH, Grodstein F. 2003 Total hip replacement due to osteoarthritis: the importance of age, obesity, and other modifiable risk factors. Am J Med 2003;114:93–8.
9. Felson DT, Zhang Y, Anthony JM, Naimark A, Anderson JJ. Weight loss reduces the risk for symptomatic knee osteoarthritis in women: the Framingham Study. Ann Intern Med 1992;116:535–9.
10. Messier SP, Gutekunst DJ, Davis C, DeVita P. 2005 Weight loss reduces knee-joint loads in overweight and obese older adults with knee osteoarthritis. Arthritis Rheum 2005;52:2026–32.
11. Beynnon BD, Johnson RJ, Abate JA, Fleming BC, Nichols CE. Treatment of anterior cruciate ligament injuries, part 2. Am J Sports Med 2005;33:1751–67.
12. Beynnon BD, Johnson RJ, Abate JA, Fleming BC, Nichols CE. Treatment of anterior cruciate ligament injuries, part I. Am J Sports Med 2005;33:1579–602.
13. Dugan SA. Sports-related knee injuries in female athletes: what gives? Am J Phys Med Rehabil 2005;84:122–30.
14. Roos EM. Joint injury causes knee osteoarthritis in young adults. Curr Opin Rheumatol 2005;17:195–200.
15. American College of Rheumatology Subcommittee on Osteoarthritis Guidelines. Recommendations for the medical management of osteoarthritis of the hip and knee: 2000 update. Arthritis Rheum 2000;43:1905–15.
16. Brandt KD. A critique of the 2000 update of the American College of Rheumatology recommendations for management of hip and knee osteoarthritis. Arthritis Rheum 2001;44:2451–5.
17. Hochberg MC, Altman RD, Brandt KD, Clark BM, Dieppe PA, Griffin MR, et al. Guidelines for the medical management of osteoarthritis. Part II. Osteoarthritis of the knee. American College of Rheumatology. Arthritis Rheum 1995;38:1541–6.
18. Hochberg MC, Altman RD, Brandt KD, Clark BM, Dieppe PA, Griffin MR, et al. Guidelines for the medical management of osteoarthritis. Part I. Osteoarthritis of the hip. American College of Rheumatology. Arthritis Rheum 1995;38:1535–40.
19. Jordan KM, Arden NK, Doherty M, Bannwarth B, Bijlsma JW, Dieppe P, et al. EULAR Recommendations 2003: an evidence based approach to the management of knee osteoarthritis: report of a task force of the Standing Committee for International Clinical Studies Including Therapeutic Trials (ESCISIT). Ann Rheum Dis 2003;62:1145–55.
20. Zhang W, Doherty M, Arden N, Bannwarth B, Bijlsma J, Gunther KP, et al. EULAR evidence based recommendations for the management of hip osteoarthritis: report of a task force of the EULAR Standing Committee for International Clinical Studies Including Therapeutics (ESCISIT). Ann Rheum Dis 2005;64:669–81.
21. Mazieres B, Bannwarth B, Dougados M, Lequesne M. EULAR recommendations for the management of knee osteoarthritis: report of a task force of the Standing Committee for International Clinical Studies Including Therapeutic Trials. Joint Bone Spine 2001;68:231–40.
22. Felson DT. Clinical practice: osteoarthritis of the knee. N Engl J Med 2006;354:841–8.
23. Felson DT, Lawrence RC, Hochberg MC, McAlindon T, Dieppe PA, Minor MA, et al. Osteoarthritis: new insights. Part 2: treatment approaches. Ann Intern Med 2000;133:726–37.
24. Carr A. Barriers to the effectiveness of any intervention in OA. Best Pract Res Clin Rheumatol 2001;15:645–56.
25. Edworthy SM, Devins GM. Improving medication adherence through patient education distinguishing between appropriate and inappropriate utilization. Patient Education Study Group. J Rheumatol 1999;26:1793–801.
26. Belza B, Topolski T, Kinne S, Patrick DL, Ramsey SD. Does adherence make a difference? Results from a community-based aquatic exercise program. Nurs Res 2002;51:285–91.
27. Allegrante JP, Marks R. Self-efficacy in management of osteoarthritis. Rheum Dis Clin North Am 2003;29:747–68, vi–vii.
28. Schneider JP. Chronic pain management in older adults: with coxibs under fire, what now? Geriatrics 2005;60:26–8, 30–1.
29. Rosenstein ED. Topical agents in the treatment of rheumatic disorders. Rheum Dis Clin North Am 1999;25:899–918, viii.
30. Bruhlmann P, Michel BA. Topical diclofenac patch in patients with knee osteoarthritis: a randomized, double-blind, controlled clinical trial. Clin Exp Rheumatol 2003;21:193–8.
31. Bradley JD, Brandt KD, Katz BP, Kalasinski LA, Ryan SI. Comparison of an antiinflammatory dose of ibuprofen, an analgesic dose of ibuprofen, and acetaminophen in the treatment of patients with osteoarthritis of the knee. N Engl J Med 1991;325:87–91.

32. Towheed T, Maxwell L, Judd M, Catton M, Hochberg M, Wells G. Acetaminophen for osteoarthritis. Cochrane Database Syst Rev 2006(1): CD004257.

33. Schnitzer TJ, Kamin M, Olson WH. Tramadol allows reduction of naproxen dose among patients with naproxen-responsive osteoarthritis pain: a randomized, double-blind, placebo-controlled study. Arthritis Rheum 1999;42:1370–7.

34. Caldwell JR, Rapoport RJ, Davis JC, Offenberg HL, Marker HW, Roth SH, et al. Efficacy and safety of a once-daily morphine formulation in chronic, moderate-to-severe osteoarthritis pain: results from a randomized, placebo-controlled, double-blind trial and an open-label extension trial. J Pain Symptom Manage 2002;23:278–91.

35. Caldwell JR, Roth SH. A double blind study comparing the efficacy and safety of enteric coated naproxen to naproxen in the management of NSAID intolerant patients with rheumatoid arthritis and osteoarthritis. Naproxen EC Study Group. J Rheumatol 1994;21:689–95.

36. Lee C, Straus WL, Balshaw R, Barlas S, Vogel S, Schnitzer TJ. A comparison of the efficacy and safety of nonsteroidal antiinflammatory agents versus acetaminophen in the treatment of osteoarthritis: a meta-analysis. Arthritis Rheum 2004;51:746–54.

37. Hooper L, Brown TJ, Elliott R, Payne K, Roberts C, Symmons D. The effectiveness of five strategies for the prevention of gastrointestinal toxicity induced by non-steroidal anti-inflammatory drugs: systematic review. BMJ 2004;329:948.

38. Brown GJ, Yeomans ND. Prevention of the gastrointestinal adverse effects of nonsteroidal anti-inflammatory drugs: the role of proton pump inhibitors. Drug Saf 1999;21:503–12.

39. Hawkey CJ, Karrasch JA, Szczepanski L, Walker DG, Barkun A, Swannell AJ, et al. Omeprazole compared with misoprostol for ulcers associated with nonsteroidal antiinflammatory drugs. Omeprazole versus Misoprostol for NSAID-induced Ulcer Management (OMNIUM) Study Group. N Engl J Med 1998;338:727–34.

40. Graham DY, Agrawal NM, Roth SH. Prevention of NSAID-induced gastric ulcer with misoprostol: multicentre, double-blind, placebo-controlled trial. Lancet 1988;2:1277–80.

41. Peura DA. Prevention of nonsteroidal anti-inflammatory drug-associated gastrointestinal symptoms and ulcer complications. Am J Med 2004;117(Suppl 5A):63S–71S.

42. Geba GP, Weaver AL, Polis AB, Dixon ME, Schnitzer TJ. Efficacy of rofecoxib, celecoxib, and acetaminophen in osteoarthritis of the knee: a randomized trial. JAMA 2002;287:64–71.

43. Schnitzer TJ, Weaver AL, Polis AB, Petruschke RA, Geba GP. Efficacy of rofecoxib, celecoxib, and acetaminophen in patients with osteoarthritis of the knee. A combined analysis of the VACT studies. J Rheumatol 2005;32:1093–105.

44. Watson DJ, Harper SE, Zhao PL, Quan H, Bolognese JA, Simon TJ. Gastrointestinal tolerability of the selective cyclooxygenase-2 (COX-2) inhibitor rofecoxib compared with nonselective COX-1 and COX-2 inhibitors in osteoarthritis. Arch Intern Med 2000;160:2998–3003.

45. Silverstein FE, Faich G, Goldstein JL, Simon LS, Pincus T, Whelton A, et al. Gastrointestinal toxicity with celecoxib vs nonsteroidal antiinflammatory drugs for osteoarthritis and rheumatoid arthritis: the CLASS study: a randomized controlled trial. Celecoxib Long-term Arthritis Safety Study. JAMA 2000;284:1247–55.

46. Schmidt H, Woodcock BG, Geisslinger G. Benefit-risk assessment of rofecoxib in the treatment of osteoarthritis. Drug Saf 2004;27:185–96.

47. Bombardier C, Laine L, Reicin A, Shapiro D, Burgos-Vargas R, Davis B, et al. Comparison of upper gastrointestinal toxicity of rofecoxib and naproxen in patients with rheumatoid arthritis. VIGOR Study Group. N Engl J Med 2000;343:1520–8.

48. Fitzgerald GA, Cheng Y, Austin S. COX-2 inhibitors and the cardiovascular system. Clin Exp Rheumatol 2001;19(6 Suppl 25):S31–6.

49. Savage R. Cyclo-oxygenase-2 inhibitors: when should they be used in the elderly? Drugs Aging 2005;22:185–200.

50. Klag MJ, Whelton PK, Perneger TV. Analgesics and chronic renal disease. Curr Opin Nephrol Hypertens 1996;5:236–41.

51. Perneger TV, Whelton PK, Klag MJ. Risk of kidney failure associated with the use of acetaminophen, aspirin, and nonsteroidal antiinflammatory drugs. N Engl J Med 1994;331:1675–9.

52. Ahmad SR, Kortepeter C, Brinker A, Chen M, Beitz J. 2002 Renal failure associated with the use of celecoxib and rofecoxib. Drug Saf 2002;25:537–44.

53. Matheson AJ, Perry CM. Glucosamine: a review of its use in the management of osteoarthritis. Drugs Aging 2003;20:1041–60.

54. Clegg DO, Reda DJ, Harris CL, Klein MA, O'Dell JR, Hooper MM, et al. Glucosamine, chondroitin sulfate, and the two in combination for painful knee osteoarthritis. N Engl J Med 2006;354:795–808.

55. McAlindon T, Formica M, LaValley M, Lehmer M, Kabbara K. Effectiveness of glucosamine for symptoms of knee osteoarthritis: results from an internet-based randomized double-blind controlled trial. Am J Med 2004;117:643–9.

56. Towheed TE, Maxwell L, Anastassiades TP, Shea B, Houpt J, Robinson V, et al. Glucosamine therapy for treating osteoarthritis. Cochrane Database Syst Rev 2005;(2):CD002946.

57. Hochberg MC. Nutritional supplements for knee osteoarthritis—still no resolution. N Engl J Med 2006;354:858–60.

58. Reginster JY, Deroisy R, Rovati LC, Lee RL, Lejeune E, Bruyere O, et al. Long-term effects of glucosamine sulphate on osteoarthritis progression: a randomised, placebo-controlled clinical trial. Lancet 2001;357:251–6.

59. Ravaud P, Moulinier L, Giraudeau B, Ayral X, Guerin C, Noel E, et al. Effects of joint lavage and steroid injection in patients with osteoarthritis of the knee: results of a multicenter, randomized, controlled trial. Arthritis Rheum 1999;42:475–82.

60. Raynauld JP, Buckland-Wright C, Ward R, Choquette D, Haraoui B, Martel-Pelletier J, et al. Safety and efficacy of long-term intraarticular steroid injections in osteoarthritis of the knee: a randomized, double-blind, placebo-controlled trial. Arthritis Rheum 2003;48:370–7.

61. Brandt KD, Block JA, Michalski JP, Moreland LW, Caldwell JR, Lavin PT. 2001 Efficacy and safety of intraarticular sodium hyaluronate in knee osteoarthritis. ORTHOVISC Study Group. Clin Orthop Relat Res 2001;385:130–43.

62. Hochberg MC. Role of intra-articular hyaluronic acid preparations in medical management of osteoarthritis of the knee. Semin Arthritis Rheum 2000;30(2 Suppl 1):2–10.

63. Petrella RJ. Hyaluronic acid for the treatment of knee osteoarthritis: long-term outcomes from a naturalistic primary care experience. Am J Phys Med Rehabil 2005;84:278–83.

64. Fidelix TS, Soares BG, Trevisani VF. Diacerein for osteoarthritis. Cochrane Database Syst Rev 2006;(1):CD005117.

65. Brandt KD, Mazzuca SA, Katz BP, Lane KA, Buckwalter KA, Yocum DE, et al. Effects of doxycycline on progression of osteoarthritis: results of a randomized, placebo-controlled, double-blind trial. Arthritis Rheum 2005;52:2015–25.

66. Spector TD, Conaghan PG, Buckland-Wright JC, Garnero P, Cline GA, Beary JF, et al. Effect of risedronate on joint structure and symptoms of knee osteoarthritis: results of the BRISK randomized, controlled trial. Arthritis Res Ther 2005;7:R625–33.

67. Bingham CO III, Buckland-Wright JC, Garnero P, Cohen SB, Dougados M, Adami S, et al. Risedronate decreases biochemical markers of cartilage degradation but does not decrease symptoms or slow x-ray progression in patients with medial compartment osteoarthritis of the knee: results of the two-year multinational Knee OA Structural Arthritis (KOSTAR) Study. Arthritis Rheum (In Press).

68. van Baar ME, Dekker J, Oostendorp RA, Bijl D, Voorn TB, Lemmens JA, et al. The effectiveness of exercise therapy in patients with osteoarthritis of the hip or knee: a randomized clinical trial. J Rheumatol 1998;25:2432–9.

69. Ettinger WH Jr, Burns R, Messier SP, Applegate W, Rejeski WJ, Morgan T, et al. A randomized trial comparing aerobic exercise and resistance exercise with a health education program in older adults with knee osteoarthritis. The Fitness Arthritis and Seniors Trial (FAST). JAMA 1997;277:25–31.

70. Torry MR, Decker MJ, Viola RW, O'Connor DD, Steadman JR. Intra-articular knee joint effusion induces quadriceps avoidance gait patterns. Clin Biomech (Bristol, Avon) 2000;15:147–59.

71. Hurley MV, Newham DJ. 1993 The influence of arthrogenous muscle inhibition on quadriceps rehabilitation of patients with early, unilateral osteoarthritic knees. Br J Rheumatol 1993;32:127–31.

72. Berth A, Urbach D, Awiszus F. 2002 Improvement of voluntary quadriceps muscle activation after total knee arthroplasty. Arch Phys Med Rehabil 2002;83:1432–6.

73. Hurley MV, Jones DW, Newham DJ. 1994 Arthrogenic quadriceps inhibition and rehabilitation of patients with extensive traumatic knee injuries. Clin Sci (Lond) 1994;86:305–10.

74. Stevens JE, Mizner RL, Snyder-Mackler L. Quadriceps strength and volitional activation before and after total knee arthroplasty for osteoarthritis. J Orthop Res 2003;21:775–9.

75. Brandt KD, Heilman DK, Slemenda C, Katz BP, Mazzuca SA, Braunstein EM, et al. Quadriceps strength in women with radiographically progressive osteoarthritis of the knee and those with stable radiographic changes. J Rheumatol 1999;26:2431–7.

76. Slemenda C, Brandt KD, Heilman DK, Mazzuca S, Braunstein EM, Katz BP, et al. Quadriceps weakness and osteoarthritis of the knee. Ann Intern Med 1997;127:97–104.

77. Sharma L, Hayes KW, Felson DT, Buchanan TS, Kirwan-Mellis G, Lou C, et al. Does laxity alter the relationship between strength and physical function in knee osteoarthritis? Arthritis Rheum 1999;42:25–32.

78. Sharma L, Dunlop DD, Cahue S, Song J, Hayes KW. Quadriceps strength and osteoarthritis progression in malaligned and lax knees. Ann Intern Med 2003;138:613–9.

79. Bennell K, Hinman R. Exercise as a treatment for osteoarthritis. Curr Opin Rheumatol 2005;17:634–40.

80. Fitzgerald GK, Piva SR, Irrgang JJ. Reports of joint instability in knee osteoarthritis: its prevalence and relationship to physical function. Arthritis Rheum 2004;51:941–6.

81. Lewek MD, Rudolph KS, Snyder-Mackler L. Control of frontal plane knee laxity during gait in patients with medial compartment knee osteoarthritis. Osteoarthritis Cartilage 2004;12:745–51.

82. Fitzgerald GK, Piva SR, Irrgang JJ, Bouzubar F, Starz TW. 2004 Quadriceps activation failure as a moderator of the relationship between quadriceps strength and physical function in individuals with knee osteoarthritis. Arthritis Rheum 2004;51:40–8.

83. Fitzgerald GK, Childs JD, Ridge TM, Irrgang JJ. Agility and perturbation training for a physically active individual with knee osteoarthritis. Phys Ther 2002;82:372–82.

84. Talbot LA, Gaines JM, Huynh TN, Metter EJ. A home-based pedometer-driven walking program to increase physical activity in older adults with osteoarthritis of the knee: a preliminary study. J Am Geriatr Soc 2003;51:387–92.

85. Buckwalter JA, Lane NE. Athletics and osteoarthritis. Am J Sports Med 1997;25:873–81.

86. Thompson JA, Jennings MB, Hodge W. Orthotic therapy in the management of osteoarthritis. J Am Podiatr Med Assoc 1992;82:136–9.

87. Brouwer RW, Jakma TS, Verhagen AP, Verhaar JA, Bierma-Zeinstra SM. Braces and orthoses for treating osteoarthritis of the knee. Cochrane Database Syst Rev 2005;(1):CD004020.

88. Kerrigan DC, Lelas JL, Goggins J, Merriman GJ, Kaplan RJ, Felson DT. Effectiveness of a lateral-wedge insole on knee varus torque in patients with knee osteoarthritis. Arch Phys Med Rehabil 2002;83:889–93.

89. Kirkley A, Webster-Bogaert S, Litchfield R, Amendola A, MacDonald S, McCalden R, et al. The effect of bracing on varus gonarthrosis. J Bone Joint Surg Am 1999;81:539–48.

90. Matsuno H, Kadowaki KM, Tsuji H. Generation II knee bracing for severe medial compartment osteoarthritis of the knee. Arch Phys Med Rehabil 1997;78:745–9.

91. Blount WP. Don't throw away the cane. J Bone Joint Surg Am 1956;38-A:695–708.

92. Chan GN, Smith AW, Kirtley C, Tsang WW. Changes in knee moments with contralateral versus ipsilateral cane usage in females with knee osteoarthritis. Clin Biomech (Bristol, Avon) 2005;20:396–404.

93. Chang A, Hayes K, Dunlop D, Song J, Hurwitz D, Cahue S, et al. Hip abduction moment and protection against medial tibiofemoral osteoarthritis progression. Arthritis Rheum 2005;52:3515–9.

94. Sharma L, Song J, Felson DT, Cahue S, Shamiyeh E, Dunlop DD. The role of knee alignment in disease progression and functional decline in knee osteoarthritis. JAMA 2001;286:188–95.

95. Jackson BD, Wluka AE, Teichtahl AJ, Morris ME, Cicuttini FM. Reviewing knee osteoarthritis—a biomechanical perspective. J Sci Med Sport 2004;7:347–57.

96. Mundermann A, Dyrby CO, Hurwitz DE, Sharma L, Andriacchi TP. Potential strategies to reduce medial compartment loading in patients with knee osteoarthritis of varying severity: reduced walking speed. Arthritis Rheum 2004;50:1172–8.

97. Basford JR. Physical agents and biofeedback. In: DeLisa JA, editor. Rehabilitation medicine: principles and practice. Phildaelphia: Lippincott; 1988. p. 257–75.

98. Osiri M, Welch V, Brosseau L, Shea B, McGowan J, Tugwell P, et al. Transcutaneous electrical nerve stimulation for knee osteoarthritis. Cochrane Database Syst Rev 2000;(4):CD002823.

99. Weinberger M. Telephone-based interventions in outpatient care. Ann Rheum Dis 1998;57:196–7.

100. Weinberger M, Tierney WM, Cowper PA, Katz BP, Booher PA. Cost-effectiveness of increased telephone contact for patients with osteoarthritis: a randomized, controlled trial. Arthritis Rheum 1993;36:243–6.

101. Creamer P, Hochberg MC. The relationship between psychosocial variables and pain reporting in osteoarthritis of the knee. Arthritis Care Res 1998;11:60–5.

102. Rejeski WJ, Craven T, Ettinger WH Jr, McFarlane M, Shumaker S. Self-efficacy and pain in disability with osteoarthritis of the knee. J Gerontol B Psychol Sci Soc Sci 1996;51:P24–9.

103. Wu LR, Parkerson GR Jr, Doraiswamy PM. Health perception, pain, and disability as correlates of anxiety and depression symptoms in primary care patients. J Am Board Fam Pract 2002;15:183–90.

104. Hawker GA, Wright JG, Badley EM, Coyte PC. Perceptions of, and willingness to consider, total joint arthroplasty in a population-based cohort of individuals with disabling hip and knee arthritis. Arthritis Rheum 2004;51:635–41.

105. Messier SP, Loeser RF, Miller GD, Morgan TM, Rejeski WJ, Sevick MA, et al. Exercise and dietary weight loss in overweight and obese older adults with knee osteoarthritis: the Arthritis, Diet, and Activity Promotion Trial. Arthritis Rheum 2004;50:1501–10.

106. van Gool CH, Penninx BW, Kempen GI, van Eijk JT, Pahor M, et al. 2005 Determinants of high and low attendance to diet and exercise interventions among overweight and obese older adults. Results from the arthritis, diet, and activity promotion trial. Contemp Clin Trials 2006;27:227–37.

107. Minor MA, Brown JD. Exercise maintenance of persons with arthritis after participation in a class experience. Health Educ Q 1993;20:83–95.

108. van Gool CH, Penninx BW, Kempen GI, Rejeski WJ, Miller GD, van Eijk JT, et al. Effects of exercise adherence on physical function among overweight older adults with knee osteoarthritis. Arthritis Rheum 2005;53:24–32.

109. Halbert J, Crotty M, Weller D, Ahern M, Silagy C. 2001 Primary care-based physical activity programs: effectiveness in sedentary older patients with osteoarthritis symptoms. Arthritis Rheum 2001;45:228–34.

110. Creamer P, Lethbridge-Cejku M, Hochberg MC. 2000 Factors associated with functional impairment in symptomatic knee osteoarthritis. Rheumatology (Oxford) 2000;39:490–6.

111. Moseley JB, O'Malley K, Petersen NJ, Menke TJ, Brody BA, Kuykendall DH, et al. A controlled trial of arthroscopic surgery for osteoarthritis of the knee. N Engl J Med 2002;347:81–8.

112. Pfahler M, Lutz C, Anetzberger H, Maier M, Hausdorf J, Pellengahr C, et al. Long-term results of high tibial osteotomy for medial osteoarthritis of the knee. Acta Chir Belg 2003;103:603–6.

113. Tria AJ Jr. Advancements in minimally invasive total knee arthroplasty. Orthopedics 2003;26(8 Suppl):s859–63.

114. Malik MH, Chougle A, Pradhan N, Gambhir AK, Porter ML. Primary total knee replacement: a comparison of a nationally agreed guide to best practice and current surgical technique as determined by the North West Regional Arthroplasty Register. Ann R Coll Surg Engl 2005;87:117–22.

115. Garbuz DS, Xu M, Duncan CP, Masri BA, Sobolev B. 2006 Delays worsen quality of life outcome of primary total hip arthroplasty. Clin Orthop Relat Res 2006;447:79–84.

116. Lingard EA, Katz JN, Wright EA, Sledge CB. Predicting the outcome of total knee arthroplasty. J Bone Joint Surg Am 2004;86-A:2179–86.

117. Bullock DP, Sporer SM, Shirreffs TG Jr. Comparison of simultaneous bilateral with unilateral total knee arthroplasty in terms of perioperative complications. J Bone Joint Surg Am 2003;85-A:1981–6.

118. Mangaleshkar SR, Prasad PS, Chugh S, Thomas AP. 2001 Staged bilateral total knee replacement—a safer approach in older patients. Knee 2001;8:207–11.

119. Beaupre LA, Lier D, Davies DM, Johnston DB. 2004 The effect of a preoperative exercise and education program on functional recovery, health related quality of life, and health service utilization following primary total knee arthroplasty. J Rheumatol 2004;31:1166–73.

CHAPTER 21

Osteoporosis

MICHAEL J. MARICIC, MD

Osteoporosis is "A disease characterized by low bone mass and microarchitectural deterioration of bone tissue leading to enhanced bone fragility and a consequent increase in fracture risk" (1) (Figure 1).

ETIOLOGY, PATHOGENESIS, AND INCIDENCE

Osteoporosis is a major medical, economic, and social health problem in the United States that results in significant pain, functional disability, and increased mortality. Approximately 1.2 million fractures attributable to osteoporosis occur each year in persons age >45 years (2). This includes 600,000 vertebral crush fractures and 250,000 fractures of the hip. Forty to fifty percent of white women older than 50 years will suffer an osteoporotic fracture and one-sixth will sustain a fracture of the hip. The risk of hip fracture begins to rise after age 45 and then rises exponentially, doubling for every 5 years of age.

After an elderly person suffers a hip fracture, mortality rate increases by 12–20% in the next year due to complications of immobilization (pneumonia, pulmonary embolus). Approximately 50% of elderly patients with hip fractures never regain the same level of functional independence, and 25% require long-term institutional care. The total direct and indirect annual costs for osteoporosis approach $14 billion.

The etiology of osteoporosis is multifactorial. Genetics accounts for 80% of the variance in bone mass. Peak bone mass is usually attained by age 20–30 years, and then remains relatively stable until menopause. A 2–3% decline in bone mass (mainly trabecular) may then occur for a period of ~5 years. In addition to gonadal deficiency, lifelong calcium deficiency, chronic alcohol and nicotine use, immobilization, and medications (such as glucocorticoids, anticonvulsants, and excessive thyroid supplementation) all may contribute to accelerated bone loss (Table 1).

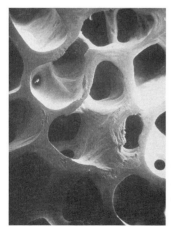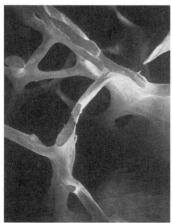

Figure 1. The image on the left shows normal bone. The image on the right displays decreased bone density and microfractures. Reproduced with permission from ACR Slide Collection on the Rheumatic Diseases, copyright American College of Rheumatology.

PREVENTION AND TREATMENT

The ultimate goal of prevention and treatment is to minimize the incidence of osteoporotic fractures. A number of important pharmacologic advances have improved our ability to both prevent and manage osteoporosis. The current challenges are to identify which patients are candidates for treatment, to choose the most appropriate therapy based on the complete patient profile, and to ensure long-term compliance with therapy.

An essential component of diagnosis and prediction of future fracture risk involves bone density measurement. Dual-energy x-ray absorptiometry is currently the gold standard because of its high accuracy and precision. Bone density measurement is essential for the diagnosis of low bone mass (3) and is an excellent method for assessing future fracture risk and monitoring efficacy of therapy (4).

If a postmenopausal woman has already suffered a fragility fracture, one would usually prescribe a drug that has an approved therapeutic indication based on its documented efficacy for reducing fracture risk. Intervention before the first fracture is a more complex decision that involves consideration not only of the patient's bone density (T-score less than or equal to −2.0 in the absence of additional risk factors and less than or equal to −1.5 if risk factors are present, according to National Osteoporosis Foundation guidelines) (2), but also a number of non-density–related risks for fracture, including maternal history of a hip fracture, current smoking, body weight <127 pounds, ever taken glucocorticoids, etc. (2). The cost, adverse effects of the medication, and likelihood of long-term adherence must also be taken into consideration in the decision to treat or not.

Successful management of osteoporosis is based on a combination of nonpharmacologic and pharmacologic approaches. Reductions of modifiable risk factors, along with adequate calcium and vitamin D intake, should be considered essential prior to pharmacologic intervention. Pharmacologic agents approved for the prevention or treatment of osteoporosis are listed in Table 2.

Nonpharmacologic Management

Although few prospective, well-controlled studies document a beneficial effect of physical activity on bone mass, weight-bearing exercise nonetheless plays an adjunctive role in the prevention and treatment of osteoporosis by maintaining muscle mass and promoting strength, coordination, and balance. For long-term adherence, it is prudent to individualize the exercise to the patient's overall physical ability, health status, and preferences. Lifestyle modifications that help counteract osteoporosis are summarized in Table 3.

Reducing the likelihood of falls may be accomplished through:
- Treatment of comorbidities—dementia, gait disorders, decreased vision, and decreased strength, for example—that predispose the patient to falls.
- Reduction in the use of such drugs as sedatives, tranquilizers, and other medications affecting central nervous system function that may increase the risk of falling.

Table 1. Selected secondary causes of diminished bone density

Endocrine disorders
  Cushing's disease
  Hyperparathyroidism
  Hyperthyroidism
  Prolactinoma
  Hypogonadism
Celiac disease and other causes of malabsorption
Vitamin D deficiency
Hepatic or renal dysfunction
Genetic disorders, e.g., osteogenesis imperfecta
Systemic inflammatory disease, e.g., rheumatoid arthritis
Malnutrition, anorexia nervosa
Malignancies, e.g., multiple myeloma

- Adjustments to the home environment, such as removing throw rugs, installing sturdy railings along stairways and in bathrooms, and assuring adequate lighting.
- Education of patients about their risk of falling and strategies to improve home safety.

Calcium and Vitamin D

The role of dietary calcium in the prevention and treatment of osteoporosis has been investigated in a number of studies (5–7). The National Institutes of Health has formulated recommendations for the optimal daily intake of bioavailable calcium, which vary with age and sex (5). The elderly need more calcium as a result of altered calcium homeostasis, including an age-related decline in intestinal calcium absorption (6).

Because the recommended dosage of calcium is usually not obtained through diet alone, calcium supplementation is often required. Calcium supplements are available in several different salt forms, dosage forms, and strengths. Calcium carbonate and calcium citrate contain a calcium composition of 40% and 22%, respectively. Calcium carbonate is well absorbed when taken after an acid-generating meal, and is usually the preparation of choice due to its low cost. In patients who are achlorhydric, calcium citrate would be preferred because calcium carbonate would not be absorbed.

The physiologic effects of vitamin D include an increase in calcium and phosphorus absorption from the small intestine, a reduction in urinary calcium excretion, and maintenance of muscle strength, which plays a very important role in protection against falls. Elderly patients are often deficient in vitamin D because of low intake and inadequate sunlight exposure.

Consumption of 400–800 IU/day of vitamin D improves calcium balance and reduces the risk of fractures in the elderly (6,7). In a study by Dawson-Hughes and colleagues that evaluated the effect of calcium and vitamin D_3 in 445 community-dwelling men and women $\geq$65 years of age, 500 mg of calcium and 700 IU of vitamin D_3 moderately reduced bone loss measured in the femoral neck, spine, and total body and reduced the incidence of nonvertebral fractures (6). Chapuy and colleagues (7) studied the effects of 1,500 mg calcium and 800 IU vitamin D per day versus placebo in a large population of assisted-care residents in France. After 18 months, hip fractures were reduced by 43%. Because a substantial proportion of the French population was vitamin D deficient, it was speculated that the results may not be applicable to the population of the United States. However, a study of 1,536 postmenopausal women in the United States receiving pharmacologic treatment for osteoporosis revealed that 52% had inadequate 25-OH vitamin D levels (<30 ng/ml), suggesting that widespread inadequacy is a common problem in this country as well (8).

Estrogen and Hormone Therapy

Estrogen therapy is approved for the prevention of bone loss in postmenopausal women, but is no longer approved for the treatment of osteoporosis. The Women's Health Initiative study did demonstrate the effectiveness of hormone therapy in reducing both vertebral and hip fracture (34% each) (9), however due to effects on the incidence of breast cancer and cardiovascular disease, neither combined hormone therapy (estrogen plus progesterone) nor estrogen therapy alone are indicated for the treatment of long-term disease. In the patient taking estrogen or hormone therapy for vasomotor symptoms, it is recommended that the lowest dosage be given for the shortest amount of time (10).

Raloxifene

Raloxifene belongs to a class of drugs known as selective estrogen receptor modulators (SERMs) and appears to have tissue-specific estrogen agonist and antagonist actions. Raloxifene was the first SERM approved for the prevention and treatment of osteoporosis. Its approval as a preventive agent is based on studies in perimenopausal women demonstrating prevention of bone loss (11).

The study demonstrating the efficacy of raloxifene in the treatment of women with osteoporosis was the Multiple Outcomes of Raloxifene Evaluation (MORE) study (12), a double-blind, placebo-controlled trial of >7,700 patients with osteoporosis. Approximately one-third of patients entered the study with prevalent vertebral fractures; the others had low bone mass without fractures. The primary study endpoint was the occurrence of new vertebral fractures. The 3-year final analysis of the MORE study results showed that raloxifene, 60 mg/day, reduced the relative risk for new vertebral fractures by 30% in postmenopausal

Table 2. FDA-approved agents for the prevention and treatment of postmenopausal osteoporosis*

Prevention	Treatment
Estrogens	Calcitonin-salmon nasal spray 200 IU/day
Raloxifene 60 mg orally once per day	Raloxifene 60 mg orally once per day
Alendronate 35 mg orally once per week	Alendronate 70 mg orally once per week
Risedronate 35 mg orally once per week	Risedronate 35 mg orally once per week
Ibandronate 150 mg orally once per month or 3 mg intravenously once every 3 months	Ibandronate 150 mg orally once per month or 3 mg intravenously once every 3 months
	Teriparatide 20 μg subcutaneously once per day

* FDA = Food and Drug Administration.

Table 3. National Osteoporosis Foundation risk factors for osteoporotic fractures

Nonmodifiable
- **Personal history of fracture as an adult**
- **History of fracture in first-degree relative**
- Caucasian race
- Advanced age
- Female sex
- Dementia
- Poor health/fragility

Potentially modifiable
- **Current cigarette smoking**
- **Low body weight (<127 lbs)**
- Estrogen deficiency
- Early menopause (age <45 years) or bilateral ovariectomy
- Prolonged premenopausal amenorrhea (>1 year)
- Low calcium intake (lifelong)
- Impaired eyesight despite adequate correction
- Recurrent falls
- Inadequate physical activity
- Poor health/frailty

women who had at least 1 baseline vertebral fracture and by 50% in those who had no prevalent vertebral fracture. There was no significant reduction of hip or nonvertebral fractures; however, the study was not powered to demonstrate these endpoints.

The MORE study demonstrated a significant decrease in the risk of new breast cancers in patients exposed to raloxifene compared with placebo (13); however, risk reduction for breast cancer was not a primary endpoint of that study. The results of a prospective, double-blind study comparing raloxifene to tamoxifen for breast cancer prevention have recently confirmed this observation. Raloxifene does not cause endometrial proliferation and has a beneficial effect on the lipid profile, decreasing total and low-density lipoprotein cholesterol (14). However, a prospective, double-blind study comparing raloxifene to placebo demonstrated no difference in cardiovascular events or mortality.

The most common adverse events associated with raloxifene include hot flashes (which are more common in perimenopausal rather than late postmenopausal women) and leg cramps. Raloxifene also increases the risk of venous thromboembolic events, and therefore should not be used in patients with an active or past history of these disorders.

Raloxifene is administered as a single daily dose of 60 mg/day with adequate calcium and vitamin D supplementation.

Calcitonin

Calcitonin-salmon nasal spray is indicated for osteoporosis treatment in women who are at least 5 years postmenopausal. Calcitonin-salmon nasal spray reduces postmenopausal bone loss as well as the risk of new vertebral fractures. The Prevent Recurrence of Osteoporotic Fractures (PROOF) study (15) evaluated the efficacy and safety of calcitonin-salmon nasal spray in reducing the rate of new vertebral fractures in 1,255 postmenopausal women with osteoporosis over a 5-year period.

The 5-year final analysis of results showed a 33% reduction ($P = 0.03$) in risk of new vertebral fractures in patients receiving 200 IU calcitonin-salmon nasal spray versus placebo. The PROOF study was not designed to assess the effect of calcitonin-salmon nasal spray on hip or other nonvertebral fractures.

Calcitonin is generally well tolerated and there are no contraindications other than allergy to calcitonin or any of its components. Adverse events include local irritation of the nasal mucosa, such as rhinitis and other nasal symptoms.

The recommended dosage of calcitonin-salmon nasal spray in postmenopausal women with osteoporosis is 200 IU/day (1 spray) administered intranasally in alternate nostrils.

Bisphosphonates

Bisphosphonates bind to the surface of bone undergoing active resorption, and inhibit the differentiation, function, and lifespan of osteoclasts. Nitrogen-containing bisphosphonates (alendronate, risedronate, and ibandronate) act by inhibiting the enzyme farnesyl-pyrophosphate synthetase, which is necessary for protein prenylation—a process necessary for cytoskeleton organization, vesicle transport, membrane ruffling, and apoptosis of osteoclasts.

As a drug class, bisphosphonates are poorly absorbed when taken orally (oral bioavailability with an overnight fast and dosing 2 hours before breakfast with water is <1%). Strict adherence to the dosing regimen is necessary to maximize absorption. Alendronate or risedronate, for example, must be taken on an empty stomach following an overnight fast with 6–8 ounces of plain water only. The patient must not consume anything for 30 minutes following dosing, and must remain upright for at least 30 minutes to reduce the risk of esophageal irritation. Patients taking oral ibandronate must wait at least 60 minutes before food or drink.

Alendronate, risedronate, and ibandronate are approved for the prevention and treatment of postmenopausal osteoporosis. Alendronate is also indicated for the prevention of bone loss in men with osteoporosis. Both alendronate and risedronate are indicated for the treatment of glucocorticoid-induced osteoporosis, and risedronate is also approved for its prevention.

Alendronate. In an initial study, alendronate reduced the relative risk of spine fracture by 48% ($P = 0.003$) compared with placebo over 3 years (16). A subsequent study, the vertebral fracture arm of the Fracture Intervention Trial, assessed the effect of alendronate in 2,027 women with low bone mineral density (BMD) and at least 1 preexisting vertebral fracture (17). Alendronate reduced the risk of new vertebral fractures by 47% ($P < 0.001$). The risks of hip and wrist fractures were reduced by 51% ($P = 0.047$) and 48% ($P = 0.013$), respectively.

The therapeutic equivalency of alendronate taken at 10 mg/day (the initially approved dosage of alendronate) and 70 mg once weekly has been demonstrated (18). In this study, increases in lumbar, hip, and total body BMD were identical among the patient groups receiving these dosages, and the rate of bone turnover suppression was also

---

Rehabilitation Considerations in Osteoporosis

- Beware of potential for fracture among men and women who complain of sudden-onset pain.
- Exercise interventions should be modified and structured based on patient age, severity of disease, medications, general fitness, and other comorbid conditions.
- Aquatic exercises help strengthen muscles without over-stressing the bone.
- Walking programs and Tai Chi are helpful to increase endurance and strength.
- Coordination and core stability are important aspects of an exercise program for adults with osteoporosis.

---

identical. The incidence of gastrointestinal (GI) side effects with once-weekly alendronate was similar to that with daily administration.

In addition to being indicated for the prevention and treatment of postmenopausal osteoporosis, alendronate has been approved for the treatment of osteoporosis in men and for the treatment of glucocorticoid-induced osteoporosis, based upon studies demonstrating its efficacy to preserve bone density at the hip and spine (19,20).

Alendronate should not be given to patients with active, symptomatic upper GI disease or esophageal abnormalities that delay esophageal emptying, such as stricture of achalasia.

Risedronate. Risedronate is approved for the prevention and treatment of both glucocorticoid-induced (21) and postmenopausal osteoporosis. In a randomized, double-blind, placebo-controlled trial of 2,458 postmenopausal women who had at least 1 vertebral fracture at baseline (22), risedronate reduced the risk of new vertebral fractures by 41% compared with placebo over 3 years ($P = 0.003$). Vertebral fracture reduction of 65% was observed as early as 12 months in this trial ($P < 0.001$). The cumulative incidence of nonvertebral fractures was reduced by 39% ($P = 0.02$) over 3 years. Risedronate also significantly increased BMD compared with placebo in the lumbar spine, femoral neck, and radius.

In a large study of almost 10,000 postmenopausal women, risedronate showed a 30% reduction of hip fractures compared with placebo ($P = 0.001$) in a subgroup of patients <80 years old who had low femoral neck BMD (T-score less than −3.0) (23). A second subgroup of women at least 80 years old were entered into the study on the basis of clinical risk factors for hip fracture, rather than low bone density. No significant reduction in hip fractures was observed in this group.

In all trials, the adverse event profile of risedronate (including GI events) was similar to that of placebo. However, the same prescribing precautions apply as for alendronate. The patient must take risedronate with 8 ounces of water on an empty stomach 30 minutes before the first meal. Caution should be utilized in patients with active reflux disease or esophageal dysmotility. Risedronate is given at a dosage of 5 mg/day or 35 mg once weekly.

Ibandronate. Ibandronate is indicated for the prevention and treatment of osteoporosis. The pivotal vertebral fracture study leading to the approval of ibandronate was the BONE (oral iBandroante Osteoporosis vertebral fracture trial in North America and Europe) study of 2,946 postmenopauusal women with osteoporosis assigned to placebo, oral ibandronate (2.5 mg/day), or an intermittent oral regimen of 20 mg orally every other day for the first 24 days every 3 months (24). After 3 years, a significant 62% reduction in incident vertebral fractures was demonstrated for the 2.5-mg daily dose compared with placebo. Overall, no significant reduction in nonvertebral fractures was seen; however, a retrospective analysis of a high-risk group (those patients with a femoral neck T-score of less than −3.0) demonstrated a 69% reduction in nonvertebral fractures with the 2.5-mg/day dose compared with placebo.

Similar to bridging studies of alendronate and risedronate demonstrating bone density noninferiority with the once-weekly doses compared to the daily doses, a bridging study of daily versus once-monthly study of ibandronate was performed (the MOBILE study: **M**onthly **O**ral I**B**andronate **I**n **L**adi**E**s Study) (25). This study demonstrated superior increases in bone density at all sites examined with ibandronate (150 mg once monthly compared to 2.5 mg once daily) with similar overall and GI adverse effects.

Ibandronate is also available as a preparation administered by a 3-mg intravenous injection every 3 months. This preparation could prove to be useful in patients with GI intolerance to oral bisphosphonates.

Parathyroid Hormone

Subcutaneous injectable parathyroid hormone (teriparatide) is indicated for the treatment of postmenopausal women with osteoporosis at high risk for fractures and men with low bone mass. In a trial of 1,637 women with postmenopausal osteoporosis, subjects were given placebo or recombinant parathyroid hormone containing amino acids 1–34 (teriparatide) at a dosage of 20 μg/day for a mean of 21 months (26). Bone mineral density was increased by 9% at the lumbar spine and 3% at the total hip, and a significant 65% reduction in new vertebral fractures and 63% reduction in nonvertebral fractures for the 20 μg teriparatide compared to placebo was demonstrated. The most common adverse effect was leg cramps (2.6% versus 1.3% in controls).

Combination Therapy

Several combinations of the above therapies have been tried. Combinations of estrogen with risedronate or alendronate, and alendronate with raloxifene have all been demonstrated to increase bone density in an additive or synergistic fashion compared to either single agent alone (27). No study has yet demonstrated additive fracture protection. A study examining the concurrent use of parathyroid hormone and alendronate offered no advantage over monotherapy in terms of changes in BMD (28). In fact, the concurrent use of alendronate blunted large parathyroid hormone-induced increases in trabecular bone mineral density. At the current time, combination therapy is not generally recommended.

GLUCOCORTICOID-INDUCED OSTEOPOROSIS

Glucocorticoid-induced osteoporosis (GIOP) is the most common form of secondary osteoporosis, and the most common adverse effect of glucocorticoid use is fracture (29). Glucocorticoids induce osteoblast apoptosis (30), leading to a marked decrease in bone formation and a decrease in bone remodeling. Glucocorticoids also increase apoptosis of osteocytes, cells thought to participate in the detection and healing of bone microdamage. Glucocorticoid enhancement of osteoclastogenesis is mediated by an increase in the expression of the receptor activator of nuclear factor-κB ligand (RANKL) and a decrease in osteoprotegerin (OPG) expression in osteoblasts and stromal cells, leading to rapid bone loss.

An average dosage of prednisolone of 5 mg/day significantly increases the risk of spine and hip fracture (31). Fracture risk rises within 3 months of starting glucocorticoids, and falls after discontinuation; however, it does not fall back to baseline irrespective of the cumulative dose.

The American College of Rheumatology (ARC) Ad Hoc Guidelines Committee (32) recommends prophylactic bisphosphonates with either alendronate or risedronate for all new glucocorticoid users expected to continue prednisone ≥5 mg/day for >3 months. For patients already receiving long-term glucocorticoids (prednisone doses of ≥5 mg/day) who have a T-score less than −1.0, the ACR also recommends bisphosphonate therapy. Followup bone density measurement annually or biannually is recommended. Nonpharmacologic interventions outlined above are also recommended for all patients.

FUTURE THERAPIES

A phase-2 study to examine the effect of intravenous zoledronic acid on bone density and bone turnover in postmenopausal women has been published (33). In this study, 351 postmenopausal women age 45–80 years with a lumbar spine T-score that was −2.0 or lower were entered into a 1-year randomized, double-blind, placebo-controlled trial. Women received placebo or intravenous zoledronic acid in doses of 0.25 mg, 0.5 mg, or 1 mg at 3-month intervals. In addition, 1 group received a total annual dose of 4 mg as a single dose, and another received 2 doses of 2 mg each, 6 months apart.

Throughout the study, lumbar spine and hip bone density increases achieved with all zoledronic acid regimens were significantly higher than those in the placebo group ($P < 0.001$), and there were no significant differences among the zoledronic acid groups. Biochemical markers of bone resorption were significantly suppressed throughout the study in all zoledronic acid groups. Studies to demonstrate fracture reduction are currently underway.

Bone turnover is mediated by an increase in the expression of the RANKL, secreted by osteoblasts (34). RANKL binds and activates its receptor RANK on the surface of osteoclast precursors and induces osteoclast differentiation and subsequent activation. Osteoprotegerin is a natural inhibitor of RANKL, preventing RANKL from binding to its osteoclast receptor.

The efficacy and safety of subcutaneously administered denosumab, a fully human monoclonal antibody to RANKL, were evaluated in a phase-2 trial of 412 postmenopausal women with low BMD over a period of 12 months (35). Denosumab treatment for 12 months resulted in a significant increase in BMD at the lumbar spine and total hip, and significant reductions and in levels of serum C-telopeptide (a marker of bone resorption) compared to placebo throughout the trial. Studies to evaluate the efficacy of denosumab in reducing fracture risk are underway.

REFERENCES

1. NIH Consensus Development Panel on Osteoporosis Prevention, Diagnosis, and Therapy. Osteoporosis prevention, diagnosis, and therapy. JAMA 2001;285:785–95.
2. National Osteoporosis Foundation. Physician's guide to prevention and treatment of osteoporosis. Washington (DC): National Osteoporosis Foundation; 1998.
3. Genant HK, Engelke K, Fuerst T, Gluer CC, Grampp S, Harris ST, et al. Noninvasive assessment of bone mineral and structure: state of the art. J Bone Miner Res 1996;11:707–30.
4. Miller PD, Bonnick SL, Rosen CJ. Consensus of an international panel on the clinical utility of bone mass measurements in the detection of low bone mass in the adult population. Calcif Tissue Int 1996;58:207–14.
5. Kitchin B, Morgan S. Nutritional considerations in osteoporosis. Curr Opinion Rheumatol 2003;15:476–80.
6. Dawson-Hughes B, Harris SS, Krall EA, Dallal GE. Effect of calcium and vitamin D supplementation on bone density in men and women 65 years of age or older. N Engl J Med 1997;337:670–6.
7. Chapuy MC, Arlot ME, Duboeuf F, Brun J, Crouzet B, Arnaud S, et al. Vitamin D$_3$ and calcium to prevent hip fractures in elderly women. N Engl J Med 1992;327:1637–42.
8. Holick MF, Siris ES, Binkley N, et al. Prevalence of vitamin D inadequacy among postmenopausal North American women receiving osteoporosis therapy. J Clin Endocrinol Metab 2005;90:3215–24.
9. Rossouw JE, Anderson GL, Prentice RL, LaCroix AZ, Kooperberg C, Stefanick ML, et al., Writing Group for the Women's Health Initiative Investigators. Risks and benefits of estrogen plus progestin in healthy postmenopausal women: principal results from the Women's Health Initiative randomized trial. JAMA 2002;288:321–3.
10. U.S. Food and Drug Administration. FDA approves new labels for estrogen and estrogen with progestin therapies for postmenopausal women following review of Women's Health Initiative data. FDA News, January 8, 2003. Accessed June 28, 2006. URL: http://www.fda.gov/bbs/topics/NEWS/2003/NEW00863.html
11. Delmas PD, Bjarnason NH, Mitlak BH, Ravoux AC, Shah AS, Huster WJ, et al. Effects of raloxifene on bone mineral density, serum cholesterol concentrations, and uterine endometrium in postmenopausal women. N Engl J Med 1997;337:1641–7.
12. Ettinger B, Black DM, Mitlak BH, Knickerbocker RK, Nickelsen T, Genant HK, et al., Multiple Outcomes of Raloxifene Evaluation (MORE) Investigators. Reduction of vertebral fracture risk in postmenopausal women treated with raloxifene. JAMA 1999;282:637–45.
13. Cummings SR, Eckert S, Krueger KA, Grady D, Powles TJ, Cauley JA, et al. The effect of raloxifene on risk of breast cancer in postmenopausal women: results from the MORE randomized trial. Multiple Outcomes of Raloxifene Evaluation. JAMA 1999;281:2189–97.
14. Walsh BW, Kuller LH, Wild RA, Paul S, Farmer M, Lawrence JB, et al. Effects of raloxifene on serum lipids and coagulation factors in healthy postmenopausal women. JAMA 1998;279:1445–51.
15. Chesnut CH 3rd, Silverman S, Andriano K, Genant H, Gimona A, Harris S, et al. A randomized trial of nasal spray salmon calcitonin in postmenopausal women with established osteoporosis: the prevent recurrence of osteoporotic fractures study. Am J Med 2000;109:267–76.
16. Liberman UA, Weiss SR, Broll J, Minne HW, Quan H, Bell NH, et al., the Alendronate Phase III Osteoporosis Treatment Study Group. Effect of oral alendronate on bone mineral density and the incidence of fractures in postmenopausal osteoporosis. N Engl J Med 1995;333:1437–43.
17. Black DM, Cummings SR, Karpf DB, Cauley JA, Thompson DE, Nevitt MC, et al., Fracture Intervention Trial Research Group. Randomised trial of effect of alendronate on risk of fracture in women with existing vertebral fractures. Lancet 1996;348:1535–41.
18. Schnitzer T, Bone HG, Crepaldi G, Adami S, McClung M, Kiel D, et al., Alendronate Once-Weekly Study Group. Therapeutic equivalence of alendronate 70 mg once-weekly and alendronate 10 mg daily in the treatment of osteoporosis. Aging (Milano) 2000;12:1–12.
19. Orwoll E, Ettinger M, Weiss S, Miller P, Kendler D, Graham J, et al. Alendronate for the treatment of osteoporosis in men. N Engl J Med 2000;343:604–10.
20. Saag KG, Emkey R, Schnitzer TJ, Brown JP, Hawkins F, Goemaere S, et al., Glucocorticoid-Induced Osteoporosis Intervention Study Group. Alendronate for the prevention and treatment of glucocorticoid-induced osteoporosis. N Engl J Med 1998;339:292–9.
21. Cohen S, Levy RM, Keller M, Boling E, Emkey RD, Greenwald M, et al. Risedronate therapy prevents corticosteroid-induced bone loss: a 12-month multicenter, randomized, double-blind, placebo-controlled, parallel group study. Arthritis Rheum 1999;42:2309–18.
22. Harris ST, Watts NB, Genant HK, McKeever CD, Hangartner T, Keller M, et al., Vertebral Efficacy With Risedronate Therapy (VERT) Study Group. Effects of risedronate treatment on vertebral and nonvertebral fractures in women with postmenopausal osteoporosis: a randomized controlled trial. JAMA 1999;282:1344–52.
23. McClung MR, Geusens P, Miller PD, Zippel H, Bensen WG, Roux C, et al., Hip Intervention Program Study Group. Effect of risedronate on the risk of hip fracture in elderly women. N Engl J Med 2001;344:333–40.
24. Chesnut CH III, Skag A, Christiansen C, Recker R, Stakkestad JA, Hoiseth A, et al., Oral Ibandronate Osteoporosis Vertebral Fracture Trial in North America and Europe (BONE). Effects of oral ibandronate administered daily or intermittently on fracture risk in postmenopausal osteoporosis. J Bone Miner Res 2004;19:1241–9.
25. Miller PD, McClung MR, Macovei L, Stakkestad JA, Luckey M, Bonvoisin B, et al. Monthly oral ibandronate therapy in postmenopausal osteoporosis: 1-year results from the MOBILE study. J Bone Miner Res 2005;20:1315–22.
26. Neer RM, Arnaud CD, Zanchetta JR, Prince R, Gaich GA, Reginster JY, et al. Effect of parathyroid hormone (1-34) on fractures and bone

mineral density in postmenopausal women with osteoporosis. N Engl J Med 2001;344:1434–41.

27. Wimalawansa SJ. Prevention and treatment of osteoporosis: efficacy of combination of hormone replacement therapy with other antiresorptive agents. J Clin Densitom 2000;3:187–201.

28. Black DM, Greenspan SL, Ensrud KE, Palermo L, McGowan JA, Lang TF, et al., PaTH Study Investigators. The effects of parathyroid hormone and alendronate alone or in combination in postmenopausal osteoporosis. N Engl J Med 2003;349:1207–15.

29. Saag KG, Koehnke R, Caldwell JR, Brasington R, Burmeister LF, Zimmerman B, et al. Low dose long-term corticosteroid therapy in rheumatoid arthritis: an analysis of serious adverse events Am J Med 1994;96:115–23.

30. Weinstein RS, Jilka RL, Parfitt AM, Manolagas SC. Inhibition of osteoblastogenesis and promotion of apoptosis of osteoblasts and osteocytes by glucocorticoids: potential mechanisms of their deleterious effects on bone. J Clin Invest 1998;102:274–82.

31. Van Staa TP, Leufkens HG, Abenhaim L, Zhang B, Cooper C. Use of oral corticosteroids and risk of fractures. J Bone Miner Res 2000;15:993–1000.

32. American College of Rheumatology Ad Hoc Committee on Glucocorticoid-Induced Osteoporosis. Recommendation for the prevention and treatment of glucocorticoid-induced osteoporosis: 2001 update. Arthritis Rheum 2001;44:1496–503.

33. Reid IR, Brown JP, Burckhardt P, Horowitz Z, Richardson P, Trechsel U, et al. Intravenous zoledronic acid in postmenopausal women with low bone mineral density. N Engl J Med 2002;346:653–61.

34. Tanaka S, Nakamura K, Takahasi N, Suda T. Role of RANKL in physiological and pathological bone resorption and therapeutics targeting the RANKL–RANK signaling system. Immunol Rev 2005;208:30–49.

35. McClung MR, Lewiecki EM, Cohen SB, Bolognese MA, Woodson GC, Moffett AH, et al., AMG 162 Bone Loss Study Group. Denosumab in postmenopausal women with low bone mineral density. N Engl J Med 2006;354:821–31.

Pediatric Rheumatic Diseases

SANGEETA SULE, MD

Rheumatic illnesses may present in childhood. Some diseases, such as systemic-onset juvenile rheumatoid arthritis and pauciarticular juvenile rheumatoid arthritis, are more common in children than adults. Special considerations apply to childhood illnesses because clinical and treatment decisions are influenced by the child's growth and development; furthermore, the impact of these rheumatic diseases extends beyond the child to the entire family.

JUVENILE RHEUMATOID ARTHRITIS

Juvenile rheumatoid arthritis (JRA) is the most prevalent rheumatic disease in children. The overall prevalence of JRA is ~30–150 per 100,000 with 70,000–100,000 inactive and active cases of JRA in the United States (1). This is approximately the same number of children as those with juvenile diabetes and at least 4 times as many children as have sickle cell anemia or cystic fibrosis (2). The course of JRA can vary widely, with some children recovering fully and others experiencing lifelong symptoms.

Classification of JRA

The diagnostic criteria for JRA include disease onset at <16 years of age, defined as persistent arthritis in 1 or more joints for 6 weeks or longer, and exclusion of other types of childhood arthritis (such as reactive arthritis, inflammatory bowel disease, or systemic lupus erythematosus) (3). The disease-onset subtype of JRA is defined by clinical symptoms that appear in the first 6 months of disease. JRA is divided into 3 subtypes: pauciarticular, polyarticular, or systemic.

A recent classification system developed by the International League Against Rheumatism is being used to more rigorously define arthritis (4). The term juvenile idiopathic arthritis is used in this classification system, which separates the idiopathic arthritidies of childhood into 8 separate categories: systemic arthritis; oligoarthritis-persistent, with <5 joints involved at any time during the onset or course of disease; oligoarthritis-extended, with arthritis in <5 joints in the first 6 months of disease but affecting a cumulative total of ≥5 joints after the first 6 months; polyarthritis-rheumatoid factor negative; polyarthritis-rheumatoid factor positive; enthesitis-related arthritis; psoriatic arthritis; and other.

Pauciarticular JRA

Pauciarticular JRA is defined by involvement of <5 joints after 6 months of disease. It is further subdivided into early-onset or late-onset. Children with early-onset pauciarticular JRA typically are <5 years old, are more often girls, and are more often antinuclear antibody (ANA) positive. A positive ANA is associated with an increased risk of uveitis. Early-onset pauciarticular JRA has the highest prevalence of uveitis, with eye involvement reported in 30–50% (5). The uveitis usually begins in the anterior chamber of the eye and is usually not associated with any systemic symptoms. If the uveitis progresses, children may suffer from serious complications, including cataracts, glaucoma, and cystoid macular edema. Ophthalmologic screening for children diagnosed before age 7 with a positive ANA is recommended every 3 months. If children <7 years old at diagnosis have had normal eye exam results for 7 years, or were diagnosed at ≥7 years and have normal eye examination results for 4 years, the frequency of eye exams can be decreased to once every 12 months (6).

Late-onset pauciarticular JRA is more common in boys and 50% are HLA–B27 positive. These children are more likely to have enthesitis or tendinitis. The arthritis typically involves the large joints, such as the hips, knees, or ankles. The differential diagnosis includes the spondyloarthropathies (including ankylosing spondylitis), arthritis secondary to inflammatory bowel disease, and psoriatic arthritis. Eye involvement is less common than in early-onset JRA and, in contrast, is usually associated with significant pain, photophobia, and sudden onset.

Polyarticular JRA

Polyarticular JRA is defined as involvement of >5 joints after 6 months of illness. It is the second most common subtype of JRA with a prevalence of 30–40%. There is a bimodal distribution of age of onset, with the first peak at 2–5 years and the second peak at 10–14 years. Girls are more commonly affected than boys. Two distinct subgroups of children can be defined based on the presence or absence of rheumatoid factor (RF). RF-positive children are usually older (>8 years) with a female predominance. Children with RF are at increased risk of developing joint erosions and rheumatoid nodules, because disease manifestations are similar to those found in adult RA.

Systemic-Onset JRA

Systemic-onset JRA accounts for ~10% of cases. It is characterized by daily or twice-daily fever spikes >101°F (quotidian fever) as well as a salmon-colored, blanching, nonpruritic rash. The rash and joint symptoms may wax and wane during febrile episodes. The rash of systemic-onset JRA is often present on the trunk and proximal extremities and may involve the palms and soles. Superficial trauma or pressure to the skin may cause eruption of the rash. Children may initially present with significant arthralgias, rather than frank arthritis, at the onset of systemic JRA. Serositis, pleuritis, pericarditis, hyperbilirubinemia, elevated liver enzyme levels, leukocytosis, and anemia may be part of the initial presentation, making exclusion of infectious or hematologic causes of fever and systemic symptoms critical.

Complications of JRA

Linear growth retardation is seen in children with active JRA, particularly with systemic or polyarticular onset. The degree of linear growth retardation depends on the severity and duration of inflammation as well as the use of corticosteroids. Pauciarticular JRA may lead to localized growth abnormalities, such as leg-length discrepancy. Leg-length measurements should be recorded at each visit and if discrepancies are noted, orthotic shoe inserts should be used to avoid a compensatory scoliosis. Early in the course of disease, bony development is accelerated due to increased blood flow to the growth plate, and the affected leg may appear longer. However, later in the course of the illness, after the epiphyseal junction has fused, the opposite may be true. Micrognathia and malocclusion are also common sequelae of localized growth defects in the temporomandibular joint in JRA. Orthodontic consultation is recommended.

Osteopenia, or low bone mass for age, may be seen in children with JRA. Both the cortical appendicular skeleton and axial trabecular bone may be involved. The degree of osteopenia correlates with disease activity and severity. Medications, such as corticosteroids, may also contribute to osteopenia. Therapy includes weight-bearing exercises, appropriate nutrition, as well as calcium and vitamin D supplementation.

Cardiac involvement may occur in up to one-third of systemic-onset JRA patients. Pericarditis, myocarditis, or endocarditis may occur, with pericarditis being the most common. Chest pain, dyspnea on exertion, or a friction rub on examination should prompt further testing, including x-ray or echocardiography. These episodes may last for weeks to months and are generally associated with arthritis flares. Treatment includes antiinflammatory medications, including corticosteroids.

Adequate nutritional status is critical for children with JRA to minimize growth abnormalities. Protein stores, iron, selenium, vitamin C, and zinc have been reported to be low in children with JRA. In addition, some patients may have mechanical problems with feeding due to jaw involvement. Medications may also impact nutritional status. For example, corticosteroids may increase appetite, elevate blood sugar, and lead to excessive weight gain.

Treatment of JRA

The optimal treatment of JRA involves physical, social, and pharmacologic strategies. Physical modalities include range-of-motion exercises for involved joints and splints to minimize joint deformity or to correct joint contractures. Active participation in physical and occupational therapy is often essential for maintaining joint mobility and physical functioning in JRA.

Social programs should involve the entire family, as family factors greatly influence a child's ability to cope with this chronic illness. Some studies have concluded that there is an increased risk of psychosocial problems in children with JRA and that chronic family difficulties predicted these problems more so than disease severity. Positive family factors also influence adherance to medications. A highly cohesive family structure that stresses individual freedom with eventual self-mastery of medications seems best suited to transition the pediatric patient into adulthood. The Arthritis Foundation and the American Juvenile Arthritis Organization are excellent resources for educational programs in family coping skills.

Pharmacologic therapy is tailored to disease severity. In pediatrics, the dose of the medicine is based on the weight of the child, with the maximum being the standard adult dose. This applies for all medicines, but has particular importance for cytotoxic medications in which the risk of side effects is high.

Often in patients with mild arthritis, such as pauciarticular JRA, nonsteroidal antiinflammatory drugs (NSAIDs) alone are sufficient. Treatment requires a full antiinflammatory dose, which is often larger than that needed for pain control alone (7). Methotrexate, at dosages of 10 mg/m², is used primarily for treatment of polyarticular or systemic-onset JRA. Approximately 70% of patients show clinical improvement while taking methotrexate, although the rate of response is lower in systemic-onset JRA patients with significant systemic symptoms (8).

In patients who do not respond to methotrexate at dosages of 10 mg/m², higher dosages of up to 1 mg/kg/week (maximum of 50 mg/week) have been shown to be well tolerated and beneficial. At doses >20 mg/m², oral absorption of methotrexate may be unpredictable and subcutaneous parenteral administration is recommended (9). Therapeutic benefit of methotrexate may not be evident for 3–4 weeks and the maximal response is not reached for 3–6 months. Methotrexate side effects include nausea, oral ulcers, decreased appetite, and abdominal pain. The gastrointestinal side effects may be minimized with subcutaneous administration or oral folate administration.

Tumor necrosis factor α (TNFα) antagonists have also been used effectively in JRA. In a randomized, prospective, placebo-controlled trial in children with methotrexate-resistant polyarticular JRA, treatment with etanercept resulted in a clinically significant improvement in joint exam, sedimentation rate, and C-reactive protein (10). Infliximab, another TNFα antagonist, has been shown to be effective for treatment of the uveitis associated with JRA (11). Other biological agents, including an interleukin-1 (IL-1) receptor antagonist, have also been studied in JRA. In children with systemic-onset JRA, investigators have demonstrated increased IL-1 in peripheral blood mononuclear cells (12). In systemic-onset patients who had failed to receive benefit with methotrexate and TNF-receptor antagonists, treatment with an IL-1 receptor antagonist resulted in dramatic improvement in systemic symptoms and arthritis.

SYSTEMIC LUPUS ERYTHEMATOSUS

Systemic lupus erythematosus (SLE) is a complex autoimmune disease with a diverse array of presentations. As in adults, SLE in children can involve any organ system. The American College of Rheumatology criteria for the classification of SLE applies to children; however, the natural history of disease may be quite variable (13). Pediatric SLE may present insidiously, making diagnosis difficult, or may present acutely with rapid progression, leading to death.

SLE accounts for 10% of patients with pediatric rheumatic diseases, with an estimated prevalence of 5,000–10,000 children in the United States (14). SLE is much more common in adolescent girls. Girls are affected 5 times more frequently than boys, and disease prevalence is higher in African Americans, Asians, and Hispanics. The disease is rare in children younger than 5 years; before menarche, the female-to-male ratio is equal.

Although available immunologic tests have made the diagnosis of SLE easier, a high index of suspicion is required for obtaining the necessary tests. Early symptoms of pediatric SLE, including fever, fatigue, anorexia, and weight loss, may be quite nonspecific and can mimic viral syndromes. Infants may also develop an SLE-like syndrome. SS-A antibody of the IgG class may pass from the mother across the placenta to the fetus, leading to positive serologies and diagnosis of neonatal SLE. Infants present with rash, thrombocytopenia, hemolytic anemia, or congenital heart block. With the exception of congenital heart block, the symptoms of neonatal SLE are transient and resolve over a few months as the antibodies are cleared.

Cutaneous manifestations of SLE occur in ~80% of pediatric patients at some time in the course of disease. The malar rash (butterfly rash) can be seen in one-third of patients and presents with erythema, with possible whitish scale and sparing of the nasolabial folds. Alopecia can occur in 20% of patients and may present as patchy, scaling areas on the scalp, leading to scarring and permanent baldness. Mucocutaneous ulcerations in the oral or nasal cavity can also be seen in pediatric SLE.

SLE arthritis is usually more transient and episodic compared with that seen in JRA. Jaccoud arthropathy in SLE is a nondeforming, reversible, soft-tissue arthritis that can mimic the boutonniere (flexion of proximal interphalangeals [PIPs], hyperextension of distal interphalangeals [DIPs]) and swan-neck (hyperextension of PIP, flexion of DIP) deformities seen in JRA. Arthralgias are usually a more prominent symptom in SLE compared to the frank arthritis and morning stiffness noted in JRA.

One of the most commonly involved organs in pediatric SLE is the kidney. Approximately two-thirds of children with SLE will have some degree of renal involvement. This often manifests early in the course of disease, but may occur years after the diagnosis has been made. Renal involvement is classified using the World Health Organization classification of lupus nephritis used in adult SLE. The glomeruli, tubules, interstitium, or blood vessels can become involved and treatment is tailored to the severity of inflammation.

Treatment of SLE

The treatment of SLE varies depending on the severity of symptoms. Corticosteroids are effective in reducing systemic inflammation but are associated with significant side effects, such as weight gain, acne, cataracts, accelerated atherosclerosis, and growth retardation. For patients with organ involvement, immunosuppressive therapy has dramatically improved survival in pediatric SLE. Ten-year survival for pediatric SLE has improved from 30% to 70% with intravenous cyclophosphamide for renal disease (15). However, treatment with cyclophosphamide can result in premature ovarian failure and amenorrhea (16). Recent studies have shown that treatment with a gonadotropin-releasing hormone (GnRH) analog was beneficial, with fewer patients developing premature ovarian failure. The GnRH agonist was given once a month, ~10 days prior to the monthly bolus of intravenous cyclophosphamide (17).

Trials of immunosuppressive therapy for pediatric SLE are ongoing. Recognition of early symptoms, initiation of treatment, and meeting medical and psychosocial needs in pediatric SLE remains a high priority for pediatric rheumatologists.

SCLERODERMA

Scleroderma, or "tight skin," is rare in children. The localized forms of scleroderma are more common in childhood than the diffuse systemic subtype. Boys and girls are affected equally when younger than 8 years; however, there is a 3:1 female predominance after age 8.

Localized scleroderma is a group of disorders in which fibrosis is limited to the skin, subcutaneous tissue, or muscle. An erythematous, pruritic border characterizes early scleroderma lesions. Morphea may occur as plaques, whereas linear scleroderma affects a single dermatome. If the linear scleroderma affects skin around joints, contractures and growth arrest may occur. When linear scleroderma occurs on the

face or scalp, it is referred to as "en coup de sabre" because it resembles a sword wound.

The ultimate prognosis of children with scleroderma depends on the extent of visceral involvement. Localized forms of scleroderma often resolve without treatment. However, systemic sclerosis may involve multiple organ systems, including gastrointestinal (gastroesophageal reflux, esophageal dysmotility), cardiac (heart block, pericardial effusion, congestive heart failure), and renal (renal crisis). Treatment is directed toward the organ system involved, such as proton-pump inhibitors for gastroesophageal reflux. Although currently available immunosuppressive treatments have shown variable effect in halting skin fibrosis, ongoing research directed at pathogenic pathways in collagen formation may hold promise.

DERMATOMYOSITIS

Dermatomyositis (DM) accounts for ~5% of all childhood rheumatic diseases. The etiology remains unknown; however, environmental or infectious triggers are thought to play a role. There is a female predominance, with a 2:1 ratio, and DM is more prevalent in the 5–14-year age group.

Children may present with varying skin manifestations, including a facial rash (heliotrope) characterized by a violaceous color around the eyes and malar region, with involvement of the nasolabial fold, erythema and pale atrophic skin changes over the interphalangeal joints (Gottron papules), and nail-bed telangiectasias. Pediatric DM patients are at an increased risk for nodular calcium deposits, particularly over pressure points and inflamed soft-tissue areas. This complication can be quite devastating, resulting in contractures and increased skin infections due to open sores. Although medications that modulate calcium are used for treatment, these have had variable success.

Patients usually present with fatigue and symmetric, proximal muscle weakness manifesting as refusal to go up or down stairs, increased desire to be carried, or clumsiness. Muscle pain can also be a prominent early symptom. Dysphagia may occur if the gastrointestinal muscles are involved, making evaluation of the gag reflex critical. A nasal voice or frequent coughing episodes should prompt further evaluation of swallowing function.

Children with DM have variable disease courses, with the majority of patients presenting insidiously rather than acutely. This may lead to a long lag time before the diagnosis is made. The clinical diagnosis of DM can be supported by laboratory tests demonstrating inflammatory muscle disease, such as elevated levels of creatine kinase, aspartate aminotransferase, alanine aminotransferase, aldolase, or lactate dehydrogenase. Only one of the muscle enzymes may be elevated during active inflammation. Magnetic resonance imaging can show edema and active inflammation in muscle.

Corticosteroid monotherapy is often effective in the treatment of DM (18). However, if the child continues to have active disease, both oral and subcutaneous methotrexate have been shown to be effective (18). There also are reports of cyclosporine, cyclophosphamide, and intravenous immunoglobulin used in the treatment of pediatric DM (19,20).

MUSCULAR DYSTROPHY

Muscular dystrophies are a group of inherited disorders resulting in progressive muscle weakness. The underlying pathology is a defect in the genes required for normal muscle function. There are many different types of muscular dystrophies, and the pattern of inheritance can vary. Two of the most common forms, Duchenne and Becker, are associated with X-linked defects in the dystrophin gene (21–23). Duchenne

Rehabilitation Considerations in Pediatric Rheumatic Diseases

- Routine strengthening exercises are important to maximize function. These activities should be play-based to promote adherence.
- Frequent assessment of leg length and assessment to determine need for orthotics is recommended.
- Weight-bearing exercises are important to maintain bone integrity.
- Routinely monitor vital signs during aerobic exercise because one-third of children with systemic-onset juvenile arthritis may have cardiac involvement. Intermittent, progressive exercise sessions (3 sets of 10 minutes) versus 30 minutes may be better tolerated as a starting point.
- Individual sports allow kids to maintain physical activities without the pressure of competition.
- Swimming and water activities allow more ease of movement and reduced joint stress.

muscular dystrophy (DMD) is associated with more severe clinical symptoms than Becker muscular dystrophy.

Children may present with proximal muscle weakness affecting the lower extremities before the upper extremities. Children may eventually manifest a characteristic waddling gait, lumbar lordosis, and calf hypertrophy. Physical examination, particularly in children with DMD, is significant for difficulty arising from the floor and having to use their hands to push themselves to an upright seated position. This is called a Gower's sign. Children may also present with elevated creatine kinase levels, even during the newborn period. Creatine kinase levels usually peak by age 2 years then progressively fall as muscle is replaced with fat and fibrosis. Treatment of DMD includes monitoring for end-organ involvement (heart, lung). Corticosteroids have also shown to be beneficial for improving muscle strength and mass in DMD (24).

GROWING PAINS

Growing pains occur in 10–20% of school-aged children. Children usually present with early-evening discomfort that may awaken the child from sleep. The discomfort is usually muscular and described as a cramping sensation in the calf, shin, or thigh area. If laboratory or x-ray evaluations are done, they are entirely normal. Physical exam is also benign, with no signs of joint tenderness or hypermobility.

The etiology of growing pains is unknown; however, there is often a family history. The treatment for growing pains is conservative. One of the hallmarks of growing pains is that they are relieved with benign measures, such as massage or moist heat. If needed, an evening dose of NSAIDs may be used to prevent attacks. The course of growing pains is usually self-limited but may persist for up to 2 years.

REFERENCES

1. Towner SR, Michet CJ Jr, O'Fallon WM, Nelson AM. The epidemiology of juvenile arthritis in Rochester, Minnesota 1960–1979. Arthritis Rheum 1983;26:1208–13.
2. Gortmaker SL, Sappenfield W. Chronic childhood disorders: prevalence and impact. Pediatr Clin North Am 1984;31:3–18.
3. Cassidy JT, Petty RE. Textbok of pediatric rheumatology. Philadelphia: Saunders; 1995.
4. Petty RE, Southwood TR, Baum J, Bhettay E, Glass DN, Manners P, et al. Revision of the proposed classification criteria for juvenile idiopathic arthritis: Durban, 1997. J Rheumatol 1998;25:1991–4.
5. Bywaters EG, Ansell BM. Monoarticular arthritis in children. Ann Rheum Dis 1965;24:116–22.
6. Cassidy J, Kivlin J, Lindsley C, Nocton J. Section on rheumatology, Section on ophthalmology. Ophthalmologic examinations in children with juvenile rheumatoid arthritis. Pediatrics 2006;117:1843–5.
7. Lovell DJ, Giannini EH, Brewer EJ Jr. Time course of response to non-steroidal antiinflammatory drugs in juvenile rheumatoid arthritis. Arthritis Rheum 1984;27:1433–7.
8. Giannini EH, Brewer EJ, Kuzmina N, Shaikov A, Maximov A, Vorontsov I, et al. The Pediatric Rheumatology Collaborative Study Group and The Cooperative Children's Study Group. Methotrexate in resistant juvenile rheumatoid arthritis. Results of the U.S.A.-U.S.S.R. double-blind, placebo-controlled trial. N Engl J Med 1992;326:1043–9.
9. Wallace CA, Sherry DD. Preliminary report of higher dose methotrexate treatment in juvenile rheumatoid arthritis. J Rheumatol 1992;19:1604–7.
10. Lovell DJ, Giannini EH, Reiff A, Cawkwell GD, Silverman ED, Nocton JJ, et al. Pediatric Rheumatology Collaborative Study Group. Etanercept in children with polyarticular juvenile rheumatoid arthritis. N Engl J Med 2000;342:763–9.
11. Kahn P, Weiss M, Imundo LF, Levy DM. Favorable response to high-dose infliximab for refractory childhood uveitis. Ophthalmology 2006;113: 864.e1, 864.e2.
12. Pascual V, Allantaz F, Arce E, Punaro M, Banchereau J. Role of interleukin-1 (IL-1) in the pathogenesis of systemic onset juvenile idiopathic arthritis and clinical response to IL-1 blockade. J Exp Med 2005;201:1479–86.
13. Tan EM, Cohen AS, Fries JF, Masi AT, McShane DJ, Rothfield NF, et al. The 1982 revised criteria for the classification of systemic lupus erythematosus. Arthritis Rheum 1982;25:1271–7.
14. Lehman TJ. Systemic lupus erythematosus in children and adolescents. In: Wallace DA, Hahn B, editors. Dubois' lupus erythematosus. 5th ed. Philadelphia: Saunders; 1997.
15. Gonzalez B, Hernandez P, Olguin H, Miranda M, Lira L, Toso M, et al. Changes in the survival of patients with systemic lupus erythematosus in childhood: 30 years experience in Chile. Lupus 2005;14:918–23.
16. Boumpas DT, Austin HA 3rd, Vaughan EM, Yarboro CH, Klippel JH, Balow JE. Risk for sustained amenorrhea in patients with systemic lupus erythematosus receiving intermittent pulse cyclophosphamide therapy. Ann Intern Med 1993;119:366–9.
17. Somers EC, Marder W, Christman GM, Ognenovski V, McCune WJ. Use of a gonadotropin-releasing hormone analog for protection against premature ovarian failure during cyclophosphamide therapy in women with severe lupus. Arthritis Rheum 2005;52:2761–7.
18. Ansell BM. Management of polymyositis and dermatomyositis. Clin Rheum Dis 1984;10:205–13.
19. Lang BA, Laxer RM, Murphy G, Silverman ED, Roifman CM. Treatment of dermatomyositis with intravenous gammaglobulin. Am J Med 1991;91:169–72.
20. Girardin E, Dayer JM, Paunier L. Cyclosporine for juvenile dermatomyositis. J Pediatr 1988;112:165–6.
21. Ervasti JM, Ohlendieck K, Kahl SD, Gaver MG, Campbell KP. Deficiency of a glycoprotein component of the dystrophin complex in dystrophic muscle. Nature 1990;345:315–9.
22. Kunkel LM, Hejtmancik JF, Caskey CT, Speer A, Monaco AP, Middlesworth W, et al. Analysis of deletions in DNA from patients with Becker and Duchenne muscular dystrophy. Nature 1986;322:73–7.
23. Worton R. Muscular dystrophies: diseases of the dystrophin-glycoprotein complex. Science 1995;270:755–6.
24. Mendell JR, Moxley RT, Griggs RC, Brooke MH, Fenichel GM, Miller JP, et al. Randomized, double-blind six-month trial of prednisone in Duchenne's muscular dystrophy. N Engl J Med 1989;320:1592–7.

Periarticular Rheumatic Diseases

PASHA SARRAF, MD, PhD, and ANTHONY M. REGINATO, MD, PhD

The majority of patients who present to their primary health care provider with musculoskeletal symptoms have a soft-tissue disorder rather than less common forms of articular rheumatism. Soft-tissue rheumatism is one of the most common and misunderstood categories of disorders, but it usually has a benign course and an excellent response to therapy (1). They include tendinopathies, structural disorders, neurovascular entrapment syndromes, and regional myofascial or generalized pain syndromes. These conditions may involve such anatomic regions as the hand, wrist, elbow, shoulder, spine, hip, knee, ankle, heel, midfoot, and forefoot. Overuse, repetitive strain or trauma, acute and chronic infections, foreign bodies, entrapment neuropathies, aging, and crystal deposition disease play important pathologic roles in their development.

The keys to diagnosis of soft-tissue rheumatism are the history and, more importantly, the precise physical examination of the anatomic structures involved and identification of precipitating and aggravating factors. Our understanding of the pathology of these conditions is improving since significant advances in magnetic resonance imaging (MRI) and recent application of musculoskeletal ultrasonography have allowed us to determine periarticular soft-tissue integrity and improve the accuracy of needle placement for diagnostic and therapeutic purposes (2).

The practitioner should not overlook clues to systemic disorders, because conditions as varied as infection (gonococcemia, secondary syphilis, mycobacterial and fungal infections), rheumatoid arthritis (RA), ankylosing spondylitis, reactive arthritis, psoriatic arthritis, crystal-induced arthritis, sarcoidosis, and amyloidosis can lead to quite similar soft-tissue rheumatism syndromes, as outlined in Table 1.

BURSITIS

Bursae are closed sacs, often with a lining that resembles the synovial membrane lining of the diarthrodial joints, which secrete and absorb bursal fluid. The bursae provide the gliding mechanism between adjacent musculoskeletal structures, such as skin over bone, muscle over muscle, and tendon over bone (3). There are ~150 such structures in the body, and new ones, called *adventitious bursae*, may develop at pressure points, such as bunions or the site of amputation. A diagnosis of bursitis is based on the clinical findings of exquisite local tenderness and swelling at the sites of bursae, pain on motion and at rest, and occasional loss of active movement. Reduced active range of motion with preserved passive range of motion on physical exam is suggestive of a soft-tissue disorder, such as bursitis, but may also be consistent with tendinopathy or muscle injury.

Bursal inflammation is broadly classified into septic and nonseptic bursitis. Anatomic classification divides bursitis into superficial (subcutaneous) or deep according to the location of the bursa. Superficial bursae include the olecranon, prepatellar, and superficial infrapatellar bursae (Figure 1); deep bursae include the posterior shoulder, subacromial, iliopsoas, trochanteric, ischial, deep infrapatellar, popliteal, anserine, retrocalcaneal, and metatarsophalangeal. Bursitis is rarely seen in patients younger than 20 years and becomes common in middle-aged

and older individuals. The superficial location of the olecranon, prepatellar, and superficial infrapatellar bursae makes them more vulnerable to bacterial infection because they are interposed between the skin and the underlying bony structures. It is presumed that local cutaneous trauma causes translocation of the normal skin flora into the bursae or by local cellulitic spread into already traumatized subcutaneous bursae. The various etiologic types of subcutaneous bursitis are summarized in Table 1.

The development of bursitis is a function of repetitive physical stresses and the condition of the bursae and surrounding tissues. Idiopathic or traumatic bursitis is characterized by noninflammatory effusion from repetitive local trauma. In septic bursitis, reduced skin gliding over bony prominences results in the abrasion, fissuring, and translocation into the bursal sac of bacteria normally present in the skin. The same mechanical factors favor formation of tophaceous deposits in crystal-induced arthritis and rheumatoid nodules. In fact, superficial bursae and independent adjacent diarthrodial joint synovitis may coexist in such conditions as RA and crystal-induced arthritis.

Certain bursae stand out as more common sites of inflammation than others. In the upper extremity, the most frequently affected are the subacromial and the olecranon bursae (Figure 1A). In the lower extremity,

Table 1. Etiology of acute and chronic bursitis and tendonitis

Common
  Bacterial
    Staphylococcus aureus
    S pyogens
  Crystal-induced
    Monosodium urate
    Calcium pyrophosphate
    Apatite
  Traumatic
  Rheumatoid arthritis
Uncommon
  Fungal
    Sporothrix scheckii
  Mycobacterial
    Mycobacterium tuberculosis
    M marinum
    M gordonae
    M leprae
  Spirochetal
    Syphilis
  Dialysis elbow
  Foreign bodies
  Reiter's syndrome
  Seronegative spondyloarthropathy
  Scleroderma
  Systemic lupus erythematosus
  Amyloidosis
  Sarcoidosis
  Hemochromatosis
  Hypertrophic osteoarthropathy
  Giant cell tumor
  Pigmented villonodular synovitis
  Synovial sarcoma

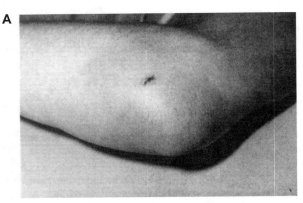

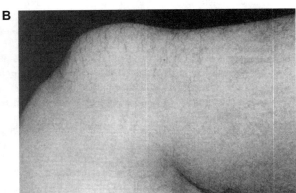

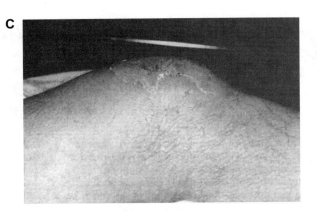

Figure 1. A, Staphylococcal olecranon septic bursitis showing skin abrasion, redness, and edema. **B,** Traumatic prepatellar bursitis showing noninflammatory changes. **C,** Prepatellar septic bursitis showing skin abrasion, erythema, and skin desquamation.

trochanteric, prepatellar (Figure 1B), anserine, gastrocnemius-semimembranosus (Baker's cyst) (Figure 2A), and retrocalcaneal bursae are most frequently involved. Inflammation of the deeper bursae may impinge on vascular or neural structures and result in limb edema, ischemia, and compression neuropathies. Alternatively, inflammation may cause rupture of the bursa to the soft tissues, inducing a pseudo-thrombophlebitis syndrome. These are well-known complications of iliopsoas and popliteal bursitis, or Baker's cyst (Figure 2B). Isolated bursal effusions are usually limited to children. Several deep bursae connect to the adjacent joints, and the bursitis might represent a pathologic process secondary to the neighboring joint. This is true for the subacromial, iliopsoas, and Baker's cyst.

Patients with acute bursitis present with abrupt onset of localized pain aggravated by any movement of the structures adjacent to the bursae. The pain is usually described as a deep, aching discomfort. Features that suggest bursitis include sudden onset of swelling, redness, or tenderness after repetitive activity that is localized to the bursa and not the joint. Imaging studies are expensive and typically not helpful in the acute setting. However, if the bursitis is traumatic in origin, an infectious etiology needs to be considered by assessing for the presence of fever, chills, and fluctuant swelling of the bursae, in association with redness, local heat, exquisite point tenderness, and sometimes significant edema over the underlying skin (Figure 1A). Fever should suggest infection, but it can also be present with crystal-induced bursitis. The absence of fever does not exclude infection, as only one-third of patients with olecranon septic bursitis present with fever (4).

Aspiration, which is easily accomplished when the bursa is superficial, can rule out infection and crystal identification. Bursal or joint fluid with white blood cell counts >1,000 cells/mm^3 indicates inflammation; <1,000 white blood cells is characteristic of traumatic and noninflammatory fluids. Olecranon bursal infections tend to give higher white cell counts (though not as high as those seen with septic arthritis) with a mean of 13,500 white cells/mm^3 (5). In about 40% of these patients, the count is below 10,000 white cells (6). Bursitis due to RA and gout can produce similarly elevated white blood cell counts.

Gram and acid-fast stains, pertinent cultures, and examination of fresh preparation of bursal fluid under polarized light are essential to identify infectious agents and different crystals (7). Patients presenting with fever and chills should also have blood cultures. Most cases of septic bursitis are caused by *Staphylococcus aureus*, but the Gram stain is positive in only 65% (4). If the stain shows no bacteria, or if gram-positive cocci are found, then a penicillinase-resistant antistaphylococcal drug should be used. If gram-negative organisms are found, an extrabursal site of infection should be sought.

The choice of an antibiotic should be based on the most likely organism causing the extrabursal infection. Penicillin-resistant *S aureus* should always be considered in a patient with diabetes, intravenous drug abuser, or immunocompromised patient. Septic bursitis always requires therapy with systemic antibiotics. Patients with more serious underlying conditions may require hospitalization for intravenous antibiotics and, rarely, surgical drainage and bursectomy. At initiation of therapy, the bursal contents should be drained through a 16- or 18-gauge needle—a process that may need to be repeated 2–3 times over the course of the first week of treatment. The duration of antibiotic therapy averages 3–4 weeks. Antibiotics should be continued for an additional 5 days after the bursal fluid has cleared or become sterile. Nonseptic bursitis can be managed with rest, cold compresses, nonsteroidal antiinflammatory drugs (NSAIDs), and corticosteroid injections. Because septic bursitis may occur with a noncharacteristic clinical presentation and clear noninflammatory bursal fluid, any corticosteroid injection should be delayed until the results of the bursal fluid cultures show no growth for at least 48 hours.

A

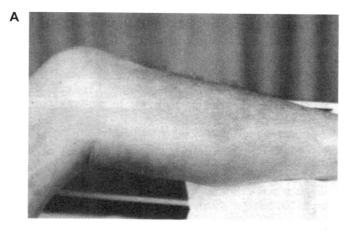

B

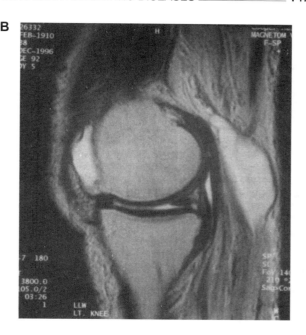

Figure 2. **A,** Inflamed and ruptured Baker's cyst in the calf of a patient with rheumatoid arthritis. **B,** Magnetic resonance image showing knee effusion and leaking of cyst into the calf.

TENDINOPATHIES

Primary disorders of tendons are common and constitute a high proportion of referrals to rheumatologists and physical therapists. Certain tendons are particularly vulnerable to degenerative pathology; these include the Achilles, patella, elements of the rotator cuff, forearm extensors, biceps brachii, and tibialis posterior tendons. These disorders are often chronic and difficult to successfully manage in the long term. The term *tendinitis* has been used to describe chronic pain relating to symptomatic tendons. It is deeply ingrained in the literature and implies that inflammation is the central pathologic process in tendinitis. However, histologic studies together with advances in imaging techniques have been able to demonstrate a degenerative rather than inflammatory etiology. Animal models suggest that an inflammatory reaction is present in acute situations, but the degenerative process soon supersedes and therefore the appropriate pathologic term of *tendinosis* should be considered (8).

Tenosynovitis refers to inflammation of the peritendinous tissues or synovial sheaths, and most often occurs from exercise, overuse, unaccustomed activity, puncture wound, or foreign body penetration. When tenosynovitis is identified in the absence of trauma, a systemic disease should always be suspected as part of a systemic inflammatory process, as seen in bursitis (Table 1; Figure 3). If these diseases are present, the recommended therapy for them should be followed. Disseminated gonococcemia or secondary syphilis should be suspected in sexually active individuals with inflammation involving the tendons of the ankle or wrist in the setting of monarthritis or polyarthritis, fever, and skin rash (Figure 3A). Needle aspiration of the tendon sheath might yield a few drops of fluid for culture and crystal analysis. The correct point of aspiration can be easily detected using ultrasonography (9).

REGIONAL MYOFASCIAL PAIN

Myofascial trigger points mark myofascial pain syndrome. The myofascial trigger points are defined as small areas within a tight band of skeletal muscle fiber that give rise to characteristic referred pain.

Spraying with ethyl chloride, followed by active or passive stretching exercises for the involved muscles, may be beneficial. Trigger point injections of a local anesthetic, such as lidocaine, should be considered in highly irritable trigger points.

GENERALIZED PAIN DISORDERS

Generalized pain disorders cause widespread pain, and in some cases disability, and include hypermobility syndrome, fibromyalgia, clencher syndrome, polymyalgia rheumatica, and somatoform disorders.

REGIONAL FORMS OF BURSITIS AND TENDINOPATHY

Several forms of bursitis and tendinopathy are particularly common; their unique aspects will be described using a regional approach.

Hand and Wrist

Dupuytren's Contracture. Dupuytren's contracture, a fibrous thickening of the palmar fascia, affects predominantly middle-aged men and older individuals of Northern European decent. It is inherited as an autosomal dominant trait with variable penetrance and is associated with tobacco smoking, diabetes mellitus, local trauma, heavy manual work, alcohol abuse, and the long-term use of antiepileptic medications with or without associated reflex sympathetic dystrophy. It usually is bilateral and involves proliferation of the hand palmar fascia with thickening and formation of tender fibrotic nodes and cords. As the disease progresses, flexion contracture of the metacarpophalangeal (MCP), proximal interphalangeal (PIP), and rarely, distal interphalangeal joints can occur. The ring and little fingers are most commonly involved.

In some patients, the disease progresses with rapid palmar fibrosis and fibrotic lesions elsewhere. These patients tend to exhibit disease earlier

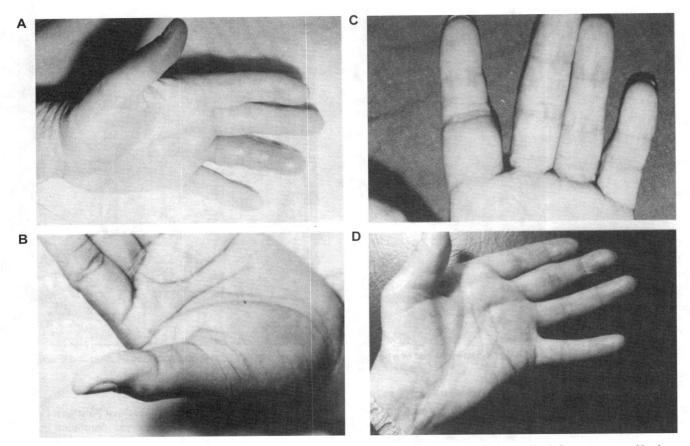

Figure 3. A, Acute staphylococcal annular finger flexion tenosynovitis showing swelling and erythema. **B,** Acute thumb flexor tenosynovitis observed in a patient with disseminated gonococcemia. **C,** Granulomatous index finger tenosynovitis in a patient with lupus pernio due to sarcoidosis. **D,** Giant cell tumor or pigmented villonodular synovitis of the middle finger flexor tendon sheath in a patient with rheumatoid arthritis.

in life (in their 20s or 30s), have a positive family history, and show bilateral involvement. In patients with diabetes mellitus, Dupuytren's contracture has been described in association with trigger fingers, carpal tunnel syndrome, lateral epicondylitis, and frozen shoulder. It can also develop in the aftermath of complex regional pain syndrome (CRPS).

Progression of Dupuytren's contracture is unpredictable, and multiple medical treatments have been tried without much success (10). Selective fasciectomy is the surgical procedure most commonly used, with results depending upon the stage and severity of the disease (11). Although surgical excision does not cure the disease, it may delay progression. Recurrences are more frequent in patients with nodular stage disease. Indications for surgery can be guided by a positive *table top test*, i.e., when the patient can no longer place the hand completely flat on a hard surface, correlated with >30° flexor contractures at the PIP joints. As the disease becomes more aggressive, complete surgical correction becomes less likely.

Trigger Finger or Finger-Stenosing Tenosynovitis. *Trigger finger* is the locking of one or several fingers in flexion, resulting in painful clicking and popping during extension of the digit. On physical examination, the patient usually localizes the pain to the volar aspect of the MCP joint. The trigger may be subtle (a simple give in the tendon) or dramatic (permanent locking of the finger in flexion). Trigger finger is common in young children, middle-aged women, and older individuals. When more than 3 digits are affected, the condition may be idiopathic or may indicate other systemic conditions. Trigger finger should be distinguished from tendon involvement seen in systemic inflammatory conditions, such as RA and psoriatic arthritis, in which the sheath is diffusely thickened and the trigger phenomenon is unusual.

Spontaneous improvement occurs in only 15–20% of cases. If untreated, permanent contracture can develop. Nonsurgical treatment includes splinting, NSAID administration, and corticosteroid injections. These injections into the tendon sheath provide pain relief in >95% of cases (12); however, they have a lower rate of success in diabetic patients (13). Such complications as infection and tendon rupture are rare, but subcutaneous fat atrophy and depigmentation may occur at the site of injection. After 2 injections without relief of symptoms, surgical release of the pulley system is highly successful, with minimal morbidity and low recurrence rate (14,15).

De Quervain's Tenosynovitis. De Quervain's tenosynovitis, or stenosing tenosynovitis of the first dorsal compartment of the hand, is a common cause of wrist and thumb pain in women 30–50 years of age (16). Patients report disabling pain in the radial aspect of the wrist or forearm over several weeks to months, often associated with recent pregnancies or repetitive use of the thumb or wrist. The patients drop objects from their hands, and activities such as lifting a baby or changing diapers cause excruciating pain.

Diffuse or localized swelling over the first extensor compartment along the radial styloid is seen on physical exam. The patients may notice crepitation during adduction/abduction motions of the thumb. A positive Finkelstein's test usually reproduces the pain when the examiner performs ulnar flexion of the wrist while the remaining 4 fingers encircle and grasp the thumb. This condition can be confused with osteoarthritis or chondrocalcinosis of the first carpometacarpal joint, which can coexist with De Quervain's tenosynovitis. Swelling and tenderness are noted along the sheath of the abductor pollicis longus, which spreads distally over the base of the first metacarpal, and the extensor pollicis brevis, which inserts at the base of the distal phalanx of the thumb.

Nonsurgical treatment includes NSAIDs, a splint that partially or totally immobilizes the thumb during certain activities that exacerbate pain, and corticosteroid injections. The injection may be repeated twice, if necessary. Lack of response may be due to anatomic variation of the sheath (17). If symptoms persist, surgical release of the first compartment is indicated.

Acute, Subacute, and Chronic Digital Flexor Tenosynovitis. Digital flexor tenosynovitis results from inflammation of the synovial sheath of the flexor digital tendon (Figure 3). Acute septic tenosynovitis is usually caused by *S aureus* or *Streptococcus pyogenes* from direct inoculation. Abrasions, fissures, puncture injuries, and foreign-body penetration is likely to cause suppurative tenosynovitis (18). Gonococcemia, meningococcemia, and secondary syphilis (19) may give rise to acute or subacute synovial and tenosynovial infection of the fingers and wrist. Mycobacteria or fungi (especially sporotrichosis) may cause subacute or chronic tenosynovitis. Calcific tenosynovitis due to apatite crystal deposition often occurs idiopathically or in patients with scleroderma, mixed connective tissue disease, or systemic lupus erythematosus (SLE). Patients with digital ulcers have an increased risk of developing a suppurative tenosynovitis.

The patient usually presents with exquisite tenderness over the entire flexor sheath, while the digit is maintained in an antalgic, semiflexed position, with pain on extension of the finger, and swelling of the digit (Figures 3A and 3B). If untreated, suppurative tenosynovitis may spread to the palmar spaces and wrist when the first and fifth digits are involved. Hand surgery consultation should immediately be obtained for surgical drainage, debridement, and biopsy. Wide-spectrum parenteral antibiotics must be administered pending Gram stain and cultures. Subacute tenosynovitis with intact skin and calcific tendinitis may be treated conservatively with NSAIDs and splints. Failure to improve should trigger surgical drainage and biopsy, with further workup and treatment as suppurative or proliferative tenosynovitis. Calcific tendinitis improves slowly, and the hand should be protected for 1–2 weeks.

Proliferative tenosynovitis. Chronic, multiple-sheath tenosynovitis usually results from systemic disease, such as RA, rheumatoid nodulosis, scleroderma, mixed connective tissue disease, SLE, and psoriatic arthritis. Single-sheath tenosynovitis usually represents foreign-body tenosynovitis (most commonly seen in children, farmers, gardeners, fishermen, and divers), pigmented villonodular synovitis (PVNS) or giant cell tumors (20) (Figure 3C), tuberculosis, sarcoidosis (Figure 3D), synovial chondromatosis, and even the deadly synovial sarcomas. Proliferative synovitis may also be caused by mycobacterias, fungi, algae, and tophaceous crystalline deposits, mainly monosodium urate crystals (21). Patients witness the slow growth of a small eccentric, elongated painless lump. Some of these conditions may cause erosive damage of adjacent bones and joints.

Local corticosteroid injections are useful in treating tenosynovitis caused by systemic diseases. In single-sheath tenosynovitis, surgical exploration is mandatory for both tissue diagnosis and treatment. The tissue requires proper bacteriologic studies for indolent microorganisms such as acid-fast organisms and fungi, as well as absolute alcohol fixation and compensated polarized light microscopy to look for crystals and foreign bodies. Tenosynovectomy is curative for PVNS or giant cell tumor, fibroma of the tendon sheath, and synovial chondromatosis; it is diagnostic for synovial sarcoma.

Carpal Tunnel Syndrome (CTS). CTS, one the most common compression neuropathies, is caused by impingement of the median nerve at the carpal tunnel (22). It occurs more frequently in women and often accompanies pregnancy, menopause, Colles' fracture, RA, diabetes mellitus, and trauma (23). CTS results from an increase or change in pressure within the carpal tunnel, which encloses the median nerve. Increased pressure with flexion or extension of the joint (Phalen's sign) explains nocturnal and early morning worsening of symptoms. Acute CTS occurs in a rapidly expanding lesion within the carpal tunnels, and is seen in fractures, hematomas (anticoagulation and hemophiliac), necrotizing fasciitis, tumoral calcinosis, crystal-induced inflammation, and other systemic inflammatory conditions.

Most patients present with paresthesias or pain in one or both hands. The thumb, index, and middle finger are most commonly involved, but the whole hand may be numb. Activities that flex the wrists, such as driving or holding the telephone, may increase numbness. Clumsiness and pain radiating up the arm to the shoulder are commonly reported. Differential diagnosis includes cervical radiculopathy, diabetic neuropathy, and compression of the median nerve at proximal locations. The anterior interosseous nerve syndrome is characterized by weakness of the thumb, index, and middle fingers. In the pronator syndrome, the pain is localized on the proximal forearm, with paresthesias in the three and one-half digits supplied by the medial nerve.

Percussion at the pronator muscle may reproduce the paresthesias although the Phalen's test is negative. Provocative tests include *Tinel's sign* (light percussion at the wrist) and *Phalen's sign* (flexing of the wrist passively), resulting in increased paresthesia within 60 seconds and an electrical sensation radiating to the thumb, index finger or middle finger, respectively. Tinel's sign is less sensitive and more specific than Phalen's sign, with a 6% false-positive rate (24). *Carpal compression test*, manual pressure on the nerve at the carpal tunnel, reproduces the painful symptoms or paresthesias. Decreased sensitivity and thenar atrophy occur in patients with longstanding median nerve compression. Electrodiagnostic testing is helpful in evaluating additional compressive sites and confirms the diagnosis before surgery. Sensory abnormalities are seen earlier than motor abnormalities because the median nerve is composed mostly of sensory fibers at the level of the wrist. A positive electrodiagnostic test is often required for surgical approval in workers' compensation claims.

Conservative measures, including NSAIDs, resting volar splints that hold the wrist in a neutral position, and corticosteroid injections, are the mainstay of nonsurgical therapy. The splints should be worn at night and during activities that exacerbate the symptoms. Surgery should be considered when permanent symptoms are present and in acute CTS, with the exception of crystal-induced synovitis, which responds to conservative treatment. Both open and endoscopic carpal tunnel release are highly effective to relieve symptoms (25). Pathologic studies of wrist flexor tendon sheaths are useful to detect granulomatous synovitis, PVNS, synovial sarcomas, and amyloidosis.

Elbow

Olecranon Bursitis. Olecranon bursitis describes inflammation of the bursa that overlies the olecranon process of the ulna. It is commonly related to infection, repetitive trauma, or an underlying rheumatic process, such as gout or RA. It is directly or indirectly related to repetitive direct pressure or repetitive activities on the bursa. The patient presents with pain at the posterior aspect of the elbow that is aggravated by flexion of the elbow past 90°, local swelling or bogginess, erythema, and a tender olecranon bursa with normal extension of the elbow joint (Figure 1A). This finding may help differentiate olecranon bursitis from an effusion within the joint itself. Aspiration of the bursa is necessary to exclude infection. The most common cause of infection is *S aureus*, requiring antibiotic treatment.

A compression bandage is recommended to prevent recurrence in nonseptic bursitis. In traumatic and crystal-induced bursitis, an injection of corticosteroid should also be considered if the Gram stain and

48-hour culture results are negative. This usually induces dramatic improvement of symptoms. Periodic applications of ice and the use of an elbow pad can prevent recurrence and offer protection against infection. Rarely, if infection persists or bursitis becomes recurrent, surgical excision may be required.

Lateral Epicondylitis (Tennis Elbow). Tennis elbow or lateral epicondylitis is common in middle-aged people. It is more often related to work (electricians, machine operators, and bricklayers) than to tennis. Tennis elbow results from overuse of the extensor carpi radialis brevis, the wrist dorsiflexors that span the lateral epicondyle and the base of the third metacarpal. Patients present with lateralized pain over the soft tissue just distal to the epicondyle. The pain is reproduced by resisted dorsiflexion of the wrist, and passive elbow range of motion is normal. Any degree of restriction in motion should raise the possibility of an intraarticular process, such as inflammatory synovitis, osteoarthritis, chondrocalcinosis, osteochondromas, aseptic bone necrosis, and osteochondritis dissecans. Radiographs are useful to detect these conditions as well as calcific tendinitis and exostosis.

Tennis elbow may resolve spontaneously with time and rest of the affected arm. Total immobilization is discouraged so as to reduce muscle atrophy and loss of strength. A counterforce forearm brace is widely used for pain relief and should be worn during activities. Ice packs, capsaicin cream, and NSAIDs can be used to control pain and inflammation. Isometric and range of motion exercises for the upper extremity should be implemented. Local corticosteroid injections can be added if treatment progresses slowly or if the patient is unable to participate in physical therapy due to residual inflammation and pain. Such injections are relatively safe, and >80% of patients experience short-term relief (26). About 10% of patients develop chronic symptoms despite medical treatment and may require surgery if other causes of elbow pain are excluded.

Golfer's Elbow. Similar to tennis elbow but much less common, golfer's elbow affects the medial epicondyle. Medial epicondylitis occurs in golfers as well in manual workers, such as bricklayers. The condition is caused from repetitive traction stress at the medial epicondyle attachment of the pronator teres or flexor carpi radialis muscles. Patients present with pain at the medial aspect of the elbow that increases with resistance to wrist flexion and forearm pronation. Local tenderness at the medial epicondyle or slightly distal to it confirms the diagnosis. Ulnar paresthesias from associated compressive neuropathy may be present in up to 30% of the cases.

The treatment for golfer's elbow is similar to that for tennis elbow. Because the ulnar nerve runs behind the medial epicondyle, corticosteroid injections should be administered with care to avoid nerve injury and transient hand weakness due to the anesthesia.

Shoulder

See Chapter 26 for a complete description of soft-tissue shoulder problems.

Hip and Buttock

Trochanteric Bursitis. Trochanteric bursitis results from abnormal gait caused by leg-length discrepancy; nerve paralysis; apatite deposits; painful conditions of the foot, knee, and hip; spinal disorders; lumbar spondylosis; and dorsal scoliosis. Iliotibial band shortening may be a contributing factor. Patients present with pain over the greater trochanter while walking and lying in bed on the affected side. Pain is aggravated by internal rotation of the hip. Trochanteric bursitis may be secondary to or associated with hip disease. Resisted abduction reproduces the pain in

a minority of cases. The classic finding is point tenderness at the posterior aspect of the greater trochanter.

Treatment includes local measures for symptom relief, rest, heat or cold applications, NSAIDs, and corticosteroid injections. Failure to respond to conservative treatment should be evaluated by the orthopedist for simple longitudinal release of the iliotibial band or arthroscopic bursectomy.

Ischial Bursitis. Patients with ischial bursitis report buttock pain that persists throughout the day and find it difficult to sit on one side of the buttock. On physical examination, point tenderness is demonstrated at the ischial tuberosity. Treatment consists of NSAIDs, hamstring stretching exercises, aspiration of the bursa, and corticosteroid injections.

Iliopsoas Bursitis. Iliopsoas bursitis involves a variety of pain syndromes and compressive syndromes caused by distention of the iliopsoas bursa. The iliopsoas bursa is the largest bursa in humans and separates the anterior aspect of the coxofemoral joint from the iliopsoas muscle. The bursa may become distended in hip conditions, such as RA, osteoarthritis, synovial chondromatosis, and septic arthritis.

Small bursal distention may be asymptomatic; however, larger distention can compress adjacent structures, such as the femoral vein, artery, or nerves. The resulting symptoms of leg edema, limb ischemia, quadriceps weakness, and sensory deficits can be appreciated in the anterior thigh. Radiographs aid in recognition of chronic hip joint abnormalities. Ultrasonography and MRI may be helpful in patients with compressive syndromes. Patients with septic arthritis of the hip may also develop an iliopsoas bursal abscess.

Irritative iliopsoas bursitis features groin pain that radiates to the buttock or anterior thigh, mimicking coxofemoral arthritis. Passive hip flexion triggers the pain. Unlike in hip arthritis, passive hip rotation is painless. Obturator nerve entrapment syndrome is an important cause of hip pain in athletes and should be considered in the differential diagnosis. The pain occurs on the adductor origin of the pubic bone and is aggravated by exercise. As the patient exercises, the pain radiates down the medial aspect of the thigh toward the knee. The patient has adductor muscle weakness, spasm, and paresthesias along the medial distal thigh. Irritative iliopsoas bursitis resolves with rest and NSAIDs. In recalcitrant cases, a corticosteroid injection may be considered under fluoroscopy. Large distended iliopsoas bursae may be treated indirectly by treating the hip condition responsible for the effusion.

Knee

See Chapter 17 for a complete description of soft tissue knee problems.

Ankle and Foot

Achilles Tendinitis. Pain associated with tenderness and swelling of the Achilles tendon or near its attachment is often seen in chronic strain resulting from recreational athletics. It may be associated with spondyloarthropathy, such as ankylosing spondylitis, psoriatic arthritis, or reactive arthritis, but is rarely seen with gout. All patients should be examined to rule out associated systemic conditions. Examination reveals localized swelling or thickening of the Achilles tendon and tenderness on palpation. Loss of dorsal flexion strength or discomfort with resisted motion can occur. Peritendinitis can be distinguished from Achilles tendinitis by the painful arc sign. Peritendinitis involves the tendon sheath, and as the foot is moved through dorsiflexion to plantar flexion, the area of tenderness is unchanged; whereas with tendinitis, the area of tenderness moves with the foot.

Treatment includes the use of a heel lift in the shoe and avoidance of irritating activity. Occasionally, a short course of cast immobilization provides symptom relief. A removable walking cast can be employed. Once symptoms resolve, the patient should follow a gentle program of gastrocnemius-soleus stretching and strengthening. Injections are generally not recommended due to the possibility of tendon rupture. Surgical intervention is rare, with the exception of tendon rupture. Surgical debridement of the degenerated thickened tendon may be indicated in patients who fail to respond to 6 months of conservative treatment.

Plantar Fasciitis and Heel Pain. Heel pain is a frequent complaint in medical practice and can be frustrating to treat. Plantar fasciitis is associated with disabling plantar heel pain, which is worse with weight bearing and usually severe during the first steps in the morning or after prolonged sitting. The pain may be sharp, dull, or burning in nature. Tenderness is typically located over the plantar aspect of the medial calcaneal tuberosity, and sometimes, the anterior plantar fascia may be tender. Calcaneal spurs may or may not be present. Plantar fasciitis may be a clinical clue to underlying spondyloarthropathy.

Time often relieves this condition, and use of soft silicone heel pads with a gel insert may be all that is needed. Initial treatment includes stretching, a heel cup, and NSAIDs. Patients should be taught to stretch the heel cord by leaning against a wall, feet flat and turned slightly inward, for 30 seconds with multiple repetitions. Orthotic devices may help correct anatomic or biomechanical abnormalities. However, when disability is pronounced, injection of the tender spot with a mixture of corticosteroid and lidocaine, using a medial or lateral approach to avoid heel fat-pad atrophy, can result in rapid cure. Multiple injections increase the chance of rupture of the plantar fascia. Cast immobilization may be used to break the chronic pain cycle. The American Orthopaedic Foot and Ankle Society recommend 6–12 months of conservative treatment before considering surgery. More than 90% of patients respond to medical treatment within this time frame (27). Surgical procedures consist of partial plantar fascia release with or without decompression of the nerve of the abductor digiti minimi.

REFERENCES

1. Canoso JJ. Musculoskeletal conditions. In: Rheumatology in primary care. Philadelphia: WB Saunders; 1997. p. 20–96.
2. Canoso JJ. Ultrasound imaging: a rheumatologist's dream. J Rheumatol 2000;27:2063–2064.
3. Zimmermann B 3rd, Mikolich DJ, Ho G Jr. Septic bursitis. Semin Arthritis Rheum 1995;24:391–410.
4. Ho G Jr, Tice AD, Kaplan SR. Septic bursitis in the prepatellar and olecranon bursae: an analysis of 25 cases. Ann Intern Med 1978;89:21–27.
5. Canoso JJ. Bursal membrane and fluid. In: Cohen AS, editor. Laboratory diagnostic procedures in rheumatic diseases. New York: Grune and Stratton; 1985. p. 55–76.
6. Ho G Jr, Mikolich DJ. Bacterial Infection of the superficial subcutaneous bursae. Clin Rheum Dis 1986;12:437–457.
7. Schumacher HR, Reginato AJ. Atlas of synovial fluid analysis and crystal identification. Philadelphia: Lea & Febiger; 1991.
8. Rees JD, Wilson AM, Wolman RL. Current concepts in the management of tendon disorders. Rheumatology (Oxford) 2006;45:508–21.
9. Koski JM. Ultrasound guided injections in rheumatology. J Rheumatol 2000;27:2131–2138.
10. Hurst LC, Badalamente MA. Nonoperative treatment of Dupuytren's disease. Hand Clin 1999;15:97–107, vii.
11. Benson LS, Williams CS, Kahle M. Dupuytren's contracture. J Am Acad Orthop Surg 1998;6:24–35.
12. Anderson B, Kaye S. Treatment of flexor tenosynovitis of the hand ('trigger finger') with corticosteroids. A prospective study of the response to local injection. Arch Intern Med 1991;151:153–156.
13. Chammas M, Bousquet P, Renard E, Poirier JL, Jaffiol C, Allieu Y. Dupuytren's disease, carpal tunnel syndrome, trigger finger, and diabetes mellitus. J Hand Surg 1995;20:109–114.
14. Benson LS, Ptaszek AJ. Injection versus surgery in the treatment of trigger finger. J Hand Surg 1997;22:138–144.
15. Turowski GA, Zdankiewicz PD, Thomson JG. The results of surgical treatment of trigger finger. J Hand Surg 1997;22:145–149.
16. Bahm J, Szabo Z, Foucher G. The anatomy of de Quervain's disease. A study of operative findings. Int Orthop 1995;19:209–211.
17. Nagaoka M, Matsuzaki H, Suzuki T. Ultrasonographic examination of de Quervain's disease. J Orthop Sci 2000;5:96–99.
18. Reginato AJ, Ferreiro JL, O'Connor CR, Barbasan C, Arasa J, Bednar J, et al. Clinical and pathologic studies of twenty-six patients with penetrating foreign body injury to the joints, bursae, and tendon sheaths. Arthritis Rheum 1979;22:170–176.
19. Reginato AJ, Schumacher HR, Jimenez S, Maurer K. Synovitis in secondary syphilis. Clinical, light, and electron microscopic studies. Arthritis Rheum 1990;33:1753–1762.
20. Reginato A, Martinez V, Schumacher HR, Torres J. Giant cell tumour associated with rheumatoid arthritis. Ann Rheum Dis 1974;33:333–341.
21. Kostman JR, Rush P, Reginato AJ. Granulomatous tophaceous gout mimicking tuberculous tenosynovitis: report of two cases. Clin Infect Dis 1995;21:217–219.
22. Allieu Y, Chammas M. Carpal tunnel syndrome. Etiology, diagnosis. Rev Prat 2000 15;50:661–666.
23. Stevens JC, Beard CM, O'Fallon WM, Kurland LT. Conditions associated with carpal tunnel syndrome. Mayo Clin Proc 1992;67:541–548.
24. Gellman H, Gelberman RN, Tan Am, Botte MJ. Carpal tunnel syndrome: an evaluation of the provocative diagnostic tests. J Bone Joint Surg Am 1986;68:735–737.
25. Brown RA, Gelberman RH, Seiler JG 3rd, Abrahamsson SO, Weiland AJ, Urbaniak JR, et al. Carpal tunnel release. A prospective, randomized assessment of open and endoscopic methods. J Bone Joint Surg Am 1993;75:1265–1275.
26. Hay EM, Paterson SM, Lewis M, Hosie G, Croft P. Pragmatic randomised controlled trial of local corticosteroid injection and naproxen for treatment of lateral epicondylitis of elbow in primary care. BMJ 1999;319:964–968.
27. Chou LB, Oloff LM, Bocko AP. The painful foot and ankle; viewpoints from orthopaedics and podiatry. In: Harris ED Jr, Genovese MC, editors. Primary care rheumatology. Philadelphia: WB Saunders; 2000. p. 213–217.

CHAPTER 24

Polymyalgia Rheumatica

STEPHEN A. PAGET, MD, FACP, FACR, and ROBERT F. SPIERA, MD, FACP, FACR

Polymyalgia rheumatica (PMR) is a systemic inflammatory disorder that occurs in individuals older than 50 years of age and is commonly associated with an elevated erythrocyte sedimentation rate (ESR) and anemia. Patients often report constitutional symptoms, proximal aches and pains, and stiffness and soreness in the neck, shoulders, and pelvic girdle. The syndrome is defined by its clinical presentation and by the exclusion of other disorders that can mimic it, including hypothyroidism; malignancy; connective tissue disorders, such as systemic lupus erythematosus; rheumatoid arthritis (RA) of the elderly; and infectious diseases. The diagnosis is confirmed by the rapid and nearly miraculous response to low-dose corticosteroids (1–4).

PMR is one part of a spectrum of inflammatory disorders, with the other component being a systemic vasculitis known as giant cell arteritis (GCA) or temporal arteritis (see chapter 30, Vasculitis). GCA is a granulomatous vasculitis of the large- and medium-sized vessels and can, in its most virulent form, lead to occlusive vascular disease and its attendant ischemic aftermaths, such as blindness and stroke. Approximately 50% of patients with GCA have the aches and pains characteristic of PMR; conversely, 10% of PMR patients either have or develop concomitant GCA. This scope of possible disease presentations has important diagnostic, therapeutic, and pathogenetic implications (5,6).

INCIDENCE

PMR is a descriptive term that was first suggested by Barber in 1957 to describe a syndrome of aching in elderly patients that could not be attributed to defined rheumatic, infectious, or neoplastic disorders. It is estimated to affect ~1 in 1,000 adults in the US older than 50 years of age, with peak incidence between the ages of 60 and 80. However, there are well-documented reports of PMR (usually in association with GCA) in patients in their 40s. Sixty percent of patients are women. Although the ESR is usually elevated, this is not invariable and the diagnoses of PMR and GCA are *clinical* ones, supported by, but not totally defined by, laboratory tests (1–4).

PATHOPHYSIOLOGY

PMR is probably a multifactorial disease, with both environmental and genetic factors contributing to susceptibility and severity. To date, the only genetic associations found relate to genes in the HLA complex (HLA–DR4). Environmental factors, such as infectious agents, have been hypothesized in the development of PMR and GCA. Immunologic senescence may also play a role in a disorder that presents primarily in the elderly. Musculoskeletal symptoms appear to be linked to a nonerosive articular and extraarticular synovitis. The specific cytokine production by involved tissues may influence clinical disease and may be different in PMR and GCA. Better understanding of these and other immunologic findings in these syndromes will help to establish the actual defects causing PMR and GCA, and eventually will lead to better understanding of the disease pathogenesis and more focused therapeutic options (7,8).

CLINICAL ASPECTS

Patients with PMR frequently report malaise and fatigue, as if they had a severe viral illness. Indeed, viral illnesses can often cause a self-limited PMR-like syndrome; and conversely, patients with PMR often complain of feeling like they have the flu. Both PMR and GCA can present with fevers of unknown origin. Fever is usually low in PMR, but temperatures may reach 102°F, especially with GCA. Anorexia and weight loss may be prominent features, but should raise vigilance regarding the possibility of underlying malignancy. Although no direct association between PMR and neoplasm has been proven, malignancy can mimic PMR. An age-appropriate and symptom- and sign-focused malignancy assessment is mandatory (3).

Other symptoms of PMR include chronic, symmetric aching and stiffness of the proximal muscles, soft tissues, and joints. These symptoms are most prominent in the shoulder, pelvic girdle, and neck. Aching and stiffness are worse in the morning and on exertion, and can be incapacitating. Muscles may be tender; disuse may lead to atrophy, and contractures can occur. Muscle strength is often difficult to evaluate because pain is present; however, it should be normal when pain is taken out of the picture (9,10).

The majority of patients have poorly localized tenderness over their joints, which is especially prominent over the shoulders, hips, low back, and buttocks. The original description of PMR excluded synovitis as a feature; however, while proximal symptoms and signs dominate the clinical picture, synovitis of the hands, wrists, and knees can be present and patients can have carpal tunnel syndrome due to flexor tenosynovitis. Inflammatory joint disorders in the elderly have many overlapping features. One-third of individuals diagnosed with RA are >60 years of age. In that age group, joint presentation can be either the characteristic symmetric polyarthritis of the small joints of the hands and feet or proximal findings more characteristic of PMR. In fact, some rheumatologists have speculated that PMR and RA in the elderly are the same disorder (11,12).

LABORATORY STUDIES

An elevated Westergren ESR is a laboratory hallmark of PMR; it is usually in excess of 50 mm/hour and may exceed 100 mm/hour. Some physicians monitor levels of C-reactive protein (CRP) as their marker to the state of the inflammatory process. It must be noted, however, that the diagnosis of PMR is a clinical one and is only supported, not defined, by an elevated ESR or CRP. A low or normal ESR may be seen in patients who are treated with corticosteroids for another disorder. The ESR should normalize within 7–10 days after initiating therapy with low-dose steroids. As steroids are tapered, the ESR may gradually rise again. However, treatment changes should be based on the return of clinical signs and symptoms of disease activity and not solely on increased ESR (13).

Normocytic normochromic anemia is seen in ~50% of patients and may serve as an indicator of clinical response to corticosteroids or of disease exacerbation when steroids are tapered. Thrombocytosis is commonly seen when disease is active, normalizes when steroids have suppressed the clinical manifestations, and can be similarly employed

Clinical Features

- Shoulder and thigh girdle pain and stiffness
- Peripheral synovitis of knees and hands possible
- Fatigue and constitutional symptoms common
- Elevated sedimentation rate, anemia, thrombocytosis common
- Dramatic, prompt response to low-dose corticosteroids expected

Treatment Guidelines

- If response to low-dose corticosteroids is not dramatic, consider alternate diagnoses (giant cell arteritis, infection, malignancy)
- Taper corticosteroids to lowest dosage that adequately controls inflammatory symptoms
- Do not chase the sedimentation rate; increased ESR in the absence of clinical symptoms does not warrant increase of steroid dosage
- Monitor for and address corticosteroid-related side effects

as a sign of active or inactive disease. Leukocytosis is common, with white blood cell counts in the 12,000–16,000 cells/mm³ range. Counts >25,000–30,000 cells/mm³ should alert the clinician to the possibility of an infection or malignancy.

The frequency of rheumatoid factors, antinuclear antibodies, and other autoreactive antibodies is not higher than that of age-matched controls. When the clinical picture is between PMR and RA, a positive rheumatoid factor or cyclic citrulline peptide IgG may support the latter.

Although muscle *pain* is a characteristic symptom, PMR is not an inflammatory myositis. Muscle enzyme levels (creatine kinase) are normal, as are electromyogram readings. Muscle biopsies may show type-II fiber atrophy, but do not show evidence of an inflammatory cell infiltrate. The latter 2 tests are not commonly performed in the setting of a diagnosis of PMR.

Bone scintigraphy has demonstrated high uptake in the region of the shoulders, consistent with joint or periarticular inflammation. Plain x-rays do not reveal erosions as might be seen with RA, but often show age-associated degenerative changes. Synovial fluid analysis may show a mildly elevated white blood cell count of 1,000–8,000 cells/mm³ with a lymphocyte predominance. Mild synovial proliferation with a slight lymphocytic infiltration has been found on biopsy of synovial tissue. Other studies frequently obtained in the workup of suspected PMR

include thyroid-stimulating hormone to rule out hypothyroidism and immunoelectrophoresis to exclude multiple myeloma and paraprotein-emias. An age-appropriate malignancy evaluation is mandatory in this age group, due to the rare malignancy as the cause of the syndrome.

DIFFERENTIAL DIAGNOSIS

When symptoms suggestive of PMR are present, clinical entities such as neoplasias, infections, muscle diseases, and other rheumatic disorders must be considered and ruled out with the appropriate clinical and laboratory testing (Figure 1) (3,13). The clinician should be guided by a complete individual and family history and physical exam. Not every patient needs an extensive workup for each differential diagnosis.

TREATMENT

The initial treatment for PMR is 10–15 mg/day of prednisone or its equivalent, sometimes initiated in divided doses. A prompt and

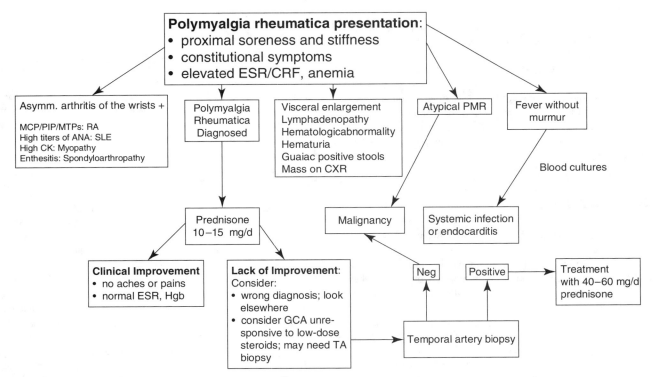

Figure 1. The diagnosis and management of a patient presenting with polymyalgia (adapted from reference 3). ESR = erythrocyte sedimentation rate; asymm. = asymmetric; MCP = metacarpophalangeal; PIP = proximal interphalangeal; MTP = metatarsophalangeal; RA = rheumatoid arthritis; ANA = antinuclear antibodies; SLE = systemic lupus erythematosus; CK = creatine kinase; CXR = chest x-ray; PMR = polymyalgia rheumatica; Hgb = hemoglobin; GCA = giant cell arteritis; TA = temporal artery; neg = negative.

Rehabilitation Considerations for PMR

- PMR usually occurs in the elderly; concurrent degenerative disease is common
- Contractures in the shoulder girdle can occur; usually resolve with medication, but assisted range-of-motion and strengthening exercises can be helpful
- Frailty related to immobility and steroid myopathy can be seen; attention to strengthening, gait training, and core/stability training are important, especially in the context of concomitant osteopenia
- Regular evaluation of joint stiffness and pain is important to determine whether the patient is having a flare and needs referral back to the rheumatologist for further assessment

---

Nursing Considerations for PMR

- Corticosteroids have many potential side effects, particularly in the elderly
- Monitor for hyperglycemia
- Monitor for hypertension
- Monitor for osteopenia/osteoporosis
- Obtain baseline bone mineral density measurement and add antiresorptive therapy when appropriate
- Recommend calcium and vitamin D supplementation
- Skin fragility is common; watch for bruising or breakdown
- Warn patient of symptoms of gastrointestinal ulceration
- Recommend ophthalmologic screening for cataracts

---

dramatic clinical response is considered by some to be an absolute criterion for the diagnosis. Most symptoms resolve in 48–72 hours and the ESR, anemia, and thrombocytosis should normalize after 7–10 days. If the anticipated dramatic improvement does not occur within a week's time, alternative diagnoses should be considered, such as RA, underlying GCA that is not responsive to low-dose prednisone, malignancy, or infection. Symptoms and signs that may indicate GCA include headache, visual symptoms (however mild and transient), scalp tenderness, and abnormal temporal arteries on examination. Malignancy may be associated with prominent weight loss; physical findings, such as a breast mass or visceral symptoms; or laboratory findings, such as guaiac-positive stools or hematuria. Infections may present with a prominent fever with chills and leukocytosis, as well as local symptoms, such as cough or dysuria. Because significant clinical overlap occurs between these disorders, PMR and GCA patients can present as diagnostic enigmas (4,5,13).

Once disease manifestations are controlled, the corticosteroid dose should be slowly tapered to the lowest level that controls the symptoms. A typical tapering schedule would be to decrease prednisone by 1–2.5 mg every 7–10 days with close observation for symptom return. Although serial ESR or CRP measures and complete blood counts are part of the monitoring, therapeutic decisions are based on signs and symptoms, not solely on an elevation of the ESR or CRP. Thus, the dose of prednisone should be increased only for recurrence of symptoms.

In most patients, PMR lasts for 1–2 years, and during that time the dosage of corticosteroids needed to control symptoms may fluctuate. Up to 40% of PMR patients have their disease for as long as 7 years. Although the dosage of steroid will inexorably decrease during the course of the illness, minor elevations of prednisone of 1–2.5 mg/day may be necessary to recapture control of the inflammatory process should a clinical flare occur. Guidelines for the treatment of PMR include the following:

1. The optimal dosage of steroid is the lowest that controls the disorder. The cumulative negative effect of steroid therapy should always be considered, especially in elderly women who are likely to have postmenopausal osteoporosis.
2. PMR patients should be made aware that they could develop GCA during the year after their PMR diagnosis was made. Thus, they should report to the physician immediately any visual symptoms, severe and persistent headache, scalp tenderness, jaw pain with eating, or limb claudication. Such symptoms may reflect impending vascular occlusion due to inflammation and may demand an immediate increase in corticosteroid dosage to 60 mg/day or more.
3. When long-term steroids are prescribed, prophylaxis against the likely long-term side effects of these drugs in an elderly

patient population with many comorbidities must be considered, including:

- Immunizations against influenza and pneumococcus.
- Close monitoring for infections, diabetes, hypertension, depression, steroid myopathy, and gastrointestinal problems such as ulcers and diverticulitis. Remember that an elevated ESR could be due to causes other than PMR and thus an increase in steroid dose based on an elevated ESR may further suppress a cholecystitis, diverticulitis, or urinary tract infection.
- Osteoporosis monitoring and treatment. This includes annual bone density measurements, the daily institution of 1,500 mg of calcium and 800 units of vitamin D, and consideration for the prophylactic or therapeutic use of antiresorptive agents, such as bisphosphonates.
- As steroids are tapered, patients often redevelop significant aches, pains, and fatigue that limit function. Increasing the dosage of steroid by a few milligrams usually controls the inflammation. If patients continue to need prednisone dosages >10 mg/day or develop increasing side effects from the cumulative doses, steroid-sparing drugs are considered. These include nonsteroidal antiinflammatory drugs (NSAIDs)—be aware of an increased rate of side effects in this elderly population, especially gastrointestinal toxicity when NSAIDs and steroids are combined—or weekly methotrexate (14). Although there is little in the literature to support the use of methotrexate in PMR, rheumatologists sometimes use it in the setting where one cannot easily differentiate between PMR and elderly-onset RA.
- Close partnership with a rheumatologist is helpful when treating patients with more refractory disease, those who have GCA, and patients with many side effects from chronic steroid use.

REFERENCES

1. Spiera H, Davison S. Long-term follow-up of polymyalgia rheumatica. Mt Sinai J Med 1978;45:225–9.
2. Bahlas S, Ramos-Remus C, David P. Clinical outcome of 149 patients with polymyalgia rheumatica and giant cell arteritis. J Rheumatol 1998;25:99–104.
3. Gonzalez-Gay MA, Garcia-Porrua C, Salvarani C, Olivieri I, Hunder GG. Polymyalgia manifestations in different conditions mimicking polymyalgia rheumatica. Clin Exp Rheumatol 2000;18:755–9.
4. Chuang TY, Hunder GG, Ilstrup DM, Kurkland LT. Polymyalgia rheumatica: a 10-year epidemiologic and clinical study. Ann Intern Med 1982;97:672–80.
5. Leibowitz E, Paget S. Giant cell arteritis. 2001; emedicine.com.
6. Hamiliton CR Jr, Shelly WM, Tumulty PA. Giant cell arteritis: including temporal arteritis and polymyalgia rheumatica. Medicine (Baltimore) 1971;50:1–27.
7. Weyand CM, Hicok KC, Hunder GG. Tissue cytokine patterns in patients with polymyalgia rheumatica and giant cell arteritis. Ann Intern Med 1994;121:484–91.

8. Wagner AD, Goronzy JJ, Weyand CM. Functional profile of tissue-infiltrating and circulating CD68+ cells in giant cell arteritis. Evidence for two components of the disease. J Clin Invest 1994;94:1134–40.

9. Salvarani C, Cantini F, Macchioni P, Olivieri I, Niccoli L, Padula A, et al. Distal musculoskeletal manifestations in polymyalgia rheumatica: a prospective followup study. Arthritis Rheum 1998;41:1221–6.

10. Salvarani C, Cantini F, Olivieri I, Hunder GS. Polymyalgia rheumatica: a disorder of extraarticular synovial structures? J Rheumatol 1999;26:517–21.

11. Healey LA, Sheets PK. The relation of polymyalgia rheumatica to rheumatoid arthritis. J Rheumatol 1988;15:750–2.

12. Healey LA. Polymyalgia rheumatica and seronegative rheumatoid arthritis may be the same entity. J Rheumatol 1992;19:270–2.

13. Stern R. Polymyalgia rheumatica and temporal arteritis. In: Paget SA, Gibofsky A, Beary JF III. Manual of rheumatology and outpatient orthopedic disorders: diagnosis and therapy. 4th ed. Philadelphia: Lippincott Williams & Wilkins; 2000. p. 181–6.

14. Caporali R, Cimmino MA, Ferraccioli G, Gerli R, Klersy C, Salvarani C, et al. Prednisone plus methotrexate for polymyalgia rheumatica: a randomized, double-blind, placebo-controlled trial. Ann Intern Med 2004;141:493–500.

Rheumatoid Arthritis

ANTHONY M. TURKIEWICZ, MD, and LARRY W. MORELAND, MD

Rheumatoid arthritis (RA) is a chronic, systemic inflammatory disorder of unknown etiology. It frequently is referred to as an autoimmune disease and is characterized by symmetric polyarticular pain and swelling, morning stiffness, malaise, and fatigue. RA has a variable course, often with periods of exacerbations and less frequently true remissions. Outcomes are variable as well, ranging from a remitting disease (rare) to a severe disease bringing disability and even premature death. The progression of joint damage without treatment in the majority of patients results in significant disability within 10–20 years.

EPIDEMIOLOGY

RA is a worldwide problem, with a prevalence of 0.5–1% of the adult population (1) and an annual incidence of 0.03% (2), with substantial variation across different studies and time periods. Overall, RA appears to be less common in Asia and Africa than in the United States and Europe (3), and it has been suggested that the incidence of RA decreases from northern to more southern European countries (4). The disease affects individuals at any age, including infants and the elderly; however, it presents most commonly in women aged 40–50 years. RA is not very common in men under 45 years of age, but the incidence rises steeply with increasing age. In women, the incidence rises to age 45, plateaus until age 75, and then declines (5). Numerous studies have demonstrated increased mortality in patients with RA compared with the general population. There are reports of increased risk of death from gastrointestinal, cardiovascular, respiratory, hematologic, and infectious diseases (6–9).

ETIOLOGY AND PATHOGENESIS

The pathophysiology of RA has undergone intensive investigation over the past 25 years. It is well known that an individual's genetic background plays a critical role in the susceptibility to and severity of RA (10). Careful studies have revealed a 15% concordance in monozygotic twins, which is ~4 times greater than the rate in dizygotic twins, which supports a genetic component (11). Disease transmission is complex and likely involves many genes. The genes with the greatest impact lie in the class II major histocompatibility (MHC) locus. There is a strong association of RA with a specific sequence on the beta chains of select HLA–DR haplotypes. This "shared epitope" contains amino acids 70–74 (glutamine-leucine-arginine-alanine-alanine) and is also known as QKRAA (12).

Although the search for a specific etiologic agent has been intense, the cause of RA has not been discovered. Its pathogenesis is likely multifactorial, with genetic background contributing to susceptibility, along with exposure to unknown environmental factors. Many theoretical and experimental arguments have supported infection as the triggering event in autoimmune disease, although no pathogens have yet been proven to initiate synovitis in RA.

Infectious agents may invade the target organ directly, or infection outside the joint may trigger the arthritis through stimulation of autoimmunity, resulting in a sterile or "reactive" arthritis (13). This extraarticular infection possibly triggers disease through the mechanism known as molecular mimicry, which proposes that similarities in antigenic proteins between infecting agents and host tissues might result in the immune response against the pathogen becoming misdirected against the host tissue—in the case of RA, the joint. Similar theories propose an autoimmune response directed at "superantigens" in the joint that can activate multiple clones of T cells through a largely MHC-independent process. Examples of antigens that have been implicated are type II collagen, proteoglycans, heat shock proteins, cartilage protein gp39, and immunoglobulins (14,15). It is possible that RA may be multiple diseases, now defined by some common clinical manifestations, and there may not be a single predominant mechanism of initiation or perpetuation.

A current concept is that inflammation and tissue destruction in the rheumatoid synovium result from complex cell—cell interactions. The process may be initiated by an interaction between antigen-presenting cells (APC) and CD4+ T cells. APC display complexes of class II MHC molecules and peptide antigens that bind to specific receptors on the T cells. With an appropriate "second signal" or costimulation delivered by the APC to the T cell, a clonal expansion of T-cell subsets occurs. This stimulates synovial macrophages to secrete proinflammatory cytokines, such as interleukin-1 (IL-1) and tumor necrosis factor α (TNFα) (16), to activate multiple inflammatory and destructive pathways.

Joint damage in RA results from proliferation of the synovial intimal layer to form a pannus that overgrows, invades, and destroys adjacent cartilage and bone, evident on radiographs as loss of joint space and juxtaarticular bone erosion. Fibroblast-like synoviocytes and macrophages are the predominant cellular components of the invading pannus. Extracellular matrix damage resulting from synovial expansion is caused by several families of enzymes, including serine proteases and cathepsins. Matrix metalloproteinases, produced mostly by synoviocytes in the intimal lining, are also important mediators of tissue destruction.

DIAGNOSIS AND CLINICAL HISTORY

Diagnosing a chronic illness, such as RA, and separating it from other conditions that may be self-limited or have different outcomes can be difficult. There are no early-onset, disease-specific features, and the characteristic hallmarks of the disease develop over time. There is no single diagnostic test that enables a diagnosis of RA to be made with certainty. Instead, diagnosis depends on the accumulation of characteristic symptoms, signs, laboratory data, and radiologic findings.

The clinical manifestations of RA are highly variable. The typical illness begins insidiously with slowly progressive development of symptoms over a period of weeks to months. Less often, the onset is acute, usually polyarticular. Symmetric arthritis affecting the metacarpophalangeal (MCP) joints and proximal interphalangeal (PIP) joints of both hands is the most characteristic early clinical feature. There is swelling with associated stiffness, warmth, tenderness, and pain, with a characteristic morning accentuation of symptoms. Edema and proliferation of the synovium contribute to stiffness by mechanically interfering with joint motion.

The number of involved joints is highly variable, but the process is eventually polyarticular in most. Almost any joint may be affected but there is a predilection for peripheral joints with sparing of the axial

4 OF THE FOLLOWING MUST BE PRESENT
WITH 1 THROUGH 4 PRESENT A MINIMUM OF 6 WEEKS

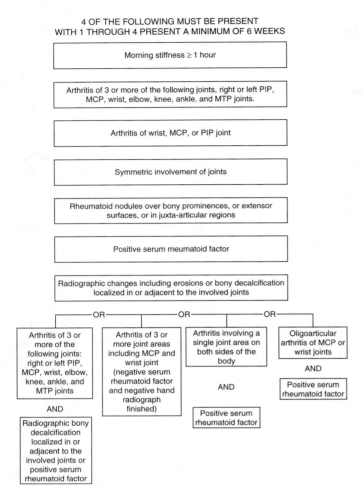

Morning stiffness ≥ 1 hour

Arthritis of 3 or more of the following joints, right or left PIP, MCP, wrist, elbow, knee, ankle, and MTP joints.

Arthritis of wrist, MCP, or PIP joint

Symmetric involvement of joints

Rheumatoid nodules over bony prominences, or extensor surfaces, or in juxta-articular regions

Positive serum meumatoid factor

Radiographic changes including erosions or bony decalcification localized in or adjacent to the involved joints

OR — OR — OR

Arthritis of 3 or more of the following joints: right or left PIP, MCP, wrist, elbow, knee, ankle, and MTP joints

AND

Radiographic bony decalcification localized in or adjacent to the involved joints or positive serum rheumatoid factor

Arthritis of 3 or more joint areas including MCP and wrist joint (negative serum rheumatoid factor and negative hand radiograph finished)

Arthritis involving a single joint area on both sides of the body

AND

Positive serum rheumatoid factor

Oligoarticular arthritis of MCP or wrist joints

AND

Positive serum rheumatoid factor

Figure 1. Classification criteria for the diagnosis of rheumatoid arthritis (18). PIP = proximal interphalangeal; MCP = metacarpophalangeal; MTP = metatarsophalangeal.

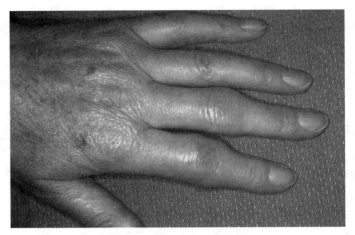

Figure 2. Swelling in the hand due to synovial hypertrophy.

skeleton, with the exception of the cervical spine. The joints involved most often are the PIP and MCP joints of the hands, wrists, elbows, ankles, metatarsophalangeal (MTP) joints, and temporomandibular joints. Involvement of shoulder, hip, sternoclavicular, and cricoarytenoid joints is less common (17).

Although RA is manifested primarily by joint involvement, it is a systemic inflammatory disease. Most patients experience such nonspecific systemic symptoms as fatigue, malaise, low-grade fever, and depression. These symptoms may precede overt arthritis by weeks or months. Because symptoms characteristically wax and wane, especially at the beginning of the illness, it is not unusual that the proper diagnosis is delayed for months.

Classification criteria for RA were drafted in 1956 by the American College of Rheumatology (ACR, formerly the American Rheumatism Association) and revised in 1987 (18) in an effort to provide guidelines for epidemiologic studies and clinical trials, but not primarily intended for clinical diagnosis (Figure 1). Disease features that initially fulfill the diagnostic criteria for RA may evolve or differentiate over time into other connective tissue diseases and other forms of inflammatory arthritis.

PHYSICAL EXAMINATION

A complete physical examination is indicated in all patients with RA, not only to make the diagnosis but to establish a baseline against which to assess disease progression. Pain and swelling are the key features

that occur in joints affected by RA. Swelling may be due to synovial hypertrophy (detected by a "boggy" feel to a swollen joint) or effusion, demonstrated by fluctuation. This is most evident in the small joints of the hands and feet, where the outline of the base of the proximal phalanx may become indistinct (Figure 2). In contrast to gout or septic arthritis, heat and redness are not prominent features of RA, although an involved joint is often warm on careful exam.

When effusion contributes to swelling and is under increased pressure with joint flexion, a portion of the synovium may become trapped and separated from the rest of the joint, forming a cyst. The cyst may be seen in many peripheral joints but is most commonly recognized in the knee (Baker's cyst), which, when ruptured, may resemble acute thrombophlebitis.

Tenderness and pain on passive motion are the most sensitive signs of inflammation, so it is important to apply gentle but firm pressure when examining a joint. A lateral squeeze of the MCP and MTP joint rows and assessment of grip strength are useful in detecting tenderness and restricted range of movement.

Visible changes include hyperflexion or hyperextension of the joints of the fingers (boutonniere and swan neck deformities), volar subluxation and ulnar deviation, hallux valgus (bunion), and hammer toes. These changes occur in the majority of patients with disease lasting more than 10 years (19). The characteristic joint deformities are late manifestations of disease that result from the physical stresses and local anatomy of involved joints. More than 10% of RA patients will develop deformity of the small joints of the hands within the first 2 years of disease, and at least one-third develop such deformities over time (20).

Subcutaneous nodules occur in ~30% of patients with RA, usually after the disease is established. They are not attached to underlying bone or overlying skin and are most commonly found over the extensor aspect of the proximal ulna, but they also occur at other pressure locations.

LABORATORY TESTS

No test is necessary to establish a diagnosis of RA, and all laboratory results may be normal in certain patients. Routine tests are often not characteristic and lack specificity; however, certain data may contribute to the diagnosis and assessment of the severity of RA in an individual.

Rheumatoid factor (RF) was identified as an antibody (typically IgM but also IgG or others) that binds to the Fc fragment of immunoglobulin G. It is detectable in the serum of 70–80% of patients with RA but may not be present in early disease. It is unclear whether the production of RF is of pathologic relevance to RA, because RF production also frequently occurs in patients with systemic lupus erythematosus; Sjögren's syndrome; endocarditis; sarcoidosis; liver and lung diseases, including hepatitis B and C infection; and other conditions (21). In addition, RF may be detected in the serum of apparently healthy individuals, especially people older than 50 and in smokers. In an individual patient, the titer does not correlate with disease activity, but it does appear that patients with very severe erosive arthritis or with extraarticular disease are likely to have relatively high titers. The presence of a positive serum RF does not establish a diagnosis of RA, but when combined with a typical clinical picture, it does help to confirm the clinical impression.

Antibodies to cyclic citrullinated peptide (anti-CCP) have been identified as a more specific marker for RA. Anti-CCP antibodies, detected using enzyme-linked immunosorbent assay, have a much higher specificity (>95%) than RF with similar sensitivity (68–80%) (22). These antibodies, which can be detected several years before the development of clinical RA (and before the development of rheumatoid factors), can be helpful in diagnosing RA in patients with RF-negative (seronegative) arthritis. They also appear to mark more severe outcomes, such as radiographic joint damage and poor prognosis (23–25). Because of their higher specificity for RA, anti-CCP antibodies may be useful in differentiating RA from other conditions with positive rheumatoid factors, including Sjögren's, infection, and hepatitis.

A mild anemia commonly occurs in RA. It is usually a normochromic, normocytic anemia of chronic disease; however, true iron deficiency anemia may also develop. The white blood cell count generally is normal, but occasionally may be elevated in patients with significant inflammatory disease; alternatively, it may be low in Felty's syndrome. Patients often have thrombocytosis, usually in association with active joint disease or extraarticular manifestations.

Acute phase reactants, such as erythrocyte sedimentation rate and C-reactive protein, are usually elevated in the presence of active inflammation, but are not specific for the diagnosis of RA. They are useful in distinguishing RA from such noninflammatory conditions as osteoarthritis or fibromyalgia. However, a significant number of RA patients have normal values of these tests, despite clinical evidence of joint inflammation. Antinuclear antibodies (ANA) can be present in 20–40% of patients with RA, commonly those with extraarticular manifestations and high RF titers.

Synovial fluid analysis is usually not necessary when the diagnosis is already established, but arthrocentesis should be performed to rule out infection or crystalline arthopathy in patients who develop disproportionate discomfort and swelling of one joint.

RADIOLOGY

Radiographic findings vary depending on the duration and severity of the illness. A normal radiograph does not exclude a diagnosis of RA; in fact, early in the disease radiographs may show nothing other than soft-tissue swelling. More than half of patients develop radiographic changes within the first 2 years of disease. The relationship between radiologic change and the consequences of RA for the patient has not yet been fully established. It is assumed, rather than proven, that the radiographic picture correlates with long-term disability.

Radiographic joint damage in RA has several features, including periarticular osteoporosis; joint-space narrowing due to generalized cartilage loss; and juxtaarticular erosions, generally at the point of attachment of the joint capsule or at the cartilage-pannus junction (Figure 3).

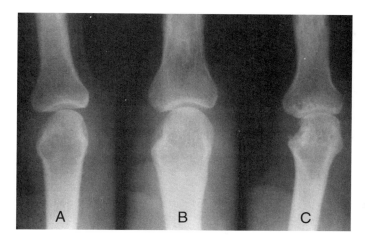

Figure 3. Erosive changes of a proximal interphalangeal joint.

In end-stage disease, large cystic erosions of bone may be seen together with bony proliferation, ankylosis, and marked deformities. Erosions, typically in the MCP and PIP joints, are present in 15–30% of patients in the first year of disease. In some patients, erosions occur first in the ulnar styloid or MTP joints. It is therefore important to evaluate both hands (including the wrists) and feet in all patients for whom a diagnosis of RA is suspected.

Cervical spine involvement is common. Joint destruction may lead to atlantoaxial (C1–C2) and subaxial malalignment (subluxation), vertebral endplate erosions, spondylodiscitis, and disc-space narrowing without osteophytes. Anterior C1–C2 subluxation is the most frequent radiographic abnormality. The earliest and most common symptom is pain radiating toward the occiput; however, the correlation between the degree of subluxation and symptoms is poor. Plain radiographic views of the cervical spine (lateral, with the neck in flexion) should be considered for all RA patients scheduled for procedures requiring manipulation of the neck. Unrecognized C1–C2 disease may lead to cord compression, irreversible paralysis, and even death.

SYSTEMIC AND NONARTICULAR MANIFESTATIONS

Extraarticular manifestations of RA usually occur in patients with relatively more severe disease, but rarely prior to the onset of arthritis. It is sometimes difficult to separate disease manifestations from drug-induced side effects. In contrast to the predilection of classic RA for women, extraarticular manifestations of the disease are more common in men. This is especially true for pleural involvement, vasculitis, and pericarditis. Systemic involvement occurs more frequently in patients who are RF positive.

Cutaneous Manifestations

The most common cutaneous manifestation is *rheumatoid nodules.* They may arise within tendons or ligaments and can result in joint dysfunction and tendon rupture. Rarely, nodules may arise in visceral organs, such as the lungs, heart valves, sclera, and vocal cords. Although effective in treating arthritis, methotrexate may concomitantly cause an increase in the size and number of rheumatoid nodules (26). The differential diagnosis of nodules should include gouty tophi, which may be found in similar locations. Very rarely, biopsy of the nodule may be necessary if the diagnosis is uncertain. Occasionally, the nodules may ulcerate or breakdown, requiring surgical excision and debridement.

About 10–15% of patients with RA develop *Sjögren's syndrome*, characterized by impaired secretion of saliva and tears, dry mouth (xerostomia), and dry eyes (keratoconjunctivitis). Laboratory findings in Sjögren's may include positive ANA, anti-Ro, anti-La, and polyclonal gammopathy. Patients with Sjögren's are at increased risk of developing lymphomas, especially low-grade B-cell lymphoma.

Ocular Manifestations

Episcleritis, a self-limited process, and *scleritis*, a more serious problem that can lead to perforation of the globe and loss of vision, occur in <5% of RA patients. The distinction between episcleritis and scleritis is difficult, and all patients with suspected scleritis should be referred to an ophthalmologist.

Pulmonary Involvement

Pulmonary involvement in RA may present with several clinical scenarios. Pleurisy with or without effusion is the most common form of pulmonary disease, occurring in up to 70% of patients. Most cases are asymptomatic, and a small pleural effusion may be discovered incidentally on a routine radiograph. The effusion is usually exudative, and the glucose concentration of the fluid is often very low. Interstitial lung disease is a common long-term manifestation of severe RA that usually follows the onset of joint symptoms by up to 5 years. It is more common in men, and smoking is a significant risk factor. Because of limited physical activity in patients with RA, it is often asymptomatic, but restrictive abnormalities on pulmonary function tests are common even in the absence of symptoms. The diagnosis should be suspected in any patient with RA with shortness of breath or dyspnea on exertion. Acute methotrexate pneumonitis may be seen occasionally, and long-term methotrexate therapy is also associated with pulmonary fibrosis. Other rare pulmonary manifestations include bronchiolitis obliterans, pneumothorax, or rheumatoid pneumoconiosis (Caplan's syndrome).

Cardiac Involvement

Atherosclerotic heart disease is the most common cardiovascular manifestation associated with RA and is the leading cause of death. Possibly related to the chronic inflammatory state of the disease, it is notable that recent studies indicate that more aggressive treatment of disease may be contributing to decreasing incidence of cardiovascular morbidity (27, 28). Pericarditis and myocarditis are other major forms of cardiac involvement in RA. Up to 30% of patients have echocardiographic evidence of pericardial effusion, but symptomatic pericarditis is rare, usually developing during a generalized disease flare. Restrictive pericarditis with tamponade is unusual. Myocarditis and conduction abnormalities secondary to nodule formation in the heart have been reported rarely and may be linked to amyloid infiltration.

Renal Involvement

Renal involvement as an intrinsic part of the rheumatoid disease process is suggested but unproven. It is usually related to amyloidosis, vasculitis, or drug toxicity. Among drugs used in RA, those most commonly implicated in renal dysfunction include cyclosporine, gold, penicillamine, and nonsteroidal antiinflammatory drugs (NSAIDs).

Felty's Syndrome

This syndrome is characterized by the triad of neutropenia, splenomegaly, and deforming RA and may occur in about 1% of patients with RA. Patients are usually older than 50 years, have a high RF titer, and often have a positive ANA and relatively severe arthritis with other extraarticular manifestations. When splenomegaly is not present, the diagnosis may be difficult. Recurrent bacterial infections, most commonly affecting the lungs and urinary tract, and chronic refractory leg ulcers are the major complications. Large granular lymphocyte (LGL) syndrome shares many clinical and laboratory features of Felty's syndrome but is not exclusive to RA. In fact, LGL syndrome may represent a process that facilitates development of RA, rather than being a result of the disease itself. Up to 14% of patients with LGL syndrome may progress to having leukemia; exacerbation, rather than improvement, frequently follows splenectomy.

Vasculitis

Inflammation involving the blood vessels is found in as many as 25–30% of patients with RA on whom autopsies are performed. However, clinically evident disease is much less common. Classification of rheumatoid vasculitis is difficult because of the variability in both the size of the vessel involved and the histologic findings. Skin vasculitis is the most common manifestation, presenting as small digital infarcts along the nail beds, palpable purpura, and petechiae. Vasculitis of the vaso vasorum, which supply blood to nerves, can lead to a mild distal sensory neuropathy or mononeuritis multiplex.

DIFFERENTIAL DIAGNOSIS

The diagnosis of RA, especially in its initial stages, can be difficult. The basic laboratory tests lack adequate sensitivity and specificity, and clinical assessment is subject to bias. Atypical early presentation with fluctuating symptoms, absence of rheumatoid factor, or single or asymmetric joint involvement makes it more difficult to distinguish RA from other causes of acute or chronic polyarthritis.

The *spondyloarthropathies* (including Reiter's syndrome, reactive arthritis, and inflammatory bowel disease) may appear similar to RA. Careful history and physical examination to look for heel pain and ocular or urethral symptoms are of greatest importance. The joint involvement in reactive arthritis is typically asymmetric oligoarthritis, usually of the weight-bearing joints, with or without sacroiliac and spinal involvement. The characteristics of enthesopathy, such as inflammation at tendon insertion sites and "sausage" appearance of the fingers, may point to the diagnosis. Morning stiffness is unusual and RF is rare.

Inflammatory bowel disease (ulcerative colitis and Crohn's disease) may be associated with peripheral arthritis in up to 20% of patients. Not infrequently, arthritis is the first clinical symptom, and abdominal complaints may not be prominent. Lower extremity joints are involved predominantly, and large joint effusions are common. Involvement is usually asymmetric and erosions are not found.

Psoriatic arthritis may closely resemble RA, and joint symptoms may precede the onset of skin disease by many years. In a majority of patients, involvement of DIP joints, psoriatic skin lesions or family history of psoriasis, and characteristic nail changes (onychodystrophy, pitting) all point toward psoriatic arthritis. The presence of dactylitis, enthesitis, spinal involvement, and a characteristic radiographic picture with new bone formation or ankylosis clarify the diagnosis. Many cases of psoriatic arthritis may, however, present with an RA-like picture characterized by a symmetric arthritis involving the MCPs and PIPs.

Osteoarthritis (OA) is most commonly confused with RA when it involves the hands, particularly the PIP joints. OA typically affects DIP joints, with characteristic Heberden's nodes, and the carpometacarpal joint of the thumb. Stiffness is most bothersome after joint immobility, but in a small number of patients it may last for several hours. In general, OA is not associated with constitutional symptoms, RF, or abnormal levels of acute phase reactants. Radiographs show narrowing of the joint space and osteophytes without erosions or cysts.

Gout, known as "the great masquerader," must always be considered before a diagnosis of RA is made. Features of gouty arthritis that mimic RA include polyarthritis, symmetric involvement, fusiform swelling of joints, and subcutaneous nodules. Radiographic findings may be similar, with overlapping appearance of the subcortical erosions of RA resembling small osseous tophi. Serologic tests may be misleading as well; often diagnosis of gout can be made only by arthrocentesis.

Polymyalgia rheumatica (PMR) can usually be distinguished from RA by the absence of persistent small-joint synovitis and by localization of symptoms in proximal muscles of the shoulders and pelvic girdle. Patients will have difficulty performing such activities as rising from a chair, climbing, or combing hair; whereas RA-associated difficulties include buttoning or opening jars. Occasionally, PMR may also be accompanied by an RA-like synovitis in the hands and feet but often is accompanied with significant pitting edema.

Viral infections, such as rubella and parvovirus, can present as an acute polyarthritis, which differs from RA by the typically self-limited nature of symptoms. Furthermore, patients with viral arthritis may present with rash, low-grade fever, and a recent history of viral exposure. Other viral infections accompanied by polyarthritis include hepatitis B and human immunodeficiency virus.

Some typical findings in *fibromyalgia* may be seen in RA patients as well. These include morning stiffness, diffuse arthralgias and myalgias, subjective joint and soft-tissue swelling, fatigue, and sleep disturbances. In fact, both of these conditions may be present simultaneously in a patient. In RA, sleep disturbances from pain are common, leading to concomitant fibromyalgia.

Other conditions that may simulate RA include systemic lupus erythematosus, systemic sclerosis, myositis, and less commonly, Lyme disease, hypertrophic osteoarthropathy, hemochromatosis, hypothyroidism, bacterial endocarditis, hemoglobinopathies, sarcoidosis, and rheumatic fever.

TREATMENT

The ultimate goals of RA management are to reduce pain and discomfort; prevent deformities and loss of normal joint function; and maintain normal physical, social, and emotional function and capacity to work. Management begins with effective communication between physician and patient. It is very important to educate the patient and his or her family about the nature and course of the disease—the specific causes of the discomfort and the goals, problems, and expectations of treatment. Misunderstandings about the disease may lead to frustration, depression, and withdrawal.

Nonpharmacologic therapeutic options include reduction of joint stress, and physical and occupational therapy. Local rest of an inflamed joint can reduce joint stress, as can weight reduction, splinting, and use of walking aids and specially designed assistive devices. Vigorous

activity should be avoided during disease flares, although full range of motion of joints should be maintained by a graded exercise program to prevent contractures and muscle atrophy (See Chapter 32, Exercise and Physical Activity).

The former pharmacologic approach to the treatment of RA was to begin with symptomatic treatment of inflammation using NSAIDs in addition to rest and corticosteroid injections. If the disease did not significantly improve, more potent disease-modifying antirheumatic drugs (DMARDs) were started. This is no longer the recommended approach for the treatment of RA. Maintaining normal joint structure and anatomy can only be achieved by controlling the disease before any irreversible damage has occurred. Studies have revealed that DMARD therapy early in the course of RA slowed disease progression more effectively than did delayed use (29). Effective, aggressive treatment can improve both signs and symptoms, and radiographic progression, even in long-standing disease. This has led to a general agreement that the inflammation of RA should be controlled as completely as possible, as soon as possible, and that this control should be maintained for as long as possible. The currently available pharmacologic and biologic agents used to treat RA will be briefly reviewed, but more information about these medications can be found in Chapters 34 and 35.

Nonsteroidal Antiinflammatory Drugs

NSAIDs are probably the most frequently used drugs in the treatment of RA, at least early in the disease process. They reduce joint pain and swelling and improve function, but they have no effect on the underlying disease process, and exacerbation of symptoms occurs quickly after metabolic elimination of the drugs. They are rarely, if ever, used alone for treatment of RA.

The major therapeutic effect of NSAIDs relates to their ability to suppress the synthesis of prostaglandins by inhibiting the enzyme cyclooxygenase, which exists in 2 isoforms: cyclooxygenase-1 and cyclooxygenase-2 (COX-1 and COX-2) (30). COX-1 is expressed in many tissues and is primarily responsible for the production of prostaglandins by endothelium and gastric mucosa, leading to homeostatic and cytoprotective effects. COX-2 is undetectable in most tissues; its expression increases during development and inflammation and can be induced by several proinflammatory stimuli. It is hypothesized that the antiinflammatory effects of NSAIDs are mainly the result of COX-2 inhibition and that inhibition of COX-1 is responsible for most of the gastrointestinal (GI) toxicity.

There are a large number of NSAIDs from which to choose, and their antiinflammatory potential is approximately equal. However, there is an unpredictable and varied individual response to different NSAIDs. Titration upward to the maximally approved doses may be required in RA, and if there is no clinical response after 2–3 weeks, another drug should be initiated.

The major side effects limiting the usefulness of NSAIDs are GI and renal toxicity. GI disturbance is secondary to direct damage to the gastric mucosa and suppression of gastroprotective prostaglandins. Ulcers, bleeding, and perforation occur in ~2–4% of patients who use NSAIDs for 1 year (31)—a risk further increased in patients taking concomitant aspirin and steroids. Therefore, periodic assessment of hematocrit in patients taking NSAIDs for an extended duration is recommended. Concomitant administration of proton-pump inhibitors may decrease risk of peptic ulceration. NSAIDs interfere with fluid and electrolyte homeostasis, resulting in fluid retention and hyperkalemia. Patients with pre-existing renal disease or diminished effective renal blood volume are at risk for effects of NSAIDs on glomerular perfusion; therefore, careful monitoring of creatinine and potassium levels is indicated.

Selective COX-2 inhibitors have been approved for use in RA. Their principal benefit is the lower risk of serious GI adverse reactions compared with the nonselective NSAIDs (32–34). Limited data are available concerning whether they are safer with regard to renal toxicity. Recent concerns regarding cardiovascular and dermatologic adverse events of the COX-2 inhibitors rofecoxib and valdecoxib, respectively, led to their removal from the market. Currently, celecoxib and meloxicam are the 2 available COX-2 inhibitors in the United States.

Corticosteroids

Corticosteroids have a long history in the treatment of many rheumatic diseases and they are still a key element in the management of RA. They produce rapid and potent suppression of inflammation with improvement in fatigue, joint pain, and swelling. One controlled study demonstrated a decrease in progression of joint erosion in patients treated with low-dose daily prednisolone (35). The use of steroids as monotherapy for RA is not a recommended strategy. Prednisone is most frequently used for RA in a dose of 5–10 mg/day to minimize adrenal suppression. The therapy is often initiated in patients with significant functional decline and active disease while awaiting the full therapeutic effect of DMARDs. Once started, corticosteroid therapy may be difficult to discontinue. Tapering should be gradual to avoid disease flares, e.g., 0.5–1.0 mg/day every few weeks to months.

A short course or even a single, high dose of corticosteroid can be administered in situations when rapid control of inflammation is desired. Occasionally, intraarticular injections may be used to control a local flare in joints with disproportionate involvement. The effects are sometimes dramatic but may be temporary.

All potential adverse effects of steroids should be fully discussed with the patient before initiating therapy. The immunosuppressive and catabolic consequences associated with corticosteroids limit their long-term use in high doses and dictate the need for careful surveillance and preventive interventions to avoid undesired complications. Periodic assessment for steroid-induced osteoporosis has become a standard of care for patients on long-term corticosteroid therapy. Patients with and without osteoporosis risk factors should undergo bone densitometry to assess fracture risk. Bisphosphonates or other strategies to prevent steroid-induced osteoporosis are recommended for many patients.

Disease-Modifying Antirheumatic Drugs

All patients with RA are candidates for DMARD therapy. DMARDs lack analgesic effect, and it may take weeks or months before any clinical benefit is recognized. They often only moderate the disease process, and some level of chronic inflammation usually persists. The disease generally recurs after the drug is discontinued. These agents may affect laboratory tests that measure acute-phase reactants, and most have now been shown to slow the rate of progression of joint erosions and disability (36–38).

Antimalarial Drugs. Antimalarials (chloroquine and hydroxychloroquine) are commonly used drugs with a favorable toxicity/benefit profile. There is no data, however, to prove that hydroxychloroquine alone reduces or prevents radiographic damage from RA. Chloroquine is more popular in Europe and appears to be more potent but more toxic than hydroxychloroquine (39), which is often used in early, mild disease and as background therapy when another DMARD is started. Although very uncommon in the doses used in treating RA (200–400 mg daily), hydroxychloroquine may rarely cause ocular toxicity. Opinions differ with regard to the appropriate frequency of monitoring; nevertheless, patients should undergo ophthalmologic examination before starting therapy, and semiannually thereafter (40).

Methotrexate. As a result of its favorable efficacy and toxicity profile, low cost, and predictable benefit, methotrexate has become the most commonly used DMARD for RA. More than 50% of patients taking methotrexate continue the drug beyond 5 years, longer than any other DMARD (41). At lower doses, methotrexate has immunomodulatory and significant antiinflammatory effects. Initial dosages range from 7.5 to 15 mg/week, and may be increased to 25 mg/week. In recent clinical trials of early RA, methotrexate was started at 15 mg/week and rapidly escalated to 20 mg/week within 3 months. Methotrexate may also be administered as a subcutaneous injection, thus avoiding GI complaints experienced by some with oral administration and assuring bioavailability in patients with compromised oral absorption.

Mucositis, bone marrow suppression, and hepatocellular injury are the primary toxicities associated with use of methotrexate. Concomitant use of trimethoprim/sulfamethoxazole may increase the risk for bone marrow suppression. Less common complications include interstitial pneumonitis and fibrosis, nephritis, and neurocognitive impairment. Opportunistic infections rarely occur. Alopecia, headache, and stomatitis are also side effects. Many GI symptoms can be avoided by the concomitant use of folic acid, or changing to parenteral administration. For side effects refractory to folic acid supplementation, leucovorin (5 mg) 12 and 24 hours after methotrexate dosing is recommended.

Clinically significant drug-related hepatic dysfunction is less frequent when patients with preexisting liver disease, alcohol abuse, or hepatic dysfunction are excluded from treatment. Use of methotrexate in patients with renal insufficiency or on dialysis should be avoided.

Guidelines for monitoring patients with RA while on methotrexate have been established (42). Baseline tests for all patients prior to therapy initiation should include a complete blood count (CBC), serum creatinine, liver function tests, and hepatitis B and C serologies. Recommendations for monitoring for hepatic safety have been published (43). Women of childbearing age must be warned to practice effective birth control, as methotrexate is potentially teratogenic.

Sulfasalazine. Sulfasalazine is a combination of a salicylate and a sulfapyridine molecule. In addition to an antiinflammatory effect due to its salicylate component, sulfasalazine appears to have immunomodulatory effects similar to those of methotrexate. It is frequently used in combination with other DMARDs. The usual starting dosage is 500 or 1000 mg/day, raised slowly to 2 or 3 gm/day over 4–6 weeks. GI symptoms are the most common side effects and are often resolved with dose attenuation or enteric-coated formulations. Glucose-6-phosphate dehydrogenase levels should be checked before the use of sulfasalazine to decrease the risk of hemolysis. Hematologic consequences may include aplastic anemia, agranulocytosis, or hemolytic anemia. Avoidance in patients with sulfa allergy is also important because skin reactions and hypersensitivity may be severe. Regular monitoring of the CBC is recommended.

Leflunomide. The active metabolite of leflunomide inhibits an enzyme that mediates synthesis of pyrimidines, with significant inhibitory effects on lymphocyte proliferation. Leflunomide is effective in decreasing signs and symptoms and in slowing radiographic progression, similar to methotrexate (44). It takes ~7–8 weeks for this drug to reach steady-state levels in the blood. To decrease this time, a loading dose of 100 mg/day for 2–3 days is sometimes used, followed by a maintenance dosage of 10–20 mg/day.

Adverse events include reversible alopecia, skin rash, stomatitis, diarrhea, and elevation in liver enzymes. Routine monitoring of CBC and liver function are required. Leflunomide is teratogenic. It may take up to 2 years after discontinuation for complete elimination, during which time pregnancy should be avoided. Excretion may be achieved more quickly by giving cholestyramine (8 grams) 3 times a day for 10–11 days, with levels of the metabolite checked and possible repeat administration of the cholestyramine required to achieve full washout.

Nursing Considerations in Rheumatoid Arthritis

- Ensure current medication list at each patient visit—medications and doses vary often
- Assess and document activities of daily living and pain scores at each visit
- Keep an updated log on laboratory toxicity monitoring—essential for patients taking DMARDs (i.e., methotrexate, azathioprine)
- Provide patient education materials on medications, disease overview, and community-based resources for exercise and physical activity

---

Biologic Agents

Tumor Necrosis Factor Antagonists. TNF is known to play a central part in the pathogenesis of RA. This proinflammatory cytokine triggers several important events that lead to the synovitis and tissue destruction exhibited in RA. It stimulates production of other proinflammatory cytokines, induces production of metalloproteinases, regulates cell proliferation and apoptosis, and increases expression of adhesion molecules.

In the past few years, 3 biologic response modifiers capable of neutralizing TNF have been developed, tested, and approved for patients with RA. The anti-TNF drugs etanercept, infliximab, and adalimumab inhibit inflammation by binding TNF before it reaches its cell-bound receptor. Infliximab and adalimumab also bind to cell-bound TNF.

Etanercept is a genetically engineered molecule containing 2 human soluble TNF receptors attached to the Fc portion of the human IgG. The clinical utility of etanercept in adults with RA has been assessed in multiple clinical trials involving >500 patients (45–48). Etanercept produced significant improvements in all measures of disease activity, including the rate of progression of joint damage. Approved dosages for adults are 25 mg twice weekly or 50 mg weekly by subcutaneous injection.

Infliximab is a chimeric (part-mouse, part-human) monoclonal antibody to TNF administered by intravenous infusion at a recommended starting dosage of 3 mg/kg every 8 weeks. Dose and frequency escalation are also possible. Infliximab reduces inflammatory activity and improves quality of life (49), and in combination with methotrexate, inhibits radiographic progression over 1 year in up to 50% of patients (50, 51). Administration of methotrexate with infliximab significantly reduces the formation of antibodies directed against the murine portion (52). Infliximab is currently recommended for use only with concomitant methotrexate therapy.

Adalimumab is a fully human IgG monoclonal antibody against TNFα administered as a 40-mg subcutaneous injection every 2 weeks, which may be increased to 40 mg every week. Patients receiving adalimumab in conjunction with either methotrexate or corticosteroids were able to reduce methotrexate and/or corticosteroid dosages without adversely affecting long-term efficacy (53–55). Like infliximab and etanercept, the combination of adalimumab with methotrexate significantly slowed radiographic progression.

Initiation of therapy with a TNF inhibitor should be accompanied by a complete physical examination and careful evaluation to rule out underlying infections, including tuberculosis (TB). Current recommendations for a purified protein derivative test (PPD) are for 5TU intradermal administration with a positive result at 5 mm of induration. Some have also advocated a second-step PPD 2 weeks after the first to increase the sensitivity for detecting latent TB. There have been reports of patients receiving all 3 agents who developed severe infections, including sepsis and disseminated tuberculosis, some of which were fatal. There are no established protocols for use of TNF antagonists in patients with a positive PPD regarding coadministration with anti-TB therapies. Patients taking TNF antagonists should be periodically reassessed for new TB exposure.

To date, overall tolerance to these agents has been acceptable. In published trials, there were no serious adverse events for any anti-TNF agent. Postmarketing surveillance data has yielded rare reports of demyelination with TNF inhibitors, although a true association remains to be determined. Injection-site reactions consisting of erythema, itching, pain, or swelling are the most common adverse effects during administration of etanercept and adalimumab. These generally occur during the first month and do not preclude continuation of therapy. It is mandatory to withhold therapy in the setting of acute bacterial infection, resuming treatment only after the infection has resolved. Patients should be reminded to call their physician immediately if they develop any signs or symptoms of infection. Anti-DNA and anticardiolipin antibodies have been seen in patients receiving both therapies, but their significance have not been fully defined. There is no clear answer as to what level of disease activity would be most appropriate to initiate or discontinue TNF-blocking therapy. Due to their cost and restrictions in insurance coverage, the biologic agents have been used primarily in patients with RA whose symptoms are resistant to DMARD treatment.

Abatacept. Beyond specific cytokine action, T-cell costimulation is believed to be crucial in orchestrating immune responses that lead to inflammation and destruction in RA (56). Abatacept, a recombinant CTLA4Ig fusion protein that selectively modulates costimulation via interrupting the CD28:CD80/86 pathway, results in downregulation of T-cell activation and multiple ensuing effector mechanisms. Abatacept has been shown to be efficacious, either when given alone or in combination with methotrexate, in patients with active RA—including those who did not receive relief from anti-TNF therapy. Improvements in clinical signs and symptoms, slowing of radiologic progression, and enhancement in patient function and pain have been reported in clinical trials (57, 58). RA patients who had long-standing disease (mean disease duration of 11.8 years), significant disease activity, moderate-to-severe disability, and inadequate response to TNF blockers (etanercept, infliximab, or both) received abatacept in a 24-week study. Abatacept was superior to placebo in all response measures, with difference between arms being significant from day 15 (59). Abatacept users had significantly higher rates of remission, lower levels of disease activity, and clinically meaningful improvements in physical functioning and disability measures. Data from the open-label extension showed continued efficacy at 18 months with results similar to the original 6-month trial (60).

Rituximab. In addition to T cells, evidence has emerged supporting the pivotal role of B cells in the pathogenesis of RA. Rituximab, a chimeric monoclonal antibody to a specific marker for mature B cells (CD20) that has been FDA approved for treatment of refractory non-Hodgkin's lymphoma, has recently gained FDA approval for the treatment of RA refractory to anti-TNFα therapy. Randomized pilot studies suggested B-cell depletion was an effective and safe approach to RA management (61, 62). The B-cell depletion with rituximab is rapid and may be prolonged for periods of >1 year. From these preliminary data, a number of clinical trials have highlighted the efficacy of rituximab. In a study of 465 RA patients with long-standing disease, significant joint damage, and an inadequate response to methotrexate, (25% of whom also had an inadequate response to anti-TNFα therapy), rituximab—at 500 mg and 1000 mg for 2 infusions given 2 weeks apart—was superior to placebo at achieving clinical response (63). A second trial of 520 RA patients with an inadequate response to one or more anti-TNFα therapies showed that significantly more patients

Rehabilitation Considerations in Rheumatoid Arthritis

- It is important to consider the stage of disease and level of disease activity in designing a rehabilitation intervention.
- Rehabilitation programs for patients with active disease should include range-of-motion exercises, isometric exercises, joint checks, and recommendations for positioning (e.g., splints).
- Dynamic strengthening exercises should be avoided in the presence of popliteal cysts or malaligned joints.
- Patients with RA are at risk for cardiopulmonary vascular complications from the disease and from medical interventions. These factors should be assessed and taken into consideration when designing exercise regimens.
- When the disease is stable, dynamic strengthening and aerobic exercises, such as walking and aquatic exercises, should be initiated.
- The type of medication and time to onset of medication effectiveness are essential factors in determining the frequency and mode of exercise used.
- Muscle weakness and fatigue is often underappreciated and should be a major factor in the design in the rehabilitation interventions. Muscle weakness can be a direct as well as indirect manifestation of the disease.
- Certain medications, such as steroids, can impact skin integrity. Careful assessment of skin integrity, particularly with the use of splints and other assistive devices, is warranted.
- Appropriate whole-body and joint-specific rest should be incorporated into the patient education program.

randomized to the rituximab arm achieved clinical response at 24 weeks compared with placebo (64). In these studies, rituximab was generally well tolerated, with safety comparable to that of methotrexate, except for increased infections. Infusion-related reactions, sometimes severe, were the most common adverse event. These reactions were decreased with intravenous corticosteroid pretreatment at the time of the infusion. Because of unknown effects on immune responses, all immunizations should be completed before beginning therapy and live virus vaccines should be avoided.

Anakinra. Similar to TNF, IL-1 is a key proinflammatory cytokine with pleiotropic effects on cartilage, bone, and effector cells. These effects contribute to the synovial inflammation, acute phase response, and osteoclast-mediated bone destruction observed in RA. An IL-1 receptor antagonist (IL-1ra) is a natural antiinflammatory cytokine released by mononuclear cells at inflammatory sites. In RA, synovial IL-1ra levels are elevated but in insufficient quantities to significantly attenuate the proinflammatory effects of IL-1. Anakinra is a recombinant human IL-1ra that has been shown to effectively reduce the signs and symptoms of disease activity in patients with RA. A phase III, randomized controlled trial showed that RA patients treated with anakinra in combination with methotrexate reached significant disease response (46%) compared with those randomized to placebo (19%) (65). Results from a large, placebo-controlled safety study demonstrated that anakinra is safe and well tolerated in a diverse population of patients with RA, with the rate of serious adverse events similar between anakinra and placebo (66). Although the frequency of serious infection was slightly higher in the anakinra group, no infection was attributed to opportunistic microorganisms or resulted in death. Anakinra's use in RA is limited due in part to the necessity of daily subcutaneous dosing.

Combination Therapy

The use of combinations of DMARDs when a single agent fails to control clinical symptoms of RA is generally accepted (67), although the most effective way of providing combination therapy is under debate. Some propose initiating treatment in a "step-up" approach by adding new agents in patients whose disease has failed to respond to a single drug, whereas others recommend beginning with combination therapy early in the disease and using a "step-down" method once disease is under control. Clinical trials have shown promising results with increased efficacy and acceptable toxicity using a triple combination of methotrexate, sulfasalazine, and hydroxychloroquine (68, 69).

Combination therapy with methotrexate and leflunomide has also been investigated (70–73). In a 24-week randomized, double-blind, placebo-controlled study of RA patients with persistent disease activity despite at least 6 months of methotrexate, the addition of leflunomide provided statistically significant clinical benefit compared with the addition of placebo; the leflunomide-methotrexate combination was generally well tolerated (72). In the open-label extension of this trial, response to active combination therapy (signs and symptoms, quality of life, and functional assessments) was maintained at 48 weeks. Response rates were similar, and adverse events (nausea, diarrhea, and elevated transaminases) were fewer in patients switched from placebo to leflunomide without a loading dose at the initiation of the extension than in patients who received a loading dose of leflunomide (100 mg/day for 2 days) at initial randomization. Specifically, patients who switched from placebo to leflunomide for the second 24 weeks of treatment without a loading dose exhibited an incidence of elevated transaminases (alanine aminotransferase [ALT] 14.6%, aspartate aminotransferase [AST] 13.7%) that was lower compared with those initially randomized to leflunomide with a loading dose (ALT 31.5%, AST 16.9%) but higher than in patients initially randomized to placebo (ALT 6.8%, AST 4.6%) (73). Elevated transaminases were reversible and no patient initiating leflunomide at the extension discontinued the study due to elevated transaminases during the open-label phase.

The combinations of biologic agents with methotrexate have been studied and found to be beneficial as well. The TEMPO study, by Klareskog and colleagues, enrolled 682 patients with moderately severe RA and showed that the combination of etanercept plus methotrexate was more effective for reducing symptoms and disease activity than monotherapy with either agent (74). Similarly, the ASPIRE study of 1,049 patients with early active RA showed that combination therapy with methotrexate and infliximab provides greater clinical, radiographic, and functional benefits than treatment with methotrexate alone (75). Finally, in the recent 2-year PREMIER study of 799 methotrexate-naïve RA patients with early and active disease, combination therapy with adalimumab plus oral methotrexate was superior to both monotherapy arms in all outcomes measured, including radiographic progression and disease remission measures (76).

Adverse event profiles were similar in all groups. Combination therapy with biologic DMARDs should be avoided. Studies have now demonstrated an increase in infections with TNF antagonists administered with anakinra, and with abatacept administered with biologic DMARDS.

Although the efficacy of combination therapy is clearly supported and current treatment guidelines suggest that early diagnosis and initial treatment with DMARDs are necessary to limit damage and functional loss (77), determining which patients will respond to DMARD monotherapy versus those who will require combination therapy remains an unmet need in the treatment of RA. Identifying reliable predictors of an individual's response will be a critical goal to help guide therapeutic decision making.

Other Agents

Gold Compounds. Due to their effectiveness in suppressing synovitis, gold compounds were the most popular remission-inducing agents in the 1970s and early 1980s. Preparations currently in use are aurothioglucose, administered parenterally, and auranofin, an oral preparation that is less effective and rarely used. The exact mechanism of action has not been established. The administration of intramuscular gold requires regular office visits to monitor for toxicity and efficacy. If there is a favorable response, therapy can be maintained with 50 mg/month.

The most common adverse effects are mucocutaneous reactions including stomatitis, pruritis, and various forms of dermatitis. Proteinuria may occur; it is usually mild, and rarely in nephrotic range. Leukopenia, thrombocytopenia, and aplastic anemia are rare but potentially fatal consequences. Blood counts and urinalysis should be performed prior to each injection during the first year of treatment. Due to their toxicity and existence of many new alternatives, gold compounds are less often used in today's practice.

Cytotoxic and Immunosuppressive Drugs. Cytotoxic drugs, including azathioprine, cyclophosphamide, and cyclosporine, are generally reserved for patients with refractory RA who have failed to receive benefit from conventional therapy. Despite their efficacy profile, use of these drugs in RA is limited due to their toxicity and the existence of new alternatives. They should be reserved only for patients with aggressive disease and life-threatening extraarticular manifestations.

REFERENCES

1. Heath CW Jr, Fortin PR. Epidemiologic studies of rheumatoid arthritis: future directions. J Rheumatol Suppl 1992;32:74–7.
2. Lawrence RC. Rheumatoid arthritis: classification and epidemiology. In: Klippel JH, Dieppe PA, editors. Rheumatology. London: Mosby-Year Book; 1994.
3. Mijiyawa M. Epidemiology and semiology of rheumatoid arthritis in Third World countries. Rev Rhum Engl Ed 1995;62:121–6.
4. Guillemin F, Briancon S, Klein JM, Sauleau E, Pourel J. Low incidence of rheumatoid arthritis in France. Scand J Rheumatol 1994;23:264–8.
5. Symmons DP, Barrett EM, Bankhead CR, Scott DG, Silman AJ. The incidence of rheumatoid arthritis in the United Kingdom: results from the Norfolk Arthritis Register. Br J Rheumatol 1994;33:735–9.
6. Gabriel SE, Crowson CS, O'Fallon WM. Mortality in rheumatoid arthritis: have we made an impact in 4 decades? J Rheumatol 1999;26:2529–33.
7. Prior P, Symmons DP, Scott DL, Brown R, Hawkins CF. Cause of death in rheumatoid arthritis. Br J Rheumatol 1984;23:92–9.
8. Wallberg-Jonsson S, Ohman ML, Dahlqvist SR. Cardiovascular morbidity and mortality in patients with seropositive rheumatoid arthritis in Northern Sweden. J Rheumatol 1997;24:445–51.
9. Gabriel SE, Crowson CS, O'Fallon WM. Comorbidity in arthritis. J Rheumatol 1999;26:2475–9.
10. Stastny P. Association of the B-cell alloantigen DRw4 with rheumatoid arthritis. N Engl J Med 1978;298:869–71.
11. Silman AJ, MacGregor AJ, Thomson W, Holligan S, Carthy D, Farhan A, et al. Twin concordance rates for rheumatoid arthritis: results from a nationwide study. Br J Rheumatol 1993;32:903–7.
12. Nepom GT, Byers P, Seyfried C, Healey LA, Wilske KR, Stage D, et al. HLA genes associated with rheumatoid arthritis. Identification of susceptibility alleles using specific oligonucleotide probes. Arthritis Rheum 1989;32:15–21.
13. Ebringer A, Wilson C, Tiwana H. Is rheumatoid arthritis a form of reactive arthritis? J Rheumatol 2000;27:559–63.
14. Albani S, Carson DA, Roudier J. Genetic and environmental factors in the immune pathogenesis of rheumatoid arthritis. Rheum Dis Clin North Am 1992;18:729–40.
15. van Eden W. Heat-shock proteins as immunogenic bacterial antigens with the potential to induce and regulate autoimmune arthritis. Immunol Rev 1991;121:5–28.
16. Arend WP, Dayer JM. Inhibition of the production and effects of interleukin-1 and tumor necrosis factor alpha in rheumatoid arthritis. Arthritis Rheum 1995;38:151–60.
17. Fleming A, Benn RT, Corbett M, Wood PH. Early rheumatoid disease. II. Patterns of joint involvement. Ann Rheum Dis 1976;35:361–4.
18. Arnett FC, Edworthy SM, Bloch DA, McShane DJ, Fries JF, Cooper NS, et al. The American Rheumatism Association 1987 revised criteria for the classification of rheumatoid arthritis. Arthritis Rheum 1988;31:315–24.

19. Komusi T, Munro T, Harth M. Radiologic review: the rheumatoid cervical spine. Semin Arthritis Rheum 1985;14:187–95.
20. Fuchs HA, Sergent JS. Rheumatoid arthritis: the clinical picture. In: Koopman WJ, editor. Arthritis and allied conditions. Baltimore: Williams & Wilkins; 1997.
21. Koopman WJ, Schrohenberg RE. Rheumatoid factor. In: Utsinger PD, Zvaifler NJ, Ehrlich GE, editors. Rheumatoid arthritis: etiology, diagnosis and therapy. Philadelphia: JB Lippincott; 1985.
22. Jansen LM, van Schaardenburg D, van der Horst-Bruinsma I, van der Stadt RJ, de Koning MH, Dijkmans BA. The predictive value of anti-cyclic citrullinated peptide antibodies in early arthritis. J Rheumatol 2003;30:1691–5.
23. Jansen TL, Bruyn GA. Diagnostic value of anticyclic citrullinated peptide antibody in rheumatoid arthritis. J Rheumatol 2004;31:1012–3.
24. Schellekens GA, Visser H, de Jong BA, van den Hoogen FH, Hazes JM, Breedveld FC, et al. The diagnostic properties of rheumatoid arthritis antibodies recognizing a cyclic citrullinated peptide. Arthritis Rheum 2000;43:155–63.
25. van Gaalen FA, Linn-Rasker SP, van Venrooij WJ, de Jong BA, Breedveld FC, Verweij CL, et al. Autoantibodies to cyclic citrullinated peptides predict progression to rheumatoid arthritis in patients with undifferentiated arthritis: a prospective cohort study. Arthritis Rheum 2004;50:709–15.
26. Kerstens PJ, Boerbooms AM, Jeurissen ME, Fast JH, Assmann KJ, van de Putte LB. Accelerated nodulosis during low dose methotrexate therapy for rheumatoid arthritis: an analysis of ten cases. J Rheumatol 1992;19:867–71.
27. Del Rincon I, Williams K, Stern MP, Freeman GL, Escalante A. High incidence of cardiovascular events in a rheumatoid arthritis cohort not explained by traditional risk factors. Arthritis Rheum 2001;44:2737–45.
28. Boers M, Dijkmans B, Gabriel S, Maradit-Kremers H, O'Dell J, Pincus T. Making an impact on mortality in rheumatoid arthritis: targeting cardiovascular comorbidity. Arthritis Rheum 2004;50:1734–9.
29. Egsmose C, Lund B, Borg G, Pettersson H, Berg E, Brodin U, et al. Patients with rheumatoid arthritis benefit from early 2nd line therapy: 5 year followup of a prospective double blind placebo controlled study. J Rheumatol 1995;22:2208–13.
30. Masferrer JL, Zweifel BS, Seibert K, Needleman P. Selective regulation of cellular cyclooxygenase by dexamethasone and endotoxin in mice. J Clin Invest 1990;86:1375–9.
31. Borgini MJ, Paulus HE. Treatment of rheumatoid arthritis. In: Weisman MH, Weinblatt ME, Louie JS, editors. Practical Rheumatology, 2nd ed. Philadelphia: WB Saunders; 2002.AQ:5
32. Simon LS, Weaver AL, Graham DY, Kivitz AJ, Lipsky PE, Hubbard RC, et al. Anti-inflammatory and upper gastrointestinal effects of celecoxib in rheumatoid arthritis: a randomized controlled trial. JAMA 1999;282:1921–8.
33. Emery P, Zeidler H, Kvien TK, Guslandi M, Naudin R, Stead H, et al. Celecoxib versus diclofenac in long-term management of rheumatoid arthritis: randomised double-blind comparison. Lancet 1999;354:2106–11.
34. Bombardier C, Laine L, Reicin A, Shapiro D, Burgos-Vargas R, Davis B, et al. Comparison of upper gastrointestinal toxicity of rofecoxib and naproxen in patients with rheumatoid arthritis. N Engl J Med 2000;343:1520–8.
35. Kirwan JR. The effect of glucocorticoids on joint destruction in rheumatoid arthritis. N Engl J Med 1995;333:142–6.
36. Iannuzzi L, Dawson N, Zein N, Kushner I. Does drug therapy slow radiographic deterioration in rheumatoid arthritis? N Engl J Med 1983;309:1023–8.
37. Weinblatt ME, Polisson R, Blotner SD, Sosman JL, Aliabadi P, Baker N, et al. The effects of drug therapy on radiographic progression of rheumatoid arthritis: results of a 36-week randomized trial comparing methotrexate and auranofin. Arthritis Rheum 1993;36:613–9.
38. Smolen JS, Kalden JR, Scott DL, Rozman B, Kvien TK, Larsen A, et al. Efficacy and safety of leflunomide compared with placebo and sulphasalazine in active rheumatoid arthritis: a double-blind, randomised, multicentre trial. Lancet 1999;353:259–66.
39. Felson DT, Anderson JJ, Meenan RF. The comparative efficacy and toxicity of second-line drugs in rheumatoid arthritis: results of two metaanalyses. Arthritis Rheum 1990;33:1449–61.
40. Bernstein HN. Ophthalmologic considerations and testing in patients receiving long-term antimalarial therapy. Am J Med 1983;75:25–34.
41. Alarcon GS, Tracy IC, Blackburn WD Jr. Methotrexate in rheumatoid arthritis: toxic effects as the major factor in limiting long-term treatment. Arthritis Rheum 1989;32:671–6.
42. Kremer JM, Alarcon GS, Lightfoot RW Jr, et al. Methotrexate for rheumatoid arthritis: suggested guidelines for monitoring liver toxicity. Arthritis Rheum 1994;37:316.
43. Kremer JM, Alarcon GS, Lightfoot RW Jr, Willkens RF, Furst DE, Williams HJ, et al. Methotrexate for rheumatoid arthritis: suggested guidelines for monitoring liver toxicity. Arthritis Rheum 1994;37:316–28.

44. Sharp JT, Strand V, Leung H, Hurley F, Loew-Friedrich I. Treatment with leflunomide slows radiographic progression of rheumatoid arthritis: results from three randomized controlled trials of leflunomide in patients with active rheumatoid arthritis. Arthritis Rheum 2000;43:495–505.

45. Moreland LW, Baumgartner SW, Schiff MH, Tindall EA, Fleischmann RM, Weaver AL, et al. Treatment of rheumatoid arthritis with a recombinant human tumor necrosis factor receptor (p75)-Fc fusion protein. N Engl J Med 1997;337:141–7.

46. Moreland LW, Schiff MH, Baumgartner SW, Tindall EA, Fleischmann RM, Bulpitt KJ, et al. Etanercept therapy in rheumatoid arthritis: a randomized, controlled trial. Ann Intern Med 1999;130:478–86.

47. Weinblatt ME, Kremer JM, Bankhurst AD, Bulpitt KJ, Fleischmann RM, Fox RI, et al. A trial of etanercept, a recombinant tumor necrosis factor receptor:Fc fusion protein, in patients with rheumatoid arthritis receiving methotrexate. N Engl J Med 1999;340:253–9.

48. Bathon JM, Martin RW, Fleischmann RM, Tesser JR, Schiff MH, Keystone EC, et al. A comparison of etanercept and methotrexate in patients with early rheumatoid arthritis. N Engl J Med 2000;343:1586–93.

49. van der Heide A, Jacobs JW, Bijlsma JW, Heurkens AH, van Booma-Frankfort C, van der Veen MJ, et al. The effectiveness of early treatment with "second-line" antirheumatic drugs: a randomized, controlled trial. Ann Intern Med 1996;124:699–707.

50. Lipsky PE, van der Heijde DM, St Clair EW, Furst DE, Breedveld FC, Kalden JR, et al. Infliximab and methotrexate in the treatment of rheumatoid arthritis. N Engl J Med 2000;343:1594–602.

51. Maini R, St Clair EW, Breedveld F, Furst D, Kalden J, Weisman M, et al. Infliximab (chimeric anti-tumour necrosis factor alpha monoclonal antibody) versus placebo in rheumatoid arthritis patients receiving concomitant methotrexate: a randomised phase III trial. Lancet 1999;354: 1932–9.

52. Maini RN, Breedveld FC, Kalden JR, Smolen JS, Davis D, Macfarlane JD, et al. Therapeutic efficacy of multiple intravenous infusions of anti-tumor necrosis factor alpha monoclonal antibody combined with low-dose weekly methotrexate in rheumatoid arthritis. Arthritis Rheum 1998;41:1552–63.

53. Weinblatt ME, Keystone EC, Furst DE, Moreland LW, Weisman MH, Birbara CA, et al. Adalimumab, a fully human anti-tumor necrosis factor alpha monoclonal antibody, for the treatment of rheumatoid arthritis in patients taking concomitant methotrexate: the ARMADA trial. Arthritis Rheum 2003;48:35–45.

54. Bang LM, Keating GM. Adalimumab: a review of its use in rheumatoid arthritis. BioDrugs 2004;18:121–39.

55. Weinblatt ME, Keystone EC, Furst DE, Kavanaugh AF, Chartash EK, Segurado OG. Long-term efficacy and safety of adalimumab plus methotrexate in patients with rheumatoid arthritis: ARMADA 4-year extended study. Ann Rheum Dis 2006;65:753–9.

56. Goronzy JJ, Weyand CM. T-cell regulation in rheumatoid arthritis. Curr Opin Rheumatol 2004;16:212–7.

57. Teng GG, Turkiewicz AM, Moreland LW. Abatacept: a costimulatory inhibitor for treatment of rheumatoid arthritis. Expert Opin Biol Ther 2005;5:1245–54.

58. Kremer JM, Dougados M, Emery P, Durez P, Sibilia J, Shergy W, et al. Treatment of rheumatoid arthritis with the selective costimulation modulator abatacept: twelve-month results of a phase iib, double-blind, randomized, placebo-controlled trial. Arthritis Rheum 2005;52:2263–71.

59. Genovese MC, Becker JC, Schiff M, Luggen M, Sherrer Y, Kremer J, et al. Abatacept for rheumatoid arthritis refractory to tumor necrosis factor alpha inhibition. N Engl J Med 2005;353:1114–23.

60. Sibilia J, Schiff M, Genovese MC, Becher JP, Li T, McCann T, et al. Sustained improvements in disease activity score 28(DAS28) and patient-reported outcomes (PRO) with abatacept in rheumatoid arthritis: the long-term extension of the ATTAIN trial. Poster presentation at 2006 European League Against Rheumatism Annual Congress. Amsterdam, Netherlands, June 21–26, 2006.

61. Edwards JC, Szczepanski L, Szechinski J, Filipowicz-Sosnowska A, Emery P, Close DR, et al. Efficacy of B-cell-targeted therapy with rituximab in patients with rheumatoid arthritis. N Engl J Med 2004;350:2572–81.

62. Higashida J, Wun T, Schmidt S, Naguwa SM, Tuscano JM. Safety and efficacy of rituximab in patients with rheumatoid arthritis refractory to disease modifying antirheumatic drugs and anti-tumor necrosis factor-alpha treatment. J Rheumatol 2005;32:2109–15.

63. Emery P, Filipowicz-Sosnowska A, Szechinski J, Racewicz A, Schechtmann J, Fleischmann RM. Primary analysis of a double-blind, placebo-controlled, dose-ranging trial of rituximab, an anti-CD20 monocloncal antibody, in patients with rheumatoid arthritis receiving methotrexate (DANCER trial). Ann Rheum Dis 2005;64(Suppl III):434.

64. Cohen S, Greenwald M, Dougados M, Emery P, Furie R, Shaw TM, et al. Efficacy and safety of rituximab in active RA patients who experienced an inadequate response to one or more anti-TNF-alpha therapies (REFLEX study). Arthritis Rheum 2005;52(9 Suppl):1830.

65. Cohen S, Hurd E, Cush J, Schiff M, Weinblatt ME, Moreland LW, et al. Treatment of rheumatoid arthritis with anakinra, a recombinant human interleukin-1 receptor antagonist, in combination with methotrexate: results of a twenty-four-week, multicenter, randomized, double-blind, placebo-controlled trial. Arthritis Rheum 2002;46:614–24.

66. Fleischmann RM, Schechtman J, Bennett R, Handel ML, Burmester GR, Tesser J, et al. Anakinra, a recombinant human interleukin-1 receptor antagonist (r-metHuIL-1ra), in patients with rheumatoid arthritis: a large, international, multicenter, placebo-controlled trial. Arthritis Rheum 2003; 48:927–34.

67. Pincus T, O'Dell JR, Kremer JM. Combination therapy with multiple disease-modifying antirheumatic drugs in rheumatoid arthritis: a preventive strategy. Ann Intern Med 1999;131:768–74.

68. O'Dell JR, Haire CE, Erikson N, Drymalski W, Palmer W, Eckhoff PJ, et al. Treatment of rheumatoid arthritis with methotrexate alone, sulfasalazine and hydroxychloroquine, or a combination of all three medications. N Engl J Med 1996;334:1287–91.

69. O'Dell J, Leff R, Paulsen G, Haire C, Mallek J, Eckhoff PJ, et al. Methotrexate(M)-Hydroxychloroquine(H)-Sulfasalazine(S) versus M-H or M-S for rheumatoid arthritis: results of a double-blind study. Arthritis Rheum 1999;42(9 Suppl):S117.

70. Mroczkowski PJ, Weinblatt ME, Kremer JM. Methotrexate and leflunomide combination therapy for patients with active rheumatoid arthritis. Clin Exp Rheumatol 1999;17(6 Suppl 18):S66–8.

71. Weinblatt ME, Kremer JM, Coblyn JS, Maier AL, Helfgott SM, Morrell M, et al. Pharmacokinetics, safety, and efficacy of combination treatment with methotrexate and leflunomide in patients with active rheumatoid arthritis. Arthritis Rheum 1999;42:1322–8.

72. Kremer JM, Genovese MC, Cannon GW, Caldwell JR, Cush JJ, Furst DE, et al. Concomitant leflunomide therapy in patients with active rheumatoid arthritis despite stable doses of methotrexate: a randomized, double-blind, placebo-controlled trial. Ann Intern Med 2002;137:726–33.

73. Kremer J, Genovese M, Cannon GW, Caldwell J, Cush J, Furst DE, et al. Combination leflunomide and methotrexate (MTX) therapy for patients with active rheumatoid arthritis failing MTX monotherapy: open-label extension of a randomized, double-blind, placebo controlled trial. J Rheumatol 2004;31:1521–31.

74. Klareskog L, van der Heijde D, de Jager JP, Gough A, Kalden J, Malaise M, et al. Therapeutic effect of the combination of etanercept and methotrexate compared with each treatment alone in patients with rheumatoid arthritis: double-blind randomised controlled trial. Lancet 2004;363:675–81.

75. St Clair EW, van der Heijde DM, Smolen JS, Maini RN, Bathon JM, Emery P, et al. Combination of infliximab and methotrexate therapy for early rheumatoid arthritis: a randomized, controlled trial. Arthritis Rheum 2004;50:3432–43.

76. Breedveld FC, Weisman MH, Kavanaugh AF, Cohen SB, Pavelka K, van Vollenhoven R, et al. The PREMIER study: a multicenter, randomized, double-blind clinical trial of combination therapy with adalimumab plus methotrexate versus methotrexate alone or adalimumab alone in patients with early, aggressive rheumatoid arthritis who had not had previous methotrexate treatment. Arthritis Rheum 2006;54:26–37.

77. Guidelines for the management of rheumatoid arthritis: 2002 Update. Arthritis Rheum 2002;46:328–46.

Shoulder Disorders

HAMMAD A. BAJWA, MD, ANGELA M. DAHLE, MD, and MAREN MAHOWALD, MD

The prevalence of shoulder pain ranges from 20% to 50% (1–4). Shoulder pain causes significant morbidity and disability, and has a substantial impact on health care consumption and ability to work. This highlights the importance of appropriate evaluation and treatment. Shoulder pain is the third most common cause of musculoskeletal consultation in primary care. Shoulder pain is categorized as one of the following: shoulder region joint problem (glenohumeral joint, acromioclavicular joint, and sternoclavicular joint), periarticular problems, or referred pain. Shoulder pain history and physical examination are the cornerstones for the diagnosis of shoulder disorders. Identification of the specific shoulder disorder requires a thorough knowledge of the anatomy and complex muscle actions that produce motion and stability. Physical examination based on the knowledge of structural and functional anatomy of the shoulder permits accurate diagnosis in many patients. Analysis of shoulder motion and maneuvers that reproduce the patient's pain permit selection of mechanism-based treatment and therapeutic rehabilitation. The goals of therapy are to decrease pain, improve function, and prevent recurrences and disability.

More than 90% of shoulder pain involves rotator cuff tendinitis, tears, or contracture. Site-specific prevalence rates for shoulder tendinitis is 4.5% in men and 6.1% in women, and for adhesive capsulitis it is 8.2% in men and 10.1% in women (2). Limitation of motion due to pain from rotator cuff problems predisposes to adhesive capsulitis (frozen shoulder) as a secondary complication, which further increases pain and loss of motion. Prompt initiation of physical therapy or home exercises to put the arm through its full range of motion (ROM) passively or actively will decrease the likelihood of developing this contracture.

ETIOLOGY OF SHOULDER PAIN

Causes of shoulder disorders are generally distributed by age, work and recreational activities, and trauma. Young people and vigorous athletes are more likely to experience abrupt severe stress forces causing acute supraspinatus tendinitis, bicipital tendinitis, rotator cuff tear, dislocation, or fracture. Middle-aged adults who engage in intermittent repetitive vigorous activities (weekend jocks and do-it-yourselfers) are susceptible to acute inflammatory supraspinatus and bicipital tendinitis. In elderly patients, normal activity superimposed on chronic degenerative or inflammatory arthritis is associated with tendinitis or a contracted rotator cuff (frozen shoulder). The elderly may develop shoulder pain from polymyalgia rheumatica or another comorbid condition.

SHOULDER REGION ANATOMY

There are 3 synovial joints (sternoclavicular, acromioclavicular, glenohumeral) and a bone-muscle-bone scapulothoracic articulation in the shoulder. The glenohumeral joint is a diarthrodial joint that is only minimally constrained by the bony components (Figure 1). The joint is supported by the rotator cuff and joint capsule (5). The rotator cuff (RC) is made up of the tendons of 4 muscles: the subscapularis, supraspinatus, infraspinatus, and the teres minor. Forces generated by contraction of the RC muscles depress the humeral head and stabilize it in the shallow glenoid, thus permitting abduction of the humerus by the deltoid. The scapula is stabilized by 6 muscles: trapezius, major and minor rhomboids, levator scapulae, serratus anterior, and pectoralis minor (Figure 2).

The weight of the arm and load being carried, plus the forces generated by the muscles that move the arm, must not dislocate the glenohumeral articulation. The glenohumeral joint has both static stabilizers (anterior, middle, and inferior glenohumeral ligaments; posterior capsule; and labrum) and dynamic stabilizers (the muscles for each planar movement and the cocontracting stabilizer muscles acting to resist dislocation). The forces acting on the glenohumeral joint are the weight of the arm (~5–9% of body weight) plus the forces from the deltoid muscle contraction moving the humerus up and out, which may be as much as 8 times the weight of the arm. These forces must be counteracted by the cocontracting RC muscles. The uniplanar motions at the glenohumeral joint are given in Table 1.

EVALUATION OF SHOULDER REGION PAIN

Disorders of the shoulder joint complex cause pain; stiffness; upper arm weakness or instability; sleep disruption; and impaired activities of daily living, work, and recreation. Patients often have difficulty accurately localizing the site causing the pain. Pain originating from a site in the shoulder may be referred to the lateral mid-humerus or up into the neck. The muscles near the lesion often contract to minimize painful movement and become another source of more diffuse pain in the taut muscles.

The differential diagnosis of shoulder pain includes:

- shoulder region joint problems (glenohumeral, acromioclavicular, and sternoclavicular joints and glenoid labrum tears);
- periarticular problems (RC tendinitis, RC tear, bicipital tendinitis, RC contracture); and
- referred pain to the shoulder region from sites extrinsic to the shoulder joint complex (cervical spine, brachial plexus, peripheral nerve, tumor in the apex of the lung, lesions in or near the diaphragm [pleura, gall bladder, liver], and rarely, angina).

It should be remembered that more than one pathology often exists in the painful shoulder (6).

History

The key to the diagnosis of shoulder disorders is obtaining precise data with a focused interview. Probe for information about the exact onset

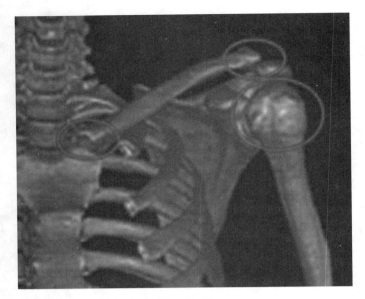

Figure 1. Skeletal anatomy of the shoulder.

increased pain with certain neck movements or postures. Patients with referred pain from lung or diaphragmatic lesions tend to have persistent gnawing or aching pain not affected by shoulder movements or position.

Physical Examination

The shoulder examination should systematically compare the affected with the unaffected side. Elements of the examination include observation, ROM and muscle-strength testing, palpation, and special/provocative testing.

Observation. Look for bony prominences and swelling over the acromioclavicular and sternoclavicular joints and the normal sulcus between the humerus and thorax anteriorly (glenohumeral joint). Note any muscle atrophy, ecchymoses, abrasions, or other signs of trauma around the shoulder.

Range-of-Motion Testing. First observe the arc (degrees) and ease of active ROM during forward flexion (raise hands up above the head), external rotation (place hands behind occiput), internal rotation (place hands behind the back), and abduction (raise arms out from the sides bringing hands together above the head). Passive ROM testing is carried out with the examiner fixing the scapula to the thorax with one hand while using the other hand to put the arm through all the motions. Greater pain with active motion compared with passive motion suggests rotator cuff problems, whereas pain with both passive and active motion suggests glenohumeral joint arthritis.

Muscle-Strength Testing. Muscle strength should be tested in the deltoid, supraspinatus, subscapularis, internal rotators, external rotators, and biceps muscles. Finding weakness may be unreliable when pain is present. Pain with weakness that is described as burning or tingling suggests an underlying neuropathic process, such as cervical radiculopathy, plexopathy, or neuropathy. Pain may be further localized by testing deep-tendon reflexes and cutaneous sensation.

Palpation of Anatomic Landmarks. Note areas of warmth. Carefully palpate for tenderness over the sternoclavicular joint, acromioclavicular joint, and glenohumeral joint beneath the coracoid process; at the insertions of the supraspinatus tendon, infraspinatus tendon, and teres minor tendon; over the anterior aspect of the rotator cuff (subscapularis tendon insertion) and the biceps tendon in the bicipital groove (Figure 3). Identify areas of focal swelling with or without

of pain and its severity, character, location, periodicity, and impact. It is important to identify activities or trauma associated with the onset of shoulder pain. Inquire about prior episodes of shoulder pain, specifically asking about cause, workup, treatment, and time course. Determine pain severity using a 0–10 scale and ask whether the pain is constant or incident to movement. If possible, have the patient point to the most painful site.

Identify impact factors by asking which positions and movements increase or relieve the pain. Determine functional impairments by asking about activities of daily living (e.g., combing hair, dressing, overhead lifting), work capabilities (e.g., how much can be lifted and carried, can the patient work full time, is job security in jeopardy?), and leisure activities that can no longer be enjoyed. Ask whether the pain is worse at night when rolling onto the affected side (a positive response indicates RC problems).

Painless and full active ROM strongly suggests referred pain. The patient with referred pain from the cervical spine may associate

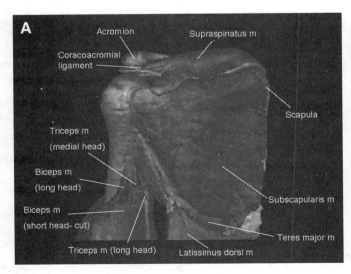

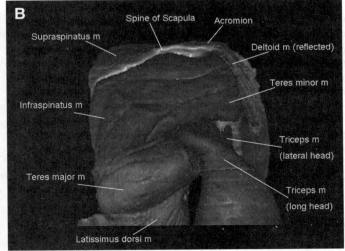

Figure 2. Shoulder anatomy. **A**, Anterior view. **B**, Posterior view.

Table 1. Uniplanar motions at the glenohumeral joint

Motion	Description	Primary muscles involved (secondary contributors)
Flexion	Shoulder elevation or forward movement of the arm in the sagittal plane	Anterior deltoid, pectoralis major and minor (medial deltoid, supraspinatus, infraspinatus, subscapularis, clavicular pectoralis)
Extension	Backward movement of the arm in the sagittal plane	Posterior deltoid, latissimus dorsi, teres major, trapezius, rhomboid, long head of triceps
Abduction	Shoulder elevation in the frontal plane = abduction of the arm away from the side of the body	Medial deltoid, supraspinatus (posterior deltoid, infraspinatus ± teres minor)
Adduction	Holding the arm to the side of the torso and moving it across the chest	Anterior and posterior deltoid, clavicular pectoralis, teres major, subscapularis, latissimus dorsi, long head of triceps
Internal rotation	Move hand behind back or across the chest	Subscapularis, anterior deltoid, pectoralis major, latissimus dorsi, teres major
External rotation	Move hand behind head and away from body with elbow near the torso	Posterior deltoid, infraspinatus, teres minor
Shoulder elevation	Shrug the shoulder	Trapezius, levator scapulae

tenderness. Palpation should be done with the fingertip pad (rather than the fingertip) applying firm direct pressure. A grinding rotation of the palpating finger may produce a misleading pain response in the absence of tissue pathology.

Special/Provocative Testing. Special tests and maneuvers to reproduce the patient's shoulder pain can be very helpful in identifying the source of pathology (Table 2). These provocative tests are designed to isolate an individual muscle action or integrated force as much as possible and deliver a counterforce or strain to reproduce the pain symptom. It is important to remember that special shoulder tests may be sensitive but are often not very specific for a single diagnosis. The maneuver to detect "impingement" is performed by forward flexing the extended arm with forearm pronation while fixing the scapula to the thorax with the other hand. This test is fairly sensitive for RC impingement between the head of the humerus and the acromion, but it is not very specific because a positive pain sign may occur with adhesive capsulitis, glenohumeral arthritis or instability, or acromioclavicular arthritis.

Shoulder pain with minimal loss of motion, no palpable tenderness, or no increase in pain with provocative tests suggests another likely cause: referred pain to the shoulder, a bone lesion, or a neuropathic process (especially if muscle atrophy is present).

Imaging Studies

Imaging studies are usually required to confirm the clinical diagnosis and to rule out other pathologic conditions. In some cases, diagnostic studies are useful to determine the size and severity of the lesion, which may direct the choice of treatment and prognosis.

Plain radiographs should be performed routinely as part of the shoulder evaluation, including the anteroposterior view (Figure 4) with internal and external rotation, lateral scapular Y view, and axillary view. These will reveal dislocation, fracture, arthritic changes, chondrocalcinosis, tendon calcifications, bone cysts, sclerosis, tumors, or avascular necrosis. The Y view will show variations in acromion morphology. A decrease in the acromiohumeral space due to upward migration of the humeral head suggests an RC tear (Figure 4). The axillary view will demonstrate dislocation of the humeral head and calcifications in the tendon of the subscapularis. Computed tomography scans provide good detail of lesions in the glenohumeral, acromioclavicular, and sternoclavicular joints. Magnetic resonance imaging (MRI) allows visualization of soft tissue lesions, bone tumors, and ischemic necrosis of bone. On MRI, muscle and tendon tears demonstrate increased signal in both T1- and T2-weighted images. MRI is sensitive for RC problems, but may not differentiate between tendinitis, partial tears, and small complete tears (7). Ultrasonography provides a noninvasive method of identifying RC lesions that has high sensitivity and

specificity when carried out by an experienced technician. Scintigraphy (bone scan) is a very sensitive, but nonspecific, method to demonstrate increased uptake due to inflammation, arthritis, infection, or bone lesions. Arthroscopy offers the opportunity for diagnosis and treatment (debridement, removal of loose bodies, cuff repair, labrum repair, excisional decompression, tenodesis and tendon transfers, subacromial decompression, and repair of some chondral lesions).

PERIARTICULAR SHOULDER DISORDERS

Rotator Cuff Tendinitis

Rotator cuff tendinitis is the most common cause of shoulder pain. Tendinitis rather than bursitis is the underlying pathologic process, which may be acute or chronic. RC tendinitis is caused by trauma, repetitive overhead activities, variations in acromion morphology, osteophytes on the undersurface of the acromion, or inflammatory processes, such as rheumatoid arthritis or microcrystalline (apatite) deposits. Symptomatic calcific tendinitis occurs when a preexisting calcific deposit begins to resorb and produces intense inflammation (see also Chapter 23, Periarticular Rheumatic Diseases).

About 25 years ago, Neer coined the term "impingement" and reported on 100 anatomic dissections of the shoulder. He described various pathologic changes associated with the impingement of the RC between the acromion, coracoid, coracoacromial ligament, acromioclavicular joint,

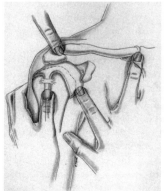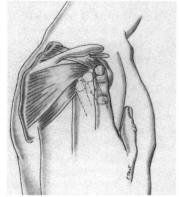

Figure 3. Landmarks for palpation of the shoulder. **A,** Anterior view of palpation landmarks for biceps tendon, acromioclavicular joint, glenohumeral joint, and sternoclavicular joint. **B,** Lateral view of palpation landmarks for supraspinatus tendon, infraspinatus tendon, and teres minor tendon insertions.

Table 2. Causes of shoulder pain: identification by physical examination*

Pathology	Palpation landmark to identify swelling and tenderness	Provocative maneuver to reproduce pain
Glenohumeral arthritis	1 cm inferior to coracoid process	Both active and passive ROM testing produce pain deep in the shoulder
Acromioclavicular arthritis	Groove lateral to distal clavicle	Adduction of arm across torso and shoulder shrug produces pain at superior aspect of the shoulder
Sternoclavicular arthritis	Groove between medial clavicle and manubrium	Shoulder shrug and rotation of torso produces pain
Periarticular structures	Rotator muscles should be tested individually	Resisted muscle contraction reproduces pain
Supraspinatus tendinitis	1 cm inferior to midlateral edge acromion	Resisted abduction of the arm positioned at 30° of abduction
Infraspinatus tendinitis (IST)	1 cm inferior to posterolateral edge of the acromion	Resisted external rotation of the arm with elbow flexed to 90°
Teres minor tendinitis	1–2 cm inferior to insertion of IST	Same as IST
Subscapularis tendinitis	Lateral to the coracoid on medial aspect of the lesser tuberosity	Resisted internal rotation with the arm at the side and the elbow flexed to 90°
Rotator cuff tendinitis	Just inferior to the anterior and lateral margins of the acromion	Pain with resisted flexion, abduction, and rotation of the arm
Rotator cuff tears	Usually cannot palpate tenderness	Pain and weakness with resisted ROM testing
Rotator cuff contracture (frozen shoulder)	Usually cannot palpate tenderness	Limited and painful ROM testing, external rotation lost first
Biceps tendinitis	Between greater and lesser tuberosity in the bicipital groove (just lateral to the coracoid)	Pain with resisted elbow flexion with hand pronated

* ROM = range of motion

and the humeral head (8). He created a staging system for impingement lesions and their characteristic features, as follows:

- *Stage I* (mild tendinitis) with edema and hemorrhage in the rotator cuff is usually seen in those under age 25 who engage in overhead activities.
- *Stage II* (chronic tendinitis) occurs in the third and fourth decade as fibrosis, thickening, and tearing of the cuff following repeated impingement and recurrent attacks of rotator cuff tendinitis.
- *Stage III* (cuff tears) develops after age 40 and includes full-thickness rotator cuff tears, biceps tendon rupture, and/or degenerative bone changes.

Acute RC impingement produces excruciating sharp pain that is exacerbated by overhead activities. Chronic lesions produce a persistent ache over the lateral upper arm that increases with active abduction. Dressing is painful, and sleep is often disrupted by pain. Pain is greater with active and resisted abduction than with passive abduction. Tenderness to palpation is localized to the greater tubercle of the humerus (the insertion of the supraspinatus tendon). Edema and swelling of the supraspinatus tendon (inflamed rotator cuff) results in impingement of the rotator cuff between the greater tuberosity and the acromion during abduction of the arm.

Neer devised a test to demonstrate the pathophysiology of rotator cuff impingement. The impingement test may also be positive with other periarticular disorders. In Neer's test, the examiner fixes the scapula to the thorax with one hand and forcefully moves the arm into forward flexion with the other hand, reproducing the patient's shoulder pain. Impingement may be confirmed if the pain is eliminated during repeat testing after an injection of lidocaine into the subacromial bursa. Hawkins sign, another impingement test, is elicited by internally rotating the arm positioned at 90° of forward flexion. External and internal rotation strength and pain response should be tested with the flexed elbow supported by the examiner and rotational force applied to the wrist. Weakness or pain during resisted external rotation from the neutral position (0° adduction) suggests inflammation or tear of the infraspinatus/teres minor tendon. Weakness or pain with resisted abduction while the arm is at 30° of forward flexion, or with resisted abduction

while the arm is at 90° of forward flexion and pronation so the thumb is pointing at the floor (empty can position), suggests a lesion in the supraspinatus tendon.

In Stage I, plain x-rays may demonstrate abnormal acromion morphology. With recurrences and progression of rotator cuff tendinitis, sclerosis and cyst formation occur in the humeral head. Spur formation develops on the undersurface of the lateral side of the acromioclavicular joint. When tears occur, the acromiohumeral distance decreases due to superior subluxation of the humeral head. Calcification in the tendon may be seen on plain x-ray (Figure 4).

With Stage I lesions, rest (but not immobilization), nonsteroidal antiinflammatory drugs (NSAIDs), and stretching are followed by progressive internal and external rotation strengthening exercises. Restoration of rotator cuff muscle strength will limit superior migration of the humeral head, reduce pain, and restore shoulder function (9,10). Corticosteroid injections often provide dramatic improvement and permit earlier physical therapy (Figures 5 and 6) (11).

With Stage II lesions, initial corticosteroid with bupivacaine injection plus NSAIDs or analgesics is preferred to permit more extensive passive, active-assisted, and active stretching and strengthening exercises to reduce contracture. Cessation of overhead activities and job modifications are necessary during the treatment period and may have to be continued to prevent recurrence.

Patients with refractory Stage II or III impingement (failure with 6 months of physical therapy) will usually need surgery. The surgical approach, called anterior acromioplasty, is designed to decompress the subacromial space (subacromial bursectomy, coracoacromial ligament section, and resection of bone at the undersurface of the acromion), repair any full-thickness cuff tears if possible, and resect the distal clavicle if it is contributing to the impingement. Surgical sectioning of the coracoacromial ligament with subacromial bursectomy or open anterior acromioplasty may be needed to prevent recurrences and disability.

Prevention of recurrences and development of disability depends on patient education. Identifying the overuse pattern or cause of repeated trauma permits development of modifications to reduce or eliminate such activities. In a deconditioned or debilitated individual, normal activities of daily living may injure the rotator cuff. Muscle strengthening and general conditioning exercises are key to preventing recurrences in these individuals.

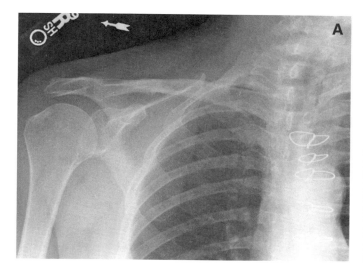
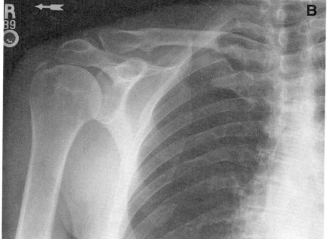
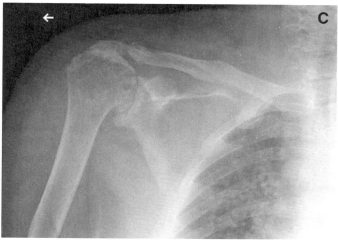

Figure 4. Shoulder radiographs. **A**, Normal anteroposterior view. **B**, Calcified supraspinatus tendon. **C**, High-riding humeral head.

Adhesive Capsulitis

Adhesive capsulitis (frozen shoulder syndrome, pericapsulitis, peri-arthritis) describes the painful or painless loss of active and passive shoulder motion in all planes. The cause may be idiopathic, as seen in patients with diabetes and thyroid disorders. It also occurs secondarily to other intrinsic shoulder lesions or extrinsic lesions that cause referred pain to the shoulder, such as cervical radiculopathy, apical lung lesions, and metastatic lesions to the shoulder region. A mild inflammatory process results in cytokine and growth factor production leading to capsular fibrosis (12). Four stages of adhesive capsulitis have been described (13).

- *Stage 1* is an early hypervascular inflammatory (lymphocytic) phase that lasts ~3 months. Shoulder pain is described as a deep aching that is present at rest and may radiate to the upper arm, back, and neck. Pain is exacerbated by any attempts at movement. Night pain is common and prevents sleeping on the affected side. On examination, there is a loss of internal and external rotation of the arm that is improved by injection of lidocaine into the glenohumeral joint (Figures 6 and 7). Flexion and extension are fairly well preserved.
- During *stage 2*, progressive loss of motion with persistent pain occurs over 3–9 months. Injection of lidocaine or a scalene block

eliminates the pain but does not improve ROM, reflecting a loss of capsule volume and flexibility. Biopsy reveals a dense proliferative synovitis and hypervascularity, as well as capsular fibroplasias without inflammation. On examination, the practitioner fixes the scapula to the thorax with one hand and is unable to abduct or internally and externally rotate the arm with the other hand.
- In *stage 3*, after 9–14 months of symptoms, patients report mild pain or pain-free stiff shoulder. No increase in ROM occurs with local anesthetic or general anesthesia. Arthroscopy reveals synovial thickening but no hypervascularity.
- *Stage 4* is called the "thawing stage" during which ROM is slowly recovered as increased motion begets increased stretching and capsule remodeling.

The primary treatment of adhesive capsulitis is physical therapy (active and passive ROM stretching) with NSAIDs and periodic corticosteroids injected into the glenohumeral joint. Treatment of stages 1 and 2 should include corticosteroid and local anesthetic injection, gentle stretching, and NSAIDs. In stages 3 and 4, analgesics and physical therapy are recommended. Patient education about the natural course and anticipated spontaneous resolution is critical to prevent discouragement and increase adherence to the exercise therapy program. Only rarely are arthroscopy or manipulation under anesthesia needed to ease the contracture (14).

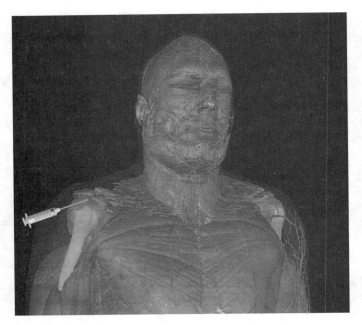

Figure 5. Subacromial injection.

Rotator Cuff Tears

Rotator cuff tears occur with trauma; they may be spontaneous in later stages of RC tendinitis or they may occur with chronic inflammation due to rheumatoid arthritis, spondyloarthropathies, or systemic lupus erythematosus. Fibers of the rotator cuff are intertwined with the glenohumeral joint capsule so that complete tears of the RC result in communication between the joint and the subacromial bursa. Rotator cuff tears are classified by size and by the involved RC tendon.

Traumatic tears are usually the result of a fall directly on the shoulder or an outstretched arm, or of lifting a heavy object. The patient often feels a snap, followed by severe pain and inability to abduct the arm. If there is a history of direct trauma, radiographs should be obtained to rule out dislocation or fracture. Many patients do not recall a specific traumatic event, suggesting gradual progressive degeneration of the rotator cuff to a complete tear or cuff attrition such that a trivial stress on the RC extends a smaller, incomplete tear. Partial tears occur in overhead athletes due to repetitive tensile overload.

Patients have pain and difficulty with upper extremity activities requiring abduction or internal and external rotation (dressing, combing

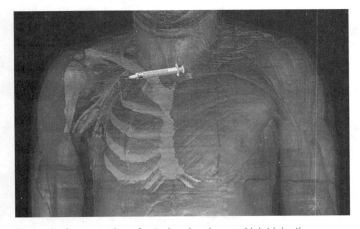

Figure 6. Cross section of anterior glenohumeral joint injection.

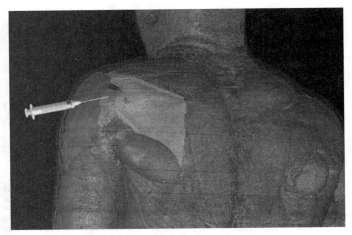

Figure 7. Posterior glenohumeral joint injection.

hair, reaching into a back pocket). On exam, the patient is unable to maintain the arm in abduction after it is passively raised (the drop arm test). Weakness of external rotation with the arm near the side of the body suggests a full-thickness tear. Symptoms of RC tear and tendinitis may be differentiated by repeating the drop arm test after injecting a local anesthetic. With tendinitis, the patient is able to maintain abduction after the pain is eliminated; however, abduction cannot be maintained by those with a complete tear.

Treatment of acute cuff tears should be conservative initially, including NSAIDs, ultrasound, or local heat before stretching exercises, and ice after overhead activity. If pain precludes physical therapy, local injection of a corticosteroid with local anesthetic can be given. When pain and motion improve, a progressive strengthening program for RC, deltoid, and scapular stabilizer muscles should be started. A gradual return to overhead activities at work and recreation is implemented when symptoms are minimal and shoulder function is restored. If pain and shoulder impairment persists after 3–6 months of conservative treatment, arthroscopic or open surgical repair is considered. Subacromial decompression and removal of acromion osteophytes usually relieve pain and improve function, even if the tear is found to be irreparable at the time of surgery (15). Earlier surgery may be indicated for full-thickness tears in a younger person with loss of function.

Bicipital Tendinitis and Rupture

The bicipital tendon has a long head and a short head. The long head of the biceps is in a groove between the lesser and greater tubercle of the humerus and passes through the glenohumeral joint to insert on the superior rim of the glenoid. The biceps is a forward flexor of the arm, a forearm flexor, and a supinator when the elbow is flexed. Bicipital tendinitis is caused by acute or chronic impingement of the tendon between the bicipital groove and the acromion, causing tenosynovitis of the long head of the biceps. Rupture of the long head of the biceps is rare in the absence of concomitant RC problems and impingement. Spontaneous rupture may occur, with sudden anterior shoulder pain and ecchymosis with a sagging prominence of the biceps belly.

Bicipital tendinitis causes anterior shoulder pain with focal tenderness to palpation in the bicipital groove. Excessive pressure of the palpating finger can readily produce a misleading pain response in the absence of tendon inflammation. Pain is provoked by resisted supination of the forearm with the elbow flexed (Yergason's supination test) and resisted forward flexion of the arm with the elbow extended (Speed's test).

Rehabilitation Considerations in Shoulder Disorders

- It is important to rule out other sources of pain (e.g., referred pain from cervical region) during the clinical examination.
- More than one pathology may exist in the painful shoulder. Careful examination and history is essential for developing an appropriate rehabilitation intervention.
- Magnetic resonance imaging is sensitive for rotator cuff problems, but may not differentiate between tendinitis, partial tears, and small complete tears.
- Early, conservative management of the tendinitis can prevent further damage, such as a rotator cuff tear.
- Stretching and strengthening exercises are key to preventing shoulder problems. Exercise even in small doses if performed frequently can be beneficial.
- Prompt initiation of motion and maintenance of shoulder range of motion can reduce the likelihood of developing adhesive capsulitis.
- Cessation of overhead activities and job modifications are necessary during the treatment period in Stage II rotator cuff tendinitis.
- Rehabilitation is an important component of postoperative management of shoulder disorders and should be conducted in collaboration with the surgeon and physical therapist.

Treatment of biceps tendinitis includes rest, NSAIDs, local corticosteroid injection, and ultrasound therapy. Tendon rupture repair is controversial, and options include tenodesis of the distal end of the tendon into the bicipital groove or tendon transfer to the coracoid process to maintain biceps power.

SHOULDER REGION JOINT DISORDERS

Acromioclavicular Disorders

Acromioclavicular arthritis produces pain at the superior aspect of the shoulder that may radiate to the neck or jaw. The pain is produced or increased by activities involving adduction of the arm, such as sleeping on the affected side, golfing, buckling a seatbelt, or doing bench presses and pushups. Acute acromioclavicular joint pain may be caused by infection, crystal-induced inflammation, or direct trauma that injures the distal clavicle or ligaments. Chronic disorders are due to repetitive trauma (e.g., heavy construction work, weightlifting, gymnastics, or swimming), chronic inflammatory disease, or idiopathic osteolysis of the distal clavicle.

On examination, there may be a visible step-off between the distal clavicle and medial acromion, indicating separation. Examination reveals tenderness to palpation of the acromioclavicular joint, and crepitus may be felt during a shoulder shrug. The pain is reproduced during forced adduction of the arm over the chest. Imaging studies should include specific acromioclavicular views because routine shoulder x-rays do not demonstrate the joint well. Radiographic changes include osteophytes, subchondral cystic changes and sclerosis, and osteopenia of the distal clavicle. Later, resorption of the distal clavicle produces widening of the joint space.

Treatment includes pain control with local heat, NSAIDs, corticosteroid injections, and shoulder rehabilitation to increase motion and strength of shoulder muscles. In refractory cases, resection of the distal clavicle via arthrotomy or arthroscopy may be required to control pain and preserve function.

Sternoclavicular Arthritis

Sternoclavicular arthritis produces pain with shoulder activities that involve movement of the clavicle or thorax. Causes of acute sternoclavicular arthritis include infection (especially in intravenous drug abusers), seronegative spondyloarthropathy, and less commonly, rheumatoid arthritis. There is focal tenderness and swelling at the sternoclavicular joint, and pain may be reproduced by a shoulder shrug or rotation of the upper thorax.

Treatment includes antibiotics and needle or surgical drainage for septic arthritis. Intraarticular corticosteroid injections are beneficial for those with underlying chronic inflammatory arthritis.

Glenohumeral Joint Disorders

Glenohumeral disorders produce variable pain with active and passive motion, often accompanied by locking and clicking. The pain is generalized over the shoulder region and may radiate into the neck, back, and upper arm. Tenderness to palpation is sought by producing direct pressure 1 cm below the coracoid process; care should be taken not to employ a rotatory motion, which will produce pain and involuntary contraction of the pectoral muscle overlying the glenohumeral joint capsule. Joint pathology and pain decrease glenohumeral ROM, which is compensated by increased scapulothoracic motion that temporarily minimizes functional losses. Periarticular contractures develop and are associated with muscle atrophy and weakness, which lead to substantial functional deficits.

Inflammatory Arthritis of the Shoulder

Rheumatoid arthritis and the spondyloarthropathies commonly cause mild to severe chronic synovitis in the glenohumeral, acromioclavicular, and sternoclavicular joints. Acute inflammation of the glenohumeral joint is seen with infection, pseudogout, gout (rare), hydroxyapatite deposition in dialysis patients, or recurrent hemarthrosis due to hemophilia or chronic anticoagulation. Synovitis in the glenohumeral joint causes rotator cuff tendinitis and may result in tears, with a cystic swelling over the anterior shoulder.

On examination, the acromioclavicular and sternoclavicular joints often have focal tenderness, swelling, and warmth. Effusion in the glenohumeral joint may be discerned by bimanual palpation of the anterior and posterior aspects of the shoulder. Radiographs reveal erosions at the greater tuberosity, humeral head osteoporosis, and uniform narrowing of the glenohumeral joint space. At the acromioclavicular joint, erosions and widening of the joint with osteoporosis of the distal clavicle are seen.

The goal of treatment is to control the underlying inflammatory process and reduce pain with NSAIDs, analgesics, and corticosteroid injections. Patients with inflammatory arthritides must develop a habit of daily stretching and strengthening exercises to prevent functional loss and increased pain (see Chapter 32, Exercise and Physical Activity). Patients with refractory disease will usually require total shoulder arthroplasty, which should be done before rotator cuff tendon attenuation or contractures are extensive.

Degenerative Disorders of the Shoulder

Degenerative changes of the shoulder increase with age and may be related to recurrent trauma associated with boxing; heavy construction; pneumatic hammer use; neuropathic conditions, such as syringomyelia, calcium pyrophosphate dihydrate crystal deposition disease, and diabetes (Charcot joints); or other conditions, such as hemochromatosis, hemophilia, and chronic dislocation of the shoulder.

The patient usually describes an insidious onset of mild-to-moderate shoulder pain. On examination, pain and crepitus occur with both active and passive ROM testing. There is greater loss of external rotation compared with internal rotation. Osteophytes are seen at the anterior and inferior joint margins, with sclerosis and subarticular cysts in the humeral head.

Symptomatic treatment is often successful with analgesics and NSAIDs, with or without corticosteroid injections. Because there is no reversible component underlying the symptoms, improvement in ROM is limited. Vigorous stretching should be avoided, as it is likely to increase pain and further limit motion. When pain is refractory, total shoulder replacement is effective.

Shoulder Instability Problems

Tears of the glenoid labrum may be associated with disruption of portions of the glenohumeral ligament, causing anterior or posterior instability or internal derangement similar to knee meniscal tears. A fall on an outstretched arm in abduction and slight forward flexion is the most common acute injury producing a SLAP (superior, labral, anterior, posterior) lesion; chronic lesions occur in athletes who throw repetitively. Patients usually describe pain associated with a catching or popping sensation during overhead activities. A SLAP lesion at the anterosuperior labrum involves injury of the long head of the biceps at its insertion to the superior glenoid labrum. *Type I* SLAP is a frayed superior labrum; *Type II* is an unstable labral biceps complex anchor to the glenoid; *Type III* is a bucket-handle tear of the labrum; and *Type IV* is a bucket-handle tear of the labrum that extends into the biceps tendon. On examination, pain is reproduced by resisting a downward force on the hand when the arm is in 90° of forward flexion, full internal rotation, and 30° of adduction (O'Brien test).

Glenohumeral instability results in recurrent transient subluxation or even dislocation of the humeral head. Anterior instability is the most common and presents with anterior shoulder pain when the arm is abducted and externally rotated. Pain may be associated with a feeling of slipping and clicking or that the joint is loose. Posterior instability typically follows unusual trauma with the arm flexed forward and internally rotated. On examination, the patient is unable to externally rotate the arm. Instability with recurrent anterior subluxation causes impingement of the rotator cuff between the subluxed humeral head and the acromion.

Glenohumeral instability can follow trauma and may be associated with generalized laxity and hypermobility, capsular tears or avulsions, and lesions in the glenoid labrum. Cuff-tear arthropathy and Milwaukee shoulder are 2 terms that likely refer to the same or similar shoulder disorders. When a large tear in the RC causes instability and permits proximal migration of the humeral head, destructive erosions and crystal deposits are seen. The primary treatment approach to glenohumeral instability is prolonged rehabilitation designed to strengthen all the muscles of the shoulder girdle.

EXTRINSIC CAUSES OF SHOULDER PAIN

Cervical radiculopathy is caused by spinal nerve compression due to foraminal stenosis, herniated disk, osteophyte, or tumor and can transmit pain to the shoulder region with altered sensation (numbness or tingling) or motor weakness. The pain is initiated or exacerbated by neck motions rather than shoulder movement and is localized to the dermatome distribution. Weakness with decreased deep-tendon reflexes localizes to the myotome distribution of C6, C7, and C8 nerves. MRI is the best test to illustrate anatomic abnormalities, and electromyogram with nerve conduction studies will provide neurophysiologic assessment of each nerve root.

Brachial plexopathy causes a deep, severe shoulder pain followed by weakness and muscle atrophy. It may be due to compression of the plexus by the first rib or muscles, tumor invasion or a paraneoplastic phenomenon, direct trauma or stretch injuries, irradiation, or various inflammatory causes (Parsonage-Turner syndrome). Spontaneous recovery occurs over months to years. Shoulder pain and loss of motion due to true weakness and atrophy in shoulder-girdle muscles occur after presumed viral infection, following immunization, or spontaneously (16). The pain is usually abrupt in onset, intense, and described as sharp, throbbing, stabbing, or aching. The pain may be bilateral and constant, worsened by arm movements, and associated with paresthesias, numbness, and objective sensory deficits. Pain may remit in a few weeks or last a few years, leaving striking weakness and muscle atrophy that gradually improve over 1–3 years. Patients should undergo MRI of the neck and shoulder region and electromyography with nerve conduction studies to localize the pathology. Treatment includes oral systemic corticosteroids or intraarticular corticosteroid injections for pain relief. During the period of weakness, a regular passive stretching exercise program is used to prevent contractures. Progression to active exercises for stretching and strengthening is recommended as soon as the patient is able.

Suprascapular neuropathy occurs secondary to direct trauma, nerve stretch injury, or compression in the suprascapular or spinoglenoid notch. The suprascapular nerve (C5, C6) innervates the supraspinatus and infraspinatus muscles and is the sensory nerve to the glenohumeral joint capsule and acromioclavicular joint. Neuropathy produces weakness on abduction and external rotation and a burning pain that increases during abduction. The pain can also be exacerbated by reaching across the chest and rotating the neck away from the painful shoulder. Deep tendon reflexes and passive ROM are normal. Atrophy of the infraspinatus muscle may occur early. The diagnosis can be confirmed by finding prolonged latency and decreased amplitude of the motor response to suprascapular nerve stimulation. Nerve entrapment in the suprascapular notch produces posterolateral shoulder pain that may radiate down the extremity or up into the neck. It is associated with weakness of abduction and external rotation and atrophy of the infraspinatus muscle. The pain is described as deep, burning, or aching and can be elicited by palpation of the suprascapular notch. The suprascapular nerve may be contused by direct trauma, compressed by a mass lesion, tethered by the suprascapular ligament, or recurrently traumatized during competitive overhead sports, such as volleyball. The diagnosis is confirmed by electromyography and nerve conduction studies. The initial approach should be to rule out a mass lesion with MRI, reduce overhead activities, and control pain with analgesics and NSAIDs or with a suprascapular nerve block. Indications for corticorsteroid and local anesthetic injection in the region of the suprascpaular notch includes uncontrolled pain, disability, and recent onset (17). The suprascapular notch is easily reached superior to the midpoint of the spine of the scapula.

Thoracic outlet syndrome is caused by compression of the neurovascular bundle (brachial plexus, subclavian artery, and vein) at the thoracic outlet. Pain, paresthesia, and numbness radiate from the neck and shoulder down the arm and into the ring and little fingers, and are worsened by activities. Associated vascular abnormalities include discoloration, temperature change, claudication, and Raynaud's phenomenon. On physical examination, the radial pulse decreases as the arm is raised above the head (hyperabduction maneuver) or when the patient holds a deep breath and turns the head to the affected side (Adson's test). However, both of these tests may be positive in healthy individuals and are therefore not conclusive. A chest x-ray may reveal a cervical rib, elongated transverse process of C7, fracture, or exostoses. An MR angiogram can demonstrate significant vascular compression.

REFERRED PAIN TO THE SHOULDER REGION

The mechanisms that lead to shoulder region pain referred from viscera are poorly understood. Nociceptive impulses from the diaphragm via the phrenic nerve produce referred pain to the trapezius area. The phrenic nerve may also be irritated by lesions in the upper thorax, mediastinum, and pericardium. Cardiac pain is referred to the axilla and left pectoral region. Irritation of intraabdominal organs can also refer pain to the top of the shoulder and scapular region. Cutaneous hypersensitivity and muscle spasm associated with referred pain may be helpful diagnostic clues. Treatment is directed at the underlying visceral disease.

REFERENCES

1. Walker-Bone K, Palmer KT, Reading I, Coggon D, Cooper C. Prevalence and impact of musculoskeletal disorders of the upper limb in the general population. Arthritis Rheum 2004;51:642–51.
2. Wofford JL, Mansfield RJ, Watkins RS. Patient characteristics and clinical management of patients with shoulder pain in U.S. primary care settings: secondary data analysis of the National Ambulatory Medical Care Survey. BMC Musculoskelet Disord 2005;6:4–10.
3. Croft P, Pope D, Silman A. The clinical course of shoulder pain: prospective cohort study in primary care. Primary Care Rheumatology Society Shoulder Study Group. BMJ 1996;313:601–2.
4. Sommerich CM, McGlothlin JD, Marras WS. Occupational risk factors associated with soft tissue disorders of the shoulder: a review of current investigations in the literature. Ergonomics 1993;36:697–717.
5. Frieman BG, Albert TJ, Fenlin JM Jr. Rotator cuff disease: a review of diagnosis, pathophysiology, and current trends in treatment. Arch Phys Med Rehabil 1994;75:604–9.
6. de Winter AF, Jans MP, Scholten RJ, Deville W, van Schaardenburg D, Bouter LM. Diagnostic classification of shoulder disorders: interobserver agreement and determinants of disagreement. Ann Rheum Dis 1999;58:272–7.
7. Iannotti JP, Zlatkin MB, Esterhai JL, Kressel HY, Dalinka MK, Spindler KP. Magnetic resonance imaging of the shoulder. Sensitivity, specificity, and predictive value. J Bone Joint Surg Am 1991;73:17–29.
8. Neer CS 2nd. Anterior acromioplasty for the chronic impingement syndrome in the shoulder: a preliminary report. J Bone Joint Surg Am 1972;54:41–50.
9. van der Heijden GJ, van der Windt DD, de Winter AF. Physiotherapy for patients with soft tissue shoulder disorders: a systematic review of randomised clinical trials. BMJ 1997;315:25–30.
10. Jobe FW, Moynes DR. Delineation of diagnostic criteria and a rehabilitation program for rotator cuff injuries. Am J Sports Med 1982;10:336–9.
11. Blair B, Rokito AS, Cuomo F, Jarolem K, Zuckerman JD. Efficacy of injections of corticosteroids for subacromial impingement syndrome. J Bone Joint Surg Am 1996;78:1685–9.
12. Rodeo SA, Hannafin JA, Tom J, Warren RF, Wickiewicz TL. Immunolocalization of cytokines and their receptors in adhesive capsulitis of the shoulder. J Orthop Res 1997;15:427–36.
13. Neviaser TJ. Adhesive capsulitis. Orthop Clin North Am 1987;18:439–43.
14. Warner JJ. Frozen shoulder: Diagnosis and Management. J Am Acad Orthop Surg 1997;5:130–40.
15. Gazielly DF, Gleyze P, Montagnon C. Functional and anatomical results after rotator cuff repair. Clin Orthop Relat Res 1994;304:43–53.
16. Tsairis P, Dyck PJ, Mulder DW. Natural history of brachial plexus neuropathy. Report on 99 patients. Arch Neurol 1972;27:109–17.
17. Torres-Ramos FM, Biundo JJ Jr. Suprascapular neuropathy during progressive resistive exercises in a cardiac rehabilitation program. Arch Phys Med Rehabil 1992;73:1107–11.

Spondyloarthropathies

MAZEN ELYAN, MD, and MUHAMMAD ASIM KHAN, MD, MACP

The spondyloarthropathies are a group of overlapping chronic inflammatory rheumatic diseases that includes ankylosing spondylitis (the prototype of this group), reactive arthritis, psoriatic arthritis, arthritis of inflammatory bowel disease, and undifferentiated spondylarthritis (1–4). There can be some overlap in the clinical features of the spondyloarthropathies, especially in their early stages (1), that may make it difficult to differentiate between them. However, this overlap does not usually influence treatment decisions.

EPIDEMIOLOGY

The prevalence of spondyloarthropathies varies among different ethnic groups and ranges from 0.5% to 1% in Europe (2,3). Spondyloarthropathies affect both sexes, although they are somewhat more common in men. They tend to cluster in families, and symptoms usually start in late teens and early 20s.

ETIOLOGY AND PATHOGENESIS

The etiology of the spondyloarthropathies is unknown; but they show a strong association with the HLA–B27 allele. The strength of this association varies among the different spondyloarthropathies and among various ethnicities (5). There is an increased incidence of spondyloarthropathies in first-degree relatives of affected individuals (6). An immune-mediated mechanism supported by the activation of T cells and macrophages results in local increase in the concentration of the proinflammatory cytokines, especially tumor necrosis factor α (TNFα), interleukin-1, and interferon-gamma (7). Inflammation may result in erosions, followed by a healing phase and ossification of the ligaments with resultant bony fusion or ankylosis, as seen in ankylosing spondylitis (AS). The primary pathologic sites include the entheses (the sites of bony insertion of ligaments and tendons) in the axial skeleton and extremities. Some nonarticular structures, such as the eye, gut, skin, and aortic valve can also be involved (1,6,8,9). Ankylosing spondylitis begins with sacroiliitis in most patients before it involves the spine.

The role of infection has been demonstrated in reactive arthritis, usually triggered by genitourinary infection with *Chlamydia trachomatis*, or enteritis due to bacteria such as *Shigella*, *Salmonella*, *Yersinia*, or *Campylobacter*. However, inflamed joints do not show evidence of active infection when fluid is cultured for bacteria (1,10). There is no evidence to support the role of infection in other forms of spondyloarthropathies.

CLINICAL MANIFESTATIONS

Ankylosing Spondylitis

AS usually presents with chronic inflammatory low back pain, which is defined by having at least 4 of the following 5 characteristics: 1) insidious onset, 2) onset before age 45 years, 3) duration of at least 3 months,

4) worsening of pain with inactivity and improving with physical exercise, and 5) stiffness on waking up in the morning (1,6,11,12). The disease usually involves the axial skeleton, including the sacroiliac joints. In very early stages, the patient may complain of alternating buttock pain due to inflammation of the sacroiliac joints. The disease can involve the hip and shoulder joints, and sometimes the more peripheral joints of the limbs can be affected, especially in the presence of associated reactive arthritis, psoriasis, or inflammatory bowel disease.

Back pain results from involvement of the discovertebral, facet, costovertebral, and costotransverse joints of the spine and the paravertebral ligaments (1,6,8). With disease progression, there is a gradual loss of mobility, flattening of the lumbar spine, and exaggerated thoracic spine kyphosis (6,8,11). Enthesitis can also result in plantar fasciitis, Achilles tendinitis, or patellar tendinitis (13).

One or more episodes of acute anterior uveitis occur in 25–40% of patients with AS (1,8,14). Involvement of the gastrointestinal tract, aorta, heart, or lungs can also be seen as a part of this disease in some patients, and they may have an increased risk of coronary artery disease (1,8,15,16).

Physical findings in AS include tenderness over the sacroiliac joints and pain with sacroiliac stress tests, such as FABERE (hip **F**lexion, **AB**duction, **E**xternal **R**otation, and **E**xtension). Enthesitis may cause tenderness over the spinal processes, the heels, iliac crest, anterior chest wall, and other bony prominences (1,8,13). There might be a decrease in chest expansion, which is normally at least 5 cm in healthy young individuals at the level of the xiphisternum. Measures of spinal mobility, such as modified Schober's test and lateral flexion, are important in the assessment of the AS (11,17). Occiput-to-wall or tragus-to-wall distances measure forward stooping deformity of the cervical spine (18). Cervical spine involvement can result in progressive limitation of the ability to turn or fully extend or laterally bend the neck.

Psoriatic Arthritis

Psoriatic arthritis is defined as an inflammatory arthritis associated with psoriasis. Inflammatory arthritis occurs in 10–30% of patients with psoriasis, and may present in different forms: monarthritis, asymmetric oligoarthritis (<5 joints), polyarthritis, arthritis of distal interphalangeal joints, arthritis mutilans, and spondylitis, although there can be significant overlap among these subtypes (1,19,20). The polyarthritis form can clinically resemble rheumatoid arthritis, although it is relatively less painful (21,22). Psoriatic arthritis is often associated with tendinitis or enthesitis. Inflammation of the entire digit involving the joints, ligaments, and the tendon sheaths (dactylitis or "sausage digits") is one of the typical features of psoriatic arthritis. Axial disease can be similar to AS, although it can sometimes be relatively asymptomatic.

It is important to extensively search the whole skin for lesions of psoriasis when evaluating a patient with any form of inflammatory arthritis or spondylitis. This search should include the scalp, ears, umbilicus, pelvic area, perineum, and perianal area. There is no correlation between the severity of skin lesions and the severity of arthritis (23).

The onset of psoriatic arthritis is usually in the fourth or fifth decade. Patients usually have had psoriasis for some time before the arthritis starts, but in about 15% of patients, arthritis precedes psoriasis (1). Nail changes of psoriasis, such as pitting or onycholysis, are more common in patients with psoriatic arthritis than in psoriasis patients without arthritis (1,19,20). Occurrence of psoriasis and psoriatic arthritis or undifferentiated spondyloarthropathy in sub-Saharan Africa has been associated with HIV infection (19,20,24,25).

Reactive Arthritis

Reactive arthritis typically occurs within 1 month of an inciting genitourinary or enteric infection. It usually manifests by acute, asymmetric oligoarthritis and is often associated with conjunctivitis, uveitis, enthesitis, dactylitis, genital psoriasiform lesions (circinate balanitis or circinate vulvitis), urethritis, or cervicits (10,16,26,27). The term Reiter syndrome has been used to describe the association of reactive arthritis with conjunctivitis and urethritis, although most patients with reactive arthritis do not have the complete triad.

Enteropathic Arthritis

Inflammatory bowel disease (ulcerative colitis and Crohn disease) can be associated with a form of inflammatory arthritis called enteropathic arthritis or spondyloarthropathy of inflammatory bowel disease (28–30). Up to 37% of patients with ulcerative colitis or Crohn disease may show sacroiliitis, spondylitis, enthesitis, or peripheral arthritis. Definite AS is seen in ~10% of these patients (28). Peripheral arthritis is usually self-limited and nondestructive; it, contrary to axial disease, parallels the activity of bowel involvement. On endoscopy, subclinical enteric mucosal inflammation is found in 26–69% of patients with AS and related spondyloarthropathies, and could be considered as one of the extraskeletal manifestations (29). The risk of developing clinical inflammatory bowel disease approaches 6% in such patients when the histology is acute and it is 15–25% in patients with histologically chronic inflammation (28–30).

Undifferentiated Spondyloarthropathies

The undifferentiated forms of spondyloarthropathies include HLA–B27-associated enthesitis, dactylitis, and rheumatoid factor-negative oligoarthritis or polyarthritis (31). The arthritis usually involves the lower extremities, without an identifiable infectious trigger or the presence of psoriasis or inflammatory bowel disease (1,31). Some patients may present with episodes of isolated acute anterior uveitis (1,14,32), which may precede the onset of the spondyloarthropathy.

RADIOGRAPHIC FEATURES

The spondyloarthropathies are characterized by the radiographic evidence of sacroiliitis, which ranges from suspicious changes to sclerotic margins, erosions, and pseudowidening to complete ankylosis of the sacroiliac joints. Spinal changes on plain films include squaring of the vertebral bodies, formation of syndesmophytes, involvement of the facet joints, spondylodiscitis, ligament ossification, and a *bamboo spine*. Spinal osteoporosis is commonly seen and it correlates with disease severity and duration (33). Conventional radiographs may also reveal soft-tissue swelling or erosive changes in the peripheral joints. Some of the classic findings of psoriatic arthritis include periosteal reactions, ankylosis, and pencil-in-cup deformities in the hands and feets.

Radiographic sacroiliitis is required for the definite diagnosis of AS according to the Modified New York Classification Criteria (34).

An anteroposterior film of the pelvis is usually adequate for detecting sacroiliitis (35). However, in the presence of high clinical suspicion but normal x-ray, a magnetic resonance image (MRI) with the STIR (Short Tau Inversion Recovery) (or a computed tomograph) can be very helpful (35–38).

LABORATORY FEATURES

There are no specific laboratory tests for spondyloarthropathies. Acute phase reactants, such as C-reactive protein (CRP) and erythrocyte sedimentation rate (ESR) can be elevated, especially when peripheral joints are inflamed; but their sensitivity and specificity are low in patients with pure axial disease (39,40). There is no association with rheumatoid factor and antinuclear antibody tests. Synovial fluid analysis is nonspecific. Stool testing may be of value in screening for inflammatory bowel disease.

Testing for HLA–B27 can be helpful in certain clinical situations, but it is not a routine test because the spondyloarthropathies can occur in the absence of HLA–B27. Moreover, HLA–B27 can be present in perfectly healthy people (4,5,41,42).

When there is a clinical suspicion of reactive arthritis, throat cultures for streptococcal infection and tests for urogenital *Chlamydia* and enteric infection, such as *Salmonella*, *Yersinia* and *Campylobacter*, are indicated (10,26). Testing for HIV should always be considered in high-risk patients (43,44).

DIAGNOSIS

The diagnosis of spondyloarthropathies is based on a combination of clinical and radiographic manifestations, and there are no validated diagnostic criteria. Instead, there are classification criteria, which are by design highly specific (to be used in clinical studies) and therefore have a relatively low sensitivity. The Modified New York Criteria (Table 1) (34) are the most commonly used classification criteria for AS.

The diagnosis of AS can be challenging due to the lack of a specific diagnostic test and the insidious onset with mild and nonspecific symptoms, especially early in its course (11). Furthermore, radiologic changes are often not apparent in the early stages (36). Thus, the diagnosis, which averages 3–11 years from the onset of symptoms, is often missed or markedly delayed. The delay can be even longer in women, children, adolescents, and HLA–B27-negative patients (2,45,46).

Table 1. The modified New York criteria for ankylosing spondylitis*

Diagnosis

Clinical criteria
- Low back pain and stiffness for >3 months that improves with exercise but not with rest
- Limitation of lumbar spine mobility in both the sagittal and frontal planes
- Limitation in chest expansion as compared with normal range for age and sex

Radiologic criteria
- Unilateral sacroiliitis of grade 3–4 OR
- Bilateral sacroiliitis of grade ≥2

Grading

Definite AS if the radiological criterion is associated with at least 1 clinical criterion

Probable AS if:
- 3 clinical criteria are present OR
- The radiological criterion is present without any signs or symptoms satisfying the clinical criteria

* Adapted with permission from reference 24.

Rudwaleit et al (47) have proposed decision trees to help primary care physicians who suspect the presence of axial spondyloarthropathy appropriately refer patients to rheumatologists in early phase of the disease. They have highlighted some of the clinically pertinent parameters (Figure 1), with each parameter having a diagnostic value, expressed as the likelihood ratio. The presence of 4 or more of these parameters in a patient with inflammatory back pain without radiographic evidence of sacroiliitis would strongly support the diagnosis of axial undifferentiated spondylarthritis (45).

CLINICAL COURSE

The course of AS varies among patients and can be characterized by spontaneous remissions and exacerbations (1,6). However, the typical spinal deformities may become noticeable within the first 10 years. The longer the diagnosis is delayed, the worse the functional outcome could be, especially in patients with juvenile-onset disease (46). Some patients have a limited disease and may never develop spinal ankylosis (1,48).

The course of psoriatic arthritis depends, in part, on the clinical presentation. Patients with symmetric polyarthritis tend to have a similar course to rheumatoid arthritis, with the development of deformities and more tendency for bony ankylosis of the proximal interphalangeal (PIP) and distal interphalangeal (DIP) joints (19,20,49). Arthritis mutilans, a rare form of psoriatic arthritis, results in osteolysis of the hand bones with severe destruction and deformity. Axial disease in psoriatic arthritis is similar to that in AS in that it may lead to spinal fusion, although it tends to be milder (19,20).

Reactive arthritis symptoms usually last for up to 5 months, although some patients may continue to have mild symptoms for >1 year (10).

Up to one-third of the patients may continue to have chronic or recurrent arthritis, sacroiliitis, or spondylitis (10,50).

TREATMENT

The treatment of spondyloarthropathies should be individualized based on the symptoms and signs, the disease activity and severity, functional status, deformities, general health status, comorbid conditions, and the patient's wishes (51).

The ASAS (Assessment in Ankylosing Spondylitis) International Society and the European League Against Rheumatism (EULAR) have recently published international recommendations for the management of AS that will be updated regularly to incorporate any future advances (51). They contain 10 key recommendations (not guidelines) based on scientific evidence and expert opinion. The optimal management requires a combination of nonpharmacologic and pharmacologic treatments, with appropriate monitoring that depends on symptoms, severity, and drug treatment (51).

Nonpharmacologic Treatment

Patient education is an essential part of the nonpharmacologic treatment in AS and should include a life-long program of regular exercise. Usefulness of individual and group physical therapy, patient associations, and self-help groups is also emphasized.

Exercise tends to improve outcome. Unsupervised recreational exercise with specific back exercises improves pain, stiffness, function, and quality of life in patients with AS (52,53). Prolonged formal physical therapy is costly and is not covered by most health insurance

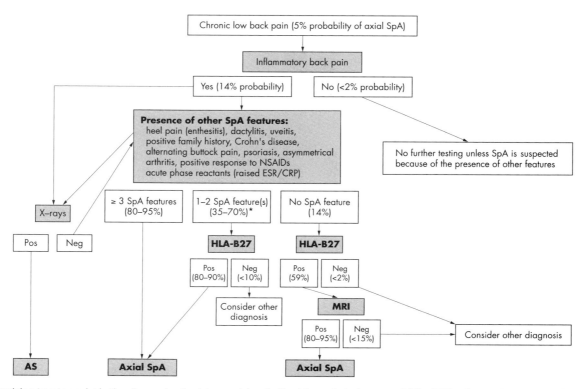

Figure 1. Decision tree to assist in the diagnosis of axial spondyloarthritis. AS = ankylosing spondylitis; CRP = C-reactive protein; ESR = erythrocyte sedimentation rate; MRI = magnetic resonance imaging; Neg = negative; NSAIDs = nonsteroidal antiinflammatory drugs; Pos = positive; SpA = spondyloarthritis. Reprinted with permission from reference 37.

plans, but a physical therapist can instruct patients about proper posture and self-administered exercise in addition to recreational sports and a regular exercise program. Written instructions and illustrations should be provided to patients. An individual therapeutic exercise program along with education significantly improves function after a few months; this improvement can be maintained by minimal maintenance therapy (54,55). Home-based exercise may decrease pain and improve spinal mobility, as well as the general sense of wellbeing (56).

Stretching exercises for different muscle groups relieve acute muscle spasm and improve mobility, chest expansion, endurance, and posture (54,57). Deep-breathing exercises should be encouraged and can be prepared for by applying local heat or taking analgesics to relieve pain from costochondritis. Patients should be advised to avoid smoking. After adequate pain and stiffness control is achieved, muscle-strengthening exercises can be initiated. Patients should exercise when their tiredness is at a minimum. They should prepare for exercise by taking a warm shower or applying local heat and engaging in a light warm-up, including gentle arm movement or walking.

Swimming and water exercises are very helpful. Warm water helps promote relaxation and reduces the discomfort of stretching. Furthermore, water exercises strengthen muscles because of the water's resistance and increase cardiovascular conditioning and endurance. Patients with heart disease should be assessed by their physician, which may require an exercise tolerance test prior to initiation of exercise. Patients with psoriasis should avoid chlorinated water (57).

Physical therapy is cost-effective and beneficial for patients with AS, although there is no clear evidence that favors a specific treatment protocol (54,55,58–60). Short-term intensive physical therapy and exercise improves mobility of the spine, hip, and shoulder (61). Group physical therapy with home exercises may be superior to individual physical therapy in terms of patient global assessment of improvement and spinal mobility (60), although results from another clinical study did not reproduce the same results (62). Intensive in-patient physiotherapy and hydrotherapy with home exercises may provide short-term advantages over home exercise alone in improving pain and stiffness (63). This form of therapy can be considered in patients with severe decline in functional capacity.

Pharmacologic Treatment

Nonsteroidal antiinflammatory drugs (NSAIDs) are the cornerstone of treatment, and they need to be taken regularly in full antiinflammatory doses to achieve the desired therapeutic effect (64–67). The traditional disease-modifying antirheumatic drugs (DMARDs), including methotrexate, leflunomide, and sulfasalazine, are not recommended for the treatment of axial disease. Sulfasalazine may be considered in patients with peripheral arthritis.

Topical corticosteroids are very effective in treating acute iritis. Intraarticular or local steroid injection can be used to achieve rapid relief of active inflammation of the peripheral joints and enthesitis in select patients in the absence of contraindications (51,68,69). Use of oral corticosteroids is not advised and the use of systemic corticosteroids in the management of AS is also not supported by evidence (51).

The use of antibiotics is not supported by evidence from the literature except for cases of reactive arthritis preceded by a known bacterial infection, especially C trachomatis. Appropriate antibiotics may reduce the duration of reactive arthritis (70), but this therapy does not seem to alter the long-term history of the disease (71).

TNF blockers (discussed extensively in Chapter 35) are remarkably effective in treating AS patients with persistently high disease activity despite conventional therapy (51,72,97). In patients with axial disease, there is no need for an obligatory use of DMARDs prior to or concomitant with anti-TNF therapy. These drugs are also dramatically effective in treating psoriasis, psoriatic arthritis, and inflammatory bowel disease. Etanercept, however, is not effective in treating inflammatory bowel disease.

Effective TNF inhibition results in rapid and dramatic improvement in the symptoms and signs of spondyloarthropathies, including back symptoms, peripheral arthritis, enthesitis, dactylitis, and psoriasis in the majority of patients. Both pain and function improve remarkably, with significant decrease in spinal inflammation as evident with MRI (72–84). TNF inhibition may also slow radiographic disease progression (78,79). Their efficacy has been shown to be persistent in the long term (78,85–89). Another advantage of TNF inhibitors may be the significant reduction in the frequency of anterior uveitis flares (90).

For initiation of anti-TNF therapy in AS, patients should fulfill the Modified New York Criteria for definitive AS. The disease must be active for at least 1 month as determined by a Bath Ankylosing Spondylitis Disease Activity Index score of ≥4. Initiation of such treatment should be decided by an expert on the subject. The patient must have failed to show adequate therapeutic response to at least 2 different NSAIDs given for at least 3 months at maximal recommended or tolerated antiinflammatory dose (unless there is intolerance, toxicity, or contraindications to the use of NSAIDs). Those with AS and peripheral arthritis must have failed to respond to adequate therapy with both NSAIDs and sulfasalazine, and those with enthesitis must have failed at least 2 local steroid injections before anti-TNF therapy is started (91). A few patients with reactive arthritis refractory to traditional therapies have responded to treatment with TNF blockers (92).

For psoriatic arthritis, TNF inhibitors can be used in combination with other therapies, such as methotrexate, the required dose of which may be reduced (1). One may switch from one anti-TNF agent to another in cases of inefficacy (primary versus secondary) or development of side effects to one agent. This should not be applied when adverse events are related to TNF inhibitors as a class (93–95).

Treatment of AS and proriatic arthritis patients with TNF inhibitors needs to be continued indefinitely to maintain therapeutic effects, because discontinuation would result in inflammation recurrence (96). Unlike infliximab, etanercept does not risk losing it efficacy if readministered after repeated discontinuations (97).

Osteoporosis is common in AS patients, and should be recognized and treated appropriately. It can occur relatively early in the disease. Spinal osteoporosis is caused partly by the ankylosis and decreased mobility and also secondary to the effect of proinflammatory cytokines (98,99). Adequate calcium and vitamin D intake should be encouraged. Prevention and treatment of osteoporosis may help decrease the risk of spinal deformities and fractures. Measurements of bone density at the spine may be unreliable when there is ligamentous ossification and formation of syndesmophytes. Thus, femoral neck measurements should be relied on for the diagnosis. Sometimes a peripheral dual-energy x-ray absorptiometry scan might be needed in patients with bilateral hip arthroplasties. Treatment for osteoporosis includes bisphosphonates or, sometimes, parathyroid hormone.

Patient Education

Patient education, behavioral therapy, counseling, and self-help programs improve patients' compliance with therapeutic regimens; decrease their pain; may have a positive impact on general health, motivation, compliance, and functional status; and may reduce the cost of conventional therapy (100–105). Patients who smoke should be urged to quit because smokers tend to have more severe illness in addition to increased incidence of respiratory complications (106).

Impact of the disease on the family should be discussed with the patient and possibly family members who are engaged in the care of the patient. Possibility of familial aggregation should be discussed, and it may help to increase the likelihood of early diagnosis in other family members.

Patients should be always encouraged to take a central role in managing their illness, and should be given information about disease-specific associations, books, pamphlets, videos, and audiotapes. Those who believe that exercise is beneficial, are followed by a rheumatologist, and are more educated are most likely to adhere to the treatment regimen (107,108). Some patients use superficial heat or cold in the form of packs, or a hot shower or bath to decrease stiffness. Patients should be encouraged to swim regularly if they can and encouraged to perform deep breathing exercises at least twice daily to maintain a good chest expansion (102).

Posture and Gait

Specific exercises, such as spinal extension, need to be performed at least twice daily to maintain good posture and spinal mobility. Patients should be advised on proper posture during activities of daily living, including walking, sitting, and sleeping. This includes sleeping on a firm mattress without a pillow, with a thin pillow, or with a contoured pillow to maintain neck extension and prevent the development of spinal deformities. They should walk erect, keeping the spine as straight as possible while maintaining normal, reciprocal arm swing and rotational movements of the lower spine and pelvis. They should avoid activities that cause strain on back muscles, such as prolonged stooping or bending. Posture can be monitored using occiput-to-wall distance, which should be measured with the patient standing against the wall with heels, buttocks, and shoulders touching the wall, and the chin parallel to the floor. Body height should also be checked on a regular basis.

Patients should avoid positions that may lead to a stooped posture, such as slouching in chairs or leaning over a desk for prolonged periods; stretches should be performed regularly. Patients who work with computers, for example, can use a slightly tilted table to avoid a bending posture. To maintain hip extension, a 15-minute period of prone lying daily is advised. A rolled towel under the forehead may help turning the head to the side (57). In case of inability to lie flat in the prone position, the patient can use a pillow under the abdomen; or the patient can lie supine with the buttocks at the edge of the bed and hips extended.

Patient Concerns

High-impact sports, or those that involve significant abrupt movement of the spine, should be discouraged because of the increased risk of spinal injury. When swimming, patients may use snorkels and masks for breathing if they have restricted motion of the neck. Badminton, walking, and cross-country (but not downhill) skiing are good options. Some modifications, such as raising the bicycle handlebars, can be applied in cases of sports that require forward-flexed posture. Footwear can be adjusted to reduce the impact of some activities on the spine and reduce the discomfort of heel spurs. Patients should always have a period of warm-up to help relieve stiffness and decrease the likelihood of injury (57). Workplace needs should be evaluated and necessary

modifications should be advised. Changing position frequently and taking breaks for stretching helps improve endurance.

Restrictions and Disability

Some functional difficulties frequently encountered include dressing, body transfers, lifting and carrying, and endurance (54). Problems in performing activities of daily living should be identified and solutions sought to compensate for loss of motion and improve functional capacity. Assistive devices, including ones for walking, can be used in certain cases—such as when there is lower-extremity joint problems. Some helpful items include long-handled devices for dressing and reaching, adjustable swivel chairs with lumbar support, and elevated and inclined writing surfaces (57).

Postural changes that affect balance because of a displacement of the center of mass of the trunk pose safety concerns (109). It is important to take measures to prevent falls. Bathrooms should have nonslippery floors and should be equipped with safety measures, such as railings, grab bars, and safety mats (57).

Decreased range of motion of the cervical spine makes driving a real challenge; however, support of the neck and back by seat and headrest can be helpful, and wide-angled mirrors help increase peripheral vision (110). Crossing roads should be done with caution due to impaired neck mobility.

Role of Surgery

Surgery may be indicated when there is severe hip and knee damage. Total hip arthroplasty deserves consideration in patients with structural damage causing refractory pain or disability, irrespective of age; and there is no need to discontinue NSAID therapy for this surgery (51). It provides pain relief and improves function (51,111). The need for future revision depends on the age and sex of the patient (112), but is not specifically higher in patients with AS. Moreover, there is no specific increase in the incidence of heterotopic bone formation and ankylosis following hip replacement in AS patients (113–115).

Elective spinal surgeries for AS patients include osteotomy to correct severe kyphosis and uncompensated loss of horizontal vision. Corrective spinal osteotomy for severe kyphosis and fusion procedures for segmental instability may provide excellent functional improvement (51,116). Spinal fusion is indicated in cases of atlantoaxial subluxation and to relieve pain and correct deformity resulting from pseudoarthrosis (117).

A challenging aspect in the care for ankylosing spondylitis patients is using general anesthesia because of intubation difficulties resulting from cervical spine ankylosis and deformity and involvement of the temporomandibular joint, which decrease the ability to open the mouth. Spinal anesthesia can even be impossible due to spinal fusion and ligament ossification. Special attention should be paid during the postoperative period to prevent pulmonary complications, which tend to increase because of decreased vital capacity from restricted chest wall expansion (118). It is wise for such patients to carry an identification bracelet (like Medic-Alert) that provides special attention to such limitations.

FOLLOWUP AND MONITORING

Patients with spondyloarthopathies should be followed on regular basis, even if their illness seems to be inactive. The frequency of monitoring in AS should be based on the clinical presentation and therapy used.

Rehabilitation Considerations for the Spondyloarthropathies

- Encourage physical activities that promote extension (e.g., reading newpaper while laying prone on floor).
- Promote use of stretching exercise for the lower back, hips, and shoulders. Stretch should be held for 30 seconds.
- Modalities, such as ulstrasound, followed by exercise may enhance benefit of exercise.
- Aerobic exercise should be encorporated to promote general fitness.
- Frequent monitoring of vitals signs and use of interval training of 3 sets of 10 minutes of exercise versus 30 minutes can be used in patients with more severe cardiovascular involvement.
- Swimming strokes, such as breast stroke and freestyle, promote extension while building strength.
- Recommend use of orthotics and proper footwear to prevent onset or exacerbation of Achilles tendinitis and plantar fasciitis.
- Encourage respiratory exercises to promote chest mobility.
- Encourage use of proper posture.

Monitoring includes following patient symptoms and signs (including axial and peripheral disease and extraskeletal manifestations), laboratory testing, and imaging studies. Specific skeletal elements to be monitored include duration of morning stiffness, severity of pain, mobility of the lumbar and cervical spine, chest expansion, enthesopathy, and changes in joint inflammation and range of motion.

Laboratory testing can be used as an adjunctive measure in monitoring response to therapy; however, CRP and ESR do not always correlate with disease activity (39,40). Other laboratory tests include complete blood count, renal function, and liver function tests to monitor for any adverse effects that might be caused by pharmacologic therapy.

Radiographic monitoring once every 2 years is usually sufficient but can be done more frequently in select cases. However, radiographs are not sensitive for changes over <1 year (119). Lateral cervical and lumbar spine films are usually sufficient, but radiographs of the thoracic spine may sometimes be needed, especially when a fracture is suspected.

Any new-onset neck or back pain in a patient with AS, even in the absence of trauma, should be carefully evaluated for spinal fracture or instability. There is high morbidity and mortality associated with transverse-displaced fractures of the neck, which can result in paraplegia or quadriplegia (120,121). Spinal pseudoarthrosis should be always kept in mind; it should be differentiated from indolent infections. Other rare neurologic complications that might be associated with AS include cauda equina syndrome, which is characterized by dull pain in the lower back and upper buttock region; analgesia in the buttocks, genitalia, or thighs (saddle area); and a disturbance of bowel and bladder function (122–124). It may result from chronic adhesive arachnoiditis, due to fibrous entrapment and scarring of the sacral and lower lumbar nerve roots. AS patients may rarely develop spontaneous atlantoaxial subluxation that may require surgery in some instances (125,126).

REFERENCES

1. Khan MA. Update on spondylarthropathies. Ann Intern Med 2002; 136:896–907.
2. Akkoc N, Khan MA. Epidemiology of ankylosing spondylitis and related spondylarthropathies. In: Weisman MH, Reveille JD, van der Heijde D, editors. Ankylosing spondylitis and the spondyloarthropathies: a companion to rheumatology. London: Mosby: Elsevier: 2006. p. 117–31.
3. Sieper J, Rudwaleit M, Khan MA, Braun J. Concepts and epidemiology of spondylarthritis. Best Pract Res Clin Rheumatol. 2006;20:401–17.
4. Elyan M, Khan MA. Diagnosing ankylosing spondylitis. J Rheumatol Suppl. In press.
5. Khan MA. Prevalence of HLA-B27 in world populations. In: Lopez-Larrea C, editor. HLA-B27 in the development of spondylarthropathies. Austin (TX): Landes; 1997. p. 95–112.
6. van der Linden S, van der Heijde, Braun J. Ankylosing spondylitis. In: Harris EJ, editor. Kelly's textbook of rheumatology. 7th ed. Philadelphia: Elsevier Saunders; 2005. p. 1125–41.
7. Smith JA, Marker-Hermann E, Colbert RA. Pathogenesis of ankylosing spondylitis: current concepts. Best Pract Res Clin Rheumatol 2006;20: 571–91.
8. Khan MA. Spondylarthropathies. In: Hunder GG, editor. Atlas of rheumatology. Philadelphia: Current Medicine; 2002. p. 141–67.
9. Francois RJ, Braun J, Khan MA. Entheses and enthesitis: a histopathologic review and relevance to spondylarthritides. Curr Opin Rheumatol 2001;13:255–64.
10. Khan MA, Sieper J. Reactive arthritis. In: Koopman WJ, Moreland LW, editors. Arthritis and allied conditions. 15th edition. Philadelphia: Lippincott Williams & Wilkins; 2004. p. 1335–55.
11. Khan MA. Ankylosing spondylitis: clinical features. In: Hochberg M, Silman A, Smolen J, Weinblatt M, Weisman M, editors. Rheumatology. 3rd ed. London: Mosby. 2003; p. 1161–81.
12. Calin A, Porta J, Fries JF, Schurman DJ. Clinical history as a screening test for ankylosing spondylitis. JAMA 1977;237:2613–4.
13. Francois RJ, Braun J, Khan MA. Entheses and enthesitis: a histopathologic review and relevance to spondylarthritides. Curr Opin Rheumatol 2001;13:255–64.
14. Banares A, Hernandez-Garcia C, Fernandez-Gutierrez B, Jover JA. Eye involvement in the spondylarthropathies. Rheum Dis Clin North Am 1998;24:771–84, ix.
15. Divecha H, Sattar N, Rumley A, Cherry L, Lowe GD, Sturrock R. Cardiovascular risk parameters in men with ankylosing spondylitis in comparison with non-inflammatory control subjects: relevance of systemic inflammation. Clin Sci (Lond) 2005;109:171–6.
16. Lautermann D, Braun J. Ankylosing spondylitis: cardiac manifestations. Clin Exp Rheumatol 2002;20(6 Suppl 28):S11–5.
17. Haywood KL, Garratt AM, Jordan K, Dziedzic K, Dawes PT. Spinal mobility in ankylosing spondylitis: reliability, validity and responsiveness. Rheumatology (Oxford). 2004;43:750–7.
18. Heuft-Dorenbosch L, Vosse D, Landewe R, Spoorenberg A, Dougados M, Mielants H, et al. Measurement of spinal mobility in ankylosing spondylitis: comparison of occiput-to-wall and tragus-to-wall distance. J Rheumatol 2004;31:1779–84.
19. Höhler T, Märker-Hermann E. Psoriatic arthritis: clinical aspects, genetics, and the role of T cells. Curr Opin Rheumatol 2001;13:273–9.
20. Gladman DD. Current concepts in psoriatic arthritis. Curr Opin Rheumatol 2002;14:361–6.
21. Buskila D, Langevitz P, Gladman DD, Urowitz S, Smythe HA. Patients with rheumatoid arthritis are more tender than those with psoriatic arthritis. J Rheumatol 1992;19:1115–9.
22. Helliwell PS, Porter G, Taylor WJ. Polyarticular psoriatic arthritis is more like oligoarticular psoriatic arthritis, than rheumatoid arthritis. Ann Rheum Dis 2006 (Jul 13). [Epub ahead of print]
23. Cohen MR, Reda DJ, Clegg DO, Department of Veteran Affairs Cooperative Study Group on Seronegative Spondylarthropathies. Baseline relationships between psoriasis and psoriatic arthritis: analysis of 221 patients with active psoriatic arthritis. J Rheumatol 1999;26:1752–6.
24. Njobvu P, McGill P. Psoriatic arthritis and human immunodeficiency virus infection in Zambia. J Rheumatol 2000;27:1699–702.
25. Mijiyawa M, Oniankitan O, Khan MA. Spondylarthropathies in sub-Saharan Africa. Curr Opin Rheumatol 2000;12:281–6.
26. Sieper J, Rudwaleit M, Braun J, van der Heijde D. Diagnosing reactive arthritis: role of clinical setting in the value of serologic and microbiologic assays. Arthritis Rheum 2002;46:319–27.
27. Leirisalo-Repo M. Early arthritis and infection. Curr Opin Rheumatol. 2005;17:433–9.
28. de Vlam K, Mielants H, Cuvelier C, De Keyser F, Veys EM, De Vos M. Spondylarthropathy is underestimated in inflammatory bowel disease: prevalence and HLA association. J Rheumatol 2000;27:2860–5.
29. Queiro R, Maiz O, Intxausti J, de Dios JR, Belzunegui J, Gonzalez C, Figueroa M. Subclinical sacroiliitis in inflammatory bowel disease: a clinical and follow-up study. Clin Rheumatol 2000;19:445–9.
30. Smale S, Natt RS, Orchard TR, Russell AS, Bjarnason I. Inflammatory bowel disease and spondylarthropathy. Arthritis Rheum 2001;44: 2728–36.
31. Olivieri I, Salvarani C, Cantini F, Ciancio G, Padula A. Ankylosing spondylitis and undifferentiated spondylarthropathies: a clinical review and description of a disease subset with older age at onset. Curr Opin Rheumatol. 2001;13:280–4.

32. Pato E, Banares A, Jover JA, Fernandez-Gutierrez B, Godoy F, Morado C, et al. Undiagnosed spondylarthropathy in patients presenting with anterior uveitis. J Rheumatol 2000;27:2198–202.

33. Barozzi L, Olivieri I, De Matteis M, Padula A, Pavlica P. Seronegative spondylarthropathies: imaging of spondylitis, enthesitis and dactylitis. Eur J Radiol. 1998;27(suppl 1):S12–7.

34. van der Linden S, Valkenburg HA, Cats A. Evaluation of diagnostic criteria for ankylosing spondylitis: a proposal for modification of the New York criteria. Arthritis Rheum 1984;27:361–8.

35. Bennett DL, Ohashi K, El-Khoury GY. Spondylarthropathies: ankylosing spondylitis and psoriatic arthritis. Radiol Clin North Am 2004;42: 121–34.

36. Oostveen J, Prevo R, den Boer J, van de Laar M. Early detection of sacroiliitis on magnetic resonance imaging and subsequent development of sacroiliitis on plain radiography: a prospective, longitudinal study. J Rheumatol 1999;26:1953–8.

37. Baraliakos X, Hermann KG, Landewe R, Listing J, Golder W, Brandt J, et al. Assessment of acute spinal inflammation in patients with ankylosing spondylitis by magnetic resonance imaging: a comparison between contrast enhanced T1 and short tau inversion recovery (STIR) sequences. Ann Rheum Dis 2005;64:1141–4.

38. Hermann KG, Landewe RB, Braun J, van der Heijde DM. Magnetic resonance imaging of inflammatory lesions in the spine in ankylosing spondylitis clinical trials: is paramagnetic contrast medium necessary? J Rheumatol 2005;32:2056–60.

39. Dougados M, Gueguen A, Nakache JP, Velicitat P, Zeidler H, Veys E, et al. Clinical relevance of C-reactive protein in axial involvement of ankylosing spondylitis. J Rheumatol 1999;26:971–4.

40. Spoorenberg A, van der Heijde D, de Klerk E, Dougados M, de Vlam K, Mielants H, et al. Relative value of erythrocyte sedimentation rate and C-reactive protein in assessment of disease activity in ankylosing spondylitis. J Rheumatol 1999;26:980–4.

41. Gran JT, Husby G. HLA-B27 and spondylarthropathy: value for early diagnosis? J Med Genet 1995;32:497–501.

42. Khan MA, Khan MK. Diagnostic value of HLA-B27 testing ankylosing spondylitis and Reiter's syndrome. Ann Intern Med 1982;96:70–6.

43. Stein CM, Davis P. Arthritis associated with HIV infection in Zimbabwe. J Rheumatol 1996;23:506–11.

44. Blanche P, Taelman H, Saraux A, Bogaerts J, Clerinx J, Batungwanayo J, et al. Acute arthritis and human immunodeficiency virus infection in Rwanda. J Rheumatol 1993;20:2123–7.

45. Rudwaleit M, Khan MA, Sieper J. The challenge of diagnosis and classification in early ankylosing spondylitis: do we need new criteria? Arthritis Rheum 2005;52:1000–8.

46. Stone M, Warren RW, Bruckel J, Cooper D, Cortinovis D, Inman RD. Juvenile-onset ankylosing spondylitis is associated with worse functional outcomes than adult-onset ankylosing spondylitis. Arthritis Rheum 2005;53:445–51.

47. Rudwaleit M, van der Heijde D, Khan MA, Braun J, Sieper J. How to diagnose axial spondylarthritis early. Ann Rheum Dis 2004;63:535–43.

48. Brophy S, Mackay K, Al-Saidi A, Taylor G, Calin A. The natural history of ankylosing spondylitis as defined by radiological progression. J Rheumatol 2002;29:1236–43.

49. Fitzgerald O, Dougados M. Psoriatic arthritis: one or more diseases? Best Pract Res Clin Rheumatol 2006;20:435–50.

50. Kanakoudi-Tsakalidou F, Pardalos G, Pratsidou-Gertsi P, Kansouzidou-Kanakoudi A, Tsangaropoulou-Stinga H. Persistent or severe course of reactive arthritis following Salmonella enteritidis infection: a prospective study of 9 cases. Scand J Rheumatol 1998;27:431–4.

51. Zochling J, van der Heijde D, Dougados M, Braun J. Current evidence for the management of ankylosing spondylitis a systematic literature review for the ASAS/EULAR management recommendations in ankylosing spondylitis. Ann Rheum Dis 2006;65:423–32.

52. Uhrin Z, Kuzis S, Ward MM. Exercise and changes in health status in patients with ankylosing spondylitis. Arch Intern Med 2000;160:2969–75.

53. Lim HJ, Lee MS, Lim HS. Exercise, pain, perceived family support, and quality of life in Korean patients with ankylosing spondylitis. Psychol Rep 2005;96:3–8.

54. Kraag G, Stokes B, Groh J, Helewa A, Goldsmith C. The effects of comprehensive home physiotherapy and supervision on patients with ankylosing spondylitis—a randomized controlled trial. J Rheumatol 1990;17:228–33.

55. Kraag G, Stokes B, Groh J, Helewa A, Goldsmith CH. The effects of comprehensive home physiotherapy and supervision on patients with ankylosing spondylitis—an 8-month followup. J Rheumatol 1994;21:261–3.

56. Lim HJ, Moon YI, Lee MS. Effects of home-based daily exercise therapy on joint mobility, daily activity, pain, and depression in patients with ankylosing spondylitis. Rheumatol Int 2005;25:225–9.

57. Helewa A, Stokes B. Spondylarthropathies. In: Robbins L, Burckhardt CS, Hannan, MT, DeHoratius RJ, editors. Clinical care in the rheumatic diseases. 2nd ed. Atlanta: Association of Rheumatology Health Professionals; 2001. p. 105–112.

58. Dagfinrud H, Kvien TK, Hagen KB. The Cochrane review of physiotherapy interventions for ankylosing spondylitis. J Rheumatol 2005;32: 1899–906.

59. van der Linden S, van Tubergen A, Hidding A. Physiotherapy in ankylosing spondylitis: what is the evidence? Clin Exp Rheumatol 2002;20(6 Suppl 28):S60–4.

60. Hidding A, van der Linden S, Boers M, Gielen X, de Witte L, Kester A, et al. Is group physical therapy superior to individualized therapy in ankylosing spondylitis? A randomized controlled trial. Arthritis Care Res 1993;6: 117–25.

61. Heikkila S, Viitanen JV, Kautiainen H, Kauppi M. Sensitivity to change of mobility tests; effect of short term intensive physiotherapy and exercise on spinal, hip, and shoulder measurements in spondylarthropathy. J Rheumatol 2000;27:1251–6.

62. Analay Y, Ozcan E, Karan A, Diracoglu D, Aydin R. The effectiveness of intensive group exercise on patients with ankylosing spondylitis. Clin Rehabil 2003;17:631–6.

63. Helliwell PS, Abbott CA, Chamberlain MA. A randomised trial of three different physiotherapy regimes in ankylosing spondylitis. Physiotherapy 1996;82:85–90.

64. Akkoc N, van der Linden S, Khan MA. Ankylosing spondylitis and symptom-modifying vs disease-modifying therapy. Best Pract Res Clin Rheumatol 2006;20:539–57.

65. Toussirot E, Wendling D. Recent progress in ankylosing spondylitis treatment. Expert Opin Pharmacother 2003;4:1–12.

66. Dougados M, Behier JM, Jolchine I, Calin A, van der Heijde D, Olivieri I, et al. Efficacy of celecoxib, a cyclooxygenase 2-specific inhibitor, in the treatment of ankylosing spondylitis: a six-week controlled study with comparison against placebo and against a conventional nonsteroidal antiinflammatory drug. Arthritis Rheum 2001;44:180–5.

67. Wanders A, Heijde D, Landewe R, Behier JM, Calin A, Olivieri I, Zeidler H, Dougados M. Nonsteroidal antiinflammatory drugs reduce radiographic progression in patients with ankylosing spondylitis: a randomized clinical trial. Arthritis Rheum 2005 Jun;52(6):1756–65.

68. Maugars Y, Mathis C, Vilon P, Prost A. Corticosteroid injection of the sacroiliac joint in patients with seronegative spondylarthropathy. Arthritis Rheum 1992;35:564–8.

69. Luukkainen R, Nissila M, Asikainen E, Sanila M, Lehtinen K, Alanaatu A, Kautiainen H. Periarticular corticosteroid treatment of the sacroiliac joint in patients with seronegative spondylarthropathy. Clin Exp Rheumatol 1999;17:88–90.

70. Lauhio A, Leirisalo-Repo M, Lahdevirta J, Saikku P, Repo H. Double blind, placebo controlled study of three months treatment with lymecycline in reactive arthritis, with special reference to Chlamydia arthritis. Arthritis Rheum 1991;24:6–14.

71. Laasila K, Laasonen L, Leirisalo-Repo M. Antibiotic treatment and long term prognosis of reactive arthritis. Ann Rheum Dis 2003;62:655–8.

72. Braun J, Brandt J, Listing J, Zink A, Alten R, Golder W, et al. Treatment of active ankylosing spondylitis with infliximab: a randomized controlled multi-center trial. Lancet 2002;359:1187–93.

73. Brandt J, Haibel H, Cornely D, Golder W, Gonzalez J, Reddig J, et al. Successful treatment of active ankylosing spondylitis with the anti-tumor necrosis factor α monoclonal antibody infliximab. Arthritis Rheum 2000;43: 1346–52.

74. Van Den Bosch F, Kruithof E, Baeten D, Herssens A, de Keyser F, Mielants H, et al. Randomized double-blind comparison of chimeric monoclonal antibody to tumor necrosis factor α (infliximab) versus placebo in active spondylarthropathy. Arthritis Rheum 2002;46:755–65.

75. Davis JC Jr, Van Der Heijde D, Braun J, Dougados M, Cush J, Clegg DO, et al. Recombinant human tumor necrosis factor receptor (etanercept) for treating ankylosing spondylitis: a randomized, controlled trial. Arthritis Rheum 2003;48:3230–6.

76. Brandt J, Khariouzov A, Listing J, Haibel H, Sorensen H, Grassnickel L, et al. Six-month results of a double-blind, placebo-controlled trial of etanercept treatment in patients with active ankylosing spondylitis. Arthritis Rheum 2003;48:1667–75.

77. Calin A, Dijkmans BA, Emery P, Hakala M, Kalden J, Leirisalo-Repo M, et al. Outcomes of a multicentre randomised clinical trial of etanercept to treat ankylosing spondylitis. Ann Rheum Dis 2004;63:1594–1600.

78. Baraliakos X, Brandt J, Listing J, Haibel H, Sorensen H, Rudwaleit M, et al. Outcome of patients with active ankylosing spondylitis after two years of therapy with etanercept: clinical and magnetic resonance imaging data. Arthritis Rheum 2005;53:856–63.

79. Baraliakos X, Listing J, Rudwaleit M, Brandt J, Sieper J, Braun J. Radiographic progression in patients with ankylosing spondylitis after 2 years of treatment with the tumour necrosis factor alpha antibody infliximab. Ann Rheum Dis 2005;64:1462–6.

80. Ory P, Sharp JT, Salonen D, Rubenstein J, Mease P, Kivitz AJ, et al. Etanercept (Enbrel) inhibits radiographic progression in patients with psoriatic arthritis. Arthritis Rheum 2002;46(suppl 9):S196.

81. Mease PJ, Goffe BS, Metz J, VanderStoep A, Finck B, Burge DJ. Etanercept in the treatment of psoriatic arthritis and psoriasis: a randomized trial. Lancet 2000;356:385–90.

82. Mease PJ, Gladman DD, Ritchlin CT, Ruderman EM, Steinfeld SD, Choy EH, et al. Adalimumab for the treatment of patients with moderately to severely active psoriatic arthritis: results of a double-blind, randomized, placebo-controlled trial. Arthritis Rheum 2005;52:3279–89.

83. Antoni C, Kavanaugh A, Kirkham B, Burmester G, Weisman M, Keystone E, et al. The infliximab multinational psoriatic arthritis controlled trial (IMPACT) [Abstract]. Arthritis Rheum 2002;46(Suppl 9):S381.

84. Antoni C, Krueger GG, de Vlam K, Birbara C, Beutler A, et al. Infliximab improves signs and symptoms of psoriatic arthritis: results of the IMPACT 2 trial. Ann Rheum Dis 2005;64:1150–7.

85. Braun J, Brandt J, Listing J, Zink A, Alten R, Burmester G, et al. Two year maintenance of efficacy and safety of infliximab in the treatment of ankylosing spondylitis. Ann Rheum Dis 2005;64:229–34.

86. Nikas SN, Alamanos Y, Voulgari PV, Pliakou XI, Papadopoulos CG, Drosos AA. Infliximab therapy in ankylosing spondylitis: an observational study. Ann Rheum Dis 2005;64:940–2.

87. Van den Bosch F, Devinck M, Kruithof E, Baeten D, Verbruggen G, de Keyser F, et al. A prospective long-term study of the efficacy and safety of infliximab in 107 patients with spondylarthropathy. Arthritis Rheum 2004;50(Suppl 9):S611.

88. Baraliakos X, Brandt J, Listing J, Rudwaleit M, Alten R, Burmester G et al. Clinical response to long-term therapy with infliximab in patients with ankylosing spondylitis—results after 3 years. Arthritis Rheum 2004;50(Suppl 9):S615.

89. Braun J, Baraliakos X, Brandt J, Listing J, Zink A, Alten R, et al. Persistent clinical response to the anti-TNF-alpha antibody infliximab in patients with ankylosing spondylitis over 3 years. Rheumatology (Oxford) 2005;44:670–6.

90. Braun J, Baraliakos X, Listing J, Sieper J. Decreased incidence of anterior uveitis in patients with ankylosing spondylitis treated with the anti-tumor necrosis factor agents infliximab and etanercept. Arthritis Rheum 2005;52:2447–51.

91. Braun J, Pham T, Sieper J, Davis J, van der Linden S, Dougados M, et al. International ASAS consensus statement for the use of anti-tumour necrosis factor agents in patients with ankylosing spondylitis. Ann Rheum Dis 2003;62:817–24.

92. Meador R, Hsia E, Kitumnuaypong T, Schumacher HR. TNF involvement and anti-TNF therapy of reactive and unclassified arthritis. Clin Exp Rheumatol 2002;20(6 Suppl 28):S130–4.

93. Wick MC, Ernestam S, Lindblad S, Bratt J, Klareskog L, van Vollenhoven RF. Adalimumab (Humira) restores clinical response in patients with secondary loss of efficacy from infliximab (Remicade) or etanercept (Enbrel): results from the STURE registry at Karolinska University Hospital. Scand J Rheumatol 2005;34:353–8.

94. Delaunay C, Farrenq V, Marini-Portugal A, Cohen JD, Chevalier X, Claudepierre P. Infliximab to etanercept switch in patients with spondylarthropathies and psoriatic arthritis: preliminary data. J Rheumatol 2005;32:2183–5.

95. Cohen G, Courvoisier N, Cohen JD, Zaltni S, Sany J, Combe B. The efficiency of switching from infliximab to etanercept and vice-versa in patients with rheumatoid arthritis. Clin Exp Rheumatol 2005;23:795–800.

96. Baraliakos X, Listing J, Brandt J, Zink A, Alten R, Burmester G, et al. Clinical response to discontinuation of anti-TNF therapy in patients with ankylosing spondylitis after 3 years of continuous treatment with infliximab. Arthritis Res Ther 2005;7:R439–44.

97. Brandt J, Listing J, Haibel H, Sorensen H, Schwebig A, Rudwaleit M, et al. Long-term efficacy and safety of etanercept after readmination in patients with active ankylosing spondylitis. Rheumatology (Oxford) 2005;44:342–8.

98. Gratacos J, Collado A, Pons F, Osaba M, Sanmarti R, Roque M, et al. Significant loss of bone mass in patients with early, active ankylosing spondylitis: a followup study. Arthritis Rheum 1999 Nov;42(11):2319–24.

99. Lange U, Jung O, Teichmann J, Neeck G. Relationship between disease activity and serum levels of vitamin D metabolites and parathyroid hormone in ankylosing spondylitis. Osteoporos Int 2001;12:1031–5.

100. Barlow JH, Barefoot J. Group education for people with arthritis. Pt Educat Counsel 1996;27:257–67.

101. de Klerk E, van der Linden S, van der Heijde D, Urquhart J. Facilitated analysis of data on drug regimen compliance. Stat Med 1997;16:1653–64.

102. Khan MA. Ankylosing spondylitis: the facts. Oxford (UK): Oxford University Press; 2002.

103. Lorig KR, Mazonson PD, Holman HR. Evidence suggesting that health education for self-management in patients with chronic arthritis has sustained health benefits while reducing health care costs. Arthritis Rheum 1993;36:439–46.

104. Basler HD, Rehfisch HP. Cognitive-behavioral therapy in patients with ankylosing spondylitis in a German self-help organization. J Psychosom Res 1991;35:345–54.

105. Krauth C, Rieger J, Bonisch A, Ehlebracht-Konig I. [Costs and benefits of an education program for patients with ankylosing spondylitis as part of an inpatient rehabilitation programs-study design and first results.] Z Rheumatol 2003;62(Suppl 2):II14–6.

106. Doran MF, Brophy S, MacKay K, Taylor G, Calin A. Predictors of longterm outcome in ankylosing spondylitis. J Rheumatol 2003;30:316–20.

107. Santos H, Brophy S, Calin A. Exercise in ankylosing spondylitis: how much is optimum? J Rheumatol 1998;25:2156–60.

108. Jensen GM, Lorish CD. Promoting patient cooperation with exercise programs: linking research, theory and practice. Arthritis Care Res 1994;7:181–9.

109. Bot SD, Caspers M, Van Royen BJ, Toussaint HM, Kingma I. Biomechanical analysis of posture in patients with spinal kyphosis due to ankylosing spondylitis: a pilot study. Rheumatology (Oxford) 1999;38:441–3.

110. Eriendsson J. Car driving with ankylosing spondylitis. The Ankylosing Spondylitis International Federation and The National Ankylosing Spondylitis Society of Great Britain.

111. Sweeney S, Gupta R, Taylor G, Calin A. Total hip arthroplasty in ankylosing spondylitis: outcome in 340 patients. J Rheumatol 2001;28:1862–6.

112. Furnes O, Lie SA, Espehaug B, Vollset SE, Engesaeter LB, Havelin LI. Hip disease and the prognosis of total hip replacements: a review of 53,698 primary total hip replacements reported to the Norwegian Arthroplasty Register 1987–99. J Bone Joint Surg Br 2001;83:579–86.

113. Brinker MR, Rosenberg AG, Kull L, Cox DD. Primary noncemented total hip arthroplasty in patients with ankylosing spondylitis: clinical and radiographic results at an average follow-up period of 6 years. J Arthroplasty 1996;11:802–12.

114. Diaz de Rada P, Barroso-Diaz JL, Valenti JR. Follow-up of the outcome of hip arthroplasty in patients with ankylosing spondylitis. Rev Ortop Traumatol 2004;48(5):340–4.

115. Sochart DH, Porter ML. Long-term results of total hip replacement in young patients who had ankylosing spondylitis. eighteen to thirty-year results with survivorship analysis. J Bone Joint Surg Am 1997;79:1181–9.

116. van Royen BJ, de Kleuver M, Slot GH. Polysegmental lumbar posterior wedge osteotomies for correction of kyphosis in ankylosing spondylitis. Eur Spine J 1998;7:104–10.

117. Chen LH, Kao FC, Niu CC, Lai PL, Fu TS, Chen WJ. Surgical treatment of spinal pseudoarthrosis in ankylosing spondylitis. Chang Gung Med J 2005;28:621–8.AQ:1

118. Carter R, Riantawan P, Banham SW, Sturrock RD. An investigation of factors limiting aerobic capacity in patients with ankylosing spondylitis. Respir Med 1999;93:700–8.

119. Spoorenberg A, de Vlam K, van der Heijde D, de Klerk E, Dougados M, Mielants H, et al. Radiological scoring methods in ankylosing spondylitis: reliability and sensitivity to change over one year. J Rheumatol 1999;26:997–1002.

120. Tico N, Ramon S, Garcia-Ortun F, Ramirez L, Castello T, Garcia-Fernandez L, et al. Traumatic spinal cord injury complicating ankylosing spondylitis. Spinal Cord 1998;36:349–52.

121. Hitchon PW, From AM, Brenton MD, Glaser JA, Torner JC. Fractures of the thoracolumbar spine complicating ankylosing spondylitis. J Neurosurg 2002;97(2 Suppl):218–22.

122. Bilgen IG, Yunten N, Ustun EE, Oksel F, Gumusdis G. Adhesive arachnoiditis causing cauda equina syndrome in ankylosing spondylitis: CT and MRI demonstration of dural calcification and a dorsal dural diverticulum. Neuroradiology 1999;41:508–11.

123. Ginsburg WW, Cohen MD, Miller GM, Bartleson JD. Posterior vertebral body erosion by arachnoid diverticula in cauda equina syndrome: an unusual manifestation of ankylosing spondylitis. J Rheumatol 1997;24:1417–20.

124. Ahn NU, Ahn UM, Nallamshetty L, Springer BD, Buchowski JM, Funches L, et al. Cauda equina syndrome in ankylosing spondylitis (the CES-AS syndrome): meta-analysis of outcomes after medical and surgical treatments. J Spinal Disord 2001;14:427–33.

125. Shim SC, Yoo DH, Lee JK, Koh HK, Lee SR, Oh SH, et al. Multiple cerebellar infarction due to vertebral artery obstruction and bulbar symptoms associated with vertical subluxation and atlanto-occipital subluxation in ankylosing spondylitis. J Rheumatol 1998;25:2464–8.

126. Thompson GH, Khan MA, Bilenker RM. Spontaneous atlantoaxial subluxation as a presenting manifestation of juvenile ankylosing spondylitis: a case report. Spine 1982;7:78–9.

CHAPTER 28

Systemic Lupus Erythematosus

MICHELLE A. PETRI, MD, MPH

Lupus represents a range of disease processes characterized by the development of autoantibodies with associated manifestations and organ damage. Some forms of lupus may be limited to the skin or occur after exposure to a drug. The prototypical form of lupus, however, is a systemic disease with protean manifestations that may be quite severe.

Systemic lupus erythematosus (SLE) is a multiorgan autoimmune disease that often presents insidiously with significant heterogeneity of expression in individuals. The disease may affect multiple organ systems at the time of presentation, but may also evolve more gradually, frequently resulting in a delay in diagnosis. The disease may range in severity from mild to life threatening, depending on the particular organ systems affected. Although disease manifestations are usually controllable with medications, the attendant morbidity associated with these medications, especially from corticosteroids, also contributes to organ damage over time.

Chronic cutaneous lupus (CCL) is a form of lupus limited to the skin but without systemic disease. Forms of CCL include discoid lupus, subacute cutaneous lupus erythematosus (SCLE), tumid lupus, and lupus panniculitis. Over time, only ~5% of CCL patients go on to develop SLE.

Drug-induced lupus erythematosus (DILE) is another form of lupus in which exposure to a medication triggers the process but in which resolution occurs after discontinuation of the drug; although resolution sometimes is delayed and requires additional therapy. Common agents implicated in the past were procainamide, hydralazine, and isoniazid. Today, minocycline and tumor necrosis factor (TNF) antagonists used to treat rheumatoid arthritis and other diseases are also potential causes of DILE.

EPIDEMIOLOGY

Systemic lupus is a disease that is seen much more frequently in women than in men, with most series reporting a female:male ratio of 9:1. In the United States, the incidence of SLE in women is 9.4 per 100,000 and in men it is 1.54 per 100,000 (1).

Disease onset is predominantly in the 20s and 30s, but may occur throughout the lifespan. In the United States, SLE is more common in African Americans than in whites, and many suspect an increased prevalence in Hispanic Americans as well.

PATHOGENESIS

As is the case with most autoimmune diseases, the exact cause of SLE is not known. Although genetic factors are contributory, as evidenced by the fact that ~10% of SLE patients have a family member with lupus, environmental factors are also important. The most recognized environmental precipitant is ultraviolet light, with patients often reporting disease onset or flare after a trip to the beach or a tanning salon. Other environmental precipitants that have been implicated include medications (trimethoprim/sulfa, Echinacea, oral contraceptives, and hormone therapy), smoking, infections (such as Epstein-Barr virus), and toxin exposure (silica and mercury).

Lupus is an autoimmune disease predominantly mediated by autoantibodies. Some autoantibodies directly contribute to disease (anti–double-stranded DNA with renal lupus, anti-Ro/La with photosensitivity, and antiphospholipid with thrombosis), whereas others may be epiphenomena (anti-RNP, anti-Sm). The binding of autoantibodies to proteins and tissue and the deposition of these immune complexes lead to an inflammatory cascade, with activation of complement and production of inflammatory cytokines.

Recent research has found that most patients with SLE have a pattern of gene expression called the "interferon signature." More than 100 genes, regulated by alpha interferon, are turned on in SLE.

DIAGNOSIS

Although a positive antinuclear antibody (ANA) test is seen in almost all cases of lupus, a positive test is not sufficient for diagnosis. A positive ANA may be seen in a number of other conditions, including other autoimmune diseases, thyroid disease, chronic infections, and malignancy; a positive test can also be due to medications. Up to 20% of otherwise healthy young women may have a positive ANA of at least low titer, but of no clinical significance. Because of the poor specificity of a positive ANA test for a diagnosis of lupus, other manifestations are required to establish a diagnosis. The presence of pain and a positive ANA, in the absence of other defining disease characteristics, may be due to fibromyalgia rather than a systemic autoimmune disease.

The diagnosis of lupus requires recognition of a systemic multiorgan illness, usually with confirmatory autoantibody tests (beyond the ANA) or low complement levels (C4, C3, or CH50). The published American College of Rheumatology classification criteria require 4 of 11 specific criteria to be present (Table 1). However, these criteria were established for disease classification rather than as diagnostic criteria. Although they serve as useful guidelines, the diagnosis of SLE for clinical management purposes may not require that 4 classification criteria be present, and recognizes the heterogeneity of disease and its variable expression.

CLINICAL PRESENTATION

The most commonly affected organ systems in SLE are musculoskeletal, dermatologic, renal, and hematologic. However, virtually any organ system can be affected.

Musculoskeletal lupus can present as isolated arthralgia (often described as joint stiffness rather than pain) or synovitis (actual joint swelling). There is usually morning accentuation of joint stiffness and sometimes the gel phenomenon following prolonged immobility. Small joints of the hands (metacarpophalangeals, proximal interphalangeals, but not distal interphalangeals) and wrists are typically involved, but other joints, including knees, can become affected. Over time, reversible ulnar deviation and swan-necking of the fingers can occur: the so-called "Jaccoud's arthropathy." In contrast to rheumatoid arthritis, the arthritis of lupus does not typically cause erosive bony changes on radiograph.

Table 1. Systemic lupus erythematosus classification criteria.*

Systemic lupus erythematosus may be classified if 4 or more of the following 11 disorders are present:

Malar rash
Discoid rash
Photosensitivity
Oral ulcers
Arthritis
Serositis
Renal disorder
    a. >0.5 gm/day proteinuria or
    b. ≥3+ dipstick proteinuria or
    c. cellular casts
Neurologic disorder
    a. seizures or
    b. psychosis (without other cause)
Hematologic disorder
    a. hemolytic anemia, or
    b. leukopenia (<4,000/μL) or
    c. lymphopenia (<1,500/μL) or
    d. thrombocytopenia (<100,000/μL)
Immunologic disorder
    a. antibody to native DNA or
    b. antibody to Sm (Smith) or
    c. anticardiolipin antibodies, lupus anticoagulant, or false-positive serologic test for syphilis
Positive antinuclear antibodies

* Adapted from Tan et al (12) and Hochberg (13).

Several different skin manifestations of lupus can be seen. The malar rash is an erythematous photosensitive rash distributed on the cheeks and bridge of nose, but sparing areas that are shaded from ultraviolet light, such as below the nares. It is important to note, however, that red cheeks do not necessarily mean a lupus rash; acne vulgaris, acne rosacea, seborrheic dermatitis, sun damage, and steroid plethora may occur in a similar distribution and are often confused with a lupus eruption. Maculopapular photosensitive lupus rashes are common on the sun-exposed V-area of the neck and extremities as well. Biopsies of the skin rashes of lupus typically demonstrate immunoglobulin and complement deposition at the dermal–epidermal junction: the so-called "lupus band" sign.

The lesions of discoid lupus involve the deeper dermis and may lead to a permanent loss of hair follicles. Upon resolution of the skin lesions, disfiguring hypo- and hyperpigmentation may occur. Discoid lupus lesions are typically found on the face (including inside the ears, above the eyebrows, on the upper palate), neck, scalp, and forearms. Subacute cutaneous lupus erythematosus is a photosensitive, nonscarring rash that occurs in both a psoriaform and an annular/polycyclic form. About half of patients with SCLE have SLE.

Lupus renal involvement may present as proteinuria alone or as both proteinuria and hematuria. Characteristic red blood cell (RBC) casts, indicating glomerular involvement, may not be found. An elevated serum creatinine can be seen, with resultant renal failure sometimes a consequence. Significant proteinuria may result in the nephrotic syndrome, with low serum albumin and elevated cholesterol. A kidney biopsy is often necessary to determine the International Society of Nephrology class: minimal mesangial (I); mesangial proliferative (II); focal proliferative (III), diffuse proliferative (IV); and membranous (V) (2). Class VI indicates that irreversible renal sclerosis has occurred. Diffuse glomerulonephritis is the most dangerous, because it can rapidly progress to renal failure. Mesangial glomerulonephritis tends to be mild. Membranous nephritis is often manifested by nephrotic syndrome.

Serositis in lupus occurs most commonly as pleurisy (pain on deep inspiration), sometimes with pleural effusion. An inspiratory and expiratory rub may be appreciated on physical examination. If a pleural effusion is tapped, it is exudative. Complaints of pleuritic chest pain in a lupus patient must be differentiated from other conditions that cause similar symptoms, including pulmonary emboli and infection. Pericarditis is also seen in lupus and may occur in isolation or can coexist with pleurisy. Pericardial pain is typically positional, worse with recumbency and better if leaning forward. Ascites in a lupus patient, although potentially due to serositis, should prompt investigation for infarcted bowel, infection, or Budd-Chiari syndrome.

The most common hematologic abnormalities in lupus are disease-related leukopenia and lymphopenia. Medications, however, may also be associated with cytopenias; corticosteroids, for example, have been associated with lymphopenia. Thrombocytopenia may be due to lupus, antiphospholipid antibodies, immunosuppressive drugs, or heparin administration for antiphospholipid antibodies. Hemolytic anemia from lupus is typically Coombs positive, with an elevated reticulocyte count and decreased haptoglobin. However, the most common anemia in a lupus patient is anemia of inflammation (formerly called anemia of chronic disease). Other common causes of anemia in SLE patients include anemia from chronic renal disease and iron-deficiency anemia.

The possible neurologic manifestations of lupus are extensive, ranging from mild to severe. These include seizures, psychosis, encephalopathy, coma, meningitis, stroke, mononeuritis multiplex, transverse myelitis, peripheral neuropathy, and cranial neuropathy. Lupus involvement of the central nervous system is only rarely attributable to vascultitis, detectable with arteriography. Rather, immune complex deposition in small vessels is more likely responsible for symptoms. Psychosis is sometimes a manifestation of lupus, but this must be differentiated from steroid psychosis. Seizures are part of the diagnositic criteria for lupus, but may also occur from thrombotic, metabolic (uremia), or toxic causes. Strokes can occur from active lupus vasculopathy, but also may be attributable to thrombosis from antiphospholipid antibodies, or be due to concomitant hypertension or accelerated atherosclerosis. A neurologic assessment includes lumbar puncture (looking for elevated protein, lymphocytes, oligoclonal bands, or high IgG index), brain magnetic resonance imaging (MRI) with gadolinium, and sometimes a central nervous system (CNS) arteriogram or electroencephalogram.

Transverse myelitis is a rare lupus complication. Cord MRI is essential to determine whether the cause is inflammation from lupus or thrombosis from antiphospholipid antibodies.

The most common neurologic complaint in lupus, cognitive impairment, is present in 80% of patients by 10 years after diagnosis. It usually represents accumulated damage, as opposed to ongoing CNS SLE and is more likely to progress in those with antiphospholipid antibodies. Formal cognitive function testing is useful in establishing the baseline and is informative in identifying comorbid conditions, such as depression.

LABORATORY TESTS

Routine laboratory tests (including complete blood count, serum creatinine, and urinalysis) are essential for both the diagnosis and management of SLE.

Autoantibodies are important in the diagnosis of SLE and also help to better define subsets of patients clinically. A positive ANA test in and of itself is not very useful, because positive ANAs can occur in healthy people, the elderly, with drugs, with localized autoimmune disease (thyroid disease, pulmonary fibrosis), and with other systemic autoimmune diseases, such as scleroderma, rheumatoid arthritis, myositis, and Sjögren's syndrome. Two autoantibodies are quite specific for SLE: anti–double-stranded DNA (anti-dsDNA) and anti-Sm (standing for Smith antigen). Other autoantibodies, referred to as extractable

---

Nursing Considerations for Systemic Lupus Erythematosus

- The Lupus Foundation of America (www.lupus.org), Arthritis Foundation (www.arthritis.org), and National Institute of Arthritis and Musculoskeletal and Skin Diseases (www.niams.nih.gov) have extensive educational material on SLE.
- SLE patients with good social support have better outcomes.
- Compliance with monitoring visits and with medications, including antihypertensive therapy, is key.
- SLE patients often need help applying for drug assistance programs, disability, Medical Assistance (Medicaid), and Medicare.
- A frequent cause of pain and fatigue in SLE is fibromyalgia. Exercise is an important part of the management and does not cause SLE flares.

---

nuclear antigens, include anti-RNP, anti-Ro (also called SSA), and anti-La (also called SSB); they occur in SLE but are also associated with other connective tissue diseases.

Patients with SLE tend to fall into 1 of 3 subset groups: those with anti-RNP and anti-Sm; those with anti-dsDNA, anti-Ro, and anti-La (more frequently associated with secondary Sjögren's syndrome); and those with anti-dsDNA and antiphospholipid antibodies (associated with antiphospholipid syndrome with thrombosis and pregnancy loss) (3).

ANTIPHOSPHOLIPID ANTIBODIES

About one-half of SLE patients will have an antiphospholipid antibody: anticardiolipin, lupus anticoagulant, or anti–β_2-glycoprotein I during the course of their disease. These autoantibodies are associated with an increased risk of thrombosis or pregnancy loss. Some patients with antiphospholipid antibodies may also have thrombocytopenia. SLE patients with antiphospholipid antibodies should avoid certain medications (estrogen, thalidomide, raloxifene) that would further contribute to hypercoagulability. If a thrombotic event does occur, life-long anticoagulation is recommended with warfarin, aiming for an international normalized ratio of 2–3.

ORGAN DAMAGE

More than half of SLE patients develop permanent organ damage over time. It is surprising that a significant burden of organ damage may be directly or partially attributable to corticosteroids in the form of obesity, diabetes mellitus, hypertension, hyperlipidemia, cataracts, glaucoma, osteoporosis, osteonecrosis, infections, depression, and psychosis.

Accelerated atherosclerosis has emerged as the major cause of death in SLE. The risk of myocardial infarction is increased 50-fold in SLE (4). Although corticosteroid use may contribute to the risk of cardiovascular disease by increasing traditional cardiovascular risk factors (diabetes, hypertension, hypercholesterolemia), the increased risk of atherosclerosis in lupus is not completely explained by these risk factors or by corticosteroids alone (5). Careful counseling and treatment of modifiable cardiovascular risk factors (e.g., cigarette smoking, cholesterol levels, hypertension, and diabetes mellitus) is thus imperative in the comprehensive management of lupus. Some have advocated earlier noninvasive diagnostic testing (carotid duplex for carotid plaque, helical computed tomography for coronary calcium) to detect early subclinical atherosclerotic disease, so these patients can be targeted for early intervention.

Progression of renal damage occurs in at least 25% of SLE patients with lupus nephritis in spite of maximal therapy. Some have

recommended that a renal biopsy may be indicated in patients with 500 mg/day or more of proteinuria to determine if active nephritis is present. Other indications for renal biopsy are active urinary sediment with or without RBC casts and rising serum creatinine. Control of hypertension is also critical in patients with lupus renal disease. Angiotensin-converting enzyme (ACE) inhibitors and angiotensin receptor blockers both control hypertension and reduce proteinuria.

Malignancy risk, for both lymphoma and solid tumors, is increased in people with lupus, even in patients who have not received cyclophosphamide (6). SLE patients with secondary Sjögren's syndrome may have a special risk of non-Hodgkin's lymphoma.

HEALTH STATUS

General health status in people with SLE is poor as measured by the Short Form 36, with levels of impairment similar to that of patients with acquired immunodeficiency syndrome. Health status may not correlate well with physician-assessed disease activity or with measures of organ damage. Secondary fibromyalgia, found in up to 30% of lupus patients, may be a significant contributory factor to the poor overall patient-assessed health status. It is important to recognize the coexistence of this condition because symptoms of fatigue and chronic pain due to fibromyalgia are not improved by treatment with corticosteroids and immunosuppressive medications.

MANAGEMENT

Education

Patient education is a critical component of the long-term treatment of the lupus patient. This education may begin at the first visit for an SLE patient to initiate a life-long effort toward patient education and empowerment. The basics of SLE pathophysiology, the chronicity of disease, its unpredictable course, and the importance for regular medical visits, medication compliance, and requisite laboratory monitoring, should be explained. Establishing an open dialogue that encourages communication of new events, complications, and early signs of flare to health care providers is also necessary. Patients should be encouraged to pursue a healthy lifestyle and to avoid potential environmental precipitants of their condition—especially sun exposure—as well as certain medications, including sulfonamide antibiotics. Other precipitants that have been described include Echinacea, melatonin, garlic, and alfalfa sprouts (7).

Health Maintenance

SLE patients are at increased risk of infection, mostly attributable to corticosteroids and immunosuppressive medication, but potentially also due to the underlying immunologic aberrations of the disease itself. Influenza vaccine is recommended yearly and pneumococcal vaccine every 5–10 years. The administration of live viral vaccines is controversial and has been associated with disease flares in some patients. Furthermore, live virus vaccines should be avoided in patients receiving certain immunosuppressive therapies. SLE patients are at increased risk of some forms of cancer. Attention to regularly scheduled colonoscopies, Pap smears, and mammograms should be enforced.

Corticosteroids significantly increase the risk of osteopenia and osteoporosis. All SLE patients should take supplemental calcium with vitamin D, especially those taking corticosteroids. Because of the

---

Rehabilitation Considerations in Systemic Lupus Erythematosus

- A physical therapist is often engaged in SLE treatment to encourage exercise and in the adjunctive management of fibromyalgia pain.
- The arthritis of SLE causes reversible deformities called Jaccoud's arthropathy. An early visit to an occupational therapist is important so that the patient can be taught joint protection and appropriate splinting, if needed.
- Carpal tunnel syndrome is the most common entrapment neuropathy in SLE. Many SLE patients will benefit from wrist splints.
- Lupus patients may have transverse myelitis with associated weakness, or experience CNS disease that presents with stroke requiring rehabilitation.
- During exercise, frequently monitor for deep vein thrombosis in those who test positive for antiphospholipid antibody or have a history of a cardiac event.
- Avoid loading of weight-bearing joints in presence of avascular necrosis; incorporate aquatic exercise.
- Use eccentric exercises with caution in presence of myositis or steroid-induced myopathy.
- Be mindful of asymptomatic coronary artery disease; beware of "pleurisy" in young patient.
- Interval training may be useful (specific duration/intensity).
- Monitor heart rate (pulsemeter) and blood pressure during exercise.
  - Intensity: 50–60% of cardiac reserve, gradually progressing to 60–70%
  - Frequency: Four to 7 days/week; start with several short daily sessions
  - Duration: Twenty to 30 minutes total per session; can also use 2, 15-minute or 3, 10-minute sessions/day based on severity of limitation

---

restricted exposure to sunlight, patients with SLE may be especially prone to vitamin D deficiency, which requires ultraviolet light for conversion to the active form. Baseline and periodic bone desitometry (dual-energy x-ray absorptiometry) for patients taking corticosteroids are recommended. Bisphosphonate treatment to prevent bone loss is an important component of comprehensive management, but cannot be given to patients with severe renal insufficiency or to women who plan later pregnancies. Patients found to be osteopenic should have assessment of vitamin D levels, with most now recommending repletion if levels of 25-OH vitamin D are <30 ng/ml. Prompt management of hypertension and screening for hypercholesterolemia is also important, as is cardiac risk factor reduction and the use of aspirin in those at greater risk for coronary artery disease. Patients who are found to be hypercoagulable should avoid multiple vitamins with vitamin K and supplements that contain vitamin K.

Pregnancy and Contraception

Pregnancy in lupus is considered high risk, but 90% are successful. Flares of lupus can occur during pregnancy. High disease activity, especially if there is also low C3 or C4 levels or high anti-dsDNA levels, is associated with fewer live births and greater preterm births. The incidence of preeclampsia is increased, especially in women with a prior history of renal disease.

If the pregnant woman has anti-Ro or anti-La antibodies, these autoantibodies can cross the placenta, leading to a 2–5% risk of congenital heart block and to a risk of a neonatal lupus rash in the baby. Four-chamber fetal cardiac ultrasounds are recommended weekly from the 16th through the 32nd week of gestation.

If the pregnant woman has medium-to-high titer anticardiolipin or anti–β2-glycoprotein I, or a lupus anticoagulant, and a history of pregnancy loss or severe preeclampsia, prophylactic heparin and low-dose aspirin are recommended during the pregnancy. Heparin should be continued for 6 weeks postpartum, the time period in which the woman with SLE is most hypercoagulable. Life-long aspirin is usually recommended.

Oral contraceptives are allowed for contraception if the woman has stable lupus and is not hypercoagulable from antiphospholipid antibodies (or other causes) (8). Depo-progesterone use has recently been limited to 2 years because of concern that longer exposure might contribute to osteopenia and osteoporosis.

Cutaneous Lupus

Avoidance of ultraviolet light—both UVA and UVB—is essential for all patients with lupus. Sunscreen with an SPF of at least 30 should be applied twice daily in photosensitive patients. Antimalarial therapy is the mainstay of therapy for cutaneous manifestations, with hydroxychloroquine dosed, on average, at 400 mg daily; yearly ophthalmic monitoring for retinopathy, a quite rare complication occurring in <1 of 5,000 exposed (and reversible if detected early), is advised. Quinacrine, 100 mg daily, can be added to hydroxychloroquine in recalcitrant cases, or the patient can be switched to 250 mg chloroquine. Chloroquine has greater ocular toxicity, and patients should be switched back to hydroxychloroquine when stable.

Cutaneous lupus that is unresponsive to antimalarial therapy may require other immunosuppressive medications, including mycophenolate mofetil, methotrexate, or azathioprine. Thalidomide, 50–100 mg, has also been used; however, because this drug is a teratogen, its use must be carefully considered in women of childbearing potential. It is also associated with sensory neuropathy and thrombosis.

Musculoskeletal Lupus

Mild arthralgias can often be managed with nonsteroidal antiinflammatory drugs (NSAIDs). With the recent awareness of potential cardiovascular risks attributed to cyclooxygenase 2 (COX-2) selective antagonists and NSAIDs, a warning has now been added concerning this risk on NSAID packaging. Because SLE is associated with accelerated atherosclerosis and in some cases hypercoagulability (e.g., antiphospholipid antibodies), the long-term use of NSAIDs and COX-2 antagonists, in particular, is a potential concern. Long-term use of NSAIDs is also associated with gastrointestinal ulceration, the risk of which is further increased with the concomitant use of corticosteroids. Thus, attention to prophylaxis with proton-pump inhibitors is important in the management of SLE patients receiving long-term NSAID therapy. Hydroxychloroquine is helpful for both arthralgias and arthritis. Low-dose prednisone (≤7.5 mg daily) is sometimes necessary to control morning stiffness. Persistent synovitis may require the addition of methotrexate (9) or leflunomide. The use of anti-TNF biologics for SLE arthritis is controversial because they can induce anticardiolipin antibodies and anti-dsDNA antibodies. Some non-SLE patients have developed a lupus-like syndrome that includes nephritis. However, some SLE patients with erosive, rheumatoid-like arthritis may require the judicious use of these agents to quell their disease and prevent further destruction. Other recently approved biologic therapeutics for the treatment of rheumatoid arthritis (abatacept, rituximab) may be additional options in the future for the treatment of recalcitrant lupus arthritis.

Serositis

Very mild serositis may respond to NSAIDs. Moderate flares of serositis may respond to a one-time intramuscular injection of 100 mg of triamcinolone. More severe flares may require a 3-day intravenous methylprednisolone pulse (1,000 mg over 90 minutes), followed by a tapering dose of oral prednisone. A maintenance immunosuppressive regimen may be necessary if serositis is recurrent.

Lupus Nephritis

A recent Food and Drug Administration-sponsored clinical trial of mycophenolate mofetil versus intravenous cyclophosphamide demonstrated superiority of mycophenolate mofetil as an induction therapy (10). It is also safer when used for maintenance therapy (11). However, lack of response to mycophenolate mofetil, or a rapidly progressive glomerulonephritis, may still require intravenous pulse cyclophosphamide monthly.

When cyclophosphamide is given, the National Institutes of Health protocol is usually followed. Cyclophosphamide is given intravenously (500–750 mg/m^2 body surface area) on a monthly basis for 6 (or more) months as induction therapy, and sometimes quarterly for 2 more years as maintenance therapy. Prehydration, posthydration, and mesna are given to reduce the chance of hemorrhagic cystitis. Antiemetics must be given before and during the infusion. A pregnancy test must be done before the infusion in any woman at risk for pregnancy. The dose of cyclophosphamide must be adjusted down if the white blood cell count, done 7–10 days later, is too low. Leuprolide acetate (Lupron) may be given 2 weeks before each infusion to reduce the risk of ovarian failure. Leuprolide does have risks, including hypercoagulability and osteoporosis.

Central Nervous System Lupus

When a lupus patient presents with neurologic or psychiatric manifestations, it is critical to first determine whether this is due to active lupus or if the symptoms are attributable to other causes, including infectious, thrombotic, metabolic, toxic, hypertensive, or atherosclerotic pathology. Severe CNS lupus manifestations, such as encephalopathy, coma, or transverse myelitis, usually require both intravenous methylprednisolone pulse therapy and the initiation of immunosuppressant drugs, typically monthly intravenous cyclophosphamide. Seizures should be managed in conjunction with a neurologist and may require additional antiepileptic drugs. Phenytoin can be used in SLE (even though it can rarely lead to a drug-induced lupus). Psychosis and disordered sensorium may require antipsychotic drugs and major tranquilizers.

Hematologic Lupus

It is unusual for SLE patients to bleed as long as the platelet count is >30,000. Mild leukopenia is common in SLE and does not require treatment. Granulocyte colony-stimulating factor should be avoided because it is associated with lupus flares. Severe hemolytic anemia and thrombocytopenia require high-dose corticosteroids, and if there is lack of response, intravenous immunoglobulin. In refractory cases in which immunosuppressive drugs have failed or if the patient cannot tolerate them, biologic treatments that target the B cell may be considered. Rituximab, an anti–B-cell directed therapy, is effective in idiopathic thrombocytopenic purpura and may have a role for recalcitrant thrombocytopenia and autoimmune hemolytic anemia.

REFERENCES

1. Uramoto KM, Michet CJJ, Thumboo J, Sunku J, O'Fallon WM, Gabriel SE. Trends in the incidence and mortality of systemic lupus erythematosus, 1950–1992. Arthritis Rheum 1999;42:46–50.
2. Weening JJ, D'Agati VD, Schwartz MM, Seshan SV, Alpers CE, Appel GB, et al. The classification of glomerulonephritis in systemic lupus erythematosus revisited. J Am Soc Nephrol 2004;15:241–50.
3. To CH, Petri M. Is antibody clustering predictive of clinical subsets and damage in systemic lupus erythematosus? Arthritis Rheum 2005; 52:4003–10.
4. Manzi S, Meilahn EN, Rairie JE, Conte CG, Medsger TA Jr, Jansen-McWilliams L, et al. Age-specific incidence rates of myocardial infarction and angina in women with systemic lupus erythematosus: comparison with the Framingham Study. Am J Epidemiol 1997;145:408–15.
5. Esdaile JM, Abrahamowicz M, Grodzicky T, Li Y, Panaritis C, du Berger R, et al. Traditional Framingham risk factors fail to fully account for accelerated atherosclerosis in systemic lupus erythematosus. Arthritis Rheum 2001;44:2331–7.
6. Bernatsky S, Boivin JF, Joseph L, Manzi S, Ginzler E, Urowitz M, et al. Race/ethnicity and cancer occurrence in systemic lupus erythematosus. Arthritis Rheum 2005;53:781–4.
7. Petri M. Diet and systemic lupus erythematosus: from mouse and monkey to woman? Lupus 2001;10:775–7.
8. Petri M, Kim MY, Kalunian KC, Grossman J, Hahn BH, Sammaritano LR, et al. Combined oral contraceptives in women with systemic lupus erythematosus. N Engl J Med 2005;353:2550–8.
9. Sato EI. Methotrexate therapy in systemic lupus erythematosus. Lupus 2001;10:162–4.
10. Ginzler EM, Dooley MA, Aranow C, Kim MY, Buyon J, Merrill JT, et al. Mycophenolate mofetil or intravenous cyclophosphamide for lupus nephritis. N Engl J Med 2005;353:2219–28.
11. Contreras G, Pardo V, Leclercq B, Lenz O, Tozman E, O'Nan P, et al. Sequential therapies for proliferative lupus nephritis. N Engl J Med 2004; 350:971–80.
12. Tan EM, Cohen AS, Fries JF, Masi AT, McShane DJ, Rothfeld NF, et al. The 1982 revised criteria for the classification of systemic lupus erythematosus. Arthritis Rheum 1982;25:1271–7.
13. Hochberg MC. Updating the American College of Rheumatology revised criteria for the classification of systemic lupus erythematosus [letter]. Arthritis Rheum 1997;40:1725.

Systemic Sclerosis

FRANCESCO BOIN, MD, and FREDRICK WIGLEY, MD

Systemic Sclerosis (SSc) is a multisystem autoimmune disease characterized by fibrosis of the skin, also referred to as scleroderma ("hard skin"), and a variable pattern of other visceral organ involvement. SSc is a relatively uncommon disease, with a prevalence in the United States general population of 0.01–0.03% and worldwide distribution. It affects women more commonly than men (3:1) and has a typical age of onset of 30–50 years. In African Americans, SSc tends to present at an earlier age, have a more aggressive course (with diffuse skin and pulmonary fibrosis), and carry a worse prognosis (1).

The clinical presentation and natural course of SSc is very heterogeneous and not infrequently has overlapping features with other autoimmune or connective tissue diseases (e.g., inflammatory arthritis, polymyositis, Sjögren's syndrome, or autoimmune thyroid disease). SSc should be distinguished from other fibrosing skin diseases including scleredema, eosinophilic fasciitis, nephrogenic fibrosing dermopathy (NFD), scleromyxedema, and localized scleroderma (including morphea and linear scleroderma). **Localized scleroderma** is characterized by isolated fibrotic skin lesions that typically begin during childhood but are not associated with internal organ involvement.

NATURAL HISTORY OF SSc

Based on the extent of clinically affected skin, 2 major SSc subsets have been identified: diffuse cutaneous scleroderma (dcSSc) and limited cutaneous scleroderma (lcSSc; Table 1) (2).

Diffuse Cutaneous SSc

After a relatively short prodromal phase characterized by constitutional symptoms, arthralgias, puffiness of the fingers, and the new onset of Raynaud's phenomenon, the diffuse cutaneous form is characterized by rapid progression of skin changes from the fingers or feet to proximal involvement of the extremities extending above the knee or elbow or to areas of the trunk. During the initial phase of the disease, the skin tends to be inflamed, appearing edematous (nonpitting) and erythematous with varying areas of hyper- or hypopigmentation (vitiligo-like). Complaints of progressive skin and soft-tissue tightness, intense pruritus, and pain

Table 1. Classification of systemic sclerosis

- **Diffuse cutaneous scleroderma:** skin thickening on the trunk in addition to the face and proximal and distal extremities
- **Limited cutaneous scleroderma:** limited skin thickening, distal to the elbow and knee; may also involve the face and neck
  CREST syndrome (subcutaneous **C**alcinosis, **R**aynaud's phenomenon, **E**sophageal dysmotility **S**clerodactyly, **T**elangiectasias)
- **Sine scleroderma:** no apparent skin thickening but characteristic visceral organ involvement, with vascular and serologic features
- **Overlap syndrome:** criteria for scleroderma coexisting with features of other connective tissue disease, such as systemic lupus erythematosus, rheumatoid arthritis, or inflammatory muscle disease
  Mixed connective tissue disease: overlap syndrome with anti—U1 RNP antibodies

typically follow the initial phase of acute inflammation. Deeper articular or periarticular inflammation or fibrosis is suggested by the detection of friction rubs (crepitus). Flexion contractures of joints (especially of the fingers, wrists, and elbows) can develop with significant associated functional impairment. The "active" inflammatory phase evolves within a period of several weeks or months into the "fibrotic" phase, characterized by sclerotic, thickened skin with areas of atrophy that can ulcerate at sites of trauma (e.g., knuckles, elbows, toes). Although highly variable, the progression of new areas of skin involvement can last, on average, up to 2 years. This active phase is followed in >95% of cases by variable degrees of improvement and, in some cases, by remission. Except in areas of severe fibrosis (e.g., the fingers), almost complete regression of fibrotic skin changes can occur.

Internal organ involvement is common in dcSSc and typically develops during the first 3 years of disease (3). At the time of diagnosis, 50% of patients complain of heartburn or dyspepsia. These symptoms are secondary to an abnormal esophageal motility due to loss of circular smooth muscle function and can result in reflux esophagitis, esophageal stricture, and progress to Barrett's metaplasia. Diminished lower gastrointestinal (GI) tract motility can cause pseudo-obstruction or milder manifestations, such as constipation or diarrhea, which can be secondary to bacterial overgrowth. Untreated bowel disease may result in profound weight loss and malnutrition. Dilatation of mucosal capillaries in the GI tract and particularly in the gastric antrum (described as "watermelon stomach") is associated with recurrent occult bleeding that may result in a severe microcytic anemia with iron deficiency.

Interstitial lung disease (ILD) is also a frequent early manifestation of dcSSc, particularly in subjects who have anti–topoisomerase I antibodies (55–60%). Typically lung function declines rapidly early in the disease, followed by either stabilization over time or further progression to end-stage fibrotic lung disease. Approximately 20% of patients with active ILD progress to having symptomatic severe restrictive lung disease. Heart involvement is also common in dcSSc, but it is usually clinically silent until late in the disease course, remaining undiagnosed until heart failure or significant arrhythmias occur. Patients with dcSSc are at an increased risk for kidney involvement (scleroderma renal crisis), which usually occurs early in the disease course and represents a life-threatening complication in 10–15% of patients (4). In most patients, after the first 4 years from the first non-Raynaud's symptom or sign, the disease process appears to stabilize without new organ involvement. However, the aggregated tissue and organ damage cause significant morbidity or decreased survival.

Limited Cutaneous SSc

Limited cutaneous SSc presents with a more benign course than dcSSc. In most patients, skin sclerosis remains limited to the fingers (sclerodactyly) and will not extend above the elbow or knees or involve the trunk (excluding the face). Although Raynaud's phenomenon is often present for years before the diagnosis, sudden worsening of the Raynaud's or new ischemic digital ulcers can herald development of new systemic signs or symptoms. A subset of lcSSc patients (rarely also in dcSSc) develops macrovascular disease with occlusive thrombotic events leading to critical digital ischemia, gangrene, and finger loss. Numerous dilated vascular skin lesions (telangiectasias) are commonly present over the fingers, face, and lips of lcSSc patients; they tend to increase in numbers and size over the lifetime of the patient. There is an increased prevalence of calcinosis, characterized by subcutaneous calcium deposits accumulating in areas of friction, trauma, or ischemia (fingers, forearms, elbows, knees, etc.). The skin overlying these areas is prone to develop hard-to-heal ulcerations caused by migration of the calcium to the surface (spontaneously or following minor trauma) that frequently are complicated by superimposed tissue infections. Similar to patients with dcSSc, GI disease is common in lcSSc with symptoms of dysphagia, gastroesophageal reflux, or changes in bowel habits. A variant of lcSSc called the CREST syndrome (subcutaneous **C**alcinosis, **R**aynaud's phenomenon, **E**sophageal dysmotility, **S**clerodactyly, and **T**elangiectasias) is associated with the presence of anticentromere antibodies and overall has a good prognosis. Isolated pulmonary arterial hypertension (PAH) can develop in ~15% of lcSSc patients and is the primary manifestation associated with poor outcome and shortened survival among these patients (5). Interestingly, PAH has a particular association with the presence of specific autoantibodies, including anticentromere antibodies.

ASSESSMENT AND DIAGNOSIS

The earliest symptoms of SSc are usually nonspecific and include fatigue, diffuse body aches, arthralgias, joint stiffness, cold sensitivity (Raynaud's phenomenon), swelling of fingers, and heartburn (Table 2). Because these complaints are common among patients in the primary care setting, the proper diagnosis of SSc is frequently overlooked. Many other diseases share symptoms and signs that are similar to the early presentation of SSc (Table 3). A delay in recognizing SSc can affect the treatment decisions that may impact disease progression or development of preventable complications. It is therefore very important for the health care provider to recognize the early stages of the disease.

When Should SSc Be Suspected?

Raynaud's phenomenon is a major and early symptom of SSc but it also occurs in ~3–5% of the general population, and in up to 15% of healthy young women (6). It is characterized by recurrent episodes of digital and cutaneous vasoconstriction triggered by cold or emotional stress. As a consequence of rapid changes in blood flow, the skin over the fingers shows characteristic color changes such as pallor (ischemic phase), cyanosis (hypoxic phase), and redness (hyperemic phase). Raynaud's phenomenon is defined as primary when no other associated disease process is detected (Table 4). A small percentage (10–20%) of patients presenting with what appears to be primary Raynaud's will eventually progress into having a more well-defined connective tissue disorder. Clinical clues for the possibility of an existing underlying rheumatic diagnosis (secondary Raynaud's) are onset of symptoms at age >20 years, male sex, asymmetric distribution,

Table 2. Early systemic sclerosis manifestations

- Constitutional symptoms: weight loss, arthralgias, myalgias
- Raynaud's phenomenon
- Heartburn and gastroesophageal reflux symptoms
- Abnormal nailfold capillaries (dilatation, capillary loss)
- Swelling of finger and hands
- Hyper or hypopigmentary skin changes
- New telangiectasias
- Tight or thick skin

Table 3. Differential diagnosis of systemic sclerosis at the time of presentation

- Primary Raynaud's phenomenon
- Other autoimmune diseases
    Systemic lupus erythematosus
    Rheumatoid arthritis
    Sjögren's syndrome
    Polymyositis, dermatomyositis
- Other fibrosing skin disease
    Scleromyxedema
    Scleredema
    Nephrogenic fibrosing dermopathy
    Eosinophilic fasciitis
    Graft versus host disease
    Generalized morphea
    Eosinophilia-myalgia syndrome
    Amyloidosis
    Bleomycin exposure
    Porphyria cutanea tarda
    Chronic reflex sympathetic dystrophy
- Chronic edema or lymphedema
- Malignant hypertension (scleroderma renal crisis "sine scleroderma")
- Paraneoplastic

worsening of painful attacks, presence of abnormal nailfold capillaries (i.e., capillary loss, dilated capillary loops), and the association with digital ischemic complications. Skin changes are a major feature that distinguishes scleroderma from other disorders. Therefore, other manifestations warranting further investigation are unexplained skin edema with increasing tightness; pain and itching involving the distal portion of extremities; rapid progression over weeks of skin thickening; new development of telangiectasias, especially on the fingertips and mucous membranes; and progression of skin changes on the extremities and face. Local skin and soft-tissue inflammation in the hands or wrists can cause or mimic carpal tunnel syndrome.

What Steps Prove a Working Diagnosis?

Physical examination. The patient should be completely examined, undressed, with a focus on recognizing the typical pattern of distribution and the characteristics of skin changes. The distal portion of the fingers (from metacarpophalangeal joints down) is invariably involved (Figure 1A). The skin is thickened and loses its elasticity; distal areas of the limbs and the face are affected first. When proximal spreading is present, the antecubital areas of the arm and midback are usually spared. Pigmentary changes are common, with darkening (pseudoacanthosis) or lightening (vitiligo-like, "salt and pepper") of the normal skin color. Visualization of nailfold capillaries by microscopy reveals the presence of dilated capillary loops, loss of capillaries, or focal areas of hemorrhages (Figure 1B). These changes can be seen when Raynaud's phenomenon is the only clinical manifestation. Telangiectasias (dilated capillaries) are present early but may be detectable only on the mucosal membranes of the lips, oral cavity, or palate. Eventually, they can also be seen on the fingertips and palms, and later in the disease they appear on the extremities and trunk. Areas of trauma such as the finger pads, elbows, and extensor surface of forearms should be examined for calcinosis. Digital "pits" are small atrophic areas on the fingertips that are a consequence of vascular disease and digital ischemia.

General laboratory screening. Scleroderma is an autoimmune disease and virtually all SSc patients have antinuclear antibodies (ANA). Although a positive ANA is nonspecific, when present at high titer and with a specific immunofluorescence pattern (centromere) or in association with specific autoantibodies, such as anti–topoisomerase I (Scl-70), this supports the diagnosis of SSc. Inflammatory parameters (erythrocyte

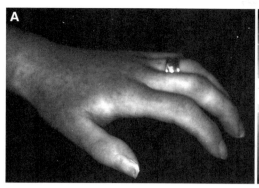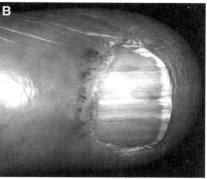

Figure 1. **A,** Fingers distal to the metacarpophalangeal joints are invariably involved in scleroderma. **B,** Visible capillary changes at the nailfold.

sedimentation rate, C-reactive protein), complete blood count, basic metabolic panel, urinalysis, thyroid function testing, and markers to investigate other overlap autoimmune disorders (e.g., rheumatoid factor, anti–cyclic citrullinated peptide antibodies, serum protein electrophoresis, muscle enzymes) are helpful to define the appropriate diagnosis and to determine specific organ involvement.

Prompt referral. Referral for specialty evaluation should not be delayed. Practitioners familiar with SSc can assist in providing a more clear diagnosis in uncertain cases, as well as a better prognostic and phenotypic characterization. Furthermore, given the uncommon nature of SSc, referral to academic centers specializing in scleroderma care and research may be very useful to establish a comprehensive, team-oriented, multidisciplinary management plan and to access the newest available therapies.

Skin biopsy. The diagnosis of scleroderma can be made by clinical examination. A skin biopsy is usually not required, but may be indicated when the overall presentation suggests another fibrosing skin disease (i.e., NFD, eosinophilic fasciitis, or amyloidosis).

Once the Diagnosis Is Proved, What Is the Routine Baseline Assessment?

A comprehensive baseline assessment is very important for 2 main reasons. First, internal organ involvement can be clinically silent at the time of diagnosis. Second, a baseline comparison of functional or imaging studies is often the only way to determine disease activity or the degree of organ dysfunction or progression of the disease overall.

Specific laboratory assessment. Serologic profiling should be completed with anti–Scl-70 and anticentromere antibodies. These are specifically associated with ILD and PAH, respectively, and therefore

have some predictive value. Other autoantibodies have been associated with specific clinical manifestations of SSc (Table 5) but most are not yet commercially available (7). Kidney function should be carefully evaluated to detect early signs of renal involvement. A renal crisis is suspected when malignant hypertension is present. However, SSc renal disease without hypertension is possible, particularly in the setting of overlap autoimmune disease. Measurement of muscle enzymes (creatine kinase, aldolase, alanine aminotransferase, aspartate aminotransferase) is recommended to exclude inflammatory or fibrosing muscle disease. Assessment of thyroid function (thyroid stimulating hormone) is also important because autoimmune thyroid disease is frequently associated with SSc. In subjects with severe Raynaud's phenomenon and ischemic manifestations, prothrombotic factors should be evaluated, such as anticardiolipin antibodies and homocysteine levels.

Pulmonary function tests (PFTs). PFTs, including total lung capacity (TLC), forced vital capacity (FVC), forced expiratory volume in 1 second (FEV_1), and diffusing capacity for carbon monoxide (DLco) are sensitive parameters to detect early lung involvement and to follow lung function over time. A decrease of TLC, FVC, and FEV_1 (<80% of predicted) suggest restrictive lung disease typical of ILD. A decline in DLco can be secondary to ILD or scleroderma vascular disease in the lung. When the DLco progressively declines out of proportion to changes in the lung volumes, pulmonary vascular disease or PAH should be suspected. PFTs are very sensitive for detecting lung disease and they should be performed routinely at baseline and yearly thereafter.

2-D Echocardiogram. Estimating the right ventricular systolic pressure (RVSP) using 2-D echocardiogram is a useful noninvasive tool to screen for PAH. However, this test is highly operator-dependent and poses a risk for false-negative or false-positive results. Nevertheless, studies have demonstrated that a 2-D echocardiogram-estimated RVSP of ≥40 mmHg had a positive predictive value of 92% and a negative predictive value of 44% for the diagnosis of PAH (8). The 2-D echocardiogram also provides important information about left ventricle function (hypertrophy, dyskynesis, dyastolic dysfunction) and possible pericardial effusion. Yearly 2-D echocardiogram is recommended in SSc patients to detect early changes.

When Is Invasive Testing Indicated?

Some clinical scenarios require invasive testing to establish an accurate diagnosis of organ involvement and to institute appropriate treatment for people with SSc.

Bronchoalveolar lavage (BAL). Declining respiratory function and detection of ground-glass opacities with underlying lung fibrosis

Table 4. Primary versus secondary Raynaud's phenomenon

Primary	Secondary*
Usually women or girls	Adult onset
Teenagers (around menarche)	Women but also men
Bilateral and symmetric	Asymmetric (dominant fingers)
No ischemic complications	Ischemic complications (ulcers, necrosis)
Normal nailfold capillaries	Loss of nailfold capillaries and dilated loops

* Raynaud's may be secondary to other autoimmune diseases, neoplasms, vasculitis, Burger's disease, cryoglobulinemia, cold agglutinin disease, hyperviscosity syndromes, atheroembolic disease, thoracic outlet syndrome, hand-arm vibration syndrome, hypothyroidism, or drug-induced (e.g., diphenhydramine, bleomycin, cisplatin, vinblastine, etc.).

Table 5. Autoantibody/phenotype association in systemic sclerosis

Antigen	Subtype	Clinical phenotype
Topoisomerase I (Scl-70)	Diffuse	Pulmonary fibrosis, cardiac involvement, and cancer
RNA polymerase III	Diffuse	Severe skin involvement, renal crisis
Centromere proteins B, C	Limited (CREST)	Ischemic digital loss, sicca symptoms
U3-RNP (fibrillarin, Mpp 10, hU3-55K)	Diffuse or limited	Pulmonary arterial hypertension, cardiac and skeletal muscle involvement
B23	Diffuse or limited	Pulmonary arterial hypertension, lung disease
Th/To-RNP	Limited	Lung disease, small bowel involvement, renal crisis
PM-Scl	Overlap	Myositis
U1-RNP	Diffuse or limited	SLE, myositis, polyarthritis

CREST = calcinosis, Raynaud's phenomenon, esophageal dysfunction, sclerodactyly, telangiectasia syndrome; RNP = ribonucleoprotein protein; SLE = systemic lupus erythematosus. Reprinted with permission from reference 7.

by chest high-resolution computed tomography may be indicative of active ILD. An elevated total cell count in BAL fluid with increased proportion of neutrophils (>3%) or eosinophils (>2%) is considered evidence for active alveolitis, warranting initiation of immunosuppressive treatment. Patients with normal BAL results or fibrosis alone may have inactive disease that requires only supportive care.

Right heart catheterization. In symptomatic patients, bedside clinical examination and noninvasive testing may under- or overestimate the presence of PAH. Therefore, to start treatment, a right heart catheterization is recommended to provide a more definitive diagnosis, to accurately assess severity, and also to obtain an estimate of cardiac function.

Kidney biopsy. The most worrisome SSc-related kidney manifestation is renal crisis. This complication should be suspected in a patient with early dcSSc (<3 years) who presents with refractory hypertension, impending renal failure, thrombocytopenia, proteinuria, or microhematuria. A kidney biopsy may help to define the type of renal involvement, since a proportion of SSc patients may have other causes of renal failure, including immune complex-mediated disease.

How Should Office Visits Be Structured?

Initial encounter. The goal of the initial evaluation is to confirm the diagnosis, to define the type of SSc, and to identify the organs and

systems affected. Careful characterization of the specific clinical features in SSc patients is essential for prognostic purposes and to design the most appropriate, individualized treatment strategy. Outside records should be carefully reviewed. If the diagnosis is secured, time should be devoted to educate the patient about the nature, clinical characteristics, and possible outcomes of the disease, encouraging patients to take notes and ask questions. Frequent misconceptions about SSc (e.g., it is an untreatable, fatal disease) should be addressed. It is important to understand the potential psychosocial burden of the disease for patients and their families. An altered self image (SSc can be disfiguring), chronic pain, sexual dysfunction, and a lack of adequate professional or family support all contribute to disrupted quality of life in SSc patients, with depression and social isolation as unfortunate consequences. These problems may not be overtly evident. A good relationship between health care providers and patients can identify these factors promptly. A comprehensive plan of care may include organ-specific treatment options and referral to pertinent specialists, such as pulmonologists, gastroenterologists, plastic surgeons, and physical therapists. SSc can be a very complex disease with serious complications and, for this reason, a team approach is important to establish an effective management program.

Subsequent visits. Regular visits with rheumatology health care professionals are very important to review routine testing (PFTs, 2-D echocardiogram) and to monitor for subjective or objective signs and symptoms suggestive of disease activation or progression. For example, unexplained high blood pressure, a recent decrease in respiratory performance, progressive weight loss, or new-onset diarrhea can all be clinical clues of specific SSc-related complications. Furthermore, the extent of scleroderma cutaneous involvement and its progression can only be assessed accurately by sequential bedside examinations. A scleroderma skin score (0 = normal and 3 = very thick) is used to follow progression by pinching the skin in 17 specific areas for a maximum score of 51 (9). SSc is a chronic systemic disease with most of the related clinical problems unremitting or recurrent with periodic exacerbations (e.g., Raynaud's phenomenon, digital ulcers, gastrointestinal motility disturbances). For this reason, easy accessibility to the health care team and prompt attention when acute problems develop are crucial for optimal care of SSc patients.

Nursing Considerations in Systemic Sclerosis

Nursing is an integral part of the team approach to effectively manage patients with systemic sclerosis (SSc). Nurses in this specialty should expect to perform case management duties such as:

- Educate patients and their family about SSc and related conditions. This should include suggestions on lifestyle modifications. Expect to provide ongoing support through disease course.
- Explain safe and correct use of prescribed medications, administration techniques, and monitoring procedures (e.g., immunosupressive agents)
- Administer questionnaires or specific disease-related scales (i.e., symptoms, pain, etc.) to assist with management and treatment plan
- Handle visits for minor issues (i.e., blood pressure adjustment, wound care)
- Coordinate multidisciplinary approach between different specialists
- Coordinate hospital admissions and home care
- Monitor functional, radiographic, and laboratory testing

TREATMENT

Therapy in SSc patients is mostly focused on organ-specific processes rather than on a global disease-modifying strategy. To date, no drug has been shown in a controlled clinical trial to change the overall course of the disease process.

Skin

The use of immunosuppressive treatments in *early active* dcSSc has been advocated to stop the autoimmune inflammatory response, which fuels the initiation and progression of the fibrosing skin process. Benefits on the skin have been reported with immunosuppressive drugs such as cyclophosphamide, mycophenolate mofetil, cyclosporine, methotrexate, thalidomide, intravenous immunoglobulin, and antithymocyte globulin. Toxicities are the major concern with all these medications, and more rigorous randomized controlled studies are necessary to confirm their usefulness. Multicenter trials of immunoablative therapy with high-dose cyclophospamide with or without stem-cell rescue are also underway. During the early inflammatory phase of the disease, the use of antihistamine drugs to control itching, and nonsteroidal antiinflammatory drugs (NSAIDs) or narcotic medications to control pain are often necessary. Routine skin care with daily emollients and protection from trauma or cuts are also important.

Raynaud's Phenomenon

The initial approach to Raynaud's should include avoidance of cold exposure, emotional stressors, cigarette smoking (active and passive), digital trauma (vibratory), and vasoconstrictive drugs (e.g., decongestants such as pseudoephedrine). Calcium-channel blockers (amlodipine, nifedipine) remain the first-line therapy. Other drugs reported to be helpful include angiotensin II receptor blockers (losartan), phosphodiesterase inhibitors (sildenafil, pentoxifylline), selective serotonin reuptake inhibitors (fluoxetine), alpha-1 adrenergic receptor blockers (prazosin), and nitrates (topical nitroglycerine). In recent clinical trials, endothelin-1 receptor inhibitors (bosentan) reduced the frequency of digital ulcers in SSc patients. Intravenous prostaglandins (epoprostenol) can be very effective in the early phase of critical digital ischemia. Local nerve sympathectomy can be considered when digital ischemic events are not responsive to medical therapy; however, the benefits are usually not permanent.

Interstitial Lung Disease

When active lung involvement (alveolitis) is detected, an immunosuppressive medication should be considered. A recent trial comparing daily oral cyclophosphamide versus placebo showed stabilization of lung function and an improvement in respiratory symptoms (10). Corticosteroids alone do not appear to be effective for SSc-related ILD. Lung transplant is an option for patients with life-threatening end-stage lung disease.

Pulmonary Hypertension

Routine management of PAH includes diuretic therapy and oxygen supplementation to maintain arterial oxygen saturation above 90%. Anticoagulation, indicated in severe cases, should be used with caution in SSc patients due to the risk of gastrointestinal bleeding. Vasodilator treatment should be initiated soon after PAH is confirmed by right heart catheterization. Several agents improve quality of life and exercise tolerance and, hopefully, may also prolong survival. Selective (sitaxsentan) and nonselective (bosentan) endothelin-1 receptor inhibitors or 5-phosphodiesterase inhibitors (sildenafil, tadalafil) can be used alone or in combination as initial therapy. Intravenous prostacyclin analogs (epoprostenol, treprostinil) can be added or used alone in severe cases. Recently, inhaled prostacyclin (iloprost) has been used in worsening or refractory cases.

Rehabilitation Considerations in Systemic Sclerosis

Limited joint motion (associated with flexion contractures)
- Activity program to prevent disuse contractures
- Finger stretching exercises (i.e., interphalangeal joint extension, "prayer position")
- Joint range of motion (e.g., shoulders and hips)
- Stretching exercise, hold for 30 seconds; slow gentle stretches

Muscular wasting (particularly shoulder girdles, deltoid muscles)
- Strengthening and isotonic exercises; progressive program
- General conditioning; monitor vitals and consider interval training as a means to build endurance

Pain management (chronic pain)
- Aerobic activities
- Coached, graded conditioning exercises
- Heat (e.g., paraffin baths)
- Biofeedback

Assistive devices (for activities of daily living)
- Custom-made handles for utensils (use and manipulation)
- Personal hygiene (e.g., bathing tools)
- Dressing (e.g., button hooks)
- Education about assistance (to patients and family members)

Rehabilitation
- After specific surgical interventions (e.g., wound care, joint replacement)
- Emotional and motivational supportt

Gastrointestinal Tract

Gastroesophageal reflux symptoms are among the earliest and most common complaints in SSc patients, requiring use of proton-pump inhibitors (omeprazole) or histamine H_2 receptor antagonists (ranitidine). Prokinetic drugs, including dopamine antagonists (metoclopramide, domperidone), erythromycin, and the newer serotonin (5-HT$_4$) receptor partial agonists (tegaserod) are useful in treating GI motility disturbances. Octreotide has been helpful in severe cases with pseudoobstruction. Persistent diarrhea secondary to malabsorption and bacterial overgrowth is usually responsive to rotational antibiotic strategies (e.g., erythromycin, ciprofloxacin, metronidazole). The use of oral probiotics (i.e., *Lactobacillus* species, *Bifidobacterium* species) is under investigation. In patients with watermelon stomach, severe anemia may develop and repeated cauterizations of bleeding gastric mucosal capillaries may be necessary.

Kidney Involvement

Scleroderma renal crisis presenting with malignant hypertension is a medical emergency that requires immediate intervention with angiotensin converting enzyme inhibitors to prevent rapidly progressive renal failure.

Musculoskeletal System

SSc patients often complain of noninflammatory articular and muscular symptoms, sometimes resulting in severe chronic pain. Effective pain control with NSAIDs and, in some cases, narcotics should always be considered. Specific immunomodulatory therapy (i.e., corticosteroids, methotrexate, tumor necrosis factor inhibitors) is indicated only when concomitant inflammatory erosive arthritis or polymyositis are present.

REFERENCES

1. Mayes MD, Lacey JV Jr, Beebe-Dimmer J, Gillespie BW, Cooper B, Laing TJ, et al. Prevalence, incidence, survival, and disease characteristics of systemic sclerosis in a large US population. Arthritis Rheum 2003;48:2246–55.
2. LeRoy EC, Medsger TA Jr. Criteria for the classification of early systemic sclerosis. J Rheumatol 2001;28:1573–6.
3. Steen VD, Medsger TA Jr. Severe organ involvement in systemic sclerosis with diffuse scleroderma. Arthritis Rheum 2000;43:2437–44.
4. Steen VD. Scleroderma renal crisis. Rheum Dis Clin North Am 2003;29: 315–33.
5. Mukerjee D, St George D, Coleiro B, Knight C, Denton CP, Davar J et al. Prevalence and outcome in systemic sclerosis associated pulmonary arterial hypertension: application of a registry approach. Ann Rheum Dis 2003;62:1088–93.
6. Weinrich MC, Maricq HR, Keil JE, McGregor AR, Diat F. Prevalence of Raynaud phenomenon in the adult population of South Carolina. J Clin Epidemiol 1990;43:1343–9.
7. Harris ML, Rosen A. Autoimmunity in scleroderma: the origin, pathogenetic role, and clinical significance of autoantibodies. Curr Opin Rheumatol 2003;15:778–84.
8. Mukerjee D, St George D, Knight C, Davar J, Wells AU, Du Bois RM et al. Echocardiography and pulmonary function as screening tests for pulmonary arterial hypertension in systemic sclerosis. Rheumatology (Oxford) 2004;43:461–6.
9. Brennan P, Silman A, Black C, Bernstein R, Coppock J, Maddison P, et al. Reliability of skin involvement measures in scleroderma. The UK Scleroderma Study Group. Br J Rheumatol 1992;31:457–60.
10. Tashkin DP, Elashoff R, Clements PJ, Goldin J, Roth MD, Furst DE et al. Cyclophosphamide versus placebo in scleroderma lung disease. N Engl J Med 2006;354:2655–66.

CHAPTER

30

Vasculitis

PHILIP SEO, MD, MHS

In its simplest sense, the word *vasculitis* refers to the histologic finding of inflammation in blood vessel walls. When rheumatologists speak of vasculitis, however, they are generally referring to the clinical syndromes associated with this pathologic finding. These syndromes are also known as the *primary systemic vasculitides*. This chapter will provide a brief introduction to the primary systemic vasculitides, and highlight common themes regarding their diagnosis, evaluation, and management.

INCIDENCE

Worldwide, the incidence of primary systemic vasculitis is ~20 cases/million/year. This single statistic fails to capture the striking diversity of patients with these diseases. The epidemiology of primary systemic vasculitis is exceedingly complex, and varies greatly among different patient populations. Giant cell arteritis, for example, is the most common form of systemic vasculitis, but almost never occurs in patients younger than 50 years old. Henoch-Schönlein purpura and Kawasaki's disease, on the other hand, are primarily diseases of childhood. Behçet's disease is common in endemic regions (predominantly in the region of Europe and Asia previously known as the Silk Road), but is uncommon in the United States. These epidemiologic associations provide important (but largely untapped) clues to the pathogenesis of these diseases.

PATHOLOGY

Inflammatory destruction of blood vessels is the pathologic hallmark of vasculitis. Activation of the immune system near a blood vessel attracts white blood cells (particularly neutrophils), a process known as *chemotaxis*. The activated neutrophils infiltrate the blood vessel walls and degranulate, releasing toxic enzymes and free oxygen radicals into blood vessel walls. This process leads to destruction of neutrophils (*leukocytoclasis*) and blood vessel walls (*fibrinoid necrosis*). Together, these findings are highly characteristic of vasculitis.

Depending on the severity of the vascular injury and the underlying nature of the blood vessel involved, 1 of 2 responses may be observed. Localized inflammation may cause the blood vessel to scar and narrow as it heals. The resulting decrease in blood flow may lead to tissue ischemia or infarction. On the other hand, the blood vessel wall may weaken and dilate to form an aneurysm. If the blood vessel wall continues to weaken, it may rupture, leading to red blood cell extravasation or localized hemorrhage.

CLASSIFICATION

The most commonly used classification system categorizes the primary systemic vasculitides by the size of the blood vessel involved (Table 1). *Large-vessel vasculitis* affects the aorta and the great vessels

(including the subclavian, carotid, and axillary arteries). *Medium-vessel vasculitis* involves the main visceral arteries (such as the renal, hepatic, coronary, and mesenteric arteries). Capillaries, venules, and arterioles (typically in the lungs, kidneys, and skin) are targeted by *small-vessel vasculitis*. Small-vessel vasculitis is further subdivided to single out forms of vasculitis associated with antineutrophil cytoplasmic autoantibodies (ANCA).

This classification system provides a useful framework for approaching these diseases, but it is not perfect. Both large-vessel and small-vessel vasculitides can affect medium-sized blood vessels. Furthermore, up to half of patients with ANCA-associated vasculitis do not have detectable levels of ANCA. Nevertheless, when assessing a patient with vasculitis for the first time, deducing the size of the blood vessels involved may be an important first step toward making a diagnosis.

CLINICAL ASPECTS

Although these diseases are clinically diverse, some general observations can be made:

- Most forms of primary systemic vasculitis have a subacute onset, typically leading to several months of nonspecific symptoms (including arthralgias, myalgias, and neuralgias) before a diagnosis is made.
- Objective evidence of inflammation—either on examination or laboratory testing—should be present; subjective complaints of pain, regardless of intensity, are not reliable to establish a diagnosis or to follow disease activity.
- Most forms of primary systemic vasculitis affect more than one organ system. When a new diagnosis of vasculitis is established, the health care practitioner must ensure that all organ systems are assessed appropriately.

The specific manifestations of any particular form of vasculitis are largely dictated by the size of the blood vessel. Inflammation of large-caliber blood vessels (such as the aorta or subclavian artery) can impair blood flow to the head or extremities. Diminished blood flow in the subclavian or axillary arteries dampens peripherally measured blood pressure or pulse amplitude (a classic finding for large-vessel

Table 1. Examples of primary systemic vasculitis

Large-vessel vasculitis	Giant cell arteritis Takayasu's arteritis
Medium-vessel vasculitis	Polyarteritis nodosa Kawasaki disease
Small-vessel vasculitis	Cryoglobulinemic vasculitis Henoch-Schönlein purpura Hypersensitivity vasculitis
ANCA-associated vasculitis	Wegener's granulomatosis Microscopic polyangiitis Churg-Strauss syndrome

---

Rehabilitation Considerations for Vasculitis

- Even after vasculitis has been effectively treated, patients may continue to have difficulty ambulating.
- Foot drop may be caused by mononeuritis multiplex; quadriceps weakness, by glucocorticoid-induced myopathy; and impaired proprioception, by peripheral sensory neuropathy.
- Some forms of vasculitis may directly damage the eyes or inner ear, which may further impair mobility.
- Routine assessment for deep vein thrombosis or ischemia in the extremities is warranted.
- Particular attention should be paid to strengthening exercises for hip- or shoulder-girdle weakness in patients taking long-term corticosteroids.
- Monitor blood pressure before, during, and after exercise.
- Gradually increase intensity of dynamic strengthening exercises to enable patients to maximize physical function.

---

vasculitis). Furthermore, patients with large-vessel vasculitis may note that repetitive upper extremity motion leads to arm pain and early fatigue, a complaint known as arm claudication. Cerebrovascular accidents, the result of carotid artery involvement, can also be seen in large-vessel vasculitis.

Manifestations of small-vessel vasculitis are typically found in organs with prominent capillary beds, including the lungs, kidneys, and skin. Inflammation of small blood vessels can cause vessel rupture. When this occurs in the lungs, patients develop pulmonary hemorrhage, which can mimic multilobar pneumonia on a chest radiograph. In the kidneys, small-vessel inflammation leads to glomerulonephritis and impaired filtration, which manifests as red blood cell casts and proteinuria.

The manifestations of medium-vessel vasculitis are determined by the territories involved. Medium-vessel vasculitis that affects blood flow to the peroneal nerve, for example, may lead to an inability to dorsiflex at the ankle, a finding that is frequently described as a "foot drop." Ischemia of the radial nerve leads to an analogous problem at the wrist, producing a "wrist drop." Occlusion of a mesenteric artery may lead to mesenteric ischemia or bowel infarction, depending on the severity of the stenosis and the extent of collateral circulation. Occlusion of the renal artery may lead to kidney infarction (but not red blood cell casts or proteinuria, which are more characteristic of a small-vessel vasculitis).

Once the size of the blood vessels involved has been determined, one can attempt to diagnose the vasculitis itself. In general, the primary systemic vasculitides are stereotyped disorders that occur in recognizable patterns. For this reason, patients with giant cell arteritis frequently have temporal artery involvement, and present with a complaint of headache. Patients with Wegener's granulomatosis, on the other hand, generally have evidence of upper respiratory disease (such as chronic sinusitis or subglottic stenosis). Recognition of these patterns is the key to putting a name to a vasculitic syndrome.

DIAGNOSTIC STUDIES

Frequently, a biopsy is the most straightforward way of confirming a diagnosis of vasculitis. When multiple organs are involved, the most accessible organ should be biopsied first. Skin biopsies, for example, are low morbidity procedures, and histologic evidence of skin vasculitis, when accompanied by evidence of involvement in other organ systems, may be sufficient to confirm the presence of a primary systemic vasculitis.

Light microscopy will demonstrate evidence of immune-mediated destruction of blood vessels. Direct immunofluorescence may help demonstrate the actual mechanism of injury. For example, IgM and C3 deposition are characteristic of cryoglobulinemia, whereas IgA deposition is seen in Henoch-Schönlein purpura. The presence of multiple immunoreactants on a biopsy is suggestive of systemic lupus erythematosus (SLE), whereas the absence of immunoreactants suggests a pauci-immune vasculitis, such as those generally associated with ANCA.

Laboratory testing may provide useful ancillary information for the diagnosis and monitoring of patients with primary systemic vasculitis. Although there is no specific serology that can be used to confirm the presence of vasculitis, blood tests may be useful to exclude other diseases that may be associated with vasculitis. Blood tests will generally demonstrate evidence of generalized inflammation. Acute phase reactants, such as the erythrocyte sedimentation rate and the C-reactive protein, will almost always be elevated in a patient with untreated vasculitis. Routine tests may also provide evidence of systemic inflammation. It would not be uncommon to find evidence of leukocytosis, normocytic anemia, or thrombocytosis, all of which may represent a nonspecific response to inflammation.

Tests for ANCA are frequently ordered but, by themselves, do not confirm or exclude the presence of systemic vasculitis. ANCA are found only in a small subset of the vasculitides and, even among patients with a relevant diagnosis, are not always present in detectable amounts. If immunofluorescence demonstrates the presence of ANCA, this should be followed by a confirmatory enzyme-linked immunosorbent assay to demonstrate antibodies directed against myeloperoxidase or proteinase 3. Antibodies against other autoantigens (such as lactoferrin)—frequently referred to as "atypical ANCA"—are not associated with vasculitis.

Tests for serum cryoglobulins, a common cause of vasculitis, are notoriously difficult to obtain because the blood and blood-drawing apparatus must be kept warm until the blood clots. Failure to take this precaution is a frequent cause of false-negative results. In many patients with cryoglobulinemic vasculitis, the presence of cryoglobulins is reflected by a positive rheumatoid factor test. A very high titer of rheumatoid factor in a patient without rheumatoid arthritis may be an important clue to the presence of cryoglobulinemia.

Once the diagnosis of vasculitis has been established, routine blood and urine testing is vital for the long-term care of the patient. Frequently, a routine urinalysis may be the first clue to incipient glomerulonephritis, long before an increase in serum creatinine is noted. Routine blood counts are also useful for monitoring for the untoward effects of immunosuppressive agents, many of which can cause bone marrow suppression. Slowly rising acute phase reactants may provide an important clue to a vasculitis flare.

DIFFERENTIAL DIAGNOSIS

Because the physical findings associated with vasculitis are generally the result of blood vessel occlusion or stenosis, one must also consider other diagnoses that are associated with blood vessel occlusion when evaluating a patient for vasculitis. Cholesterol emboli, for example, may follow cardiac catheterization, and in some cases produce findings similar to those associated with a medium-vessel vasculitis. Subacute bacterial endocarditis may also be associated with both embolic events and evidence of chronic inflammation (in this case, from chronic infection), closely mimicking the findings associated with a systemic vasculitis. Hypercoagulability states, such as the antiphospholipid antibody syndrome, can lead to blood vessel occlusion, and may produce many signs and symptoms associated with primary systemic vasculitis.

In some cases, small-vessel vasculitis is a manifestation of another primary disorder. Many medications, including penicillins and sulfonamides, can lead to a drug-induced hypersensitivity vasculitis. In these cases, withdrawal of the offending medication is the only effective treatment strategy (although antiinflammatory or short-term immunomodulatory therapy may be required as well). Malignancy can be associated with atypical forms of vasculitis, as can several chronic infections, including hepatitis B, hepatitis C, and the human immunodeficiency virus. Finally, autoantibody and complement testing may be useful for detecting evidence of SLE, which can lead to a secondary form of vasculitis.

TREATMENT

When developing a treatment strategy for vasculitis, 3 goals should be considered simultaneously. The short-term goal of therapy is to halt the inflammation that leads to active disease. The intermediate-term goal is to prevent recurrence, which may lead to more damage and require more therapy. The long-term goal is to minimize the toxicity associated with prolonged therapy.

Standard therapy of a primary systemic vasculitis generally starts with glucocorticoids, such as prednisone or prednisolone. Even with modern advances in the treatment of these diseases, nothing else works as quickly to quell active vasculitis. Unfortunately, long-term treatment with glucocorticoids can lead to a number of untoward effects, including an increased risk of myocardial infarction, osteoporosis, avascular necrosis, hypertension, cataracts, muscle atrophy, and weight gain. For this reason, a second immunosuppressive (steroid-sparing) agent is frequently started at the same time. In this way, glucocorticoids may bring active disease under control rapidly, giving the second immunosuppressive agent time to become effective.

When selecting a steroid-sparing agent, it is important to "let the punishment fit the crime." In other words, the potency (and potential toxicity) of the medication should be commensurate with the potential of the vasculitis to cause harm. For example, Henoch-Schönlein purpura is a form of small-vessel vasculitis that is typically mild and self limited, and may require no more than a short course of glucocorticoids and observation. Life-threatening forms of vasculitis, however, are typically treated with a cytotoxic drug, such as cyclophosphamide.

Although cyclophosphamide is a standard therapy for severe forms of vasculitis, it is not without risk. Cyclophosphamide can lead to hemorrhagic cystitis, bone marrow suppression, infertility, and opportunistic infection (especially *Pneumocystis* pneumonia). Long-term treatment with cyclophosphamide is associated with an increased risk of malignancy, in particular lymphoma and bladder cancer. For that reason, the modern approach to the treatment of severe forms of vasculitis entails a short course of cyclophosphamide, typically 3–6 months, followed by a longer course of treatment with an antimetabolite, such as methotrexate, azathioprine, or mycophenolate mofetil. It is not uncommon to treat non–life-threatening forms of vasculitis with antimetabolites alone, to reduce lifetime exposure to cytotoxic drugs.

Unfortunately, antimetabolite medications are also associated with risk. Less than 1% of Americans lack functional thiopurine methyltransferase (TPMT), which is critical for the metabolism of azathioprine. In patients with TMPT deficiency, administration of azathioprine can lead to significant drug accumulation, bone marrow suppression, and attendant morbidity. TPMT testing is now routinely available, and should be performed prior to initiating this medication. Both azathioprine and mycophenolate mofetil can be associated with nausea that may preclude increasing the drug to therapeutic levels. In the case of mycophenolate mofetil, this can sometimes be avoided by increasing the frequency of administration, which decreases the total concentration of proemetic metabolites present at any one time. Methotrexate should not be taken with alcohol or medications that can cause liver dysfunction, and should always be taken with folate supplementation.

Nursing Considerations for Vasculitis

• Educate patients on cyclophosphomide:
  – Be aware that alopecia (reversible) may occur
  – Increase fluid intake to avoid hemorrhagic cystitis and keep uric acid level normal
  – Report any unusual bruising or bleeding
• Educate patients on glucocorticoids:
  – Never abruptly discontinue medication
  – Advise patient of cushingoid effects
  – Monitor for hypertension
  – Monitor for depression

MINIMIZING RISKS OF THERAPY

It is important to consider proactively the potential untoward effects of therapy. This is especially important because the immunosuppressive agents used to treat vasculitis are generally needed for months to years; fast tapers and abbreviated courses of medications may increase the risk of disease flare, which ultimately increases exposure to these potentially toxic medications.

Patients who are treated with cyclophosphamide should undergo routine laboratory testing (including urinalysis) to look for early evidence of bone marrow suppression or hemorrhagic cystitis. Patients who have previously been exposed to cyclophosphamide should be monitored particularly carefully, as their bone marrow may be less resilient to the effects of cytotoxic medications. For many patients, particularly those being treated with cytotoxic medications or who have a history of pulmonary compromise, *Pneumocystis* prophylaxis may be warranted.

The list of side effects associated with chronic glucocorticoid use is daunting. Glucocorticoid-induced osteoporosis is a significant concern, and should be treated prophylactically with calcium and vitamin D supplementation, as well as bisphosphonates or other drugs as warranted. Glucocorticoid-induced myopathy is also an important consideration. The fatigue, arthralgias, and myalgias experienced by some patients with vasculitis—even when the disease is no longer active—is sometimes attributable to glucocorticoid-induced myopathy and disuse atrophy, all of which may respond slowly to gradually increasing levels of physical activity and decreasing glucocorticoid exposure. Psychiatric manifestations, ranging from depression to mania, may appear during treatment with glucocorticoids, and it is important to assess patients actively for such complaints because they may not volunteer such information. Antidepressants and other medications may be useful for managing the psychiatric complications of high-dose glucocorticoids until they can be tapered safely.

WHEN TO CALL THE DOCTOR

When a patient with vasculitis develops a new sign or symptom, determining whether it is due to the underlying vasculitis is not always straightforward. Infectious diseases may closely mimic many of the manifestations of primary systemic vasculitis. For example, a new cavitary pulmonary nodule could be the result of a fungal infection or Wegener's granulomatosis; similarly, arthralgias may be caused by a viral infection or may herald a vasculitis relapse. This issue becomes particularly challenging when a patient has been treated with immunosuppressive therapies that may mask an infection, or alter its presentation. For that reason, prior to treating a "vasculitis flare," it is always wise to consult with someone who is experienced in the assessment of these protean diseases.

SUMMARY

The primary systemic vasculitides are among the most challenging of the rheumatic diseases. They are primarily diagnosed on clinical grounds, although biopsy can be useful to confirm one's clinical suspicion. Laboratory testing by itself is not sufficient to confirm or refute the presence of a systemic vasculitis, but it can be valuable to exclude mimics of vasculitis. Lab work is also used to follow patients longitudinally for flare and for the untoward effects of medications. Treatment choices should reflect the severity of the vasculitis, because there are risks associated with both overtreatment and undertreatment. Finally, for many patients, the side effects of therapy may be worse than the disease itself. Vigilant monitoring for the untoward effects of glucocorticoids (especially diabetes, osteoporosis, myopathy, and opportunistic infection) is vital to preserve overall health and quality of life.

Recommended Reading

Jennette JC, Falk RJ, Andrassy K, Bacon PA, Churg J, Gross WL, et al. Nomenclature of systemic vasculitides: proposal of an international consensus conference. Arthritis Rheum 1994;37:187–92.

Scott DG, Watts RA. Systemic vasculitis: epidemiology, classification and environmental factors. Ann Rheum Dis 2000;59:161–3.

Seo P, Stone JH. Large-vessel vasculitis. Arthritis Rheum 2004;15:128–39.

Seo P, Stone JH. The antineutrophil cytoplasmic antibody-associated vasculitides. Am J Med 2004;117:39–50.

American College of Rheumatology classification criteria for vasculitis. Accessed July 4, 2006. URL: http://www.rheumatology.org/publications/classification/index.asp?aud=mem.

SECTION C: CLINICAL INTERVENTIONS

<table>
<tr><td>CHAPTER
31</td><td></td></tr>
</table>

CHAPTER 31

Self-Management Education and Support

TERESA J. BRADY, PhD, and MICHELE L. BOUTAUGH, BSN, MPH

Over the past decade there has been increasing recognition of the importance of self-management in the control of arthritis. According to American College of Rheumatology (ACR) guidelines, patient education and self-management programs are first-line nonpharmacologic treatments for the management of hip and knee osteoarthritis (OA), and rheumatoid arthritis (RA) (1,2). Similarly, *Healthy People 2010*, the United States' health objectives for 2010, includes an objective to increase the proportion of people with arthritis who receive evidence-based arthritis education as an integral part of their condition management (3). Although references to self-management are increasing, the term is frequently used interchangeably with patient education and with a specific form of self-management education, the Arthritis Self-Management Program (ASMP). This chapter will differentiate self-management, self-management support, and self-management education; review evidence on the impact of evidence-based arthritis education programs; and describe practical strategies for providing self-management support in clinical practice.

DEFINITIONS AND CONCEPTUAL CLARITY

There are many definitions of self-management in the literature; most definitions focus on tasks or behaviors, such as exercise, healthy eating, and appropriate medication use, necessary to live with a chronic condition. This chapter adopts the definitions of self-management and self-management support specified by the Institute of Medicine (4). The concept of self-management support is 1 of the 6 essential elements of high-quality chronic care according to Wagner's chronic care model, and self-management education is one form of self-management support (5). Table 1 lists complete definitions (4–6). Some, but not all, patient-education activities are designed to foster patient self-management. Traditional patient education that focuses primarily on transmitting information has less impact than forms of education that focus on helping patients incorporate behavior change into their lifestyles. Self-management education, designed to enhance patient self-management and foster behavior change, uses behavioral techniques to increase

patients' confidence (i.e., self-efficacy) and skills in day-to-day management of their arthritis. A meta-analysis of patient education clinical trials demonstrated that interventions including behavioral techniques produced greater changes in pain, functional disability, and tender joints than interventions that rely solely on information dissemination (7).

In short, although self-management (performing the tasks necessary to live well with one or more conditions) is the responsibility of the patient, self-management support (the provision of education and supportive interventions to increase patients' skill and confidence in managing their health problem) is the responsibility of the health care system and providers.

TYPES OF ARTHRITIS-EDUCATION PROGRAMS

Education to foster self-management can be provided through group classes or individualized instruction delivered by lay leaders or health professionals. Such programs may be combined with telephone support, print materials, exercise interventions, or cognitive behavioral therapy. (Chapter 33 describes cognitive-behavioral interventions, which will not be reviewed in this chapter.) Alternative delivery formats, such as mailed or internet-based home-study programs are showing promise. Table 2 describes common types and key features of arthritis education interventions.

SUCCESSFUL GROUP EDUCATION MODELS

Arthritis Self-Management Program (ASMP)

The pioneering group-education program is the ASMP developed by Lorig and colleagues at Stanford University. The 6-week class series is designed to be delivered in community settings by a pair of trained lay leaders who follow a standardized curriculum to enhance self-efficacy. In the United States, the Arthritis Foundation has been

Table 1. Definitions

Term	Definition
Self-management	The tasks that the individuals must undertake to live well with one or more chronic conditions. These tasks include having the confidence to deal with medical management, role management, and emotional management of their conditions (4).
Self-management support	The systematic provision of education and supportive interventions by health care staff to increase patients' skills and confidence in managing their health problems, including regular assessment of progress and problems, goal setting, and problem-solving support (4).
Patient education	Planned, organized learning experiences designed to facilitate voluntary adoption of behaviors or beliefs conducive to health (5).
Self-management education	Educational interventions specifically designed to enhance patient self-management. Self-management education focuses on building generalizable skills, such as decision-making, problem-solving, and self-monitoring (7).

Table 2. Types of educational interventions and programs

Type/ References	Characteristics	Capabilities/Advantages	Limitations
Self-management group programs (8–20)	Group class series with sessions usually lasting about 2–2.5 hours for 5–7 weeks. Emphasis on interactive methods/ experiential learning and strategies to improve self-efficacy (via goal setting, action plans, feedback, use of positive role models, reinterpretation of symptoms, persuasion). Content focuses on how to adopt new behaviors and problem-solving skills.	Promotes peer support and problem-solving skills. Ideally taught by trained lay leaders who provide modeling and can be low cost. Efficient; able to educate up to 15 patients at a time. Solid evidence on effectiveness.	Time- and labor-intensive for course leaders and participants. Classes not always available in desired locations and times. Training required for course leaders. Some patients dislike groups. Not tailored to individual needs.
Individual/one-to-one instruction (23)	Verbal instruction by individual practitioner or team of health professionals. Typical content is disease and treatment information. Effectiveness can be enhanced if combined with other educational or behavioral strategies (e.g., use of print materials and other media/technology, demonstration and practice of recommended skills, telephone support, etc.).	Can be personalized to meet needs of patients. Can be individualized to patient's readiness to change. Can be incorporated into clinical practice.	Verbal instruction alone and leaflet alone have minimal impact beyond increased knowledge. Difficult to coordinate comprehensive education if multiple providers are involved.
Exercise/education classes (skill practice) (21, 22)	Group class series that includes exercise demonstration, practice, and educational discussion. May include self-efficacy–enhancing strategies, problem-solving discussions, and other activities to promote long-term maintenance of exercise.	Can be taught in community by fitness professionals. Ongoing class series can help support long-term behavior change. Promotes peer support.	Lack of availability. Requires commitment of facilities, course leaders, and participants to time-intensive activity.
Telephone support (23, 30, 53)	Proactive, structured telephone contacts by trained laypersons or professional counselors. Content may include monitoring of symptoms, medication adherence and side effects, barriers to medical care/appointment-keeping, and self-care activities.	Can be used to reinforce professional instruction and reduce face-to-face clinical encounters. Can be low-cost when delivered by lay persons. Evidence of effectiveness.	One-to-one contact can be labor-intensive. Lack of nonverbal cues reduces ability to gauge reactions of the patients and effectiveness of communication.
Mediated instruction/ technology based (26–29, 31, 32)	Can be delivered as home or self-study programs via mail or Internet. Format may include personalized, self-paced instruction using self-instructional workbooks and audiovisual aids, computer-assisted instruction with or without computer-tailored print materials, or Internet programs. Content may be focused on one issue (such as stress management or total joint replacement) or may include a variety of self-management and/or cognitive behavioral topics and strategies.	Can reduce need for professional time; can reinforce professional instruction. Alternative delivery modes allow for broad dissemination. Tailored content is more persuasive and effective. Internet models allow for peer interaction.	Cost varies depending upon the type of media used. Media can be costly and difficult to keep up to date. Some formats do not allow for peer support; may involve minimal human interaction.

disseminating the ASMP since 1981. The Stanford trials showed significant short-term improvements in self-efficacy, frequency of self-management behaviors, and pain. A 4-year followup study showed a persistent decrease in pain and reduction in physician visits, resulting in cost savings (8). The program has been successfully disseminated in the United Kingdom, Canada, the Netherlands, Australia, New Zealand, and Hong Kong. International replication studies have resulted in similar outcomes (9–11).

Chronic Disease Self-Management Program (CDSMP)

In an attempt to more efficiently and effectively support patients with multiple chronic conditions, Lorig and colleagues developed the CDSMP. Originally tested in people with arthritis, heart disease, lung disease, or stroke, this 6-week class series is also based on self-efficacy theory and taught by trained lay leaders. Compared with controls, class participants increased their self-efficacy, improved their health behaviors and health status (e.g., disability, fatigue, and health distress), and had fewer hospitalizations and hospital days at 6 months (12). At the 1-year and 2-year followup checks, participants continued to show significant improvements in their health distress and self-efficacy and had fewer physician and emergency room visits (13). Similar results were achieved when the program was replicated within the Kaiser-Permanente health system in the US (14) and in the UK (15) and China (16).

A study comparing the relative effectiveness of the ASMP and the generic CDSMP showed that both programs produced positive outcomes among people with arthritis. At 4 months, the ASMP participants demonstrated significantly greater improvement in health distress, activity limitation, and fatigue as compared with arthritis patients participating in CDSMP, although some of these differences were lost at 1 year. The authors concluded that the disease-specific course should be considered first when there is a sufficient arthritis patient base and resources, but that the generic chronic disease course is a reasonable alternative (17).

Spanish-Language Group Programs

Both the ASMP and the CDSMP have been adapted by Stanford for Spanish-speaking communities. Participants in the original controlled trial of the Spanish-language version of the ASMP demonstrated significant positive changes in self-efficacy, exercise, pain, general health, depression, and disability at 1 year (18). Similarly, a dissemination study showed significant improvements in self-efficacy and arthritis symptoms that were maintained at 6 months (19). Participants in the Hispanic CDSMP, 15% of whom had comorbid arthritis, demonstrated significant improvements in health behavior, health status, and self-efficacy, and had fewer emergency room visits at 4 months and 1 year (20).

Combination Exercise and Education Interventions

Several studies have examined the effects of combining education with exercise programs. A pilot study compared a combined self-management education and walking program to education alone. Both groups received a 12-week version of the ASMP. The walking group also received instruction in the use of a pedometer. The combination group showed a significant increase in walking steps, muscle strength, and walking speed as compared with the education-only group (21). Dutch investigators found that combining a peer-led ASMP course series with group exercises supervised by physical therapists resulted in improved self-efficacy and pain in people with knee OA (22).

INDIVIDUAL EDUCATION STRATEGIES

Individual one-to-one instruction plays an important role in improving patient knowledge, but to be effective in fostering self-management skills, it must incorporate self-efficacy–enhancing activities and reinforcement strategies, as described in the section on Enhancing Self-Management in Clinical Practice. For example, in inner-city patients with knee OA, a brief (30–60 minute) individualized learning session provided by an arthritis nurse specialist and supplemented by 2 followup telephone calls reduced knee pain and significantly improved functional status. These benefits persisted at 12 months along with a significant reduction in primary care visits (23).

Educational booklets may be a useful adjunct to other educational interventions, but are not considered a form of self-management education when used alone. Several studies demonstrated increased knowledge at 3-week and 6-month followups, but no change in health status was noted (24). A review of print interventions in chronic disease concluded that print interventions produce modest benefits at best (25).

Alternative Delivery Methods and Use of Technology

The need to reach broader audiences and maximize program cost-effectiveness has led to the development and testing of alternative methods of program delivery. Compared with usual care, a computer-tailored and mailed education program resulted in decreased disability, improved role function, and increased self-efficacy at 1 year with decreases in global severity and doctor visits and increased self-efficacy at 2 years (26). Compared with ASMP participants, the program showed greater decreases in disability and increases in self-efficacy at 1 year, but at 3 years the ASMP participants had better role function and fewer doctor visits (27). A similar mailed intervention with customized feedback was tested among managed care organization members; the arthritis study participants had increased self-efficacy, decreased visits, and improved health status at the 30-month followup (28). A computer-assisted instruction program was found to be effective in increasing appropriate use of medication and self-efficacy in patients with hip and knee OA (29).

Self-management education has also been delivered via telephone. In a small pilot study, subjects with OA received 6 weekly 45-minute telephone support sessions conducted by a nurse, weekly educational mailings adapted from the ASMP textbook, and a relaxation audiotape. Compared with a control group, study participants experienced significant 3-month improvement in self-efficacy, functional status, and depression (30).

Lorig and colleagues have developed an Internet-based version of the ASMP as well as an e-mail discussion group for people with back pain. Participants in the back pain program demonstrated improved pain, disability, and function and decreased physician visits (31); early data from the online ASMP also showed significant changes in health status (32).

IMPACT OF ARTHRITIS SELF-MANAGEMENT EDUCATION

There is a growing body of research showing that self-management education programs can have positive benefits on knowledge, self-efficacy, performance of self-management behaviors, and aspects of health status, although effect sizes are modest and benefits may not be long lasting. Two recent reviews examined self-management education programs across chronic diseases using meta-analysis, which allows investigators to calculate effect sizes as a standardized measure of treatment efficacy. Effect sizes of <0.2 are considered small, whereas effect sizes of >0.5 are considered large (33). One review of 24 arthritis studies found a very small trend toward improvements, with effect sizes of 0.12 in pain and 0.07 in disability (34). Another review included 18 OA studies and found statistically significant but clinically modest treatment effects on pain and function (35). A recent RA-specific Cochrane review examined the differential effects of 3 types of patient education interventions: information-only (verbal communication or informational brochures), counseling (social support and problem discussion), and behavioral change programs, such as the ASMP. Neither information-only nor counseling programs showed significant effects. Behavioral treatment programs showed small but significant short-term benefits with effect sizes ranging from 0.11 to 0.32. These included improvements in disability scores (10%), patient global assessment (12%), joint counts (9%), and depression (12%). However, these effects were short-lived—no significant benefits were found at final followup (36,37). An earlier meta-analysis of 34 arthritis studies reported effect sizes ranging from 0.28 to 0.56 for pain, depression, and functional status in patients with OA. Improvement in patients with RA was much less, with effect sizes up to 0.13 (38).

Additional research is needed to determine which components of self-management education are most efficacious, how to best integrate these interventions into clinical practice, and which populations will benefit most from these interventions. One trial of the ASMP in a primary care physician network failed to show significant benefits in class participants as compared with a group that received only the course textbook. The authors suggested that their contrasting results may be due to a less-motivated study population and concluded that more studies should be conducted in a variety of practice settings to determine how best to implement these interventions (39). Reimsma and colleagues have postulated that participant recruitment may explain differing effectiveness; studies done with participants recruited by public service announcement may be healthier and more motivated (40).

Cost-Effectiveness of Arthritis Education

There is some evidence that arthritis education can affect health care utilization and costs. Studies of the ASMP have demonstrated reduction of physician visits and costs (8,41). Participants in the CDSMP had lower hospitalization rates and made fewer visits to emergency rooms and physicians over the 2-year followup period, resulting in a conservative estimated savings of $590 per participant (13); a Chinese study showed similar cost-savings (16). Another cost-benefit study evaluated 3 different education and support interventions in contrast to a usual-care group. The usual-care group had significantly greater increases in health care costs at 1 year followup than did the 3 intervention groups; these differences were maintained at year 2 and year 3. The combined cost-benefit ratio of the 3 experimental interventions was $7.46 per dollar spent on the program costs (42). Reduced physician visits were also demonstrated with an intervention of a single educational session with telephone support (23).

ENHANCING SELF-MANAGEMENT IN CLINICAL PRACTICE

Structured self-management education programs, such as the ASMP, play a vital role in assisting patients to build their self-management skills. Equally important is the self-management support provided in routine clinical practice. The time-pressured clinician is unlikely to have the time and expertise to provide sophisticated behavior change interventions in the midst of routine clinical care, but simple behavioral counseling techniques can help patients enhance their self-management. Because of both their inherent credibility and ongoing relationships with patients, clinicians have a unique opportunity to assess patients' current beliefs and behaviors, provide and reinforce health information, assist with behavior change strategies, and assure ongoing followup. Although there is a multitude of behavior change theories, the 5 A's model, originally developed to guide smoking cessation interventions, offers a simple organizing framework to guide clinicians in providing self-management support in the midst of their routine practice.

Five Critical Activities

The 5 A's model identifies a pragmatic sequence of support activities (Assess, Advise, Agree, Assist, Arrange followup) useful to guide patients to formulate a personal action plan and to develop appropriate self-management skills. This 5-step approach can be tailored to support any of the key self-management behaviors useful in arthritis. The specific content in each step may change depending on whether the focus is weight control, exercise, or another behavior, but the clinician strategies can be organized within the 5 A's framework (43,44).

Glasgow and others have outlined the 5 A's of self-management support or behavioral counseling as: 1) **Assess:** Assess both current behaviors and beliefs, such as perceived importance of making a behavior change, confidence in ability to, and intention to change; 2) **Advise:** offer clear, specific, personalized advice on need to change, benefits of change, risk of not changing; 3) **Agree:** Using collaborative goal setting, negotiate a mutually agreeable, specific, and achievable action plan for change (see Action Plan below); 4) **Assist:** Aid the patient to develop the skills and confidence to achieve their action plan (i.e., by providing educational materials, referrals to community services such as ASMP, and social support); and 5) **Arrange followup:** successful behavior change requires ongoing support and assistance, in the form of referral to more intensive services and followup telephone contact to provide ongoing assistance and support. More specific details on the using the 5 A's framework are provided in Table 3.

Theory-Based Strategies to Enhance Self-Management in Clinical Practice

Self-management support capable of truly enhancing a patient's self-management skills is likely to require both brief interventions within the context of the clinical visit, such as the 5 A's, and more intensive interventions such as the ASMP or CDSMP outside of the clinical setting. Several theory-based strategies can be useful to clinicians providing brief interventions within clinical care, and to educators developing more intensive self-management education programs.

Match Approach to the Patient's Perspective. Effective education begins with the identification of the patients' perspective: their needs and problems, goals and expectations, and relevant health beliefs and practices (45). Because readiness to learn is usually oriented to current problems, eliciting patients' key concerns or problems allows the clinician to capitalize on teachable moments and to individualize the educational mes-

sages and recommendations. A patient whose main perceived problem is pain may be more likely to adopt a recommendation, such as participating in an exercise program, if it is framed as a way to help manage pain. The Assess section of Table 3 lists additional assessment questions.

Tailor Strategy to Patient's Readiness to Change. Although systematic reviews of stage-of-change interventions have produced equivocal results, many behavior change interventions are designed to accommodate patients with varying readiness to change (46). In a study of the readiness of RA or OA patients to adopt self-management strategies, 44% were categorized as "precontemplative" (not intending to take action in the foreseeable future), 11% "contemplative" (thinking about a change but undecided about when), and 22% in "preparation" (getting ready to take action). Another 6% were classified as being in "unprepared action" (those who were making overt changes in behavior but who had not really thought about or prepared for action), and 17% were in "maintenance" (47).

A simple way to gauge a patient's readiness to change is to ask whether they have ever considered doing the behavior, are thinking about changing, or are ready for action. Having this information allows the clinician to tailor recommendations, such as prescribing exercise. Detailed instruction about how to make exercising a regular habit is irrelevant to a patient in pre-contemplation; counseling time would be better spent raising awareness of the benefits of change. Table 4 identifies clinician actions tailored to the patient's readiness to change.

Facilitate Specific Written Action Plans. The 5 A's framework of brief counseling or self-management support is oriented toward assisting the patient to formulate a personal action plan; one of the primary skills emphasized in the ASMP and CDSMP is action planning. Similarly, a Cochrane review on asthma self-management concluded that a written action plan was a hallmark of successful interventions (48). Asking a patient to write down their goal and action steps can also strengthen their commitment to the plan. To be effective, action plans need to focus on patient-identified priorities, and the patient needs to specify the what, when, how, and how often of their plans. Identifying potential barriers and strategies to overcome those barriers can be a useful part of action planning. Patient-rating of their confidence (described below) is a crucial element of an action plan.

Build Self-Efficacy. Self-efficacy refers to an individual's belief or confidence in his or her ability to successfully perform a task or execute a behavior (49). Self-efficacy is related not only to improved health outcomes, such as pain, mood, self-rated health, and function, but also to a person's willingness to initiate a self-management behavior and persist in that behavior despite obstacles (49). The addition of self-efficacy–enhancing strategies to the ASMP increased the course's effectiveness (50). Self-efficacy–enhancing strategies can easily be incorporated into clinical practice within the context of the 5 A's framework.

Experiencing success, or skills mastery, requires that skills or behaviors be broken down into easily mastered components; these can be formulated into realistic short-term goals. Patients should set short-term goals just slightly above their current level of performance. Once patients have experienced success, incrementally more ambitious goals can be set. A crucial element of developing an achievable action plan is to ask the patient to rate, on a scale of 0–10, how confident they are that they can carry out their plan (0 = not at all sure, 10 = totally sure). If the confidence rating is <7, the plan should be modified to make it more achievable. Vicarious experience and persuasion can also be used to build self-efficacy, and can be accomplished though positive role models. People with arthritis who are successfully managing their condition can be used as lay instructors or mentors. Modeling also can be provided through the media and print materials by using visuals and real-life vignettes of people that represent the patient's age and ethnic diversity. Clinician advice can also be framed by describing what "other patients like you" have done (51).

Table 3. Key actions and strategies for the 5 A's of self-management support

Step	Activities	Useful Tips, Phrases, Questions
Assess	Initially assess: • Knowledge • Self-management behaviors • Beliefs • Risk factors For action-planning, assess: • Perceived importance (of the behavior) • Confidence (in ability to make change) • Barriers (to making change) • Supports (for making change)	Tips • Use brief standardized assessments where possible • On followup, assess patient view of progress, and how choices relate to progress Questions • "What is the biggest worry you have right now?" • "Tell me what you hoped to get out of today's visit?" • "I know about treating arthritis, but you know yourself best. What should I know about how you (like to get information, manage your arthritis right now, make decisions)?" • "What do you know about…?" • "How important do you think exercise is for your arthritis?"
Advise	Provide specific personalized information on: • Health risks • Healthy behaviors • Benefits of adopting healthy behaviors	Tips • Personalize test results, health status, and how choices affect outcomes • Ascertain patient interest before making recommendations • Make the source of advice clear (medical knowledge, similar patient experience) • Have a key message for each condition or symptom • Provide level of detail patient prefers • Listen more than you talk Phrases and Questions • "I think you have…" • "The important thing about…" • "As your physician I feel I need to tell you…" • "Can you review what we just discussed so I know I said it clearly?"
Agree	Collaboratively select goals, medical and self-management treatment methods. Make sure goals are based on patient's • Priorities • Values • Confidence in their ability to change	Tips • Prioritize among potential targets; don't try to work on everything at once • Consider importance, readiness, and confidence • Goal needs to be patient's, not the clinician's goal for the patient • Restate goal so it is specific, and measurable • Shape goal to be achievable within a set period of time (3–6 months, 1 year) Questions • "Is there something you have been thinking about that you would like to do to improve your (arthritis, pain, weight, eating habits, exercise)?" • "We have been talking about several things. Which one is most important to you right now?" • "Where would you like to be in terms of your (weight, physical condition) 6 months from now?
Assist	Help the patient achieve agreed-upon goals. Use behavior change techniques to help the patient: • Acquire self-management skills • Build confidence • Develop social/environmental supports • Address barriers likely to arise	Tips • Work together to develop a specific personal action plan, with specifics defined and confidence rated • Rework action plans with confidence ratings <7 (on scale of 1–10) • Remember to use the patient's own words • Identify the patient-specific motivators • Explore and respond to ambivalence • Identify small steps that lead to success • Offer a menu of ways to achieve goal (i.e., written self-management education materials, attendance at group education class) • Provide supporting materials • Focus on problem solving to circumvent roadblocks. Questions • "Goals are large and usually take several months to accomplish. What is the first step you could take towards your goal of ___?" • "Most patients I work with have problems with ___. What problems are you having?" • "Would you like to hear what other people with similar issues have tried?" • "What is the downside of changing (i.e., becoming more active)?" • "What is the upside of changing (i.e., becoming more active)?"
Arrange followup	Provide • Specific referrals to other resources (in the community and health care system) • Schedule followup contacts for ongoing assistance • Recommendations on adjustment to the plan as needed	Tips • Make referrals as specific as possible. "Contact (the Arthritis Foundation) at (phone number) to ask about the (ASMP)." • Offer a wide variety of methods, based on patient preference (in person, phone, e-mail, groups). • Use community resources and other members of the health care team. • Make sure followup happens; patient trust can be destroyed by missed followup Questions • "What is the best method to reach you?" • "When should I check back with you on the plan?" Followup questions • "I am calling to follow up on the plan we made to ___. How is it going?" • "How did your action plan work for you?" • "Not all plans are successful—what got in the way?" • "What could you do differently next month to help you succeed?"

Table 4. Trans-theoretical model stages of change

Stage	Description	Intervention Strategy
Precontemplation	Have not considered/not intending to take any action	Provide information on benefits of taking action, risks of not taking action. Raise awareness about how action will help achieve patient goal.
Contemplation	Thinking about taking action, but undecided	Prompt description of the pros and cons of taking action, and of not taking action
Preparation	Getting ready to take action	Assist in making plans specific; encourage patient to set a start date, share plans with supportive friends and family, and identify small beginning steps.
Action	Performing the desired action	Positively reinforce progress; suggest maintenance strategies.
Maintenance	Have been performing the desired action for 6 months or more	Positively reinforce progress; address factors that may lead to relapse.

Cultivate Problem-Solving Skills. Problem solving is becoming recognized as the central self-management skill and is essential for success (43). Although providing a ready answer is the natural reaction for many clinicians, health professionals can help patients become more active partners in their care by teaching them how to solve problems rather than by providing solutions (50). When patients present a problem—for example, a situation in which they have not followed through on plans to increase their exercise—clinicians can ask them to generate a list of potential solutions, including any they have used in the past to deal with similar problems. The patient can then weigh the pros and cons of each option before selecting one to try. Generating multiple solutions is vital because no one solution is likely to work in all situations. Problem-solving practice focused on identifying potential barriers to change can be particularly useful in overcoming those barriers.

Use Multiple Learning Modes and Channels. Self-management often requires that the patient learn a variety of information and skills; multiple modes of patient engagement can facilitate this learning (51). The effectiveness of verbal instructions can be enhanced by being specific and by using lay language to provide patient information (45). Posters, anatomic models, supplementary videotapes, and other audiovisuals can be used to reinforce key messages. Summarizing conclusions and instructions at the end of the visit will help retention, as will providing supplementary print materials, such as those available from the Arthritis Foundation or Lupus Foundation of America.

Videotapes can also be useful. Preoperative anxiety was decreased by 50% in patients with knee OA who viewed a short video film on joint lavage. Tolerability of the procedure was also significantly better in those who viewed the video as compared with a group that did not see the video (52).

Multimodal interventions also show promise. A comprehensive self-management program, including classes, written handouts, audiotapes of classes, letters of support from their physician, and biweekly to monthly phone calls to assist with goal setting and problem solving was developed for inner-city primary care patients with acute low back pain. Compared with the control group, study participants reported significant improvements in anxiety, self-efficacy, and self-management behaviors and better physical function related to low back pain (53).

Web sites can provide useful information, but many lack relevance and the quality of information is often poor (54). Two studies in arthritis found that more than half of the Web sites uncovered through Web search engines were commercial sites hosted by for-profit organizations (55,56). In one study, 71% of the commercial (.com) sites promoted some form of alternative medicine (55). Ansani and colleagues demonstrated that government sites (.gov), such as the National Institute of Arthritis and Musculoskeletal and Skin Diseases (www.niams. nih.gov), and university sites (.edu), such as the Missouri Arthritis Rehabilitation Research and Training Center site (www.muhealth.org/~arthritis), generally received higher ratings on content, navigability, literacy, and currency. Selected nonprofit organization sites (.org), such as the Arthritis Foundation (www.arthritis.org), can also be valuable sources for information for patients who prefer to receive health information from the Internet.

Mobilize Support Systems. Social support can motivate and reinforce behavior change. Clinicians can nurture natural support networks by asking patients which family members or significant others are most likely to help them with their self-management and clarify what kind of help is desired (50). This may include doing the recommended behavior (i.e., exercising) with the patient, providing praise or other positive consequences, giving reminders, or engaging in other supportive activities (57).

Including significant others in group education programs has produced mixed results. In one study targeting education sessions at both patient and spouse, those receiving the couples intervention had better attendance and greater increases in self-efficacy for managing pain and other symptoms following the 6-week intervention (58). However, a similar study of a 5-week group-education program found that those who participated with their partner had decreases in self-efficacy and increases in fatigue at 12 months compared with those who participated without a partner (40).

SUMMARY

Self-management support is critical to quality arthritis care and patient self-management. Self-management education, a more behaviorally focused form of patient education, has produced significant positive changes in knowledge, behaviors, and health outcomes. Meta-analyses have demonstrated significant, although modest, effect sizes. Trends in arthritis education include more of an emphasis on theory-based programs, training in generic skill development, and more innovative, cost-effective methods of program delivery. Effective, empirically proven, and theory-based self-management support can be integrated into routine clinical practice, and provided in structured education programs in the community. Both should be considered an essential part of the management of rheumatic diseases.

The findings and conclusions in this book chapter are those of the authors and do not necessarily represent the views of the Centers for Disease Control and Prevention.

REFERENCES

1. American College of Rheumatology Subcommittee on Osteoarthritis Guidelines. Recommendations for the medical management of osteoarthritis of the hip and knee: 2000 update. Arthritis Rheum 2000;43:1905–15.
2. American College of Rheumatology subcommittee on Rheumatoid Arthritis Guidelines. Guidelines for the management of rheumatoid arthritis: 2002 update. Arthritis Rheum 2002;46:328–46.
3. U.S. Department of Health and Human Services (HHS). Healthy People 2010 summary of objectives. Accessed June 23, 2006. URL: http://www.healthypeople.gov/document/HTML/Volvume1/02Arthritis.htm.
4. Adams K, Greiner AC, Corrigan JM, editors. Report of a summit. The 1st annual crossing the quality chasm summit—a focus on communities. 2004. Washington (DC): National Academies Press.
5. Bodenheimer T, Wagner EH, Grumbach K. Improving primary care of patients with chronic illness. JAMA 2002; 288:1775–9.
6. Burckhart CS, Lorig K, Moncur C, Melvin J, Beardmore T, Boyd M, et al. Arthritis and musculoskeletal patient education standards. Arthritis Care Res 1994;7:1–4.
7. Superio-Cabuslay E, Ward MM, Lorig KR. Patient education interventions in osteoarthritis and rheumatoid arthritis: a meta-analytic comparison with nonsteroidal antiinflammatory drug treatment. Arthritis Care Res 1996;9:292–301.
8. Lorig KR, Mazonson PD, Holman HR. Evidence suggesting that health education for self-management in patients with chronic arthritis has sustained health benefits while reducing health care costs. Arthritis Rheum 1993;36:439–46.
9. Barlow JH, Turner AP, Wright CC. A randomized controlled study of the Arthritis Self-Management Programme in the UK. Health Educ Res 2000;15:665–80.
10. Osbourne R, Wilson T, McColl G. Does self-management lead to meaningful and sustainable change? Two-year follow-up of 452 Australians. In press.
11. Siu AMH, Chui DYY. Evaluation of a community rehabilitation service for people with rheumatoid arthritis. Patient Educ Couns 2004;55:62–9.
12. Lorig KR, Sobel DS, Stewart AL, Brown BW, Bandura A, Ritter P, Gonzales VM, Laurent DD, Holman HR. Evidence suggesting that a chronic disease self-management program can improve health status while reducing hospitalization: a randomized trial. Med Care 1999;37:5–14.
13. Lorig KR, Ritter P, Stewart AL, Sobel DS, Brown BW Jr, Bandura A, et al. Chronic disease self-management program: 2-year health status and health care utilization outcomes. Med Care 2001;39:1217–23.
14. Lorig K, Sobel D, Ritter P, Laurent D, Hobbs M. Effect of a self-management program on patients with chronic disease. Eff Clin Pract 2001;4:256–62.
15. Barlow JH, Wright CC, Turner AP, Bancroft GV. A 12 month follow-up study of self-management training for people with chronic disease: are changes maintained over time? Br J Health Psych 2005;10:589–99.
16. Dongbo F, Hua F, McGowan P, Yi-e S, Lizhen Z, Huiqin Y, et al. Implementation and quantitative evaluation of chronic disease self-management programme in Shanghai, China: randomized controlled trial. Bull WHO 2003;81:174–82.
17. Lorig K, Ritter PL, Plant K. A disease-specific self-help program compared with a generalized chronic disease self-help program for arthritis patients. Arthritis Rheum 2005;53:950–7.
18. Lorig K, Gonzalez VM, Ritter P. Community-based Spanish language arthritis education program: a randomized trial. Med Care 1999;37:957–63.
19. Wong AL, Harker JO, Lau VP, Shatzel S, Port LH. Spanish Arthritis Empowerment Program: a dissemination and effectiveness study. Arthritis Rheum 2004;51:332–6.
20. Lorig KR, Ritter PL, Gonzales VM. Hispanic chronic disease self-management: a randomized community-based outcome trial. Nurs Res 2003;52:361–9.
21. Talbot LA, Gaines JM, Huynh TN, Metter EJ. A home-based pedometer-driven walking program to increase physical activity in older adults with osteoarthritis of the knee: a preliminary study. J Am Geriatr Soc 2003;51:387–92.
22. Hopman-Rock M, Westhoff MH. The effects of a health educational and exercise program for older adults with osteoarthritis for the hip or knee. J Rheumatol 2000;27:1947–54.
23. Mazzuca SA, Brandt KD, Katz BP, Hanna MP, Melfi CA. Reduced utilization and cost of primary care clinic visits resulting from self-care education for patients with osteoarthritis of the knee. Arthritis Rheum 1999;42:1267–73.
24. Hill J, Bird H. The development and evaluation of a drug information leaflet for patients with rheumatoid arthritis. Rheumatology 2003;42:66–70.
25. Harris M, Smith B, Veale A. Printed patient education interventions to facilitate shared management of chronic disease: a literature review. Intern Med J 2005;35:711–5.
26. Fries JF, Carey C, McShane DJ. Patient education in arthritis: randomized controlled trial of a mail-delivered program. J Rheumatol 1997;24:1378–83.
27. Lorig KR, Ritter PL, Laurent DD, Fries JF. Long-term randomized controlled trials of tailored-print and small-group arthritis self-management interventions. Med Care 2004;42:346–54.
28. Dally DL, Dahar W, Scott A, Roblin D, Khoury AT. The impact of a health education program targeting patients with high visit rates in a managed care organization. Am J Health Promot 2002;17:101–11.
29. Edworthy SM, Devins GM. Improving medication adherence through patient education distinguishing between appropriate and inappropriate utilization. Patient Education Study Group. J Rheumatol 1999;26:1793–801.
30. Blixen CE, Bramstedt KA, Hammel JP, Tilley BC. A pilot study of health education via a nurse-run telephone self-management programme for elderly people with osteoarthritis. J Telemed Telecare 2004;10:44–9.
31. Lorig KR, Laurent DD, Deyo RA, Marnell ME, Minor MA, Ritter PL. Can a Back Pain E-mail Discussion Group improve health status and lower health care costs: a randomized study. Arch Intern Med 2002;162:792–6.
32. Lorig KR, Laurent DD, Plant K, Ritter PL. Arthritis self-management online: a randomized trial. Arthritis Rheum 2005;52(9 Suppl):S234.
33. Cohen J. Statistical power analysis for the behavioral sciences. Hillsdale (NJ): Lawrence Erlbaum, 1988.
34. Warsi A, Wang PS, LaValley MP, Avorn J, Solomon DH. Self-management education programs in chronic disease. Arch Intern Med 2004;164:1641–9.
35. Chodosh J, Morton SC, Mojica W, Maglione M, Suttorp MJ, Hilton L, et al. Meta-analysis: chronic disease self-management programs for older adults. Ann Intern Med 2005;143:427–38.
36. Riemsma RP, Kirwan JR, Taal E, Rasker JJ. Patient education for adults with rheumatoid arthritis. Cochrane Database Syst Rev 2002;(2):CD003688. Update in: Cochrane Database Syst Rev 2002;(3):CD003688.
37. Riemsma RP, Taal E, Kirwan JR, Rasker JJ. Systematic review of rheumatoid arthritis patient education. Arthritis Rheum 2004;51:1045–59.
38. Hawley DJ. Psycho-educational interventions for the treatment of arthritis. Baillieres Clin Rheumatol 1995;9:803–23.
39. Solomon DH, Warsi A, Brown-Stevenson T, Farrell M, Gauthier S, Mikels D, et al. Does self-management education benefit all populations with arthritis: a randomized controlled trial in a primary care physician network. J Rheumatol 2002;29:362–8.
40. Riemsma RP, Taal E, and Rasker JJ. Group education for patients with rheumatoid arthritis and their partners. Arthritis Rheum (Arthritis Care Res) 2003;49:556–66.
41. Krueger JM, Helmick CG, Callahan LF, Haddix AC. Cost-effectiveness of the arthritis self-help course. Arch Intern Med 1998;158:1245–9.
42. Groessl EJ, Cronan TA. A cost analysis of self-management programs for people with chronic illness. Am J Community Psychol 2000;28:455–80.
43. Glasgow RE, Goldstein MG, Ockene JK, Pronk NP. Translating what we have learned into practice: principles and hypotheses for interventions addressing multiple behaviors in primary care. Am J Prev Med 2004;27 (2 Suppl):88–101.
44. Whitlock EP, Orleans CT, Pender N, Allen JA. Evaluating primary care behavioral counseling interventions: an evidence-based approach. Am J Prev Med 2002;22:267–84.
45. Daltroy LH. Doctor-patient communication in rheumatological disorders. Baillieres Clin Rheumatol 1993;7:221–39.
46. Bridle C, Riemsma RP, Pattenden J, Sowden AJ, Mather L, Watt IS, et al. Systematic review of the effectiveness of health behaviors interventions based on the transtheoretical model. Psychol Health 2005;20:283–301.
47. Keefe FJ, Lefebvre JC, Kerns RD, Rosenberg R, Beaupre P, Prochaska J, et al. Understanding the adoption of arthritis self-management: stages of change profiles among arthritis patients. Pain 2000;87:303–13.
48. Gibson PG, Powell H, Coughlan J, Wilson AJ, Abramson M, Haywood P, et al. Self-management education and regular practitioner review for adults with asthma. Cochrane Database Syst Rev 2002;(3):CD001117.
49. Allegrante JP, Marks R. Self-efficacy in management of osteoarthritis. Rheum Dis Clin N Am 2003;29:747–68.
50. Gonzalez VM, Goeppinger J, Lorig K. Four psychosocial theories and their application to patient education and clinical practice. Arthritis Care Res 1990;3:132–43.
51. Marks R, Allegrante JP, Lorig K. A review and synthesis of research evidence for self-efficacy-enhancing interventions for reducing chronic disability: implications for health education practice (part II). Health Promotion Practice 2005;6:148–56.
52. Ayral X, Gicquere C, Duhalde A, Boucheny D, Dougados M. Effects of video information on preoperative anxiety level and tolerability of joint lavage in knee osteoarthritis. Arthritis Rheum 2002;47:380–2.

53. Damush TM, Weinberger M, Perkins SM, Rao JK, Tierney WM, Qi R, et al. The long-term effects of a self-management program for inner-city primary care patients with acute low back pain. Arch Intern Med 2003;163:2632–8.

54. Maloney S, Ilic D, Green S. Accessibility, nature and quality of health information on the Internet: a survey on osteoarthritis. Rheumatology 2005;44:382–5.

55. Suarez-Almazor ME, Kendall CJ, and Dorgan M. Surfing the Net: information on the World Wide Web for persons with arthritis: patient empowerment or patient deceit? J Rheumatol 2001;28:185–91.

56. Ansani NT, Vogt M, Fedutes Heanderson BA, McKaveney TP, Weber RJ, Smith RB, et al. Quality of arthritis information on the Internet. Am J Health Syst Pharm 2005;62:1184–9.

57. Allegrante JP, Kovar PA, MacKensie CR, Peterson MG, Gutin B. A walking education program for patients with osteoarthritis of the knee: theory and intervention strategies. Health Educ Q 1993;20:63–81.

58. Martire LM, Schutz R, Keefe FJ, Starz TW, Osial TA, Dew MA, et al. Feasibility of a dyadic intervention for management of osteoarthritis: a pilot study with older patients and their spouse caregivers. Aging Mental Health 2003;7:53–60.

CHAPTER 32

Exercise and Physical Activity

MARIE D. WESTBY, BScPT, PhD Candidate, and MARIAN A. MINOR, PT, PhD

People with arthritis often have limited range of motion, decreased muscle strength and endurance, changes in gait and posture, functional limitations, and general deconditioning. Appropriate regular physical activity and exercise can lead to improvements in these areas and can reduce pain, fatigue, and depression (1,2). Knowledgeable professionals can help the person with arthritis live actively and well.

Physical activity (PA) is any bodily movement produced by contraction of skeletal muscle that results in increased energy expenditure (3). Regular physical activity is made up of leisure-time PA, occupational PA, and daily-living PA. Physical activity is not only necessary for general health, it also reduces the risk of developing a number of diseases and decreases disability in arthritis. *Exercise*, a subcategory of physical activity, consists of planned, structured, and repetitive bodily movement designed to improve or maintain one or more components of physical fitness (3). Therapeutic exercise often is prescribed to address impaired functioning (pain, range of motion/flexibility, strength, balance, fatigue) and to maintain or improve activity and participation (activities of daily living, locomotion, leisure, work). *Physical fitness* is "the ability to carry out daily tasks with vigor and alertness, without undue fatigue, and with ample energy to enjoy leisure time and to meet unforeseen emergencies." (1996 US President's Council on Physical Fitness and Sport) (4). Physical fitness consists of different components, including cardiorespiratory and muscular endurance, muscle strength, balance, flexibility, and body composition.

This chapter presents research from systematic reviews, clinical practice guidelines, and results of important randomized controlled trials (RCT) for 5 common rheumatic conditions. Where possible, both statistical and clinical significance will be discussed and effect sizes[1] presented. Key clinical messages are suggested.

OSTEOARTHRITIS

Osteoarthritis (OA) in lower extremity joints causes activity limitation, deconditioning and disability. Thus, for people with OA, it is important to assess causes of inactivity and support physical activity to minimize health risks and unnecessary disability. Identifying exercise and physical activities that produce desired outcomes and do not exacerbate pain and stiffness can be challenging because pain often is activity related. Furthermore, more studies have been published in lower-limb OA, compared with upper-limb OA.

Evidence of joint loading and intraarticular pressures in normal and diseased joints may guide activity recommendations. Aquatic exercise,

stationary bicycling, and weight-bearing activities (such as walking, low-impact aerobic dance, and neuromuscular strengthening and conditioning) can be performed safely by persons with symptomatic joints (5). In fact, regular moderate exercise may improve cartilage health. An RCT compared exercise to no exercise in 45 subjects at risk for developing knee OA (6). After 4 months of moderate weight-bearing and strengthening exercises, the exercise group was significantly better than the nonexercise control group as measured by glycosaminoglycan (GAG) content in femoral cartilage. Additionally, there was a strong positive correlation between increased physical activity and GAG content, and a moderate positive correlation between GAG and clinical outcomes. Some weight-bearing activities do increase lower extremity joint loading and should be assessed for activity-related pain and biomechanical stress. Stair descent and ascent, one-legged stance, and carrying loads greater than 10% of body weight may significantly increase loading of the hip (7), whereas fast walking and running increase biomechanical stress at the knee.

Studies of hip OA are rare and evidence is often extrapolated from knee OA samples, or both conditions are included in a single study. Tak and colleagues (8) reported an RCT (n = 109) of 8 weeks of strength training, lifestyle advice, and a home program for people with hip OA. Benefits (small to moderate effects) at posttest and 3-month followup were found for pain, hip function, physical performance, and self-reported disability. Quality of life (QOL), observed disability, and body mass index were not affected.

In studies of exercise and knee OA, most clinical trials have reported small to moderate effects for both strengthening and aerobic exercise. Current treatment guidelines consistently recommend both types of exercise (9,10). In general, exercise of moderate intensity and frequency is associated with important benefits for the general population (10) (See Table 1). Recent research supports these recommendations.

A multicenter RCT (n = 134) compared outcomes of a 4-week home exercise program with and without 7 physical therapy sessions of supervised exercise and manual therapy (12). The exercise program included strengthening, stretching and range of motion, riding a stationary bicycle, and daily walking. Both groups improved on the primary outcome measure, the Western Ontario and McMaster's Universities Osteoarthritis Index (WOMAC), and the 6-minute walking test at the 4- and 8-week followup assessments; however, only at 4 weeks was the clinical treatment group significantly different from the home exercise group (52% versus 26% improvement). After 1 year, a similar percentage in each group had received a total knee arthroplasty (7–8%), knee arthroscopy (3%), or steroid injections (2–3%); WOMAC scores were still significantly improved from baseline (32% clinic group, 28% home group). The clinic group reported significantly less medication use and greater satisfaction.

Not all studies have reported positive effects. An RCT (n = 61) of 6 weeks of high-intensity exercise for middle-aged patients with moderate to severe radiographic knee OA demonstrated no difference between groups in pain or function at posttest or 6 months' followup (13). The exercise group attended supervised group classes twice a week and was compared with a no-exercise control group. The only significant differences between groups were in the Knee Injury and Osteoarthritis Outcome Score (KOOS) and the SF-36 Mental

---

[1] Effect size (ES) is a measure of the differences between group means or an estimate of the effect of the intervention. It allows one to compare the relative effect of the treatment across different outcomes regardless of the instrument or measurement units. Small ES = 0.20; Medium ES = 0.50 or one-half a standard deviation; Large ES ≥ 0.80. A study with a large sample size and little variability likely will have a larger ES despite small improvements in the outcome of interest. (Portney LG, Watkins MP. Foundations of Clinical Research: Applications to Practice. 2nd ed. Upper Saddle River, NJ: Prentice Hall; 2000.)

Component score at immediate posttest (exercise > control). The KOOS difference persisted at the 6-month followup assessment.

The question of high-versus low-intensity exercise for people with knee OA was investigated in an RCT of stationary cycling (14). Both intensities improved function, aerobic capacity, and pain. The subjects in this sample were older and exhibited a greater range in disease severity than the subjects in the Thorstennson et al high-intensity study (13).

The benefit of specific neuromuscular training was demonstrated in an RCT of women with knee OA (n=66) that compared a strengthening-only program to the same program with a balance/kinesthetic training component (15). After 8 weeks of supervised group sessions (3 times weekly), both groups showed significant improvements in WOMAC, SF-36 physical performance, quadriceps strength, and lower extremity proprioception. The neuromuscular training group showed significant improvement over the strength-training-only group in WOMAC and SF-36 physical function, physical performance, and isokinetic muscle strength at high angular velocity.

Currently, the synthesized evidence to support exercise in people with knee OA can be found in recommendations from the Ottawa Panel (9) and the MOVE Consensus (10), as well as publications and work group recommendations from the International Conference on Health Promotion and Disability Prevention for Individuals and Populations with Rheumatic Disease: The Evidence for Exercise and Physical Activity (16). The primary recommendations from each group are presented in Table 2.

Key clinical messages for OA:
- Current evidence demonstrates important benefits from both aerobic and lower-extremity conditioning exercise for people with hip and knee OA. Although there is notable variability within trials, it is clear that appropriate and well-tolerated exercise regimens are available for most people.
- Functional exercises to improve balance, promote neuromuscular coordination and proprioception, and increase flexibility are components of successful interventions.

- Exercise instruction, supervision, and implementation can be effective in a group setting.

RHEUMATOID ARTHRITIS

Patients with rheumatoid arthritis (RA) experience restrictions in work and leisure-time physical activity early in the disease. Exercise is a key component of management to minimize functional impairment, disability, and potential deconditioning. A Cochrane review of 6 studies concluded that regular and appropriate dynamic exercise improves pain, stiffness, joint mobility, strength, and aerobic capacity without exacerbating pain or disease activity in persons with RA (2). An RCT (n=281) of middle-aged patients with RA reported reductions in disease activity (ES=0.26), bone loss, and the rate of small-joint damage in the high-intensity weight-bearing exercise group (17,18). Patients with greater large-joint damage at baseline experienced more joint progression, with a trend toward greater damage in the exercise group. Low study withdrawal rates and high adherence to the 2-year program suggest that the high-intensity program was well tolerated by these patients.

Another RCT examined the effects of a 21-week combined strength and endurance training program on 23 women with established RA and low disease activity, and 12 matched controls (19). After completion of the supervised 1–2 times weekly progressive resistance strengthening and endurance (cycling/walking) program, participants in both groups had significant improvements in aerobic capacity (15% in RA cases, 7% in healthy controls) and maximum leg extension strength (24–26% RA, 20–23% controls) and reduction in subcutaneous fat (12% RA, 10% controls). No change was evident in disease activity, pain, or function as measured by the Health Assessment Questionnaire in the RA group. The authors suggest that intensive and progressive training of only 1.5 times a week may be able to reverse the breakdown of muscle tissue (protein catabolism) and stimulate muscle hypertrophy in people with RA.

The Ottawa Panel performed a Cochrane review of the literature up to 2002 and reported the findings of 16 trials (n=661) of differing

---

Table 1. Recommendations for health and fitness–ACSM guidelines (11)*

Physical activity for general health

Mode:	Whole body, repetitive activities
Frequency:	On most days of the week
Intensity:	Moderate; 55–70% age-predicted maximal heart rate; RPE 12–13/2–4
Duration:	30 minutes *accumulation* (three 10-minute bouts)

Exercise training for cardiovascular fitness

Mode:	Rhythmic, aerobic exercise
Frequency:	3–5 days/week
Intensity:	70–85% age-predicted maximal heart rate; RPE 14–16/4–7
Duration:	20–30 minutes continuous

Exercise training for muscular fitness (strength and endurance)

Mode:	Dynamic, resistance exercise for major muscle groups
Frequency:	2–3 days/week on alternate days
Volume:	8–10 exercises; resistance adequate to induce fatigue after 8–12 repetitions; or 10–15 repetitions if >50–60 years of age or frail

Exercise training for musculoskeletal flexibility

Mode:	Gentle stretching; static or PNF technique
Frequency:	2–3 days/week minimum
Intensity:	Stretch to a position of mild tension/discomfort
Duration:	Hold position for 10–30 seconds for static; 6-second contraction followed by 10–30-second assisted stretch for PNF
Repetitions:	3–4 repetitions for each stretch

* RPE = rating of perceived exertion (original scale 6–20/modified scale 0–10); PNF = proprioceptive neuromuscular facilitation (3).

forms of exercises in patients with RA (20). After grading the strength of the evidence, evidence-based clinical practice guidelines were developed, some with Grade A recommendations. These recommendations combined with recommendations from the 2002 Exercise and Physical Activity Conference (16) are presented in Table 3.

Key clinical messages for RA:
- Current evidence supports the effectiveness of prolonged, moderate-to-high-intensity aerobic and strength training programs in adults with stable RA.
- High-intensity exercise over 2 years can have protective effects on bone density and the rate of joint damage in RA.
- With low-frequency, high-intensity training, women with RA can have similar if not greater gains in aerobic capacity, muscle strength, and muscle hypertrophy as healthy controls.
- Minimal adverse events or clinical side effects are reported with moderate-to-high- intensity aerobic and strength training.

ANKYLOSING SPONDYLITIS

Therapeutic exercise also plays a critical role in the management of ankylosing spondylitis (AS) and related spondyloarthropathies. A Cochrane review of 3 RCTs (n=241) evaluated the effectiveness of physiotherapy (PT) interventions for AS; however, due to clinical and methodologic differences among studies, only descriptive comparisons were made (21). Group exercises including a 3-week inpatient hydrotherapy or a 9-month outpatient program were compared with individualized home exercise programs in 2 studies. Significant reductions in pain and spinal stiffness (50%; ES=2.03) and increased cervical mobility (ES=1.02) were reported after an intensive inpatient program; however, improvements were not maintained at the 6-month followup. Positive changes in chest expansion and spinal mobility were not significant. Thoracolumbar mobility improved slightly following the outpatient program. The third study compared a home-based individualized exercise with no intervention and found statistically significant improvements in fingertip-to-floor distance and physical function in the exercise group.

Sweeney et al enrolled 200 patients with long-standing AS and evaluated a home-based program delivered by mail compared with standard care for 6 months (22). The intervention group received an instructional video, educational booklet, and exercise progress wall chart. Statistically significant improvements in exercise self-efficacy and the amount of self-reported AS mobility and aerobic exercise were found for the intervention group over a 6-month period. No statistically significant between-group differences were found for other outcomes, and effect sizes could not be calculated.

More recently, a global posture re-education (GPR) program delivered by a PT was compared with a conventional exercise program over a 4-month period in 40 patients with AS (23). Both groups received weekly classes of 1-hour duration. The GPR group reported significant improvements in mobility, function, and disease activity, although effect sizes were small.

Key clinical messages for AS:
- Specific group exercises have minimal to large treatment effects on the impairments and activity limitations typical of AS.
- No one exercise type, dosage, or method of delivery has been shown to have better short-term or long-term results.
- Home-based exercise and educational videos and print materials may help to increase AS-related exercise activity.

Table 2. Guidelines and recommendations for exercise in OA*

Source	Recommendations	Strength
Ottawa Panel: evidence-based clinical practice guidelines for OA (9)	• Lower-extremity strengthening is effective for improving pain and functional status. Exercise modes include isometric, concentric, and eccentric resistance training of quadriceps and hamstrings as well as general lower-extremity exercise programs, including resistance, flexibility, mobility, and coordination training. • Whole-body functional exercise, walking, and jogging in water are effective for improving pain and functional status.	Grade A based on evidence from 1 or more RCT of a statistically significant, clinically important benefit (>15%). Most subjects had a diagnosis of knee OA.
MOVE consensus (10)	• Both strengthening and aerobic exercise can reduce pain and improve function and health status in patients with knee OA. Effect sizes from both strengthening and aerobic interventions for pain and function were small to moderate (0.22 to 0.76). • To be effective, exercise programs would include advice and education to promote a positive lifestyle change with an increase in physical activity. • Group exercise and home exercise are equally effective, and patient preference should be considered. • Strategies to improve and maintain adherence should be adopted, e.g., long-term monitoring and review, inclusion of spouse and family in exercise.	Delphi process established 10 recommendations; used systematic reviews to determine evidence. Nine of 10 received positive recommendations. Four were strongly supported (Grade A) and are reported here. For hip OA, recommendations were extrapolated from knee OA and the strength of recommendation is C.
2002 Exercise and Physical Activity conference (16)	1. Aerobic exercise and physical activity for hip or knee OA: • Accumulate 30 minutes moderate-intensity (50–70% maximal heart rate) physical activity or exercise at least 3 days a week. • Tailor type of activity and venue to individual needs. • If overweight, combine activity/exercise with diet modifications to reduce weight. • Incorporate self-management education into activity/exercise recommendations and programs. 2. Neuromuscular rehabilitation for people with knee OA: • A lower-extremity exercise program should combine strengthening, endurance, coordination and balance, and functional exercise. • Recommended programs will progress in duration, intensity, and complexity; be tailored to individual needs, abilities, and preferences; move from clinical supervision to self-directed community settings; be periodically reviewed, revised, and reinforced.	Recommendations were derived from literature reviews and expert panel consensus.

* OA = osteoarthritis; RCT = randomized controlled trial.

Table 3. Guidelines and recommendations for exercise in RA*

Source	Recommendations	Strength
Ottawa Panel: evidence-based clinical practice guidelines for RA (20)	• There is good evidence for short-term improvements in pain, function, and grip force with therapeutic exercises, including functional strengthening and low- or high-intensity exercises in adults with RA. • Therapeutic exercises reduce pain while improving periarticular muscle force, aerobic capacity, and joint mobility.	Grade A based on evidence from 1 or more RCT of a statistically significant, clinically important benefit (>15%).
2002 Exercise and Physical Activity conference (16)	• Initial assessment of fitness to determine safety and dose • Supervised or self-directed settings • Periodic review, revision, and reinforcement • Cardiovascular: intensity: 60–85% maximal heart rate, progressively adjusted; frequency: 2–3 times per week; duration: 30–60 minutes; mode: whole body, dynamic (walk, dance, water exercise, stationary cycle) • Neuromuscular: intensity: 50–80% maximal load, progressively adjusted; frequency: 2–3 times per week; volume: 8–10 exercises, 8–12 repetitions, 1–2 sets; mode: dynamic	Recommendations were derived from literature reviews and expert panel consensus.

* RA = rheumatoid arthritis; RCT = randomized controlled trial.

SYSTEMIC LUPUS ERYTHEMATOSUS

Patients with systemic lupus erythematosus (SLE) have reduced exercise and aerobic capacity due to various clinical factors, including fatigue and pulmonary and heart disease (24). (See also Chapter 28 on SLE) In a non-randomized, controlled trial, a PT-supervised cardiovascular exercise program was evaluated in 60 women (mean age 36 years) with SLE (24). Upon completion of the 12-week program (1 hour exercise session with 40 minutes of aerobic conditioning, 3 times a week), participants in the exercise group had statistically significant improvements in exercise tolerance, aerobic capacity, depression, fatigue, and most domains of the Short Form 36. Three participants in the training program experienced mild transitory joint pain. Effect sizes were not reported but, when calculated, suggest moderate treatment effects ranging from 0.44 for fatigue to 0.73 for aerobic capacity.

Key clinical messages for SLE:
• Despite numerous systemic factors contributing to reduced exercise capacity, aerobic exercise training within the American College of Sports Medicine (ACSM) parameters can have important benefits in patients with SLE.

FIBROMYALGIA

Deconditioning in fibromyalgia (FM) may be both a contributing factor to and a consequence of a sedentary lifestyle, which patients may adopt in response to the fear of exacerbating muscle and generalized pain. Yet several studies have demonstrated favorable responses to both aerobic and progressive strengthening programs. A Cochrane review of 16 RCTs of moderate-to-high methodologic quality evaluated the efficacy of exercise training in FM (25). Of the 8 studies that met ACSM criteria for sufficient training stimulus, short-term improvements were evident in aerobic fitness, physician- and patient-rated global wellbeing, and pain pressure threshold of FM tender points. Inconsistent and nonsignificant effects were evident for overall pain, fatigue, and sleep, and there was no evidence that aerobic training improves psychological function. Strength training resulted in short-term improvements in pain, musculoskeletal and psychological function, but not in fatigue or sleep.

More recently, a 21-week resistance strength training program in older women with FM resulted in a 35% increase of lower-extremity strength (26), less delayed-onset muscle soreness (DOMS), and decreased pain level (27). Neuromuscular changes and muscle pain were similar for the FM and healthy age-matched control groups, suggesting older women with FM can safely and effectively exercise.

Water-based exercises were investigated in 2 recent RCTs with both deepwater running (28) and a combined mobility/aerobic/strengthening program in waist-deep water (29). Results indicated significant improvements in pain intensity (36%), aerobic capacity (38%), and scores on the Fibromyalgia Impact Questionnaire (FIQ) (28) and statistically and clinically significant changes in lower extremity strength (20–33% increase) and quality of life (ES = 0.87) (29).

Key clinical messages for FM:
• Aerobic exercise is an effective treatment component in the management of FM.
• Clinicians are advised to stress improvements in physical fitness and general health rather than FM symptoms.
• Older patients with FM may achieve the same health-related benefits of strength training as healthy peers.
• Aquatic exercises are a safe and effective alternative to weight-bearing aerobic activities.

TYPES OF EXERCISE

Therapeutic exercises prescribed by health professionals address specific joints or body parts affected by arthritis or arthritis-related surgery. Undertaking a therapeutic exercise program may be a necessary first step for individuals who have been inactive; have joint pain; have restricted joint motion, muscle strength, or balance; or are recovering from surgery, such as a joint replacement. Patients need to understand the purpose and value of specific therapeutic exercises and recognize that subsequent improvements in the targeted body parts may facilitate the safe progression to recreational exercises and other leisure pursuits.

Recreational or general fitness exercises can range from walking and swimming to cross-country skiing and running. The most appropriate forms are those that can be done in a controlled and safe manner, have little risk of injury, and place minimal stress and impact on affected joints. In most cases, participating in recreational exercise does not eliminate the need for therapeutic exercises.

Competitive or elite-level activities are performed at higher intensities, for longer durations, require greater skill and training, and pose greater risk for musculoskeletal injury. There are limited reports of people with arthritis continuing or returning to a competitive level of sport participation. However, as a general rule, exercising at this level is not recommended for individuals with inflammatory arthritis or other joint problems (e.g., marathon running with hip or knee arthritis).

COMPONENTS OF EXERCISE

Flexibility Exercises

Arthritis, disuse, habitual or protective positioning (postures), and normal aging can all affect flexibility of contractile (muscle, tendon) and noncontractile tissues (capsule, ligaments). Resultant joint stiffness and soft-tissue shortening is relieved by regular range of motion (ROM) and stretching exercises. ROM exercises involve taking the joint through its full available range once or several times without holding the end position. Stretching exercises place gentle and controlled tension on the targeted soft tissue and require the person to hold the position for as long as 30 seconds. Fewer repetitions are typically recommended for stretching exercises.

When performed in the evening, active ROM exercise can significantly reduce morning stiffness in the person with RA (30). During acute joint inflammation, joint motion should be maintained with at least 1 complete ROM exercise daily. When joint symptoms are subacute or chronic, gentle controlled stretching should be initiated. It is important not to overstretch acutely inflamed tissues, as tensile strength can be reduced by as much as 50%, and tears and overstretching can occur. Typically, published recommendations are made for stretching rather than ROM exercises. Table 1 contains recommendations for stretching exercises.

Additional recommendations for ROM and stretching exercises include the following:

- Use moist heat or take a warm shower or bath prior to exercise to increase soft tissue elasticity.
- Do exercises daily when stiffness and pain are the least.
- Do gentle ROM in the evening to reduce morning stiffness or in the morning to limber up prior to arising.
- Use self-assistive techniques (such as overhead pulleys or wand exercises) to facilitate greater ROM and provide gentle stretch.
- Reduce the number of repetitions when joints are actively inflamed.

Muscle Conditioning Exercises

Decreased muscle strength, endurance, and power may be due to intra- and extraarticular inflammation, side effects of medication, disuse, reflex inhibition in response to pain and joint effusion, impaired proprioception leading to decreased protective muscular reflexes, and loss of mechanical integrity around the joint. Muscle conditioning programs can improve strength, endurance, proprioception, and function without exacerbating pain or disease activity (9,20,26,27).

Isometric Exercise. Isometric or static exercise involves muscle contraction without joint movement. This form of strengthening exercise is often suggested prior to or in conjunction with dynamic resistive and aerobic exercise programs. Initially, isometric exercise may be indicated to enhance awareness of muscular contraction and recruitment, improve muscle tone, and prepare adjacent joints for more vigorous activity. Isometric contractions performed at 70% of the maximal voluntary contraction, held for 6 seconds, and repeated 5–10 times

> ### Adherence Is a Complex Phenomenon that Requires Personalized and Multifaceted Approaches
>
> Keeping up-to-date on the exercise and arthritis literature is an ongoing challenge; however, with the numerous systematic reviews, clinical practice guidelines, and high-quality professional and public education resources now available, clinicians can feel confident in their ability to prescribe safe and effective recommendations for therapeutic and recreational exercise for people with arthritis. With support and guidance from knowledgeable health care providers, individuals with arthritis can integrate physical activity into their daily routine and lifestyle, and use community-based resources for much of their ongoing exercise needs.

daily can increase strength significantly and are easily performed at home. Although isometric exercise avoids the concerns associated with joint motion and mechanical irritation, it can produce other unwanted effects. When performed at >50% of maximal voluntary contraction, isometric exercise constricts blood flow through the exercising muscle, which can produce unnecessary postexercise muscle soreness. Also, the increased peripheral vascular resistance raises blood pressure. In the knee and hip, high-intensity isometric contraction has been shown to increase intraarticular pressure (7,31).

Dynamic Exercise. Dynamic (isotonic) exercise is repetitive muscle contraction and relaxation involving joint motion and changes in muscle length. It includes both shortening (concentric) and lengthening (eccentric) contractions. By varying the level of resistance, contraction speed, number of repetitions and sets, and duration of rest periods, dynamic exercise can selectively improve strength, power, and endurance. Resistance (physiologic overload) can be supplied by the weight of the body part or external resistance in the form of free weights (dumbbells, cuff weights), elastic bands, or a variety of resistive exercise equipment. An informed and cautious approach to resistance training is recommended to protect unstable or inflamed joints from damage.

Adequate neuromuscular warm-up and cool-down with gentle stretching of the exercised muscles enhance comfort and safety. If the strengthening exercise is painful in the outer muscle or joint range, the exercise should be performed within the pain-free range. A minimum of 8–10 repetitions against gravity should be well tolerated before additional resistance is added. Other methods for determining appropriate initial intensity include basing the prescription on a percentage of 1 repetition maximum (1RM) or 8–12 repetition maximum (8RM or 12RM). Both techniques are safe in elderly subjects; however, joint pain and muscle soreness are more likely with 1RM testing (32).

Gradual progression of resistance and repetitions is recommended to improve strength and endurance. Progressive resistance exercise involves performing a small number of repetitions until muscle fatigue occurs, as seen by compensatory movements or inability to complete 1 more repetition through full ROM. Although multiple sets may produce greater strength gains, one set of 8–12 repetitions of adequate intensity is recommended because ~85% of the benefits are achieved with a single set, and exercise adherence is likely to be greater (11). The ACSM provides strategies for safe and effective resistance progression in healthy adults and suggests increasing the load by 2–10% when the individual can perform the current workload for 1 or 2 repetitions more than the targeted number (33) (see www.acsm.org). Maximum benefit is achieved by incorporating functional movements and body positions in the recommended exercise routine. Table 1 provides recommendations for strength training.

Table 4. Clinical signs and symptoms of deconditioning

- Daytime tiredness
- Lack of energy and strength for usual daily activities
- Prolonged exercise recovery
- Shortness of breath with minimal exertion
- Excessive fatigue with physical exertion
- Low pain threshold
- Decreased lean muscle mass

Aerobic (Cardiovascular) Exercise

Arthritis is a common cause of limitations in physical activity and people with arthritis tend to be less fit than noninvolved peers (5,34). Indicators of deconditioning are listed in Table 4. However, consistent evidence suggests that people with arthritis can safely exercise regularly and vigorously enough to improve all components of physical fitness, including cardiovascular fitness and endurance (2,9,14,17,19,20,24,25).

Interventional studies of aerobic exercise have often incorporated the guidelines for cardiovascular fitness described in Table 3. It is important to note that the aerobic exercise interventions have been progressive and of moderate–not vigorous–intensity. Exercise modes have included walking, stationary bicycling, aerobic dance, aquatic exercise, and circuit training. Age and medical status dictate the need for exercise screening or testing. People who are medically stable, independent, and without cardiopulmonary symptoms do not generally require diagnostic exercise testing to initiate a low- or moderate-intensity aerobic exercise program. Adequate warm-up and cool-down periods, exercise that does not exceed moderate-intensity levels, and attention to signs of fatigue or distress are components of a safe and effective exercise routine. When appropriate, evaluation of cardiovascular fitness, including submaximal and functional aerobic capacity testing (6-minute walk test), can determine a starting point for exercise intensity and duration. For individuals who are currently sedentary, the physical activity recommendation for *accumulating* 30 minutes of moderate activity on most days of the week is an appropriate goal (11). As activity tolerance and fitness improve, progression to the more demanding fitness guidelines may become an option.

Body Awareness

A fourth less recognized, yet very important group of exercises is collectively referred to as body awareness exercises. These include activities to address posture, balance, proprioception, coordination, and relaxation. Although some of these components may be addressed through the first 3 types of exercise, problems in these areas often require different approaches. Exercises on a wobble board or body ball often are prescribed in a therapeutic setting. Tai Chi and yoga are examples of recreational exercises that are safe and effective for persons with arthritis and incorporate elements of body awareness. A Cochrane review examining the effects of Tai Chi on individuals with RA found statistically significant and clinically important improvements in ankle ROM and levels of participation when compared with traditional ROM exercise/rest programs (35). No adverse effects were reported in the 3 controlled clinical trials (n=206), which ranged in intensity from 1 hour of Tai Chi exercises done daily to once per week. Yoga performed as a 90-minute series of modified Iyengar yoga postures once weekly for 8 weeks improved pain and self-reported function in a small sample of patients with knee OA (36). No adverse events were reported; however, only 7 of the 11 participants completed the pilot study.

Community-Based Exercise

Although most research has evaluated exercise interventions in clinical settings under the supervision of a healthcare professional, some trials have reported the benefits of exercising in community-based settings with various levels and types of professional supervision. To maintain benefits achieved during the therapeutic phase, patients should be encouraged to seek community-based programs or participate in home exercise (37). The advantages of community-based exercise include economy, socialization, self-management, wellness focus, and variety in activities, equipment, participants, and locations. Communication between community-based providers and health care professionals facilitates positive, successful exercise experiences and continuity for clients. Arthritis-appropriate exercise programs are available through local YMCA organizations, health clubs, hospital-sponsored fitness facilities, community colleges, parks and recreation departments, senior centers, and cooperative programs between the Arthritis Foundation and local groups.

Not all community-based programs are appropriate or accessible for persons with arthritis. Guidelines for evaluating a facility or program in addition to the usual requirements of safety are provided in Table 5.

Pool-based or aquatic exercises offer an excellent alternative for individuals with arthritis, particularly those with lower-extremity involvement. Pain often decreases while in water due to a number of factors, including increased sensory input from the pressure and temperature, muscle relaxation, and decreased joint compression (5). Improvements in joint tenderness, disease activity, functional status, grip strength, exercise tolerance, and mood have been shown with aquatic fitness programs (29,34,38,39). More recently, deep-water running has been recommended and found to be helpful (28). Programs such as the Arthritis Foundation Aquatic Program in the United States and Water

Table 5. Guidelines for evaluating community-based facilities or programs*

Physical accessibility

- Proximity to parking or public transportation
- Accessible entry, changing rooms, shower, and washroom facilities

Social accessibility

- Attitude, support, and friendliness of staff and members
- Willingness and ability of instructors to respond to participants' needs
- Ongoing classes appropriate regarding time of day, size, intensity, and exercise content

Cost

- Reasonable costs with possibility of paying only for classes attended rather than a prepaid membership
- Flexibility in membership policy to allow for times when participation is medically inadvisable
- Ability to observe and participate before making a financial commitment

Qualifications of staff/instructors

- Current certification by a professional organization and CPR certification
- Training or experience in teaching exercise to people with arthritis or other special needs
- Program has an educational and a monitoring component
- Acknowledgement of individuals' prior exercise experiences and confidence in their ability to exercise in specific situations

Equipment

- Adequate choice of aerobic and strengthening equipment
- Strengthening equipment of suitable low resistance or weights
- Ability to easily adjust and modify devices to suit individual needs
- Ability to use recommended joint protection techniques and devices
- Equipment is clean and in good condition

* CPR = cardiopulmonary resuscitation.

Works in Canada are examples of pool-based programs designed specifically for people with mild-to-advanced arthritis.

Exercising at home is another alternative for individuals who prefer the convenience, minimal cost, and relative safety of their home. Several arthritis-related exercise videos are available to provide guidance. Most manufacturers of commercial exercise equipment also offer less expensive models designed for home use. Patients should be encouraged to self-monitor their progress and modify their exercises in consultation with their health professional if problems arise.

IMPLEMENTING AN EXERCISE PROGRAM

Starting a regular exercise program can be both intimidating and challenging for persons with arthritis–especially if they have negative beliefs or attitudes about exercise or have received mixed messages about its benefits and safety. The most important requirements for the successful design, implementation, and long-term maintenance of an exercise program are to do the following with your patients:

- Provide basic and accurate disease-specific information on the benefits and potential adverse effects of exercise.
- Establish reasonable short- and long-term goals.
- Monitor for effectiveness.
- Understand how and when to modify or progress the exercise program.
- Implement exercise adherence strategies.

EXERCISE CONSIDERATIONS

Rheumatology health professionals need to consider a number of factors when prescribing therapeutic exercises or recommending recreational programs for people with arthritis. Common deterrents to regular physical activity include pain, fear of pain or injury, joint or muscle stiffness, fatigue or lack of energy, and impaired balance. Disease acuity, systemic manifestations and comorbidities, previous surgeries, need for assistive devices, side effects of medications, joint damage and stability, and age-related changes must also be kept in mind to properly advise the patient.

Pain

Much can be done to alleviate exercise-related fear and anxiety about pain and minimize symptom exacerbation. Of all the physical modalities, exercise appears to be the most consistently effective in reducing arthritis-related pain (40). Pain may indicate tissue damage and should be respected and investigated in the process of prescribing exercise. However, persons who have previously experienced severe pain or who are depressed or inactive may have a lower threshold for stimuli that are interpreted as pain. The most common pain reports at the beginning of an exercise program arise from DOMS. It is important the individual understands the difference between DOMS, a typical response to initiating or progressing an exercise program (particularly eccentric exercise), and pain originating from irritation or damage to joint structures. The use of heat or cold and a sufficient warm-up period are recommended prior to an exercise session and, similarly, heat or cold and an adequate cool-down including gentle stretching can minimize pain after exercise. Additional strategies to reduce exercise-related pain include planning short periods of rest or non-weight bearing activity, moving at a slower pace, and appropriate dosage and timing of medications for optimal pain management. Although some medications may enhance exercise performance in general, others may decrease it through complex biochemical and physiologic processes and patient-reported side effects (41).

Rest

Finding the right balance between physical activity and rest is a key component of rheumatic disease care. Rest can be divided into 2 types: general (whole body) rest and local (specific joint) rest. Adequate general rest, including restorative sleep at night, is necessary for health. During periods of active systemic inflammatory disease, additional rest is recommended to offset the fatigue that may be a physiologic consequence of increased disease activity. More frequent rest periods are likely needed when starting an exercise program. Prescription for general rest should include instructions for time, place, and proper posture and positioning. (See also Chapter 45, Sleep Disturbances.)

The purpose of joint-specific or local rest is to avoid activity-related injury, provide periods of joint unloading, maintain good alignment, and encourage maintenance of function and activity in spite of isolated joint swelling or pain. (See also Chapter 39 on splinting.) This type of rest includes activity modifications, use of assistive devices and walking aids, and protective or supportive splinting. Patients should be encouraged to exercise using any assistive devices or orthoses that have been devised for them. This is particularly important when vulnerable or inflamed joints are at risk for injury, increased stress, or deforming forces–such as with the use of hand weights and other resistive equipment.

The Ottawa Panel practice guideline on RA suggests there is Grade C (or weak evidence with mixed results) supporting the role of bed rest versus physical activity on joint swelling and tenderness, ROM, grip force, and 50-foot walk time for patients with chronic RA (20). With this in mind, unnecessary or prolonged bed rest should be avoided.

Biomechanics and Joint Protection

Regular dynamic exercise is associated with improved blood flow (31) and cartilage health (6), as well as improved ROM and increased strength and endurance of surrounding muscles. Strong and fatigue-resistant muscles can reduce impact forces crossing a joint with daily activities. Weak, easily fatigued muscles cannot provide joint stability or control. An intact neuromuscular mechanism is the most important

Table 6. Strategies to minimize biomechanical stresses during exercise*

- Determine the minimal joint ROM needed to safely and correctly perform the activity or use a certain piece of equipment.
- Select activities that involve only a single plane of motion when joint instability is present.
- Change planes of motion (direction) in a slow or controlled manner or ensure the individual has adequate joint stability (static and dynamic), proprioception, and muscular strength to reduce the risk of injury.
- Select activities with minimal rotary and shearing forces, especially under conditions of joint loading.
- Avoid activities that load or generate resistance rapidly or explosively (e.g., running).
- Ensure equipment can be adjusted to accommodate limb lengths and joint restrictions.
- Use joint protection principles while exercising (positioning, alternating activities).
- Use orthoses, splints, and other external devices as prescribed.
- Select activities with low risk of injury or falling.

* ROM = range of motion.

component of shock attenuation and is vital to adequate proprioception. In addition, exercise helps maintain adequate flexibility to allow pain-free, active ROM and more normal joint kinematics.

Exercise plays an important role in joint protection. Joints can be injured by inflammatory activity, biomechanical stress, pathologic joint loading, immobilization, increased intraarticular pressure, and diminished blood flow. Although healthy articular cartilage can tolerate high and repeated compressive forces without undue negative effects, it is less able to withstand the shearing and rotary forces typical of many sporting activities. High joint forces can be created through both intrinsic factors (e.g., muscle contraction) and extrinsic factors (e.g., ground reaction force). Strategies to minimize harmful forces are provided in Table 6. Issues related to joint biomechanics also are important when designing exercise programs for individuals who have undergone joint replacement surgery.

PUBLIC HEALTH PERSPECTIVE

The bulk of evidence supporting the benefits of exercise and physical activity comes from clinical trials of targeted interventions in well-controlled settings. However, the majority of people with arthritis and their opportunities to be active occur within the community are self-selected and embedded in daily life. Access to health professionals and clinically supervised exercise are limited. Therefore, to translate the benefits of physical activity for people with arthritis, we must consider daily or lifestyle physical activity in a population-based context (42).

Sufficient levels of daily physical activity to promote and maintain health for the general population are major public health goals; now the role of physical activity in the lives of people with arthritis has been recognized in the public health arena (42). The Report of the U.S. Surgeon General on Physical Activity and Health and the U.S. Department of Health and Human Services' *Healthy People 2010* program include recommendations for people with arthritis. The Arthritis Program at the Centers for Disease Control and Prevention (CDC) was established in 1999 to promote state-level arthritis programming and evidence-based physical activity (http://www.cdc.gov/arthritis/).

Currently the CDC projects the prevalence of self-reported doctor-diagnosed arthritis in the United States will rise to nearly 67 million in 2030 (25% of the adult U.S. population). Accompanying this increase in arthritis, the number of people with arthritis-attributable activity limitations is projected to rise to 25 million (9.3% of the adult U.S. population) (43). Consequences of activity limitation in people with arthritis include increased risk for other diseases, poor QOL, functional limitations, and disability. In the U.S. adult population with arthritis, data from the 2001 Behavioral Risk Factor Surveillance Survey showed that 24% were physically inactive compared with 14% in the general population. Another 38% reported insufficient physical activity. (Insufficient activity was defined as <5 days a week or <30 minutes a day of moderate activity. Inactivity was defined as <10 minutes of moderate physical activity a week) (44). Thus, more than 60% of people with doctor-diagnosed arthritis are not active enough to meet the guidelines for adequate physical activity for general health (Table 1). Inactivity in people with arthritis is associated with poor health-related QOL (45) and increased general distress (46), in addition to cardiovascular risk and disability. Furthermore, physical inactivity predicts functional loss over time in people with arthritis (47).

In a large survey of community-dwelling older adults, a number of environmental and neighborhood characteristics were associated with higher physical activity levels, including hills, biking lanes/trails, walking/hiking trails, street lights, and seeing active people in the neighborhood (48). Current recommendations for population-based

Table 7. Recommendations for population-based approaches to health promotion and disability (49)

- Physical activity has a potent impact on multiple health outcomes in people with arthritis and other chronic conditions. Community interventions aimed at lifestyle physical activity are not individual exercise prescriptions or rehabilitation, but are critical components to clinical interventions.
- Health care professionals should assess physical activity levels, recommend physical activity as a self-management strategy, and refer people to physical activity programs.
- People with arthritis should engage in moderate physical activity on a regular basis.

approaches to health promotion and disability prevention through physical activity come from the 2002 Physical Activity and Exercise conference (49) and are presented in Table 7.

EXERCISE ADHERENCE: ROLE OF THE HEALTH CARE PROFESSIONAL

Health care professionals influence exercise and physical activity. The mode of instruction can influence both adherence and correctness of exercise performance in the short term. Face-to-face verbal instructions and supervision, together with an illustrated brochure written at the appropriate reading level, have been effective when used in older adults with OA (50). Exercise that can be performed successfully and produces desired short-term and long-term results can enhance self-efficacy, exercise satisfaction, and adherence (37). Improved outcomes are clearly related to exercise adherence (37) and amount of exercise (dosage) performed (38). Community-based programs provide exercise or promote exercise within the context of self-management, such as in the Arthritis Self-Management Program. The providers' beliefs and attitudes regarding exercise and whether they initiate discussion with the patient about the role of exercise will influence the amount of discussion and likelihood of patients with RA receiving a prescription for exercise (51). Additional strategies to foster self-efficacy and promote long-term exercise adherence are outlined in Table 8.

Table 8. Strategies for increasing long-term exercise adherence

- Initiate an exercise program under expert instruction with supervision and support available several times weekly for several months.
- Ensure that health and fitness professionals have adequate knowledge and skills regarding arthritis-related factors and exercise prescription to ensure positive behavior changes and successful outcomes.
- Provide less supervision and more community-based programs as exercise confidence improves.
- Utilize a variety of methods for enhancing exercise self-efficacy, such as making a plan or contract that assures a sufficiently high level of self-efficacy for the program (e.g., at least 80% confident that the exercise program can be carried out as prescribed).
- Set realistic short- and long-term goals.
- Recommend exercise with a friend or family member for added support and encouragement.
- Encourage use of an exercise log or calendar to monitor progress.
- Anticipate problems or barriers that are likely to interfere with the exercise program and plan ahead how to deal with them.
- Adjust exercise intensity, volume, duration, and frequency accordingly as the individual progresses.
- Provide access to regular followup or booster sessions.
- Choose activities and programs that are simple, practical, convenient, relatively inexpensive, easily modified, supportive, and fun!
- Recommend an exercise class in which other persons with arthritis are successful exercisers.

REFERENCES

1. Minor MA. Exercise in the treatment of osteoarthritis. Rheum Dis Clin North Am 1999;25:397–415.
2. Van den Ende CH, Vliet Vlieland TP, Munneke M, Hazes JM. Dynamic exercise therapy for rheumatoid arthritis. Cochrane Database Syst Rev 2000;CD000322.
3. Howley ET. Type of activity: resistance, aerobic, and leisure versus occupational physical activity. Med Sci Sports Exerc 2001;33:S364–9.
4. United States Department of Health and Human Services. Physical Activity and Health: A Report of The Surgeon General. Atlanta: U.S. Department of Health and Human Services, Centers for Disease Control and Prevention, National Center for Chronic Disease Prevention and Health Promotion, The President's Council on Physical Fitness and Sports; 1996.
5. Westby MD. A health professional's guide to exercise prescription for people with arthritis: a review of aerobic fitness activities. Arthritis Rheum (2001;45:501–11.
6. Roos EM, Dahlberg L. Positive effects of moderate exercise on glycosaminoglycan content in knee cartilage. Arthritis Rheum 2005;52:3507–14.
7. Krebs DE, Elbaum L, Riley PO, Hodge WA, Mann RW. Exercise and gait effects on in vivo hip contact pressures. Phys Ther 1991;71:301–9.
8. Tak E, Staats P, Van Hespen A, Hopman-Rock M. The effects of an exercise program for older adults with osteoarthritis of the hip. J Rheumatol 2005;32:1106–13.
9. Ottawa panel evidence-based clinical practice guidelines for therapeutic exercises and manual therapy in the management of osteoarthritis. Phys Ther 2005;85:907–71.
10. Roddy E, Zhang W, Doherty M, Arden NK, Barlow J, Birrell F, et al. Evidence-based recommendations for the role of exercise in the management of osteoarthritis of the hip or knee–the MOVE consensus. Rheumatology 2005;44:67–73.
11. American College of Sports Medicine. ACSM's guidelines for exercise testing and prescription. 6th ed. Philadelphia: Lippincott Williams & Wilkins; 2000.
12. Deyle GD, Allison SC, Matekel RL, Ryder MG, Stang JM, Gohdes DD, et al. Physical therapy treatment effectiveness for osteoarthritis of the knee: a randomized comparison of supervised clinical exercise and manual therapy procedures versus a home exercise program. Phys Ther 2005;85:1301–17.
13. Thorstensson CA, Roos EM, Petersson IF, Ekdahl C. Six-week high-intensity exercise program for middle-aged patients with knee osteoarthritis: randomized controlled trial. BMC Musculoskelet Disord 2005;6:27.
14. Mangione KK, McCully K, Gloviak A, Lefebvre I, Hofmann M, Craik R. The effects of high-intensity and low-intensity cycle ergometry in older adults with knee osteoarthritis. J Gerontol A Biol Sci Med Sci 1999;54:M184–90.
15. Diracoglu D, Aydin R, Baskent A, Celik A. Effects of kinesthesia and balance exercises in knee osteoarthritis. J Clin Rheumatol 2005;11:303–10.
16. Minor M, Stenstrom CH, Klepper SE, Hurley M, Ettinger WH. Work Group Recommendations: 2002 Exercise and Physical Activity Conference, St. Louis, Missouri. Session V: Evidence of benefit of exercise and physical activity in arthritis. Arthritis Care Res 2003;49:453–4.
17. De Jong Z, Munneke M, Zwinderman AH, Kroon HM, Jansen A, Ronday KH, et al. Is a long-term high-intensity exercise program effective and safe in patients with rheumatoid arthritis? Results of a randomized controlled trial. Arthritis Rheum 2003;48:2415–24.
18. De Jong Z, Munneke M, Zwinderman AH, Kroon HM, Ronday KH, Lems WF, et al. Long term high intensity exercise and damage of small joints in rheumatoid arthritis. Ann Rheum Dis 2004;63:1399–405.
19. Häkkinen A, Pakarinen A, Hannonen P, Kautiainen H, Nyman K, Kraemer WJ, et al. Effects of prolonged combined strength and endurance training on physical fitness, body composition and serum hormones in women with rheumatoid arthritis and in healthy controls. Clin Exp Rheumatol 2005;23:505–12.
20. Ottawa Panel. Ottawa Panel evidence-based clinical practice guidelines for therapeutic exercises in the management of rheumatoid arthritis in adults. Phys Ther 2004;84:934–72.
21. Dagfinrud H, Kvien TK, Hagen K. Physiotherapy interventions for ankylosing spondylitis. Cochrane Database Syst Rev 2004:CD002822 .
22. Sweeney S, Taylor D, Calin A. The effect of a home based exercise intervention package on outcome in ankylosing spondylitis: a randomized controlled trial. J Rheumatol 2002;29:763–6.
23. Fernandez-de-Las-Penas C, Alonso-Blanco C, Morales-Cabezas M, Miangolarra-Page JC. Two exercise interventions for the management of patients with ankylosing spondylitis: a randomized controlled trial. Am J Phys Med Rehabil 2005;84:407–19.
24. Carvalho MR, Sato EI, Tebexreni AS, Heidecher RT, Schenkman S, Neto TL. Effects of supervised cardiovascular training program on exercise tolerance, aerobic capacity, and quality of life in patients with systemic lupus erythematosus. Arthritis Rheum 2005;53:838–44.
25. Busch A, Schachter CL, Peloso PM, Bombardier C. Exercise for treating fibromyalgia syndrome. Cochrane Database Syst Rev 2002;CD003786.
26. Valkeinen H, Häkkinen K, Pakarinen A, Hannonen P, Häkkinen A, Airaksinen O, et al. Muscle hypertrophy, strength development, and serum hormones during strength training in elderly women with fibromyalgia. Scand J Rheumatol 2005;34:309–14.
27. Valkeinen H, Häkkinen A, Hannonen P, Häkkinen K, Alén M. Acute heavy-resistance exercise-induced pain and neuromuscular fatigue in elderly women with fibromyalgia and in health controls. Arthritis Rheum 2006;54:1334–9.
28. Assis MR, Silva LE, Alves AM, Pessanha AP, Valim V, Feldman D, et al. A randomized controlled trial of deep water running: clinical effectiveness of aquatic exercise to treat fibromyalgia. Arthritis Rheum 2006;55:57–65.
29. Gusi N, Tomas-Carus P, Häkkinen A, Häkkinen K, Ortega-Alonso A. Exercise in waist-high warm water decreases pain and improves health-related quality of life and strength in the lower extremities in women with fibromyalgia. Arthritis Rheum 2006;55:66–73.
30. Byers PH. Effect of exercise on morning stiffness and mobility in patients with rheumatoid arthritis. Res Nurs Health 1985;8:275–81.
31. James MJ, Cleland LG, Gaffney RD, Proudman SM, Chatterton BE. Effect of exercise on 99mTc-DTPA clearance from knees with effusions. J Rheumatol 1994;21:501–4.
32. Di Fabio RP. One repetition maximum for older persons: is it safe? [editorial]. J Orthop Sports Phys Ther 2001;31:2–3.
33. Kraemer WJ, Adams K, Cafarelli E, Dudley GA, Dooly C, Feigenbaum MS, et al. American College of Sports Medicine position stand, Progression models in resistance training for health adults. Med Sci Sports Exerc 2002;34:364–80.
34. Minor MA, Hewett JE, Webel RR, Anderson SK, Kay DR. Efficacy of physical conditioning exercise in patients with rheumatoid arthritis and osteoarthritis. Arthritis Rheum 1989;32:1396–405.
35. Han A, Robinson V, Judd M, Taixiang W, Wells G, Tugwell P. Tai chi for treating rheumatoid arthritis. Cochrane Database Syst Rev 2004; CD004849.
36. Kolasinski SL, Garfinkel M, Tsai AG, Matz W, van Dyke A, Schumacher. Iyengar yoga for treating symptoms of osteoarthritis of the knees: a pilot study. J Altern Complement Med 2005;11:689–93.
37. Marks R, Allegrante JP. Chronic osteoarthritis and adherence to exercise: a review of the literature. J Aging Phys Act 2005;13:434–60.
38. Belza B, Topolski T, Kinne S, Patrick DL, Ramsey SD. Does adherence make a difference? Results from a community-based aquatic exercise program. Nurs Res 2002;51:285–91.
39. Sanford-Smith S, MacKay-Lyons M, Nunes-Clement S. Therapeutic benefit of aquaerobics for individuals with rheumatoid arthritis. Physiother Can 1998;50:40–6.
40. Minor MA, Sanford MK. The role of physical therapy and physical modalities in pain management. Rheum Dis Clin North Am 1999;25:233–48.
41. Moore G. Arthritis. In: Durstine J, Moore G, editors. ACSM's exercise management for persons with chronic diseases and disabilities, 2nd ed. Champaign, IL: Human Kinetics; 2003. p. 210–6.
42. Brady TJ, Sniezek JE. Implementing the National Arthritis Action Plan: new population-based approaches to increasing physical activity among people with arthritis. Arthritis Rheum 2003;49:471–6.
43. Hootman JM, Helmick CG. Projections of US prevalence of arthritis and associated activity limitations. Arthritis Rheum 2006;54:226–9.
44. Fontaine KR, Heo M, Bathon J. Are US adults with arthritis meeting public health recommendations for physical activity? Arthritis Rheum 2004;50:624–8.
45. Abell JE, Hootman JM, Zack MM, Moriarty D, Helmick CG. Physical activity and health related quality of life among people with arthritis. J Epidemiol Community Health 2005;59:380–5.
46. Da Costa D, Lowensteyn I, Dritsa M. Leisure-time physical activity patterns and relationship to generalized distress among Canadians with arthritis or rheumatism. J Rheumatol 2003;30:2476–84.
47. Feinglass J, Thompson JA, Witt W, Chang RW, Baker DW. Effect of physical activity on functional status among older middle-age adults with arthritis. Arthritis Rheum 2005;53:879–85.

48. Chad KE, Reeder BA, Harrison EL, Ashworth NL, Sheppard SM, Schultz SL,et al. Profile of physical activity levels in community-dwelling older adults. Med Sci Sports Exerc 2005;37:1774–84.

49. Meenan R, Sharpe P, Boutaugh M, Brady T. Work Group Recommendations: 2002 Exercise and Physical Activity Conference, St. Louis, Missouri. Session VI: population approaches to health promotion and disability prevention through physical activity. Arthritis Rheum 2003;49:477.

50. Schoo AMM, Morris ME, Bui QM. The effects of mode of exercise instruction on compliance with a home exercise program in older adults with osteoarthritis. Physiotherapy 2005; 91:79–86.

51. Iversen MD, Eaton HM, Daltroy LH. How rheumatologists and patients with rheumatoid arthritis discuss exercise and the influence of discussions on exercise prescriptions. Arthritis Rheum 2004;51: 63–72.

CHAPTER 33

Cognitive-Behavioral Interventions for Arthritis Pain Management

FRANCIS J. KEEFE, PhD, DAVID S. CALDWELL, MD,
JESSICA TISCHNER, PhD, and ANN ASPNES

Rheumatic disease patients who have similar disease severity can vary substantially in the level of pain and pain-related disability they experience. A rheumatoid arthritis (RA) patient, for example, who feels helpless about being able to cope with his or her disease and who has little social support from friends or family may report severe pain and become quite disabled in the face of mild-to-moderate disease. Another patient with the same degree of disease severity may complain little of pain and lead an active and productive life. Such variations in response to rheumatic disease cannot be explained by biomedical models, which view arthritis pain and disability as primarily due to disease activity.

Newly developed cognitive-behavioral approaches maintain that cognitive factors (e.g., beliefs, coping strategies, or appraisals) and behavioral factors (e.g., home or work environment) may be just as important as biomedical factors in understanding how individuals adjust to pain. Cognitive-behavioral approaches are influenced by advances in pain theories (i.e., the gate control theory and the neuro-matrix theory) that recognize that pain is a complex experience and that centers of the brain responsible for cognition (e.g., thoughts, memories, and expectations) and emotions (e.g., depression, anxiety) can influence whether nociceptive signals (e.g., from an arthritic joint) are blocked at the level of the spinal cord before they reach the brain (1–4). Cognitive-behavioral approaches have led to innovative treatments that have been shown in recent controlled studies to be effective in managing pain and disability in rheumatic disease patients (5–8).

BASIC ELEMENTS OF COGNITIVE-BEHAVIORAL THERAPY

Cognitive-behavioral therapy (CBT) for managing pain in rheumatic disease has 3 basic elements: a rationale for treatment, coping skills training, and training in methods for maintaining the use of coping skills to prevent setbacks.

Rationale for Treatment

The rationale for CBT is introduced at the start of treatment and prior to any training in pain coping skills. The rationale is designed to do the following: 1) educate patients about the influence that cognitive and behavioral factors can have on pain and other arthritis symptoms, 2) emphasize the role that training in coping skills can play in managing pain and reducing pain-related physical and psychological disability, and 3) enhance a sense of control over their pain.

Most CBT programs use an adaptation model to help patients understand the interrelationships between arthritis pain and patterns of adjustment. To introduce this model, patients are typically asked to describe how pain has affected 3 major areas of functioning: 1) behavioral, 2) cognitive, and 3) affective. Patients often can identify a variety of problematic behaviors (e.g., reduced tolerance for activities, decreased involvement in pleasurable activities, and increased dependence on others), cognitions (e.g., negative thoughts about self, others, and the future), and affective responses (e.g., depression, guilt, or anxiety). In discussion with the patient, the emphasis is on increasing awareness of how problematic patterns develop and are learned over time and on helping patients recognize the connections between their thoughts, feelings, and behaviors.

An important tenet of the cognitive-behavioral model is that learned patterns of adjustment to pain can be changed by learning new cognitive and behavioral coping skills. In CBT, patients are systematically trained in the use of a variety of cognitive pain coping skills (e.g., imagery, cognitive restructuring) and behavioral pain coping skills (e.g., activity pacing, goal setting). CBT thus encourages patients to take an active role in managing and controlling their pain. Although CBT is effective in reducing pain and suffering, it will not allow patients to achieve total control over pain due to a rheumatic disease such as RA. Thus, in providing a treatment rationale, the therapist helps the patient understand that they can increase their ability to control their pain while acknowledging that, at times, there may be disease flares and pain symptoms that are beyond their control.

Coping Skills Training

In CBT, each treatment session is structured to maximize the learning of cognitive and behavioral pain coping skills. The patient is first instructed in a coping skill and is guided by the therapist through a brief practice session. After the practice session, the therapist provides corrective feedback and suggestions for how to best apply the skill in controlling arthritis pain. The coping skills are practiced in order of difficulty starting with the least difficult (e.g., relaxation training) and proceeding to the more difficult and complex (e.g., cognitive restructuring).

A hallmark of CBT is that it provides training in a wide variety of pain coping skills. The skills are grouped together on a list that is often referred to as a menu to highlight the fact that patients have multiple options for coping with pain and can mix and match skills to deal with different problem situations.

Relaxation Training. Relaxation training is one of the most important and basic coping skills included in CBT programs for managing arthritis pain. Relaxation training is typically introduced early in CBT because it is easy to learn and is very effective in controlling pain. Training in relaxation methods can help patients in several ways. First, it can reduce muscle tension that may be contributing to pain. Second, it helps make patients more aware of increases in their level of tension so they can intervene early, before tension causes increased pain. Third, when patients relax they are able to shift their attention away from pain, which often reduces pain. Finally, learning to relax can improve patients' abilities to rest and sleep, both of which can enhance pain control.

Although there are a variety of methods of teaching patients to relax (e.g., meditation, autogenic training, biofeedback), most CBT programs use a progressive relaxation method similar to that of Bernstein and Borkovec (9). Progressive relaxation involves a series of exercises in which patients are asked to alternately tense and relax major muscle groups throughout their body. The exercises focus on muscles in the legs, arms, trunk, shoulders, neck, and face. The patient repeats each exercise slowly while attending to the sensations that accompany tension and relaxation. The instructions in relaxation are often tape recorded and patients are encouraged to listen to and practice the 15–20 minute audiotape twice a day. After 2–3 weeks of daily practice, most arthritis patients show an excellent ability to relax when in a quiet and comfortable environment. Training then shifts to teaching patients to apply learned relaxation skills to more physically demanding activities, such as walking or climbing stairs. Patients can be taught abbreviated relaxation methods in which they briefly (for 30 seconds) scan major muscle groups and identify and then relax any areas of excessive tension. These abbreviated relaxation methods can be done while the patient is engaged in other activities (e.g., eating, talking on the phone, driving) and provide an excellent means of generalizing the benefits of relaxation to a wide variety of home and work activities.

Imagery Training. Imagery is a very useful method of diverting attention away from pain. Imagery is often introduced early in CBT as an adjunct to relaxation training. A variety of image types are used in CBT, but probably the most common is pleasant imagery, e.g., imagining oneself reclining on a sunny beach. The instructions for pleasant imagery emphasize the need to focus on the imagined scene for a specific period of time (e.g., 3 minutes) and encourage the individual to try to involve as many sensory modalities as possible: try to imagine feeling the warmth of the sand on the beach, seeing the blue sky, hearing the sounds of the waves breaking and seagulls flying overhead, and even tasting the slight salty taste that might be on one's lips after a brief swim. It is important to underscore that patients are in control of the image, i.e., they can select whatever scene they want and can switch to a new scene or stop focusing on the image whenever they want. This reduces patients' concerns that the therapist is controlling their thoughts or hypnotizing them. Asking patients to close their eyes and relax deeply usually helps them concentrate more fully on the imagery.

Activity–Rest Cycling. Patients with persistent pain often have difficulty pacing their activities. Many arthritis patients report a pain cycle in which they overdo daily activities, experience increased pain, and then require a prolonged period of rest to recover. When this pain cycle is repeated over the course of months and years, it has many negative consequences, including a decreased tolerance for activity, a belief that one is incapable of being active, and a tendency toward a restricted lifestyle that provides few diversions from pain. Recent research shows that arthritis patients who cope with pain by decreasing activity have substantially higher pain and psychological distress, and report that arthritis interferes more with their involvement in activities of daily living (10,11). Activity–rest cycling is designed to break this maladaptive pattern by teaching patients to plan their daily schedule so that moderate periods of activity are followed by limited periods of rest (also see chapter 32, Exercise and Physical Activity)

For example, an RA patient who experiences severe joint pain after 2 hours of working at a computer terminal can alter his work schedule so that he types no longer than 30 minutes before taking a 5 minute break. The activity–rest cycle thus consists of a period of moderate activity (30 minutes of typing) followed by limited rest (a 5 minute break). Over a period of weeks, the duration of the activity phase of the cycle is gradually increased (e.g., from 30 to 40 and then 50 minutes of typing) and the rest phase of the cycle is decreased (e.g., from 5 to 1–2 minutes). This enables patients to gradually increase their activity without increasing their pain. Benefits of pacing activities using the activity–rest cycle include a reduction in pain and fatigue, increased level of involvement in activities of daily living, and an enhanced sense of control over pain. As patients increase their activity, they are usually taught how to set goals for engaging in highly valued, pleasant activities. These activities serve to reinforce and maintain learned patterns of activity and rest.

Cognitive Restructuring. In cognitive restructuring, patients are taught to identify, challenge, and modify negative automatic thoughts that may be contributing to increased pain or emotional distress. Rheumatic disease patients who are experiencing severe pain or who are depressed or anxious typically report having negative thoughts about themselves, others, and the future. These negative thoughts represent how the individual appraises their situation and do not directly reflect the actual situation. When these thoughts are erroneous and distorted, they can trigger emotional responses such as depression or anxiety. A growing body of research shows that some arthritis patients cope with pain by engaging in catastrophizing, i.e., they focus on and exaggerate the threat value of pain stimuli, which negatively affects their ability to deal with pain (12). This tendency to *catastrophize* has been shown to be associated with much higher levels of pain, pain behavior, and psychological and physical disability (13,14). The goal of cognitive restructuring is to help the patient become aware of negative pain-related thoughts and to restructure their underlying attitudes and beliefs. Because the negative thoughts are automatic, i.e., occur spontaneously for brief periods of time, patients need to learn how to become aware of them. A common strategy to increase awareness of such thoughts is self-monitoring. One form of self-monitoring is the 3-column method that asks patients to record the situation, their thoughts, and feelings (see Table 1). Patients are encouraged to recognize the connections between increased pain, their automatic thoughts, and their feelings. The therapist works with the patient to examine the evidence for the negative thoughts and to develop alternative ways of appraising the situation (e.g., "I've been through pain flares in the past. They are difficult, but I know my symptoms will improve with time."). When patients change their negative automatic thoughts they report substantial improvements in mood. They are also better able to comply with and maintain the use of other cognitive and behavioral coping skills.

OUTCOMES OF COGNITIVE-BEHAVIOR THERAPY

A number of controlled studies have evaluated the efficacy of CBT for rheumatic disease patients. The basic design of these studies is

Table 1. Sample of a 3-column thought recording form

Situation	Automatic thoughts	Feelings
Flare in my arthritis pain	It is hopeless, I am never going to get better	Depressed and discouraged
Criticism from a coworker because had to leave work early due to pain	No one understands what it is like to have arthritis pain	Anger
Because of increased pain, inability to do housekeeping, husband had to help out	I should be able to pull my own weight	Guilt

similar. Patients are randomly assigned to CBT or one or more control conditions. The CBT interventions are typically carried out in group sessions that last from 1.5 to 2 hours for 6–10 weeks. Outcome is evaluated using a comprehensive set of pain, physical disability, and psychological disability measures administered before and after treatment. Many studies have included a long-term followup assessment to evaluate the maintenance of therapeutic improvements.

Several controlled studies have documented the efficacy of CBT in the management of *rheumatoid arthritis*. RA patients receiving CBT have shown significant reductions in pain, pain behavior, anxiety, and depression when compared with patients in a social support control condition (15). RA patients undergoing CBT have also been found to improve significantly in terms of pain relief, coping, and function (5,6,16–21). Many of the controlled studies of CBT have been carried out with patients who met stringent inclusion criteria. Interestingly, a recent study tested the effectiveness of CBT in 63 unselected RA patients who were consecutive referrals to a rheumatology clinic. These patients were randomly assigned to a CBT intervention or a routine-care control condition. Results indicated that following treatment, patients receiving CBT showed lower levels of disease progression, medication intake, depression, anxiety, and helplessness. Long-term followup studies (16,22) have revealed that many RA patients are able to maintain their gains over 12 months. Long-term improvements in pain and functional status are most clearly apparent in patients who continued to practice coping skills on a frequent basis (16).

Controlled research has also tested the effects of CBT for *osteoarthritis* (OA) patients. Research conducted in our own lab has demonstrated that CBT is more effective than an arthritis education condition and standard care control condition in reducing pain and psychological disability in patients with OA of the knees (23). The efficacy of an intervention that combined CBT with educational information about arthritis has been tested in a large sample of patients, 85% of whom had OA (24). Results indicated significant reductions in pain and psychological disability. A followup study of patients who had undergone this intervention found they were able to maintain improvements in pain and depression up to 4 years after completing treatment (25).

Over the past 10 years, the effects of CBT on *fibromyalgia* have been evaluated in controlled studies. A recent systematic review of this literature identified a number of studies showing that CBT can produce improvements in pain and functional disability (5,26). As noted in the reviews, however, few controlled studies have compared CBT interventions to a condition that controls for therapist attention and other nonspecific factors. Only 2 studies found that CBT was more effective than an attention control condition (27,28). One limitation of systematic reviews is that they provide a qualitative, rather than quantitative analysis of studies. Because many studies in the fibromyalgia treatment literature have small sample sizes, such a review may obscure potentially significant treatment effects. Meta-analysis is a useful strategy to deal with this problem because it provides a quantitative estimate of effect sizes by pooling results across multiple studies. A meta-analysis of 49 treatment outcome studies conducted by Rossy et al compared the effects of nonpharmocologic treatments for fibromyalgia to those of pharmacologic treatments (e.g., antidepressants, muscle relaxants, and nonsteroidal antiinflammatory drugs) (29). The results showed that nonpharmacologic treatments (psychologically based treatments, such as biofeedback, relaxation, and CBT; physically based treatments, such as aerobic exercise, muscle strengthening, and stretching; and combination treatments, such as combined psychological and physical treatment) were superior to pharmacologic treatments in reducing fibromyalgia symptoms and improving function. Nonpharmacologic treatments and pharmacologic treatments,

however, did not differ significantly on such outcomes as physical status (e.g., tender point index, myalgic score, or grip strength) or psychological status (depression or anxiety).

PRACTICAL ISSUES IN THE USE OF CBT

Referring Patients for CBT

CBT therapists typically are clinical psychologists who have graduate training in cognitive and behavioral psychology and are experienced in working with medical patients. CBT is one of the most popular therapeutic techniques used with medical populations and, thus, many teaching hospitals have CBT therapists on their faculty or staff. Many of the psychologists listed in the Membership Directory of the Association of Rheumatology Health Professionals, a division of the American College of Rheumatology, have experience in CBT and accept referrals for CBT. The membership directory is available on the Internet at http://www.rheumatology.org/arhp/index.asp. The Association for Behavioral and Cognitive Therapies (http://www.abct.org) also maintains a referral service that can provide the names of CBT therapists in the patients' local area, along with guidelines on choosing a therapist.

Barriers to Cognitive-Behavioral Pain Management

We recently have identified barriers that reduce the likelihood of patients accepting a referral for CBT (7). These barriers occur at several levels. The first level of barriers is related to *attitudes of patients* themselves. Rheumatic disease patients themselves may be reluctant to accept a referral to a psychologist or mental health professional because they view this as a sign that their symptoms are not being taken seriously. Thus, it is important to prepare the patient before making the referral. Patients should be reassured about the reality of their diagnosis and symptoms, and told that CBT is designed to help them cope with their disease. It is often helpful to emphasize that CBT focuses on coping in the here and now, and does not dwell on early childhood conflicts or underlying unconscious conflicts. We usually encourage patients who are overly skeptical or otherwise concerned about CBT to pursue treatment on a 3-session trial basis. At the end of the trial, most of these patients have become quite involved in treatment and choose to continue their CBT program.

A second level of barriers involves *attitudes of the patients' families* and significant others (7). A spouse or family member may be overly negative regarding psychological treatment based on stereotypes and/or personal experience and, because of this, may convince the patient not to pursue a CBT intervention. For this reason, it is often helpful to discuss the reasons for referral for CBT with both the patient and the patient's spouse or significant other and to provide information on the complementary role that psychosocial intervention and traditional medical treatments can play in pain management.

A third level of barriers is the *attitudes of health care professionals* (7). Some health care professionals are skeptical or dismissive of the role of CBT in pain management. This often is due to a lack of awareness of recent research demonstrating benefits of CBT in pain management. Educational efforts are needed to address these negative attitudes. It is encouraging to see that there is growing emphasis on CBT approaches to pain management in clinical guidelines for arthritis pain management (30) and in offerings at rheumotologic scientific meetings.

Providing Patients with a Rationale for CBT

One problem for some rheumatic disease patients is that they tend to view their pain from either a purely medical or purely psychological viewpoint. Patients who see their pain as simply a medical problem are willing to pursue medical treatment options but view psychological treatments as irrelevant. Conversely, patients who respond quite well to CBT or other psychological based treatments may downplay the significance of medical treatments. To circumvent this problem it is important to help patients adopt a biobehavioral model of their pain. Such a model acknowledges the relevance of both biological and behavioral factors in the understanding and treatment of pain.

In our own work on arthritis pain management, we have used a simplified version of the gate control theory (1) to help patients adopt a more biobehavioral perspective on their pain. We begin our presentation by drawing a schematic diagram that illustrates basic elements of the traditional pain pathway, such as pain receptors in a joint, a neural pathway through the spinal cord, and sensory centers in the brain. We then discuss how this traditional model of pain sensation fails to account for many clinical pain phenomena, such as the persistence of pain following amputation, the absence of pain during sports or wartime injuries, or the fact that surgical interruption of the pathway often fails to abolish persistent pain. The gate control theory is then introduced as an alternative explanation. This theory maintains that there is a gating mechanism in the spinal cord that serves to regulate the flow of neural impulses from the site of disease or injury to the brain. When the gate is closed, pain signals are blocked at the level of the spinal cord and thus do not reach the brain. When the gate is open, however, the signals are free to pass through to centers of the brain responsible for pain sensation. In discussing the functioning of the gate, we emphasize that thoughts, feelings, and behaviors can influence whether the gate is open or closed (2,3). The role that the patient's own coping efforts can play in controlling problematic cognitive and emotional responses is then discussed. Arthritis patients respond quite positively to the gate control theory and report that it helps them better understand the connections between CBT interventions and their own arthritis pain.

CBT in the Context of Ongoing Medical Treatment

CBT is designed to complement the medical treatment of rheumatic diseases, not replace it. Although some rheumatic disease patients may reduce their use of pain medications during treatment, most patients continue with important components of their treatment regimen, such as the use of disease-modifying antirheumatic drugs or physical therapy.

CBT methods may actually be useful in enhancing rheumatic disease patients' compliance with medical regimens. Consider, for example, the RA patient who becomes depressed during a major flare and decides to stop taking methotrexate. By applying coping methods, such as cognitive restructuring and relaxation, the patient may be able to calm himself or herself, reduce emotional distress, and make a more rational choice about the need for arthritis medication.

Involving the Spouse and Family Members in CBT

In treating arthritis patients, it is important to remember that their pain and pain-related disability occur in a social context. The way that a spouse or family member responds to the patient's pain can have an important impact on treatment outcome. Recently, there has been growing interest in involving a spouse or significant other in CBT treatment

programs. Involving these individuals in treatment can help the patient acquire coping skills, increase the frequency of coping skills practice, and enhance treatment outcome.

When the patient's spouse or family member is included in treatment, it is important to have him or her serve as active participants rather than passive witnesses to the treatment process. The spouse, for example, can be taught relaxation techniques along with the patient and the couple can be encouraged to practice together at least once a week. Family members can also be encouraged to prompt and reinforce the use of pain coping skills. A family member, for example, could accompany the patient to an exercise session and encourage the patient to use activity–rest cycling to pace their exercise or to use imagery techniques to reduce pain following vigorous exercise. Training in communication skills can be provided to help patients and family members communicate more effectively about newly learned pain coping techniques.

Although there are few controlled studies of the effects of involving spouses or family members in CBT programs for arthritis, available evidence suggests that this approach may be quite effective. For example, some of the largest effects of CBT on pain and pain behavior were obtained in a study that incorporated spouses or family members in the treatment program (31). We conducted a study (32) that directly compared a spouse/family-assisted CBT intervention for OA patients with an arthritis information control condition that involved a spouse or family member. Results indicated that the spouse-assisted CBT intervention was significantly more effective in reducing the severity of pain and number of swollen joints posttreatment. At 12 months' followup, patients receiving spouse-assisted CBT had significantly higher levels of self-efficacy and tended to show improvements in physical disability when compared with patients in the control group (33). In another recent study of OA patients, we found that the combination of spouse-assisted CBT and exercise training produced significant improvements in pain coping, physical fitness, strength, and self-efficacy (34). Taken together, these studies suggest that involving spouses in pain coping interventions may have benefits for patients with arthritis pain.

Training in Maintenance-Enhancement Methods

The daily use of coping strategies appears to be an important mediator of the long-term outcome of CBT. RA patients who use pain coping skills frequently have had much better outcomes 12 months after completing CBT than those who did not (16). However, rheumatic disease patients who are faced with flares in disease activity or other stressful life events may question the effectiveness of their coping abilities and may reduce or curtail their coping efforts. To prevent such setbacks, most CBT programs for pain management include some training in maintenance-enhancement methods. Comprehensive programs for training in maintenance enhancement have been used to prevent relapse from such disorders as smoking, obesity, and alcoholism, and have recently been extended to rheumatic disease patients (35). These programs have several important features. First, they use cognitive therapy methods to increase patients' awareness of potential relapse situations. These methods include developing a list of high-risk situations likely to lead to setbacks, identifying early warning signs of relapse, and cognitively rehearsing how one might cope with different relapse situations. Second, comprehensive maintenance enhancement programs use behavioral rehearsal to enhance patients' sense of self-efficacy in managing arthritis pain. In behavioral rehearsal, the patient identifies a high-risk situation (e.g., an emotionally demanding life event) that might lead to a setback or relapse. The therapist then models coping strategies that could be used, has the patient rehearse these strategies, and then provides feedback. Third, maintenance enhancement emphasizes training in self-control skills for maintaining frequent practice with pain coping skills. Patients, for example, are taught how to use diaries and calendars to monitor important target behaviors (e.g., frequency of relaxation practice or early warning signs of a setback). They are also trained how to use self-reinforcement to reward the appropriate use and practice of coping skills.

CBT as an Early Intervention

Patients are usually referred for CBT late in the course of their disease. Most published studies of CBT, for example, have been conducted with patients who have had their disease for 6–12 years. CBT need not, and probably should not, be reserved as a treatment of last resort. Early intervention with CBT methods could have many benefits in the management of rheumatic disease. These include reducing pain and emotional distress, enhancing the effects of ongoing treatment, improving treatment compliance, and possibly even slowing the progression of disease. Two studies have systematically evaluated the efficacy of CBT in patients with recent-onset RA (20,36). In the first study, 53 recent-onset RA patients were randomly assigned to a CBT intervention or a routine-care control condition (20). Data analyses revealed that, following treatment, patients receiving CBT had a significant reduction in depressive symptoms and C-reactive protein levels (a marker of disease activity). At 6 months' followup, CBT patients showed improvements in scores on the Ritchie Articular Index, a measure of the number of actively inflamed joints. In the second study (36), a CBT intervention was found to be effective in increasing active coping and perceived social support and decreasing fatigue and depression. Taken together, these findings suggest that CBT may have a role to play in the early treatment of RA pain.

Alternative Approaches to Delivering CBT

CBT is typically delivered by psychologists who have extensive experience in cognitive and behavioral therapies. Researchers have begun to explore alternative ways to deliver CBT. First, several of the pain coping skills used in CBT are also taught at an introductory level by lay leaders in the Arthritis Foundation Self-Help Program or other variations of the Arthritis Self-Management Program. This course offers a low-cost way of introducing patients to CBT and thus may provide another option for referral. Following completion of the course, patients who require additional intervention can be referred to a therapist who has more extensive formal training in CBT. Second, Lorig et al (37) have explored an Internet-based intervention for introducing pain self-help methods. In a study of patients with persistent low back pain, they found that individuals receiving the Internet-based intervention had significant reductions in pain, disability, and physician office visits and improvements in their sense of self-efficacy. Finally, telephone-based educational interventions have shown promise in the management of arthritis pain (38) and could provide a very cost-effective approach for delivering CBT.

CONCLUSIONS

CBT is a promising treatment approach that has much to offer rheumatic disease patients. CBT systematically educates patients about the role that they can take in managing their pain, and provides practical training in pain coping skills. Although CBT is relatively new, it represents an important addition to the list of therapeutic strategies for managing pain in patients with rheumatic disease.

REFERENCES

1. Melzack R, Wall P. Pain mechanisms: a new theory. Science 1965;50:971–9.
2. Melzack R. The challenge of pain. London: Penguin Press, 1999.
3. Keefe FJ, France CR. Pain: biopsychosocial mechanisms and management. Curr Dir Psych Sci 1999;8:137–41.
4. Melzack R. Pain: an overview. Acta Anaesthesiol Scand 1999;43:880–4.
5. Bradley LA, Alberts KR. Psychological and behavioral approaches to pain management for patients with rheumatic disease. Rheum Dis Clin North Am 1999;25:215–32.
6. Keefe FJ, Smith SJ, Buffington ALH, Gibson J, Studts JL, Caldwell DS. Recent advances and future directions in the biopsychosocial assessment and treatment of arthritis. J Consult Clin Psychol 2002;70:640–55.
7. Keefe FJ, Abernathy AP, Campbell LC. Psychological approaches to understanding and treating disease-related pain. Ann Rev Psychol 2005;56:601–30.
8. Newman S, Steed L, Mulligan K. Self-management interventions for chronic illness. Lancet 2004;364:1523–37.
9. Bernstein DA, Borkovec TD. Progressive relaxation training: a manual for the helping professions. Champaign, IL: Research Press; 1973.
10. Van Lankveld W, Naring G, van't Pad Bosch P, Van de Putte L. The negative effect of decreasing the level of activity in coping with pain in rheumatoid arthritis: an increase in psychological distress and disease impact. J Behav Med 2000;23:377–91.
11. James NT, Miller CW, Brown KC, Weaver M. Pain disability among older adults with arthritis. J Aging Health 2005;17:56–69.
12. Sullivan MJL, Thorn B, Haythornthwaite J, Keefe F, Martin M, Bradley LA, et al. Theoretical perspectives on the relation between catastrophizing and pain. Clin J Pain 2001;17:52–64.
13. Keefe FJ, Lefebvre JC, Egert JR. The relationship of gender to pain, pain behavior, and disability in osteoarthritis patients: the role of catastrophizing. Pain 2000;87:325–34.
14. France CR, Keefe FJ, Emery CF, Affleck G, France JL, Waters S, et al. Laboratory pain perception and clinical pain in post-menopausal women and age-matched men with osteoarthritis: relationship to pain coping and hormonal status. Pain 2004;112:274–81.
15. Bradley LA, Young LD, Anderson KO, Turner RA, Agudelo CA, McDaniel, et al. Effects of psychological therapy on pain behavior of rheumatoid arthritis patients: treatment outcome and six-month followup. Arthritis Rheum 1987;30:1105–14.
16. Parker JC, Frank RG, Beck NC, Smarr KL, Buescher KL, Phiullips LR, et al. Pain management in rheumatoid arthritis patients: a cognitive-behavioral approach. Arthritis Rheum 1988;31:593–601.
17. Astin JA, Beckner W, Soeken K, Hochberg MC, Berman B. Psychological interventions for rheumatoid arthritis: a meta-analysis of randomized controlled trials. Arthritis Rheum 2002;47:291–302.
18. Evers AW, Kraaimaat FW, van Riel PL, de Jong AJ. Tailored cognitive-behavioral therapy in early rheumatoid arthritis for patients at risk: a randomized controlled trial. Pain 2002;100:141–53.
19. Applebaum KA, Blanchard EB, Hickling EJ, Alfonso M. Cognitive behavioral treatment of a veteran population with moderate to severe rheumatoid arthritis. Behav Ther 1988;19:489–502.
20. Sharpe L, Sensky T, Timberlake N, Ryan B, Brewin CR, Allard S. A blind, randomized, controlled trial of cognitive-behavioral intervention for patients with recent onset rheumatoid arthritis: preventing psychological and physical morbidity. Pain 2001;89:275–83.
21. Sharpe L, Sensky T, Timberlake N, Ryan B, Allard S. Long-term efficacy of a cognitive behavioural treatment from a randomized controlled trial for patients recently diagnosed with rheumatoid arthritis. Rheumatology (Oxford) 2003;42:435–41.
22. Bradley LA, Young LD, Anderson KO, Turner RA, Agudelo CA, McDaniel, et al. Effects of cognitive-behavior therapy on rheumatoid arthritis pain behavior: one year follow-up. In: Dubner R, Gebhart G, Bond M, editors. Proceedings of the Vth World Congress on Pain. Amsterdam: Elsevier; 1988. pp. 310–4.
23. Keefe FJ, Caldwell DS, Williams DA, Gil KM, Mitchell D, Robertson D, et al. Pain coping skills training in the management of osteoarthritic knee pain: a comparative study. Behav Ther 1990;21:49–62.
24. Lorig K, Lubeck D, Kraines RG, Seleznick M, Holman HR. Outcomes of self-help education for patients with arthritis. Arthritis Rheum 1985;28:680–5.
25. Holman H, Mazonson P, Lorig K. Health education for self-management has significant early and sustained benefits in chronic arthritis. Trans Assoc Am Physicians 1989;102:204–8.
26. Williams DA. Psychological and behavioural therapies in fibromyalgia and related syndromes. Best Prac Res Clin Rheumatol 2003;17:649–65.

27. Buckelew SP, Coway R, Parker J, Deuser WE, Read J, Witty TE, et al. Biofeedback/relaxation training and exercise interventions for fibromyalgia: a prospective trial. Arthritis Care Res 1998;11:196–209.

28. Keel PJ, Bodoky C, Gerhard U, Muller W. Comparison of integrated group therapy and group relaxation training for fibromyalgia. Clin J Pain 1998;14:232–8.

29. Rossy LA, Buckelew SP, Dorr N. A meta-analysis of fibromyalgia treatment interventions. Ann Behav Med 1999;21:180–91.

30. Simon L, Lipman AG, Caudill-Slosberg M, Gill LH, Keefe FJ, et al. Guideline for the management of pain in osteoarthritis, rheumatoid arthritis and juvenile chronic arthritis. Glenview, IL: American Pain Society; 2002.

31. Radjovec V, Nicassio PM, Weisman MH. Behavioral intervention with and without family support for rheumatoid arthritis. Behav Ther 1992; 23:13–30.

32. Keefe FJ, Caldwell DS, Baucom D, Salley A, Robinson E, Timmons K, et al. Spouse-assisted coping skills training in the management of osteoarthritic knee pain. Arthritis Care Res 1996;9:279–91.

33. Keefe FJ, Caldwell DS, Baucom D, Salley A, Robinson E, Timmons K, et al. Spouse-assisted coping skills training in the management of knee pain in osteoarthritis: long-term followup results. Arthritis Care Res 1999;12:101–11.

34. Keefe FJ, Blumenthal J, Baucom D, Affleck G, Waugh R, Caldwell DS, et al. Effects of spouse-assisted coping skills training and exercise training in patients with osteoarthritic knee pain: a randomized controlled study. Pain 2004;110:539–49.

35. Keefe FJ, Van Horn Y. Cognitive-behavioral treatment of rheumatoid arthritis pain: maintaining treatment gains. Arthritis Care Res 1993;6:213–22.

36. Evers AW, Kraaimaat FW, van Riel PL, de Jong AJ. Tailored cognitive-behavioral therapy in early rheumatoid arthritis for patients at risk: a randomized controlled trial. Pain 2002;100:141–53.

37. Lorig KR, Laurent DD, Deyo RA, Marnell ME, Minor MA, Ritter PL. Can a back pain e-mail discussion group improve health status and lower health care costs?: a randomized study. Arch Intern Med 2002;162:792–6.

38. Weinberger M. Telephone-based interventions in outpatient care. Ann Rheum Dis 1998;57:196–7.

CHAPTER 34

Pharmacologic Interventions: Small Molecules

DONALD R. MILLER, PharmD, and LEE S. SIMON, MD

In recent years, significant strides have been made in the management of rheumatic diseases. The increased number of effective drugs has permitted early and aggressive therapy of autoimmune disease, especially rheumatoid arthritis (RA). The evidence is now clear that early use of disease-modifying antirheumatic drugs (DMARDs) in RA can delay joint damage and prevent loss of function. On the other hand, nonsteroidal antiinflammatory drugs (NSAIDs) are now regarded as palliative adjunctive therapies in RA, with recognized toxicities. Current strategies rely less on controlling symptoms alone and more on altering progressive joint destruction and other long-term complications. American College of Rheumatology (ACR) guidelines stress starting DMARDs within 3 months for patients with an established diagnosis of RA and ongoing symptoms despite NSAID treatment (1). ACR guidelines are available for osteoarthritis (OA) as well, suggesting initial use of simple analgesics (2). All health care professionals need to recognize the expected therapeutic and adverse effects of antirheumatic drugs so they can participate in patient assessment and monitoring of drug effects.

Consideration of the expected ratio of risk versus benefit is important in evaluating any drug for use in a specific patient. The intensity of treatment should reflect the type and severity of disease. It is inappropriate to use systemic glucocorticoids in OA, for example, but these drugs are essential in treating many manifestations of systemic lupus erythematosus (SLE). Drug regimens should be used in adequate doses and for a long enough time to see benefits before changing or adding another. Some drugs may require up to 3–6 months to show full efficacy. Successful therapy often combines drugs having different mechanisms of action, with additive or synergistic efficacy and sometimes toxicities.

ANALGESICS

Because a cardinal manifestation of most types of arthritis is pain, analgesic drugs play an important role in therapy. Analgesics alone are a therapeutic mainstay in less inflammatory arthritides, such as OA, but they may be insufficient when significant inflammation is prominent.

Acetaminophen

In the treatment of OA, according to ACR guidelines, nonprescription acetaminophen (as needed up to 4 gm/day), should be the first-line pharmacologic therapy (2). Acetaminophen has been found to be slightly less effective than NSAIDs when used in OA patients in some studies, but its safety and low cost make it the logical first choice. Doses higher than 4 gm/day can risk liver toxicity with no increase in benefit. Because there are many brand names for acetaminophen and combination products also contain it (especially cold medications and narcotic pain relievers), accidental overdose from multiple products is a leading cause of acute liver failure (3). However, therapeutic doses of acetaminophen do not cause gastrointestinal bleeding and have minimal toxicity. Acetaminophen can also be used as an adjunct to NSAID therapy. Unfortunately, acetaminophen has no antiinflammatory effect.

Narcotics

Weak narcotic drugs, such as propoxyphene (Darvon), codeine, and oxycodone (OxyContin, Percocet) are frequently used for acute musculoskeletal pain or as long-term adjunct therapy with NSAIDs. Tramadol (Ultram and generic forms) is a drug with some opioid properties that is not scheduled as a controlled substance. The ACR guidelines for OA suggest that tramadol, propoxyphene, codeine, or oxycodone can be appropriate for long-term use in patients with moderate-to-severe pain and poor response or contraindications to other oral therapy (2). Tramadol should be used first due to lower risk of abuse but should be carefully titrated upward in dose.

Opioids reduce the perception of pain in the central nervous system. They are additive to NSAIDs in analgesia and have no ceiling effect. Thus their mechanism is different from, and complementary to, the peripheral mechanism of other analgesics. Occasional doses may induce sleepiness, dizziness, or constipation but otherwise are relatively safe for short-term use.

Long-term narcotic use is controversial due to the potential for inducing physical and psychological dependence. However, in 1997, the American Academy of Pain Management and the American Pain Society (APS) published a joint consensus statement that encouraged a more liberal role of opioids in chronic nonmalignant pain. The American Geriatric Society guidelines for chronic nonmalignant pain and the APS guideline for the treatment of chronic pain in chronic arthritis (2002) also address the underuse of opioids to treat chronic pain. The guidelines emphasize that fear of tolerance or addiction for patients with physiologic pain is grossly exaggerated and leads to undertreatment.

A decision to prescribe and take these drugs regularly should be based on the severity of pain, lack of effect of other drugs, and a clear understanding by the patient of permissible maximum daily doses. Preferably, opioids should be prescribed in controlled-release dosage forms that do not contain other analgesics so that dosage titration is simplified. Individual dosage titration and appropriate management of side effects are important components of therapy. With careful supervision, use of these drugs is a reasonable option for certain patients.

Capsaicin

Capsaicin, available in a topical cream in 0.025%, 0.075%, and 0.25% concentrations (Zostrix, Dolorac, and others), is a derivative of red chili peppers that depletes peripheral sensory nerves of a neurotransmitter called substance P. Initially, capsaicin causes stinging or burning sensations that may be severe and extremely uncomfortable as it displaces substance P. After a few days, however, pain perception is usually reduced. One study in OA demonstrated that capsaicin decreased pain and tenderness by ~40% when applied to specific joints 4 times daily for a month (4). A high-strength (0.25%) formulation of capsaicin can be applied twice a day and has been shown to provide faster and stronger pain relief than a 0.025% preparation. However, care needs to be taken in the application of these topical agents; if the patient touches her mucous membranes after application before hands are washed, an important irritant adverse event may occur.

NONSTEROIDAL ANTIINFLAMMATORY DRUGS (NSAIDs)

The NSAIDS are a large group of drugs that have peripheral analgesic and antiinflammatory effects. These drugs are often divided into several classes based on chemical category, but such classification is arbitrary and is not helpful in choosing a specific drug. Selectivity for the cyclooxygenase (COX) enzyme is a more useful classification (5). The prototype NSAID is aspirin (acetylsalicylic acid), which is converted to salicylic acid after absorption. Several other nonacetylated salicylate derivatives are available. A complete list of NSAIDs currently available in the United States is provided in Table 1.

NSAIDs inhibit COX, which converts a precursor molecule into various prostaglandins. Prostaglandins are ubiquitous, locally synthesized chemicals that have a role in inflammation as well as numerous other body processes, such as serving as an early signal of pain processing in the spinal cord and thalamus. The nonspecific inhibition of prostaglandin synthesis throughout the body explains the wide range of adverse effects that are caused by NSAIDs. The nonacetylated salicylates are only very weak inhibitors of prostaglandin synthesis.

In 1990 it was discovered that 2 different forms of COX exist. COX-1 is present at low levels in many organs, including platelets, kidneys, and the gastrointestinal (GI) tract, whereas under basal conditions COX-2 is present in a much more limited distribution. However, COX-2 is induced up to 20-fold by inflammatory cytokines during tissue injury, and thus generates prostaglandins that influence pain sensation and inflammation. Therefore, it appears that the therapeutic activity of NSAIDs is due primarily to COX-2 inhibition, whereas certain potential adverse effects (particularly GI and antiplatelet effects) are primarily the result of COX-1 inhibition. All of the older nonselective NSAIDs have activity against both forms of COX. Some drugs, including nabumetone, etodolac, and meloxicam, appear to be somewhat COX-2 preferential. Celecoxib is currently the only NSAID available that is COX-2 selective in the United States—meaning it spares COX-1 activity at therapeutic doses; thus in vivo there are no antiaggregatory effects in platelets (5).

The analgesic action of NSAIDs occurs at lower dosages than those that are antiinflammatory. Thus, lower dosages may be adequate for some patients with OA, with dose titration upward to the minimal effective dose. The analgesia occurs peripherally and perhaps centrally by inhibition of prostaglandin synthesis. Prostaglandins sensitize afferent sensory nerves to the effect of pain-inducing chemical stimuli. Antiinflammatory effects of NSAIDs occur near the higher end of their dosage range; however, NSAIDs should always be used at the lowest effective dosage. The antiinflammatory mechanism may be due to several effects in addition to inhibiting prostaglandin synthesis. Although NSAIDs provide symptomatic relief of arthritis, they have no effect on underlying disease processes.

When NSAIDs are compared in clinical trials, there is little difference between them in effectiveness or tolerance. Superiority of one versus another has been difficult to demonstrate. However, patient response is variable and highly individual. A patient may respond to one drug in the class despite no benefit from another. This unpredictability means that drug selection is essentially a trial-and-error process. Although pain relief will be obtained quickly with NSAIDs, it may take 2–4 weeks before full antiinflammatory effect is achieved. Thus, patients are usually given a 1-month trial before deciding to alter therapy.

Two areas in which NSAIDs differ are duration of action and frequency of dosing. Longer-acting drugs may be useful for patients who

Table 1. Nonsteroidal antiinflammatory drugs*

Drug	Starting dose	Maximum approved dose	Half-life (hours)	Generic/OTC	COX selectivity
Aspirin	650 mg qid	1300 mg qid	3–20†	yes/yes	COX-1
Celecoxib	200 mg qd	200 mg bid	5–11	no/no	COX-2
Choline salicylate	870 mg qid	1,740 mg qid	3–20†	yes/yes	COX-2
Diclofenac	50 mg bid	75 mg tid	2	yes/no	None
Diflunisal	250 mg bid	500 mg tid	12	yes/no	None
Etodolac	300 mg bid	400 mg tid	7	yes/no	COX-2 preferential
Fenoprofen	300 mg tid	800 mg qid	3	yes/no	None
Flurbiprofen	50 mg qid	300 mg tid	6	yes/no	None
Ibuprofen	300 mg qid	800 mg qid	2	yes/yes	None
Indomethacin	25 mg bid	50 mg qid	4	yes/no	None
Ketoprofen	50 mg qid	75 mg qid	3	yes/yes	None
Meclofenamate	50 mg tid	100 mg qid	2	yes/no	None
Meloxicam	7.5 mg qd	15 mg qd	20	yes/no	COX-2 preferential
Nabumetone	1 gm qd	1 gm bid	24	yes/no	COX-2 preferential
Naproxen	250 mg bid	500 mg tid	13	yes/yes	None
Oxaprozin	600 mg qd	1,800 mg qd	42	yes/no	None
Piroxicam	10 mg qd	20 mg qd	45	yes/no	None
Salsalate	500 mg tid	1,000 mg tid	3–20†	yes/no	COX-2
Sulindac	150 mg bid	200 mg bid	18	yes/no	None
Tolmetin	200 mg tid	400 mg tid	1–5†	yes/no	None

* OTC = over-the-counter; COX = cyclooxygenase; qid = four times daily; qd = once daily; bid = twice daily; tid = three times daily. Adapted with permission from Miller DR. Osteoarthritis. In: Pharmacotherapy self-assessment program. 4th ed. Kansas City: American College of Clinical Pharmacy; 2001 (book 3). p. 225–6.
† Dose-related half-life.

have difficulty remembering to take frequent doses. All NSAIDs are well absorbed; taking with food may delay but does not reduce absorption. Normally, NSAIDs are taken with meals to reduce GI distress. These drugs also differ significantly in cost. Because they are comparably effective, it is reasonable to try a lower-cost generic NSAID in most patients before moving to more expensive drugs.

GI problems are the most common side effect of NSAID use. Nausea and abdominal distress may be reduced by taking medication with food and may not be mediated through inhibition of COX-1 activity. All NSAIDs may cause GI ulcers and bleeding, but bleeding does not always correlate with subjective patient reports and may occur without premonitory symptoms. Gastrointestinal bleeding may be due to 2 separate effects. First, almost all NSAIDs are weak organic acids capable of disrupting GI mucosa by direct topical actions. Second, NSAIDs inhibit synthesis of prostaglandins in the GI tract, rendering it less able to protect and repair itself. COX-2–selective drugs have been shown to cause bleeding from ulcers less frequently than older NSAIDs (6–8). However, concurrent use of even low-dose aspirin negates much of the advantage of a COX-selective drug.

Patients at high risk of GI ulcers include patients older than 65 years of age, those with a previous history of ulcers, smokers, those taking concurrent corticosteroids or anticoagulants, and those with severe arthritis or other disability (8). Higher NSAID doses also increase risk. Patients with 2 or more risk factors for GI bleeding should receive a COX-2–selective drug or take a concurrent therapy to prevent GI bleeding. Misoprostol, an orally active prostaglandin analog, and proton-pump inhibitors (such as omeprazole or lansoprazole) have been shown to prevent both gastric and duodenal ulcers, although they have not been proven to alter serious GI complications in the long term. Regular-dose H_2 receptor antagonists, such as cimetidine and ranitidine, may decrease development of duodenal ulcers but not gastric ones, and thus are not recommended as adequate cytoprotection. When an ulcer does develop from an NSAID, it will heal with normal ulcer therapies. If the NSAID must be continued, proton-pump inhibitors can heal most ulcers even during concomitant NSAID therapy (8).

Since the removal from the market of rofecoxib, due to an increased risk of cardiovascular complications, and valdecoxib, due to an increased risk of Stevens Johnson Syndrome and a potential risk of myocardial infarction (MI) in unique patient populations, all NSAIDs have undergone scrutiny of their cardiovascular safety. Patients taking long-term rofecoxib had more cardiovascular events, including MI, compared with nonusers. Furthermore, patients who took valdecoxib as a pain reliever after coronary artery bypass graft (CABG) surgery also suffered a short-term increase in events. The proposed mechanism remains controversial but it is possible that selective inhibition of vascular prostacyclin, an inhibitor of platelet aggregation, without concomitant inhibition of platelet thromboxane, which promotes aggregation, can tip the balance toward thrombosis. However, in the CABG trials with valdecoxib, patients who developed MIs were concomitantly treated with low-dose aspirin and clopidrogel. Thus, it is possible that other issues, such as hypertension, could be the predominant cause. There are also prospective trials that have shown nonselective NSAID users are at higher risk of cardiac events compared with nonusers, but there are no placebo-controlled, randomized studies.

Randomized trials with celecoxib have generally not supported an increased risk with usual therapeutic doses. However, analyses by the Food and Drug Administration (FDA) of the totality of the prospective trials have suggested that all NSAIDs, nonselective and selective, may increase the risk of cardiac events compared with nonusers, and all such drugs thus carry a label warning to that effect in the US. At this time, the European community regulators have chosen not to identify nonselective NSAIDs with the same risk.

Due to inhibition of renal prostaglandin synthesis, NSAIDs decrease renal blood flow and may cause fluid retention, hypertension, or even renal failure, especially in patients with intrinsic renal dysfunction or reduced renal blood flow (e.g., the elderly and patients with congestive heart failure). These effects may contribute to the increased cardiovascular risk mentioned above. NSAIDs can also induce interstitial nephritis that is unpredictable and allergic in nature. Serum creatinine level and blood pressure should be monitored in any patient at risk. COX-2 is present in renal tissue and COX-2–selective drugs have effects on renal blood flow similar to older NSAIDs (6). Even small changes in blood pressure may yield important long-term effects and increase risk for cardiovascular complications with long-term therapy.

Central nervous system toxicities may also occur with NSAID use. Dizziness, headache, drowsiness, or ringing in the ears will sometimes develop, especially with aspirin and nonacetylated salicylates. Indomethacin is particularly likely to cause headaches.

Some patients develop pseudoallergic reactions to NSAIDs. A syndrome of wheezing, nasal rhinitis, and laryngeal edema has been described and is associated with nasal polyps and asthma. This syndrome is prostaglandin mediated, so patients who react to one NSAID may react to others. A nonacetylated salicylate may be cautiously tried. A second type of reaction to aspirin involves urticaria and angioedema, and patients are more likely to cross-react to other salicylates as well as NSAIDs.

Nonsteroidal drugs cause minor elevations of liver enzyme levels in up to 15% of patients. Serious liver toxicity is rare, but both hepatocellular and cholestatic reactions, with occasional deaths, have been reported. Most NSAIDs, except nonacetylated salicylates and COX-2–selective drugs, inhibit platelet aggregation and prolong bleeding time.

Patients taking NSAIDs should be monitored regularly for efficacy and safety. If little or no benefit is obtained within 1 month, it is reasonable to try an alternative NSAID. Combining 2 or more NSAIDs is not beneficial and increases the risk of toxicity. Monitoring for safety usually includes periodic complete blood counts to watch for anemia as a sign of GI bleeding, serum creatinine and potassium levels to assess renal impairment, and possibly liver enzyme tests to watch for liver problems. Because of the recognition of sodium retention, decreases in glomerular filtration rate, and increasing concerns over cardiovascular risks, periodic monitoring of blood pressure after instituting or changing doses of NSAIDs or COX-2–selective drugs is recommended.

HYALURONIC ACID DERIVATIVES

Hyaluronic acid (HA) is a large glycosaminoglycan that forms complex molecular networks providing viscosity to synovial fluid and contributing to elasticity of the fluid to serve as a shock absorber at high shear rates. In OA, the concentration and molecular weight of HA are reduced, compromising the viscoelastic properties of joint fluid. Thus, injection of exogenous HA into the joint may restore some of the normal protective properties of endogenous HA (9). Technically, hyaluronan products are classified as medical devices because of their purported mechanism as lubricating agents. In the US, clinicians can choose between 5 proprietary products that contain either sodium hyaluronate or higher-molecular-weight polymers of hyaluronate. Sodium hyaluronate products are generally administered in a series of 5 weekly joint injections, the higher-molecular-weight preparations, in 3 or 4 injections. These products are approved for treatment of OA of the knee, although case series have been reported for injection into other joints.

Clinical trials have found that HA preparations reduce OA symptoms, and in some per-protocol or completer analyses, up to 75% of patients derived benefit lasting 8 months or more. HA normally flows through the joint with a half-life of only 12–24 hours in animals, so the reason for its long-lasting therapeutic effect is not well understood. The role of HA preparations are controversial because high placebo responses are seen even with saline injections into the knee, and some studies have found HA products to be no better than placebo. However, other clinical trials in OA of the knee have demonstrated that the products relieve pain and improve function with effect sizes similar to NSAIDs or intraarticular corticosteroids (10). Compared with intraarticular steroids, HA injections have less dramatic but longer-lasting effects. The best responses occurred in patients with milder changes on radiographs. Differences between preparations are unclear but some studies found polymeric hyaluronans to be better than sodium hyaluronate.

Hyaluronate preparations appear to be relatively safe; local reactions at the injection site (pain, swelling) are generally mild and transient. Treatment candidates include patients with residual knee symptoms despite pharmacologic therapy; those with poor adherence to oral medication; patients at risk of GI and cardiovascular complications from NSAIDs; those who need glucocorticoid injections; and patients with early, milder OA who fail to get relief from acetaminophen therapy and are not candidates for any form of NSAID. Courses of treatment can be repeated approximately every 6 months for several years if effective, although limited data are available on the effectiveness of multiple courses.

CORTICOSTEROIDS

Corticosteroids are analogs of cortisone, a natural antiinflammatory hormone first isolated in the 1940s. They were considered "wonder drugs" during the 1950s until their adverse effects became apparent. Corticosteroids are still recognized as powerful antiinflammatory drugs. However, they should be used judiciously in the lowest dose for the shortest possible time to avoid long-term adverse effects. Corticosteroids are used only for conditions in which inflammation is prominent and not responsive to NSAIDs. In certain cases when organ inflammation complicates SLE or rheumatoid vasculitis, large doses may be life saving. A list and comparison of drugs is shown in Table 2.

The mechanism of action of corticosteroids is complex (11). They alter the distribution and function of white blood cells, suppress both humoral and cell-mediated immune function, and inhibit phospholipase A2, an enzyme in cell membranes that generates a prostaglandin precursor. Furthermore, glucocorticoids have been shown to inhibit the translation of COX-2 with little effect on COX-1 activity.

A physiologic dose of systemic corticosteroid is considered to be the equivalent of the body's normal daily secretion of 20–30 mg of hydrocortisone. Thus, a physiologic dose of prednisone is 5–7.5 mg/day. Doses lower than this cause only modest suppression of endogenous

hydrocortisone secretion and few adverse effects in most patients; whereas, larger doses are likely to cause significant adverse effects (12). However, we do not know the threshold dose of gluococorticoids on bone, leaving frail, elderly, thin women at further increased risk for osteoporosis. Prednisone is usually the steroid of choice in rheumatic disease because of its intermediate duration of action, which allows once-daily dosing. However, if given in the morning, prednisone's effect will have diminished by the time the body's endogenous hydrocortisone secretion peaks early the next morning. To further minimize adrenal suppression, prednisone is sometimes given only on alternate days. However, alternate-day therapy is not maximally effective and is not suitable for initiating therapy or for controlling highly active disease, such as observed in temporal arteritis or other similar diseases. Steroids with a long duration of action, like dexamethasone, may suppress the adrenal gland even with alternate-day therapy.

Corticosteroids may be given orally, intravenously, or intraarticularly. Local injection into a joint, tendon sheath, or bursa may be used with few adverse effects when inflammation is localized, whereas systemic administration is used for generalized inflammation. A potential complication of articular injection is introduction of bacteria causing an infection. Intraarticular injections are normally not repeated more than 3–4 times per year because of potential adverse effects on joint structure, although specific data to support this are lacking (13). Additional side effects of corticosteroid injection include tendon weakening and often irreversible depigmentation of overlying skin.

Indications for systemic steroids in RA is controversial but usually include short-term treatment while waiting for slow-acting drugs to work, severe synovitis that impairs functional ability, and extraarticular inflammation. Low doses of prednisone ($\leq$7.5 mg/day) are often sufficient for articular inflammation, medium doses (10–15 mg/day) are used in polymyalgia rheumatica, and high doses (40–60 mg/day) are often required in SLE or vasculitis. Occasionally, large intravenous boluses (up to 1 gm/day methylprednisolone for 3 days) may be used in severe rheumatic diseases, including vasculitis or SLE.

The effect of corticosteroids on RA progression is controversial. The traditional view is that they do not alter the course of RA, but recent studies indicate that early use of steroids in RA does reduce radiographic joint destruction for at least 2 years (14). Thus, many rheumatologists use corticosteroids as part of an aggressive early drug regimen, with the goal of quickly gaining control of disease, then tapering the steroid and leaving patients on disease-modifying drugs alone. Continued use of steroids in RA gains little and exposes the patient to many long-term complications, including weight gain, hyperglycemia, hypertension, cataracts, glaucoma, poor wound healing, osteoporosis, and adrenal suppression. An increased risk of GI bleeding is seen, especially when combined with NSAIDs.

Clinical benefit occurs rapidly; patients usually notice improvement within 24 hours. Once improvement has stabilized, the dosage is tapered to the minimum effective dosage. Monitoring corticosteroid therapy should include periodic blood counts, serum potassium level, and glucose level. Due to the risk of osteoporosis with long-term use, calcium and vitamin D should be supplemented. Early use of a bisphosphonate in the context of calcium and vitamin D repletion may prevent most of the osteoporotic effects of the corticosteroid.

DISEASE-MODIFYING ANTIRHEUMATIC DRUGS (DMARDs)

This heterogenous group of drugs has a delayed onset of action, ranging from 3 weeks to 3 months. They have no immediate analgesic effects, but appear to work at more fundamental stages in the inflammatory

Table 2. Comparison of oral corticosteroids

Drug (trade name)	Equivalent dose (mg)	Relative antiinflammatory potency
Short acting		
Hydrocortisone (Cortef)	20	1
Cortisone (Cortone)	25	0.8
Intermediate acting		
Prednisone (Deltasone)	5	4
Prednisolone (Delta-Cortef)	5	4
Methylprednisolone (Medrol)	4	5
Triamcinolone (Kenacort)	4	5
Long acting		
Betamethasone (Celestone)	0.6	25
Dexamethasone (Decadron)	0.75	30

process than NSAIDs, and can retard progression of joint erosion; thus the name disease-modifying antirheumatic drugs (DMARDs).

Used alone at later stages of RA, beneficial effects of these drugs are often modest and short-lived, and they seldom improve disease enough to cause true remission. Even with continued treatment, only half of all patients stay on the same individual drug longer than 2 years (1). However, the apparently disappointing long-term efficacy of these drugs may be due in part to the fact that they had been started too late in the disease course. One reason for delay was fear of severe organ toxicity, but the adverse effects of these drugs are no more severe than those of NSAIDs when regularly monitored (15). The current approach is to start the drugs early in the course of RA, often in combination. The superiority of this approach is now well proven (16,17). Many of the DMARDs are also effective in other rheumatic diseases, such as psoriatic arthritis and ankylosing spondylitis. Table 3 lists the usual doses and key toxicities for the DMARD drugs discussed in this chapter.

Methotrexate

Methotrexate, an analog of folic acid, is currently the standard first DMARD prescribed for RA of any severity. Its mechanism of action is unclear. It inhibits dihydrofolate reductase, an enzyme critical to synthesis of DNA in actively dividing cells. However, other mechanisms, such as adenosine release, are probably more important, because small doses of supplemental folic acid do not interfere with methotrexate's efficacy. Methotrexate has both antiinflammatory and immunosuppressive properties, but antiinflammatory activity predominates at the low doses used in RA.

Methotrexate can be given orally or parenterally in a once-weekly dose. The typical starting dosage for RA is 7.5–15 mg once weekly, increased as needed to a maximum of about 25 mg/week. Higher dosages are sometimes used in pediatric patients and in management of myositis. Methotrexate is also effective in the treatment of psoriatic arthritis. The once-weekly dosing regimen is used to minimize liver toxicity. Several studies found that patients are likely to stay on methotrexate longer than other DMARDs (1). Another advantage is a relatively fast onset of action (3–6 weeks). Its use has been reported to reduce mortality in RA (18). A switch to subcutaneous administration will often avoid GI side effects and will increase bioavailablilty of the compound; therefore, some patients experiencing a plateau after oral administration can be improved with a conversion to the subcutaneous or intramuscular route of administration.

The adverse effects of low-dose, weekly methotrexate are usually well tolerated, although some may be life threatening. Common side effects are nausea, vomiting, diarrhea, mouth ulcers, alopecia, headache, decreased white blood cell counts, and megaloblastic anemia. Hepatotoxicity is the most worrisome long-term effect. Liver function tests should be performed regularly in patients taking methotrexate, especially after dosage increases. An increase in liver enzyme levels may occur and should first be repeated before making changes in regimen. Liver function abnormalities may return to normal with dose reduction. An extremely small number of patients may develop significant liver fibrosis or cirrhosis, with liver biopsies indicated to evaluate persistent increases in liver enzyme levels. Patients taking methotrexate should be warned to avoid alcoholic beverages, which increase liver toxicity. Other risk factors are obesity, diabetes, and impaired renal function. Another potentially fatal toxicity of methotrexate is the unpredictable development of pulmonary interstitial pneumonitis that may require high-dose steroid treatment. Long-term pulmonary fibrosis may also be seen.

Methotrexate is teratogenic and should be discontinued in women who are considering conception. Although there is empiric evidence of

Table 3. Usual doses and key toxicities for antirheumatic drugs*

Drug	Usual dose	Toxicities that require monitoring
Salicylates, NSAIDs	See Table 1	Gastrointestinal ulceration and bleeding; renal impairment
Corticosteroids	See text and Table 2	Hypertension, hyperglycemia, euphoria, depression, osteoporosis, adrenal suppression, impaired wound healing, cataracts, susceptibility to infection
Analgesics		
Acetaminophen	600 mg to 1 gm qid	Risk of hepatotoxicity in overdose or in chronic alcohol abusers
Capsaicin	topically bid–qid	Local burning sensation initially
Hyaluronates	2 ml by intraarticular injection once weekly for 3–5 weeks	Local reactions, pain
Oxycodone	5–10 mg qid as needed or 10–20 mg (sustained release) bid	Dizziness, drowsiness, nausea, low risk of physical and psychologic dependence
Propoxyphene	65 mg qid as needed	Dizziness, drowsiness, nausea, low risk of physical and psychologic dependence
Tramadol	50–100 mg qid as needed	Drowsiness, dizziness, nausea, low risk of physical and psychologic dependence
Disease-modifying drugs		
Auranofin	3 mg bid	Bone marrow suppression, proteinuria
Azathioprine	50–150 mg/day	Bone marrow suppression, liver toxicity, lymphoproliferative disorders
Cyclosporine	3–5 mg/kg/day	Renal impairment, anemia, hypertension
Gold, injectable	50 mg weekly	Bone marrow suppression, proteinuria
Hydroxychloroquine	200–400 mg/day	Retinal damage
Leflunomide	10–20 mg/day	Liver toxicity, rash
Methotrexate	7.5–15 mg weekly	Bone marrow suppression, liver toxicity, pulmonary toxicity
Minocycline	100 mg bid	Dizziness
Mycophenolate	1 gm bid	Bone marrow suppression
Penicillamine	250–750 mg/day	Bone marrow suppression, proteinuria
Sulfasalazine	1 gm bid	Bone marrow suppression, rash

* bid = twice daily; tid = three times daily; qid = four times daily.

an association with increased risk for non-Hodgkin's lymphoma, this increased risk is also recognized in patients with significant and progressive chronic inflammation and patients with RA not treated with methotrexate; so what component of risk is contributed by methotrexate versus state of disease is not known.

Although folate antagonism may not entirely account for methotrexate's therapeutic efficacy, it does cause much of the toxicity. Low-dose folic acid supplements (~1 mg/day) are recommended to lessen adverse effects without altering efficacy. On the other hand, the antibiotic trimethoprim, found in Proloprim, Septra, and Bactrim, is also a human folate antagonist and should be avoided. Many side effects of methotrexate, including alopecia, stomatitis, headache, and anemia can also be decreased with the administration of folinic acid (Leukovorin)—5 mg given 12 and 24 hours after methotrexate administration.

Leflunomide

Leflunomide (Arava) is an antimetabolite with an antiproliferative effect on T lymphocytes through inhibition of pyrimidine synthesis. The active metabolite has a half-life of about 2 weeks, so it takes some time for blood levels to build up or be reduced. Leflunomide is approved for use in RA and has also shown efficacy in psoriatic arthritis.

Trials in RA patients found leflunomide to be superior to placebo and comparable to methotrexate or sulfasalazine after 1 year (19). Improvement began as early as 1 month after treatment started. In one study, the Sharp x-ray score was essentially unchanged in leflunomide patients compared to a worsening of 1.4 points with sulfasalazine and 5.6 with placebo.

Common adverse effects include diarrhea, rash, and reversible alopecia. Liver enzyme levels increase in about 10% of patients and fatal liver toxicity can occur. Although leflunomide has been used in combination with methotrexate, the risk of liver toxicity is increased. Anaphylaxis has been reported. Occasionally, weight loss, peripheral neuropathy, or interstitial lung disease can occur. Leflunomide is also teratogenic and must be avoided in patients who may conceive. Both men and women who wish to have children must discontinue the drug and should take cholestyramine (8 gm 3 times daily for 11 days) to bind and eliminate the drug.

Because of the long half-life of its metabolite, leflunomide dosage may begin with a loading dose of 100 mg/day for 3 days, followed by a maintenance dose of 20 mg/day (or 10 mg/day if 20 mg is poorly tolerated). However, some physicians decrease or omit the loading dose because diarrhea is so common.

Sulfasalazine

Although sulfasalazine may be better known for treating inflammatory bowel disease, it has proven efficacy in RA and peripheral manifestations of spondyloarthropathies. It is also FDA approved for use in children with RA. Antibacterial, antiinflammatory, and immunomodulatory effects may contribute to its efficacy, but no predominant mechanism has been established. Like other slow-acting drugs, improvement is not seen for at least 8–12 weeks. The dosage is 2–3 gm/day in divided doses, although the starting dose is usually smaller to avoid side effects.

Sulfasalazine has been shown to prevent joint erosions in RA and is an effective alternative to methotrexate (1). Common side effects are nausea, vomiting, headache, or fever. Use of enteric-coated formulations and administration with meals may significantly increase adherence and decrease GI side effects. Other potential adverse reactions may include rash, hemolysis, blood dyscrasias, and reversible male infertility. Screening for G6PDH levels is important and the drug should also be avoided in patients with sulfa allergy.

Hydroxychloroquine

Hydroxychloroquine was used as an antimalarial drug before its antirheumatic activity was discovered. It is believed to work by raising the pH of cytoplasmic compartments in antigen-processing cells like macrophages, thus interfering with antigen presentation. More recently its effects on toll-like receptors have been described and more likely defines its effect on the immune system. It is less effective in treating the signs and symptoms of RA than methotrexate but its safety is excellent (1), so it is sometimes used in mild RA. As monotherapy, however, hydroxychloroquine has not been shown to decrease radiographic progression. It is also very useful in treating joint and skin symptoms in SLE.

Hydroxychloroquine is very well tolerated, occasionally causing significant nausea or dizziness. The major concern is ocular toxicity. The drug has a high affinity for the retina, and if early signs of retinal damage are not detected, it can become irreversible and lead to blindness. If ophthalmic exams are done every 6 months, damage is easily detected and reversible at an early stage. Patients may report poor distance vision, difficulty reading, night blindness, and small areas of vision loss. The drug may also deposit in the cornea, but this does not cause serious problems. Ocular toxicity is dose related. Consequently, dosage is limited to <6.5 mg/kg/day (typically 400 mg/day).

Gold Compounds

Gold compounds were the first disease-modifying drugs to be widely used, but are seldom prescribed today. Presently, there is 1 compound (gold sodium thiomalate) commercially available for intramuscular injection, and 1 (auranofin) given orally. The parenteral and oral drugs have different profiles of safety and efficacy.

The standard intramuscular regimen is a 50-mg injection once a week. Lower doses are often given at first to test for tolerance, and less frequent doses (50 mg every 2–4 weeks) are used for maintenance. Injectable gold can produce clinical improvement in ~70% of patients; however, it may take 3–6 months for this to occur. A major drawback to the use of gold sodium thiomalate is that of adverse effects, which occur in ~30% of patients, leading to discontinuation. The most common reactions are mucocutaneous. Less frequent reactions include stomatitis, generalized pruritus, long-term gray-blue discoloration of mucous membranes, and alopecia. Proteinuria and nephrotic syndrome may occur. Blood dyscrasias are another serious adverse effect. Leukopenia, thrombocytopenia, and aplastic anemia have all been reported. Monitoring of injectable gold should include blood counts and urinalysis every 1–2 weeks prior to the next scheduled injection.

Auranofin is an orally active gold compound. It is given twice daily in 3-mg capsules. Its effectiveness is less than that of injectable gold, which offsets its convenience. Adverse effects are similar to injectable gold except that diarrhea is very common with auranofin, whereas the incidence of renal and hematologic effects is somewhat lower. However, it may take up to 9 months to see a clinical response.

Penicillamine

Penicillamine is seldom used today because of its side effects. It has been used in the past for RA and systemic sclerosis. It is taken orally, starting at 250 mg once daily and increasing to 250 mg 3 times daily, as necessary. Because penicillamine is a metal chelator, it must be taken on an empty stomach and 2 hours apart from iron salts or antacids to assure adequate absorption. Many side effects of penicillamine are dose-related and similar to those seen with gold compounds. Blood counts and urinalysis need to be monitored regularly. Additional effects caused by penicillamine include nausea, changes in taste that may resolve with continued therapy, and, rarely, autoimmune syndromes.

Azathioprine

Azathioprine (Imuran) is an immunosuppressive purine analog believed to interfere with cell division by inhibiting metabolism and synthesis of proteins and DNA. It has been used in doses of 0.75–2.5 mg/kg/day for rheumatic diseases, including lupus, myositis, and RA. Dosage is started at the low end and gradually increased as needed. Allopurinol interferes with azathioprine metabolism, necessitating a 50% reduction in dosage.

Azathioprine is similar in effectiveness to other slow-acting drugs in the treatment of RA (1). The usual lag period is required to see an effect. Side effects include GI intolerance, reduced white blood cell counts with risk of infection, pancreatitis, hepatotoxicity, and long-term risk of malignancy.

Cyclophosphamide

Cyclophosphamide (Cytoxan) is an alkylating agent, which nonspecifically kills cells by chemically reacting with DNA and RNA molecules. It suppresses the immune system by killing lymphocytes. Oral dosage begins at 50–75 mg/day and may be cautiously increased after 8 weeks if response is poor. Large intravenous doses may be used for lupus nephritis.

Cyclophosphamide is an important part of the treatment armamentarium for SLE and vasculitis. This drug is infrequently used in RA due its considerable toxicity. Nausea, mouth sores, alopecia, and low white blood cell counts are common. Suppression of ovarian and testicular function may occur with long-term therapy. A unique problem with cyclophosphamide is hemorrhagic inflammation of the urinary bladder, due to accumulation of an irritating drug metabolite. Patients may report painful urination or blood in the urine. Bladder cancer can be a long-term adverse effect. These problems are reduced by drinking plenty of fluids and frequently emptying the bladder, especially before bedtime.

Cyclosporine

Cyclosporine is an immunosuppressive drug commonly used to prevent organ rejection. The drug is available in different dosage forms that are not interchangeable, and only the microemulsion form (Neoral) is FDA approved for treatment of severe RA. It inhibits production and utilization of interleukin-2, a growth factor for lymphocytes, and has a 6–12-week lag period before producing benefit. Renal damage, hypertension, gum hypertrophy, and increased body hair are the most common adverse effects. Recommended dosing is 2.5–4.0 mg/kg/day divided into 2 equal doses (20). Higher dosages increase the risk of nephropathy. It is reserved for severe, progressive RA unresponsive to other drugs. However, cyclosporine has also been used in other autoimmune diseases, including myositis.

Minocycline

Three double-blinded trials have shown minocycline to have a slow-acting effect in RA, although it is not FDA approved for this indication. The benefit appears modest, but may be more pronounced in early RA. Minocycline's mechanism of action is probably unrelated to its antibiotic activity. Tetracyclines are known to inhibit matrix metalloproteinases, and potentially may retard loss of joint space in OA as well. Because minocycline is well tolerated except for nausea and dizziness, it may be used in mild RA (21). There is no evidence, however, that minocycline has a disease-modifying effect in RA.

Mycophenolate Mofetil

Mycophenolate mofetil (CellCept) is a purine antimetabolite currently approved for immunosuppression to prevent organ rejection. It has been studied in ~600 RA patients with promising results. It has also been studied as an alternative to cyclophosphamide in treating lupus nephritis. The drug has no liver or renal toxicity and could provide a safer alternative to cyclosporine or azathioprine in immunosuppressive regimens. Gastrointestinal upset is the most common adverse effect. Neurologic symptoms are also seen, with paresthesias and neuropathies. It is unclear if mycophenylate is associated with an increased risk of lymphoproliferative disease in patients with underlying autoimmunity.

Combination Therapy

Combining drugs with different mechanisms of action may provide additional benefits over monotherapy, especially in the case of RA, sometimes without a significant increase in toxicity. Most DMARDs may be combined effectively with methotrexate or biologic therapies. Hydroxychloroquine and minocycline are often used together with other DMARDs. Combination therapies give clinicians more options for aggressive treatment (22).

Many rheumatologists now initiate treatment with combinations of slow-acting drugs, biologics, and/or steroids and gradually withdraw drugs as disease improvement occurs. Other rheumatologists save combination therapy for patients who fail to respond satisfactorily to methotrexate alone.

MEDICATIONS FOR GOUT

Medications used in gout can be divided into 2 groups: those used for treating acute gouty arthritis and those used to prevent long-term complications by lowering uric acid blood levels. The first group includes NSAIDs and corticosteroids, which have been discussed already, and colchicine. The second group includes probenecid, sulfinpyrazone, allopurinol, and febuxostat.

Colchicine

Colchicine has been used in plant form for centuries, but it is less often used today because of its toxicities. It inhibits neutrophil function by an effect on microtubules. Although many texts still report a traditional regimen for acute gouty arthritis using 0.5 or 0.6 mg of colchicine given orally every hour until relief is obtained, intolerable side effects of diarrhea often occur before the maximum dose of 6 mg is reached. The use of colchicine on a long-term basis (1 or 2 tablets daily) is usually tolerated without GI complaints and is commonly used to prevent gouty arthritis.

Although effective, most patients complain of significant nausea, vomiting, and diarrhea from colchicine, particularly with escalating acute therapy. Although these side effects can be partly overcome by giving the drug intravenously (up to 3 mg), administration via this route is more likely to produce organ toxicity, such as neuropathy, bone marrow depression, renal and liver toxicity, and shock. The intravenous dose should be considered only in exceedingly unusual circumstances and never in patients with renal dysfunction, even if it is mild, because fatal outcomes have been reported. The drug is predominantly cleared through the kidney. The maximum dose should be lowered for the elderly and those with renal or hepatic impairment (23).

Probenecid and Sulfinpyrazone

These 2 drugs are uricosurics, meaning they increase excretion of uric acid in the urine. The dose range is 500–2,000 mg/day for probenecid and 100–800 mg/day for sulfinpyrazone (23). The dose should start at the lower end for both drugs to avoid precipitation of renal stones, and fluid intake should be increased concomitantly. These drugs are ineffective in patients with poor renal function and can be antagonized by even low doses of aspirin. In the early weeks of therapy, any drug that lowers uric acid may actually increase the risk of gouty arthritis, so a prophylactic antiinflammatory drug, colchicine, or low-dose corticosteroid should also be prescribed. The drugs are well tolerated, with occasional rashes or GI distress reported.

Allopurinol and Febuxostat

Allopurinol and febuxostat lower formation of uric acid by inhibiting xanthine oxidase, the enzyme that converts purines to uric acid. Xanthine oxidase inhibitors are more versatile than uricosurics because they are effective at all levels of renal function and also in both overproducers and underexcretors of uric acid.

The usual dosage of allopurinol is 300 mg/day; this should be lowered to 100 mg/day in patients with renal impairment. However, allopurinol inhibits metabolism of many other drugs and can cause rashes, bone marrow suppression, and a multiorgan hypersensitivity syndrome involving fever, severe skin reactions, and renal and hepatic failure. Febuxostat is a new nonpurine xanthine oxidase inhibitor that is at least as effective as allopurinol but less allergenic (24). It has been used in dosages of 80–240 mg/day and is reported to be relatively well tolerated, with diarrhea, nausea, and headache being possible side effects. Neither uricosuric drugs nor xanthine oxidase inhibitors should be used in asymptomatic hyperuricemia unless accompanied by tophi.

MUSCLE RELAXANTS

Muscle-relaxing drugs, such as carisoprodol, cyclobenzaprine, methocarbamol, and chlorzoxazone, are used to relieve secondary muscle spasm in back pain and other chronic painful conditions. Cyclobenzaprine (Flexeril) is widely used to manage fibromyalgia. Both cyclobenzaprine and a chemically related antidepressant, amitriptyline, have been shown to improve sleep and relieve pain in patients with fibromyalgia (25). Cyclobenzaprine's dosage is 5–10 mg 1–3 times daily, and amitriptyline is used in low doses (10–50 mg) at bedtime. Both of these drugs frequently cause drowsiness and anticholinergic side effects, such as dry mouth, constipation, confusion, and urine retention.

REFERENCES

1. American College of Rheumatology Subcommittee on Rheumatoid Arthritis Guidelines. Guidelines for the management of rheumatoid arthritis: 2002 update. Arthritis Rheum 2002;46:328–46.
2. American College of Rheumatology Subcommittee on Osteoarthritis Guidelines. Recommendations for the medical management of osteoarthritis of the hip and knee: 2000 update. Arthritis Rheum 2000;43:1905–15.
3. Larson AM, Polson J, Fontana RJ, Davern TJ, Lalani E, Hynan LS, et al. Acetaminophen-induced acute liver failure: results of a United States multicenter, prospective study. Hepatology 2005;42:1364–72.
4. McCarthy GM, McCarty DY. Effect of topical capsaicin in the therapy of painful osteoarthritis of the hands. J Rheumatol 1992;19:604–7.
5. Lipsky PE, Abramson SB, Crofford L, Dubois RN, Simon LS, van de Putte LB. The classification of cyclooxygenase inhibitors. J Rheumatol 1998;25:2298–303.
6. Tannenbaum H, Bombardier C, Davis P, Russell AS. An evidence-based approach to prescribing nonsteroidal antiinflammatory drugs. Third Canadian consensus conference. J Rheumatol 2006;33:140–57.
7. Silverstein FE, Faich G, Goldstein JL, Simon LS, Pincus T, Whelton A, et al. Gastrointestinal toxicity with celecoxib vs nonsteroidal anti-inflammatory drugs for osteoarthritis and rheumatoid arthritis: the CLASS study: a randomized controlled study. JAMA 2000;284:1247–55.
8. Wolfe MM, Lichtenstein DR, Singh G. Gastrointestinal toxicity of nonsteroidal anti-inflammatory drugs. N Engl J Med 1999;340:1888–99.
9. Brandt KD, Smith GN Jr, Simon LS. Intraarticular injection of hyaluronan as treatment for knee osteoarthritis: what is the evidence? Arthritis Rheum 2000;43:1192–203.
10. Bellamy N, Campbell J, Robinson V, Gee T, Bourne R, Wells G. Viscosupplementation for the treatment of osteoarthritis of the knee. The Cochrane Database of Systematic Reviews 2005; Issue 2:CD005321.
11. Moreland LW, O'Dell JR. Glucocorticoids and rheumatoid arthritis. Back to the future? Arthritis Rheum 2002;46:2553–63.
12. Saag KG, Koehnke R, Caldwell JR, Brasington R, Burmeister LF, Zimmerman B, et al. Low dose long-term corticosteroid therapy in rheumatoid arthritis: an analysis of serious adverse events. Am J Med 1994;96:115–23.
13. Schumacher HR, Chen LX. Injectable corticosteroids in treatment of arthritis of the knee. Am J Med 2005;118:1208–14.
14. Harris ED. Prednisolone in early rheumatoid arthritis: an antiinvasive effect. Arthritis Rheum 2005;52:3324–5.
15. Fries JF. ARAMIS and toxicity measurement. J Rheumatol 1995;22:995–7.
16. Grigor C, Capell H, Stirling A, McMahon AD, Lock P, Vallance R, et al. Effect of a treatment strategy of tight control for rheumatoid arthritis (the TICORA study): a single-blind randomized controlled trial. Lancet 2004;364:263–69.
17. Tsakonas E, Fitzgerald AA, Fitzcharles MA, Cividino A, Thorne JC, M'Seffar A, et al. Consequences of delayed therapy with second-line agents in rheumatoid arthritis: a 3 year follow up on the hydroxychloroquine in early rheumatoid arthritis study. J Rheumatol 2000;27:623–9.
18. Choi HK, Herman MA, Seeger JD, Robins JM, Wolfe F. Methotrexate and mortality in patients with rheumatoid arthritis: a prospective study. Lancet 2002;359:1173–7.
19. Osiri M, Shea B, Robinson V, Suarez-Almazor M, Strand V, Tugwell P, et al. Leflunomide for the treatment of rheumatoid arthritis: a systematic review and meta-analysis. J Rheumatol 2003;30:1182–90.
20. Cush JJ, Tugwell P, Weinblatt M, Yocum D. US consensus guidelines for the use of cyclosporin A in rheumatoid arthritis. J Rheumatol 1999;26:1176–86.
21. O'Dell JR, Haire CE, Palmer W, Drymalski W, Wees S, Blakely K, et al. Treatment of early rheumatoid arthritis with minocycline or placebo: results of a randomized, double-blind, placebo-controlled trial. Arthritis Rheum 1997;40:842–8.
22. Smolen JS, Aletaha D, Keystone E. Superior efficacy of combination therapy for rheumatoid arthritis. Fact or fiction? Arthritis Rheum 2005;52:2975–83.
23. Schlesinger N. Management of acute and chronic gouty arthritis. Present state-of-the-art. Drugs 2004;64:2399–2416.
24. Becker MA, Schumacher HR, Wortmann RL, MacDonald PA, Eustace D, Palo WA, et al. Febuxostat compared with allopurinol in patients with hyperuricemia and gout. N Engl J Med 2005;353:2450–61.
25. Carette S, Bell MJ, Reynolds WJ, Haraoui B, McCain GA, Bykerk VP, et al. Comparison of amitriptyline, cyclobenzaprine, and placebo in the treatment of fibromyalgia: a randomized, double-blind clinical trial. Arthritis Rheum 1994;37:32–40.

Recommended Reading

American College of Rheumatology Ad Hoc Committee on Clinical Guidelines. Guidelines for monitoring drug therapy in rheumatoid arthritis. Arthritis Rheum 1996;39:723–31.

American Geriatrics Society Panel on Chronic Pain in Older Persons. The management of chronic pain in older persons. J Am Geriatr Soc 1998;46: 635–51.

Drugs for rheumatoid arthritis. Treat Guidel Med Lett 2005;3:83–90.

O'Dell JR. Therapeutic strategies for rheumatoid arthritis. N Engl J Med 2004;350:2591–602.

Simon LS, Lipman AG, Caudill-Slosberg M, Gill L, Keefe FJ, Kerr KL, et al. Guideline for the management of pain in osteoarthritis, rheumatoid arthritis, and juvenile chronic arthritis. Glenview (IL): American Pain Society; 2002.

Web Resources

CiaoMed.org. News on rheumatology and musculoskeletal diseases. URL: http://www.ciaomed.org.

JointAndBone.org. News on rheumatology, including drug therapy. URL: http://www.jointandbone.org.

Medscape Drug Information. Free, updated drug information. URL: http://www.medscape.com/druginfo/.

Pharmacologic Interventions: Biologic Agents

ALAN K. MATSUMOTO, MD

Biologic agents (biologic response modifiers) represent a remarkable advance for the treatment of rheumatic disease. Fulfilling the promise of research in immunology and biotechnology, these drugs are effective options for patients refractory to, or intolerant of older conventional therapies. Particularly when used early in inflammatory arthritis, these agents not only improve signs and symptoms, but also significantly prevent joint damage and may ameliorate future disease severity. By targeting specific immunologic pathways, they have revealed new insights into mechanisms of disease. The currently approved biologic agents for the treatment of rheumatic diseases are summarized in Table 1. Produced by recombinant DNA technology, all are bioengineered replicas of human proteins and must be administered by subcutaneous (SC) injection or intravenous (IV) infusion. Because they potently inhibit critical cytokines and immune cells, the most significant side effects of treatment to date have been serious infections. Open-label clinical trials and registries continue to study the long-term effects of chronic immunomodulation with these agents. With these therapies, we face new challenges to define the patients best served by these therapies, to accurately assess disease activity, and to effectively administer and monitor these new agents. At the present time, with few exceptions, biologic agents remain reserved for those patients who continue to have active disease despite treatment with conventional disease-modifying agents or who have experienced side effects while taking those agents.

Biologic agents may be classified into 3 basic structural categories: soluble receptors, monoclonal antibodies, and receptor antagonists (Figure 1). Soluble receptors are fusion proteins combining the ligand binding regions of receptors normally found on the surface of cells with an immunoglobulin Fc region. The resultant soluble receptor binds ligands, such as cytokines, in the circulation and prevents them from binding to their normal receptors on cells. Thus, the ligand is prevented from activating the cell. In the case when both ligand and target receptor are cell-bound, the soluble receptor can interfere with this cell-cell interaction.

Therapeutic monoclonal antibodies (mAbs) bind to cytokines in the circulation or proteins on the cell surface. In the case of mAbs directed against cytokines, the antibody clears the cytokine from the circulation and prevents its binding to receptors on the surface of cells. Monoclonal antibodies that bind proteins on specific immune cells can deplete those cells from the circulation, either through apoptosis, complement-mediated cell lysis, or Fc receptor-mediated clearance. Early mAbs utilized the binding regions of mouse antibodies (chimeric antibodies), but advancements have yielded more "humanized" and fully human mAbs that have reduced immunogenecity.

Bioengineered copies of naturally occurring receptor antagonists have also been developed as therapeutic agents. Mimicking the function of native proteins, these agents occupy a cell-surface receptor and prevent engagement and binding by a particular cytokine or receptor ligand.

TUMOR NECROSIS FACTOR INHIBITORS

Tumor necrosis factor α (TNFα) is a proinflammatory cytokine produced primarily by macrophages and monocytes that is involved in normal inflammatory and immune responses. It is increased in a variety of pathologic conditions, including sepsis, malignancy, heart failure, and chronic inflammatory diseases. It is found at high levels in the joint and circulation of patients with severe rheumatoid arthritis (RA). In the rheumatoid joint, TNFα recruits inflammatory cells, increases vasodilation, induces bone resorption, and stimulates production of collagenase and prostaglandins, making it an important therapeutic target in RA. Due to the central role of TNFα in chronic inflammation, TNF inhibition is effective in a variety of inflammatory diseases, including psoriatic arthritis, skin psoriasis, ankylosing spondylitis, uveitis, and Crohn's disease.

Table 1. Biologic agents approved for use in rheumatic disease*

	Etanercept (Enbrel)	Infliximab (Remicade)	Adalimumab (Humira)	Anakinra (Kineret)	Abatacept (Orencia)	Rituximab (Rituxan)
Structure	Soluble receptor	Chimeric monoclonal antibody	Human monoclonal antibody	Human IL-1 receptor antagonist	Soluble receptor	Chimeric monoclonal antibody
Target	TNFα	TNFα	TNFα	IL-1 receptor	T-cell costimulatory pathway	CD20+ B cells
Route of adminstration	Self-injection SC	IV infusion	Self-injection SC	Self-injection SC	IV infusion	IV infusion
Dosing	25 mg biweekly or 50 mg weekly	3–10 mg/kg every 4–8 weeks after loading doses at 0, 2, 6 weeks	40 mg every 2 weeks or weekly	100 mg daily	500, 750, or 1,000 mg based on weight every 4 weeks after loading dose at 0, 2, 4 weeks	1,000 mg at day 1 and 15 and repeat in 4 months if necessary
Indications	RA, PsA, AS, JRA, Ps	RA, PsA, Crohn's	RA, PsA, AS	RA	RA	RA
Need for concomitant MTX	No	Yes in RA only	No	No	No	Yes

* IL-1 = interleukin 1; TNF = tumor necrosis factor; SC = subcutaneous; RA = rheumatoid arthritis; PsA = psoriatic arthritis; AS = ankylosing spondylitis; JRA = juvenile rheumatoid arthritis; Ps = psoriasis; MTX = methotrexate.

Table 2. Recommended procedures prior to initiation of biologic therapy

History and physical exam
Complete blood count, chemistries
Purified protein derivative screening
Baseline chest x-ray
Baseline electrocardiogram (rituximab)
Immunization: pneumoccal vaccine, influenza vaccine (yearly)
Hepatitis B and C screening

Etanercept, infliximab, and adalimumab are the currently available TNF antagonists. These agents are similarly effective in the treatment of RA but differ in their efficacy for some other diseases. Notably, infliximab and adalimumab, both monoclonal antibodies, are effective in inflammatory bowel disease, whereas the soluble receptor etanercept is not, raising the possibility that structural or dosing differences may affect efficacy of particular compounds. In RA and psoriatic arthritis, all 3 agents decrease the signs and symptoms of joint inflammation and significantly inhibit joint destruction. The safety of the 3 anti-TNF agents, including risks of infection, appears to be similar (Table 3).

Etanercept

Etanercept is a dimeric fusion protein consisting of 2 binding domains of the human p75 TNF receptor attached to a human immunoglobulin IgG1 Fc region. It binds TNF and lymphotoxin alpha with high affinity and is given by SC self-injection. It is effective and approved for use in RA, juvenile rheumatoid arthritis, psoriatic arthritis, ankylosing spondylitis, and skin psoriasis. Dosing is 25 mg twice weekly or 50 mg weekly. In skin psoriasis, it is initially given 50 mg twice weekly for 3 months and then reduced to a maintenance dosage of 50 mg weekly. In RA, etanercept is effective as monotherapy but has greater efficacy when used in combination with methotrexate (1,2).

Infliximab

Infliximab is a chimeric monoclonal antibody with the binding regions for TNF derived from mouse and the remainder of the molecule of human origin. It binds TNF with high affinity and specificity and is administered by IV infusion. Approved indications are RA, ankylosing spondylitis, psoriatic arthritis, and Crohn's disease. In RA, the initial dosage is 3 mg/kg with a loading dose at 0, 2, and 6 weeks followed by

a maintenance dose every 8 weeks. In nonresponsive patients, the dosage may be incrementally increased up to 10 mg/kg every 4 weeks (3). In RA, it is recommended that infliximab be given together with methotrexate (10–20 mg weekly) to prevent the formation of human antichimeric antibodies (HACA), which can diminish efficacy and increase infusion reactions (4). HACAs are also more common if infliximab is not dosed on a regular schedule. For other indications, the starting dosage is 5 mg/kg with a dosing schedule similar to RA, but concomitant methotrexate use is optional. The lack of need for methotrexate in these indications may represent lower rates of HACA formation with the larger starting dosage of infliximab or a different tendency to develop such an immune response in different conditions.

Adalimumab

Adalimumab is a fully human monoclonal antibody with high affinity and specificity for TNF. It is given by self-administered SC injection and is approved for use in RA, psoriatic arthritis, and ankylosing spondylitis (5,6). Adalimumab has also been shown to be effective in inflammatory bowel disease (7). The starting dosage for all 3 approved indications is 40 mg every other week. If RA patients fail to respond, the approved dosage may be increased to 40 mg weekly. Adalimumab in RA is more effective when administered with methotrexate, in part due to increased serum levels of adalimumab when used in combination.

Side Effects

Infusion reactions or injection site reactions are the most common reported side effect associated with TNF antagonists, but only rarely cause serious problems or discontinuation of therapy. Acute infusion reactions with infliximab occurred in up to 20% of cases in clinical trials and included pruritis, urticaria, flushing, headache, fever, hypotension, chest pain, and dsypnea. Most reactions are mild and are treated by briefly stopping or slowing the rate of infusion. Many infusion centers pretreat with a nonsedating antihistamine prior to infusion. Occasionally, pretreatment with corticosteroids is needed. In clinical trials, 3% of patients discontinued infliximab due to infusion reactions. Local injection-site reactions (urticaria, pruritis, erythema, pain) may be seen in up to 30% of patients starting on etanercept or adalimumab. The frequency and severity of these reactions typically diminish after the first several injections and then resolve completely; however, some patients may develop urticarial eruptions that become generalized. More severe systemic allergic reactions are rare, however.

Infections are the side effect of greatest concern with TNF antagonists. Registries, case series, and long-term open-label studies have shown an increased risk for serious bacterial infections, tuberculosis and other granulomatous infections, and opportunistic infections (8). Quantifying the risk has been difficult because of the increased rates of infection associated with the underlying rheumatic diseases and the use of concomitant immunosuppressive medications, particularly prednisone.

Tuberculosis (TB) is associated with all 3 of the anti-TNF agents (9). It presents more commonly with extrapulmonary manifestations and most occur soon after the initiation of therapy, suggesting reactivation of latent TB. Screening for latent TB prior to the initiation of TNF antagonist therapy is important in identifying patients at risk. All patients starting a TNF inhibitor should undergo a 5 TU purified protein derivative (PPD) skin test, regardless if they have a history of TB vaccination with bacilli Calmette-Guerin (BCG). A ≥5-mm induration should be considered positive, regardless of BCG status. Guidelines for the administration of TNF antagonists in patients with evidence

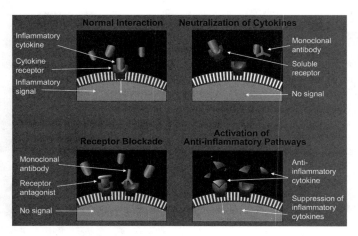

Figure 1. Inhibition of cytokines.

Table 3. Contraindictions to the use of tumor necrosis factor inhibitors

Serious active infections
Recurrent serious infections
Untreated latent tuberculosis
History/family history of multiple sclerosis
Class III or IV congestive heart failure
History of or active lymphoma

of prior TB exposure are not established. However, recommendations have been made for the treatment of latent TB with isoniazid (300 mg/day) and pyridoxine (50 mg/day) for 9 months, or if not tolerated, rifampin (600 mg/day) for 4 months (10). These recommendations have not been specifically evaluated for patients with rheumatic diseases receiving concomitant immunomodulatory therapy. Although no formal guidelines exist, most practitioners start the TNF inhibitor 1 month after initiating TB therapy to ensure that it is tolerated and that patients are adherent. A baseline chest x-ray should be obtained. Nonspecific granuloma on chest x-ray with a negative PPD skin test does not necessarily require further evaluation or testing before the initiation of anti-TNF therapy. Clinical vigilance should be maintained for the possibility of reactivation of other granulomatous diseases, such as histoplasmosis. Patients who are receiving TNF antagonists should be periodically tested for new exposure to TB, especially those with occupational risk or travel to endemic areas.

Serious bacterial infections are the most common problem associated with anti-TNF therapy. In clinical studies, when defined as infections requiring hospitalization or IV antibiotics, serious infections occur in ~4–5 patients per 100 patient-years of exposure. In most studies, the increased rate of infection is 1.5–2 times greater than in RA patients not treated with anti-TNF therapy (11). Pneumonia, cellulites, and urinary tract infections are most common. Prompt diagnosis and appropriate antibiotic treatment are most important. If patients encounter any symptoms of infection, particularly fever, they should be instructed not to take their TNF inhibitor and contact their doctor. Pneumoccal vaccination and annual influenza vaccine are recommended. Live viral vaccinations (e.g., Flumist) should not be administered.

Infections with other organisms have been reported, including *Histoplasma, Coccidioides, Listeria, Pneumocystis, Candida,* and *Aspergillus* (12). Most of these cases are sporadic. Histoplasmosis and coccidoidomycosis cases are almost exclusively found in endemic areas. Rates are estimated at ~0.05 cases per 100 patient-years exposure. No specific precautions or monitoring is required beyond clinical vigilance. Anti-TNF therapy has been used in patients with chronic hepatitis C without apparent problems, but reactivation of hepatitis B has been reported (13).

Because of the possible role of TNF in normal immunosurveillance for malignancy, concern has been generated about a potential risk of malignancy associated with anti-TNF therapy. Cases of lymphoma have been reported, but the association with TNF inhibitors remains unclear due to the increased risk of lymphoma seen in severe RA (14). To date, no clear association has been found with any solid tumors. Further studies are ongoing.

Other adverse effects associated with TNF inhibitors have also been reported. The recommendation has been made that TNF inhibitors not be used in patients with advanced heart failure because cases of worsening or new-onset congestive heart failure that improved with drug cessation have been reported, as have results of clinical trials of TNF inhibitors in congestive heart failure that showed negative outcomes (15). However, additional studies from RA clinical trials have not shown an increased risk of heart failure. Reports of demyelinating disease of the brain and spinal cord, optic neuritis, seizures, and Guillan-Barre syndrome have

been described (16). Patients with a history of multiple sclerosis or a strong family history of multiple sclerosis should be excluded from anti-TNF therapy. Autoantibody formation, including anti–double-stranded DNA (anti-dsDNA), have been associated with all 3 anti-TNF drugs, but drug-induced syndromes are generally mild and reversible. However, more significant manifestations have occurred. Some practitioners check baseline antinuclear antibodies, dsDNA, and anticardiolipin antibodies prior to the initiation of TNF antagonists so that if a patient develops a lupus-like illness in the course of therapy, it may be easier to determine if it is a drug-induced phenomenon. Cases of cytopenias, specifically neutropenia and elevated liver enzyme levels, have been reported but usually are reversible with therapy cessation. Because of these risks, complete blood count and serum chemistries should be checked on a regular basis.

INTERLEUKIN-1 INHIBITORS

Anakinra

Interleukin-1 (IL-1) is a proinflammatory cytokine with actions similar to those of TNFα. It is also found at high levels in the joints and circulation of patients with active RA. To activate inflammatory cells, IL-1 binds to a cell-surface receptor and then recruits an accessory protein necessary for cell signaling. IL-1 receptor antagonist (IL-1Ra) is a naturally occurring antiinflammatory protein that binds the IL-1 receptor and prevents the recruitment of the accessory signaling protein. Anakinra is a genetically engineered version of human IL-1Ra. It is approved for use in RA (17). However, its short half-life requires daily injections, and its modest clinical efficacy compared with the anti-TNF drugs has resulted in limited use. Anakinra has also been effective in some periodic fever syndromes and Still's disease. It should not be used in conjunction with TNF inhibitors because of a demonstrated increased risk of cytopenias and infection, and no increase in efficacy.

T-CELL INHIBITORS

Abatacept

Activated T cells are found within the rheumatoid synovium, and oligoclonal expansions are well documented. The efficacy of some non-biologic T-cell active therapies has shown a role for the T cell in RA and other autoimmune diseases. For T-cell activation to occur, antigen is presented to the T-cell receptor in the context of a major histocompatibility class I or class II molecule on the surface of an antigen presenting cell (APC). For efficient activation of the T cell, a second T-cell surface protein, CD28, must bind with the CD80/86 receptor on the APC to activate a costimulatory signaling pathway. Human cytotoxic T-lymphocyte–associated antigen (CTLA-4) is a naturally occurring T-cell surface protein that competes with CD28 for binding to CD80/86, thus preventing T-cell activation.

Abatacept is a soluble fusion protein combining the extracellular domains of 2 CTLA-4 molecules with the Fc portion of human IgG1. Abatacept binds CD80/86, preventing binding of CD28 and thus inhibiting the costimulatory pathway and T-cell activation. It is administered as a 30-minute IV infusion at weeks 0, 2, and 4 and every 4 weeks thereafter. Doses are 500 mg, 750 mg, or 1,000 mg based on body weight. Infusion reactions are rare and occurred in 0.9% of patients in clinical trials. Abatacept is approved for use in RA that has been refractory to traditional disease-modifying agents (18). It is effective in improving signs and symptoms as well as in inhibiting radiographic progression. Side effects, including infection, are similar to the TNF inhibitors. In clinical trials, patients with chronic obstructive pulmonary disease suffered more serious adverse events, making this a group at increased risk for the use of abatacept. Further studies are underway. Screening for TB is also recommended. Vaccination responses may also be impaired while taking abatacept, so immunizations should be completed before starting therapy. Abatacept should not be used concomitantly with a TNF inhibitor because of a demonstrated increased risk of infection.

B-CELL DEPLETION

Rituximab

B cells are also abundant in the rheumatoid synovium and likely play a role in antigen presentation, upregulation of such inflammatory cytokines as IL-6, and autoantibody production. Rheumatoid factor and anti-cyclic citrullinated peptide antibodies are produced by B cells locally within the joint. Thus B cells also appear to be a promising therapeutic target. Rituximab is a monoclonal antibody directed against CD20, a B-cell–specific surface protein present throughout B-cell maturation but not present on mature plasma cells. Rituximab was first approved for the treatment of B-cell lymphomas and produces profound depletion of peripheral B cells with limited effect on total serum immunoglobulin levels. It is also approved for the treatment of RA refractory to TNF inhibitors (19,20). Dosing is 1,000 mg intravenously for 2 doses, given 2 weeks apart. Patients should be treated with concomitant weekly oral methotrexate (10–20 mg/week). Patients have noted sustained benefit, some up to 1 year or longer. Patients experiencing disease flare may be retreated after 4 months, but the safety and timing of retreatment has not been demonstrated in large numbers of patients. Because of the prolonged B-cell depletion, which may persist a year or longer, the safety of subsequent immunomodulatory therapy if required is also not well studied. Long-term and retreatment experience with rituximab is limited but additional studies are underway.

Infusion reactions are the most significant side effect. Patients should receive methylprednisolone (100 mg intravenously) prior to the dose of rituximab to prevent infusion reactions. Antihistamines may also be used. Infusion reactions including fever, chills, rash, and hypotension; bronchospasm can occur in up to 30% of patients with the first dose even with pretreatment, but diminishes to ~10% with the second dose. Serious cardiac arrythmias and hypotension have been described in patients receiving rituximab for lymphoma, but to date have not been reported in patients treated for RA. Nonetheless, precautions should be taken in patients with significant cardiac history, and infusion centers need to assess the availability of appropriate care if cardiac events should occur. Rates of infection are similar to the TNF inhibitors. Cases of reactivation of hepatitis B and C have been reported. Primary immune responses are diminished with Rituximab, thus all immunization series should be completed prior to treatment (e.g., hepatitis B vaccination, pneumococcal vaccination, etc.). Live virus vaccines (e.g., Flumist) should be avoided in Rituximab-treated patients.

FUTURE DIRECTIONS

Strategies to inhibit cytokines and receptors with mAbs and soluble receptors has provided significant insight into disease pathogenesis. Active investigation is ongoing to identify downstream signaling molecules that are activated by cell-surface receptors and cytokines, which may present additional targets of therapy that can be inhibited with the use of small molecules and orally active agents. Exciting gene therapeutic approaches are in development that provide an additional way to turn off proinflammatory cytokines and growth factors. These may provide even more selective tissue-specific or time-limited inhibition, leading to fewer systemic side effects.

Multiple studies are underway assessing the use of the approved biologic agents in other rheumatic diseases and other chronic inflammatory diseases. Trials of rituximab in vasculitis and systemic lupus erythematosus are in progress and TNF antagonists are being evaluated in scleroderma, myositis, and lupus. However, chronic inflammation is a complex process and agents will not be universally effective in all diseases, demonstrated by a large negative trial of etanercept use in Wegner's vasculitis (21). The challenge will be to determine which of the agents may be the most effective for which diseases. Research, particularly the expanding fields of genomics and proteomics, is identifying new biologic targets and biologic agents offer the ability to specifically inhibit these pathways, testing the hypothesis quickly and efficiently. Studies with IL-6 antagonists and IL-12 antagonists are ongoing for the treatment of RA and appear to be promising.

Given the chronic nature of rheumatic illness, there must also be continued research regarding the long-term safety profile of these agents. Understanding the long-term safety of biologic response modifiers is necessarily limited by the fact that the longest human exposures to the first of these agents is only 10 years. It is clear that even targeted immunomodulation from a number of pathways increases the risk of infection, serious infection, and in some cases particular opportunistic infections based on the drug's mechanism of action. Because of an increased risk of certain forms of malignancies in some rheumatic diseases, only long-term exposure of larger numbers of patients will definitively determine if there is any causal relationship between exposure to these medications and a new tumor. A heightened sensitivity to these issues of safety will likely improve the care of patients with rheumatic diseases, leading to a lower threshold for evaluation of unusual complaints, and including potential drug-related adverse events in the differential diagnosis.

From a practical perspective, safe, efficient, cost-effective means of delivering these drugs must be established. Certainly formidable challenges remain, but there can be little doubt of the potential for biologic agents to further improve outcomes for patients with rheumatic diseases.

REFERENCES

1. Moreland LW, Schiff MH, Baumgartner SW, Tindall EA, Fleischmann RM, Bulpitt KJ, et al. Etanercept therapy in rheumatoid arthritis: a randomized, controlled trial. Ann Intern Med 1999;130:478–86.
2. van der Heijde D, Klareskog L, Rodriguez-Valverde V, et al. Comparison of etanercept and methotrexate alone and in combination in the treatment of rheumatoid arthritis: two-year clinical and radiographic results form the TEMPO study, a double blind randomized trial. Arthritis Rheum 2006;54:1063–74.
3. van der Heijde D, Klareskog L, Rodriguez-Valverde V, Codreanu C, Bolosiu H, Melo-Gomes J, et al, Anti-Tumor Necrosis Factor Trial in Rheumatoid Arthritis with Concomitant Therapy Study Group. Infliximab and methotrexate in the treatment of rheumatoid arthritis. N Engl J Med 2000;343:1594–602.
4. Maini RN, Breedveld FC, Kalden JR, Smolen JS, Davis D, Macfarlane JD, et al. Therapeutic efficacy of multiple intravenous infusions of anti-tumor necrosis factor alpha monoclonal antibody combined with low-dose weekly methotrexate in rheumatoid arthritis. Arthritis Rheum 1998;41:1552–63.
5. Weinblatt ME, Keystone EC, Furst DE, Moreland LW, Weisman MH, Birbara CA, et al. Adalimumab, a fully human anti-tumor necrosis factor alpha monoclonal antibody, for the treatment of rheumatoid arthritis in patients taking concomitant methotrexate: the ARMADA trial. Arthritis Rheum 2003;48:35–45.

6. Breedveld FC, Weisman MH, Kavanaugh AF, Cohen SB, Pavelka K, van Vollenhoven R, et al. The PREMIER study: a multicenter, randomized, double-blind clinical trial of combination therapy with adalimumab plus methotrexate versus methotrexate alone or adalimumab alone in patients with early, aggressive rheumatoid arthritis who had not had previous methotrexate treatment. Arthritis Rheum 2006;54:26–37.

7. Hanauer SB, Sandbom WJ, Rutgeerts P. Human anti-tumor necrosis factor monoclonal antibody (adalimumab) in Crohn's disease: CLASSIC I trial. Gastroenterology 2006;130:323–33.

8. Giles JT, Bathon JM. Serious infections associated with anti-cytokine therapies in the rheumatic diseases. J Intensive Care Med 2004;19:320–34.

9. Askling J, Fored CM, Brandt L, Baecklund E, Bertilsson L, Coster L, et al. Risk and case characteristics of tuberculosis in rheumatoid arthritis associated with tumor necrosis factor antagonists in Sweden. Arthritis Rheum 2005;52:1986–92.

10. Nuremberger E, Bishai WR, Grossett JH. Latent tuberculosis infection. Semin Respir Crit Care Med 2004;25:317–36.

11. Bongartz T, Sutton AJ, Sweety MJ. Anti-TNF antibody therapy in rheumatoid arthritis and the risk of serious infections and malignancies: systemic review and meta-analysis of rare and harmful effects in randomized controlled trials. JAMA 2006;295:2275–85.

12. Wallis RS, Broder MS, Way JY. Granulomatous infectious diseases associated with tumor necrosis factor antagonists. Clin Infect Dis 2004;38:1261–86.

13. Calabrese LH, Zein N, Vasssiloupoulos D. Safety of tumor necrosis factor therapy in patients with chronic viral infections: hepatitis C, hepatitis B and HIV infection. Ann Rheum Dis 2004;63(suppl 2):18–24.

14. Askling J, Fored CM, Baecklund E, Brandt L, Backlin C, Ekbom A, et al. Haematopoietic malignancies in rheumatoid arthritis: lymphoma risk and characteristics after exposure to tumor necrosis factor antagonists. Ann Rheum Dis 2005;64:1414–20.

15. Kwon HJ, Cote TR, Cuffe MS, Kramer JM, Braun MM. Case reports of heart failure after therapy with tumor necrosis factor antagonists. Ann Intern Med 2003;138:807–11.

16. Magnano MD, Robinson WH, Genovese MC. Demyelination and inhibition of tumor necrosis factor. Clinical Exp Rheumaatol 2004;22(suppl): S134–40.

17. Fleischmann RM, Schechtman J, Bennett R, Handel ML, Burmester GR, Tesser J, et al. Anakinra, a recombinant human interleukin-1 receptor antagonist (r-metHuIL-1ra), in patients with rheumatoid arthritis: a large, international, multicenter, placebo-controlled trial. Arthritis Rheum 2003;48:927–34.

18. Kremer JM, Dougados M, Emery P, Durez P, Sibilia J, Shergy W, et al. Treatment of rheumatoid arthritis with the selective costimulation modulator abatacept: twelve-month results of a phase iib, double-blind, randomized, placebo-controlled trial. Arthritis Rheum 2005;52:2263–71.

19. Edwards JC, Szczepanski L, Szechinski J, Filipowicz-Sosnowska A, Emery P, Close DR, et al. Efficacy of B-cell-targeted therapy with rituximab in patients with rheumatoid arthritis. N Engl J Med 2004;350: 2572–81.

20. Higashida J, Wun T, Schmidt S, Naguwa SM, Tuscano JM. Safety and efficacy of rituximab in patients with rheumatoid arthritis refractory to disease modifying antirheumatic drugs and anti-tumor necrosis factor-alpha treatment. J Rheumatol 2005;32:2109–15.

21. Wegener's Granulomatosis Etanercept Trial (WGET) Research Group. Etanercept plus standard therapy for Wegener's granulomatosis. N Engl J Med 2005;352:351–61.

Therapies from Complementary and Alternative Medicine

SHARON L. KOLASINSKI, MD

The broad field of complementary and alternative medicine (CAM) continues to contribute to the therapeutic choices available to patients with all forms of rheumatic disease. Patient interest in these therapies remains high and the literature in this area has been expanded by the publication of many well-designed clinical trials. The budget of the National Center for Complementary and Alternative Medicine within the National Institutes of Health (NIH), the major national agency funding CAM research, has more than doubled since it was established in 1999, to more than $120 million in fiscal year 2006. Furthermore, in 2005 the American College of Rheumatology (ACR) revised its position statement on CAM (1). It acknowledges that use of CAM is "extremely common" among patients with rheumatic disorders, and recommends that rheumatologists should be able to knowledgeably discuss CAM therapies with their patients and integrate those therapies that are proven safe and effective as appropriate. However, the ACR also advises caution in the use of therapies that are not validated (1). Because of the breadth of CAM interventions (Table 1), this chapter will focus on those therapies for which high-quality trials provide grounds for evidence-based discussion.

SCOPE OF USE

In a landmark 1993 article, Eisenberg and colleagues brought the previously unrecognized extent of CAM use to the attention of the traditional medical community (2). They defined CAM interventions as those not traditionally taught in US medical schools and not traditionally available in US hospitals, and reported that 34% of randomly selected telephone interviewees had used at least 1 such therapy in the preceding year. A followup study in 1997 documented that use of CAM had increased to >42% of those interviewed, with clinical encounters for alternative care exceeding visits to primary care providers (3). These studies suggested that CAM therapies are often used for chronic disease and chronic pain, a finding confirmed in a number of observational studies in the rheumatic literature in the United States, as well as in Europe, Australia, and Canada (4,5). The definition of CAM has expanded to include numerous specific interventions (Table 1), and information regarding them is now taught in >40 medical schools. PubMed uses CAM as a search category.

Subsequent research has clarified which therapies rheumatology patients are using and why. Although earlier studies suggested that

CAM users were more likely to be middle-aged, white, and have a higher level of education and income (2,3), subsequent studies in arthritis patients have shown that CAM is frequently used across racial, ethnic, education, and income groups (4). Studies in Hispanic and rural African American communities show high rates of use as well, though the spectrum of alternative therapies differs.

Among rheumatology patients, CAM therapies are often used to supplement standard medical care, rather than replace it. Those who tend to use CAM have inadequately controlled pain. In a survey of rheumatology outpatients, 87% said they used CAM to control pain and 62% had heard it helped someone else (6). The perception that CAM therapies were safe was held by 72%, but only 10% believed that they would cure arthritis. This study also confirmed that physicians asked about CAM use only 30% of the time, but that patients expected their doctors to know about the efficacy of CAM treatments, as well as potential interactions with prescription medications. A more recent survey, based on data from the National Health Interview Survey of the Centers for Disease Control and Prevention, compared the CAM use of 5,600 respondents age >45 years with arthritis to the use of 9,655 without arthritis (7). This survey noted that the most consistent predictors of CAM use in those with arthritis were joint pain and functional status. It also pointed out that older individuals with arthritis often have other chronic health concerns and frequently use CAM to treat these conditions as well.

Diet

The use of dietary interventions is appealing as a readily accessible and seemingly controllable factor in the treatment of arthritis symptoms. Although medical history is rich with descriptions of the relationship between food and drink and gout, more recent systematic study has shown that only rarely can clinical symptoms in other arthritis patients be documented to occur in relation to specific foods (8). However, certain intriguing findings suggest that this will continue to be an area of active investigation.

A variety of small studies have suggested that a diet rich in fruits and vegetables reduces the risk for or improves symptoms of rheumatoid arthritis (RA), whereas a diet high in red meat may increase the risk. However, specific nutrients that play an unequivocal role have not been identified.

Some RA patients have been shown to benefit from the use of fish or plant oil preparations. Eicosapentaenoic acid and docosahexaenoic acid are present in cold-water fish and are widely available in capsule form. Each has been shown to lead to the suppression of arachidonic acid-derived prostaglandins and leukotrienes. Some studies have suggested that cytokines, such as interleukin-1 and tumor necrosis factor α, may be reduced by omega-3 fatty acid supplementation as well. Similar in-vitro findings have been demonstrated for plants oils derived from borage (*Borago officinalis*), evening primrose (*Oenothera biennis*), and flaxseed (*Linum usitatissimum*). However, optimal patient selection criteria and appropriate dosing have not been established in controlled clinical trials (9).

Table 1.   Common complementary and alternative therapies

Acupressure	Meditation
Acupuncture	Naturopathy
Aromatherapy	Nutritional therapy
Ayurveda	Osteopathy
Chiropractic	Reflexology
Herbal medicine	Reiki
Homeopathy	Relaxation and visualization
Hypnosis	Spiritual healing
Kinesiology	Therapeutic touch
Massage	Yoga

Fasting has been demonstrated to have short-term antirheumatic efficacy. Although not a practical or recommended intervention, fasting for 7–10 days has led to reductions in pain, stiffness, evidence of inflammation on physical examination and laboratory testing, and medication requirements in studies of patients with RA. The mechanisms for this effect remain obscure, but could include a reduction in the antigenic challenge to the immune system provided by food ingestion (10). Short-term studies of vegetarian, vegan, and Mediterranean diets have suggested potential benefits in RA, including reductions in swollen and tender joints, and improved functioning and quality of life.

VITAMINS

The use of vitamin supplementation is an area of considerable interest for patients, for both health promotion and improvement of arthritis symptoms. Two epidemiologic studies noted intriguing links between vitamin D and osteoarthritis (OA). Analysis of Framingham data, including food frequency questionnaires and measurement of serum 25-$(OH)_2$ D levels, suggested that those with the lowest intake and serum levels of vitamin D were 3 times more likely to have progression of established OA, although no preventive benefit was noted (11). This trend mirrored a subgroup analysis in the Study of Osteoporotic Fractures (12), which found that those with the lowest levels of 25-$(OH)_2$D were 3 times more likely to develop OA of the hip as measured by radiographic joint-space narrowing. More recent observations include the finding that only one-third of patients with OA in the Framingham cohort were vitamin-D replete (13) and that higher vitamin-D intake is associated with a reduced risk of RA (14), suggesting a possible immunologic role for vitamin D. Despite these interesting observations, it is not known what the appropriate dosage of vitamin D might be to prevent or help treat either OA or RA.

Analysis of another Framingham population subset, again by food frequency questionnaire, revealed that high vitamin C intake was associated with a 3-fold reduction in OA disease progression. A weaker positive association was found for beta-carotene. No association could be demonstrated for vitamins E, B1, B6, niacin, or folate (15). The role of supplementation with vitamin C remains controversial, however, because of the observation that vitamin C might worsen OA in animal models.

Vitamin E may have different effects in RA and OA. In a mouse model of RA, vitamin E supplementation was associated with a reduction in joint destruction and levels of interleukin-1β, though not the severity of disease (16). It was suggested that vitamin E might uncouple joint inflammation and joint destruction. One small study in RA patients showed that vitamin E had modest analgesic benefits but did not alter the number of swollen or tender joints (17). In contrast, vitamin E appears to be of no benefit in OA. A 6-month study of vitamin E supplementation showed that it did not affect symptoms (18). A subsequent 2-year study similarly concluded that vitamin E supplementation was of no benefit for symptom control (19). In addition, it showed that vitamin E had no effect on cartilage loss due to OA.

GLUCOSAMINE AND CHONDROITIN

These building blocks of normal connective tissue have been used for OA pain relief for decades in Europe. Their increasing use in the United States followed the publication of the popular bestseller *The Arthritis Cure*, by Dr. Jason Theodosakis in 1997 (20). This book not only brought glucosamine and chondroitin to the attention of the American public, it also forced an examination of the accumulated clinical data available to evaluate these substances.

Glucosamine is an aminomonosaccharide that is a component of glycoproteins, proteoglycans, and glycosaminoglycans. It is involved in proteoglycan synthesis and, when added to chondrocytes in vitro, stimulates proteoglycan production. Glucosamine is known to be reduced in osteoarthritic cartilage. Limited laboratory studies have demonstrated glucosamine's effectiveness in reducing cellular production of inflammatory mediators, as well as in reducing inflammation in the rat adjuvant arthritis model. Pharmacokinetic data suggest that oral administration of radio-labeled glucosamine results in detectable serum levels of ^{14}C within hours of administration, but there has been no direct demonstration that the glucosamine is incorporated into cartilage. Nonetheless, rabbit data have suggested a preventive role for glucosamine. Chondroitin, too, is a normal constituent of connective tissue and appears to be capable of increasing proteoglycan synthesis in articular cartilage. Both are widely available over the counter as individual preparations, as well as in combination with each other or a variety of vitamins, minerals, and other supplements.

Early clinical trials of glucosamine were of short duration and small size. However, several randomized, double-blind, placebo-controlled trials have been carried out (21,22), suggesting benefit by some measures of pain relief. In short-term nonsteroidal antiinflammatory drug (NSAID) comparator trials, the analgesic benefits have been comparable, but the time of onset for symptom relief from glucosamine has been delayed over a period of weeks. The effects of glucosamine may also persist weeks after discontinuation. Adverse events have been minimal and comparable to placebo; gastrointestinal upset is most often mentioned. A meta-analysis of many of the early trials was intended to address some of their shortcomings in trial design and size (23). The authors identified 6 randomized, double-blind, placebo-controlled trials of glucosamine and 9 of chondroitin. Although the trials showed moderate to large effect of these nutraceuticals, interpretation of the results was limited by inconsistencies in study methods and industry sponsorship. Nonetheless, the authors concluded that glucosamine and chondroitin have some efficacy in treating OA symptoms and that they are safe. Most studies have used a daily dose of 1,500 mg of glucosamine sulfate and 1,200 mg of chondroitin sulfate.

Proponents of glucosamine and chondroitin point out that they may offer structural modification and slow the progression of OA in addition to providing symptomatic relief. This reasoning is supported by 2 trials that suggested glucosamine use was associated with a slowing in the rate of radiographic progression of OA measured by joint-space narrowing on plain radiographs over 3 years (24,25). However, these trials have been criticized on the basis of the difficulty in interpreting the radiographic technique used. The most recent Cochrane Collaboration meta-analysis of glucosamine trials identified 20 randomized, controlled trials involving 2,570 participants, but found most methodologically lacking. Overall, glucosamine favored placebo with a 28% improvement over baseline in pain and a 21% improvement in function using the Lequesne Index. However, in the 8 studies with adequate allocation concealment, glucosamine was found to be of no benefit in reducing pain or function measured by the Western Ontario and McMaster Universities Index (WOMAC) (26).

The possibility of structural modification in OA through the use of chondroitin is supported by the largest trial investigating use of chondroitin alone for OA to date (27). In this study of 300 participants, half received 800 mg of chondroitin sulfate daily for 2 years. The study failed to show a significant difference from placebo in WOMAC pain, stiffness, or function. Nonetheless, the chondroitin group showed no joint-space narrowing during the trial, whereas the placebo group worsened in both mean and minimum joint-space width.

It was hoped that some of the controversy about these nutraceuticals would be settled with the completion of a recent, large, NIH-funded multicenter trial, the Glucosamine/chondroitin Arthritis Intervention Trial (GAIT). This study included 1,583 participants in 1 of 5 arms: glucosamine alone, chondroitin alone, glucosamine plus chondroitin, celecoxib, or placebo. However, this trial failed to show analgesic efficacy for glucosamine, chondroitin, or the combination—except in a subgroup of participants with moderate-to-severe knee pain (28). This is the only trial to date that has compared glucosamine to chondroitin and to the combination of the 2 directly. Interpretation of the results of this trial are hampered by the very high placebo response and high attrition rate in all subgroups. Furthermore, the subgroup that appeared to have a response to the combination of glucosamine and chondroitin had no benefit from celecoxib, the active comparator. The radiographic data has not yet been published.

HERBAL PREPARATIONS

A visit to the local health-food store will reveal a large number of preparations devoted to the treatment of arthritis. The array of herbal ingredients present in these preparations can be quite impressive, some coming from folk tradition, others of less clear origin. A small number of clinical trials are available to help evaluate the potential role of herbal medicine in the treatment of arthritis.

Willow Bark (Salix sp.)

The bark of the willow and poplar trees has been used since antiquity for the treatment of pain, fever, and gout. Willow bark remains a popular ingredient in over-the-counter antirheumatic preparations due to its content of salicin, a source of salicylic acid. One study looked at >200 individuals with low back pain recruited from the community (29). After 6 months, patients treated with willow-bark extract had a significant increase in pain-free intervals without the need for rescue medications. A more recent study used a standardized willow-bark extract delivering 240 mg/day of salicin and compared it to diclofenac or placebo in 127 participants with OA and 26 with RA (30). This study failed to show a significant difference in WOMAC pain in OA or pain measured by visual analog scale in RA between the willow-bark extract and placebo, whereas diclofenac was confirmed to be effective.

Devil's Claw (Harpagophytum procumbens)

The medicinal roots of this native African plant have been used in folk medicine for relief of pain due to rheumatism. A handful of small but well-designed studies have shown significant improvement in pain in OA patients using devil's claw. Double-blind trials have demonstrated reductions in pain scores and increases in mobility for patients taking devil's claw over a 2-week period. Short-term tolerability was high, but long-term efficacy and side effects have yet to be determined. A 4-month trial involving 122 participants suggested that devil's claw was as efficacious as diacerhein in the treatment of OA pain, but the trial was not placebo controlled. The mechanism of action is unknown; several studies have suggested that devil's claw lacks antiinflammatory effects on prostaglandin biosynthesis.

Feverfew (Tanacetum parthenium)

A resident of many suburban backyards in the United States despite its European origins, feverfew is another herb long used to treat rheumatism. As the name implies, feverfew has been used as an antipyretic and antiinflammatory folk remedy. It is known to reduce platelet aggregation, prostaglandin synthesis, and histamine release. More recent data suggest that feverfew extract may inhibit cytokine-induced adhesion molecule expression on rheumatoid synovial fibroblasts, although studies of feverfew in patients with RA have shown little or no benefit. In a 6-week trial using a powdered extract of Tanacetum parthenium, 41 women with RA had no improvement in pain, stiffness, or the number of swollen or tender joints on physical examination. Feverfew should be avoided by those with allergies to chamomile, ragweed, or yarrow. Current investigations are focusing on the use of feverfew for migraine and rosacea, as well as on its potential antiproliferative effects.

Thunder God Vine (Tripterygium wilfordii)

The roots, leaves, and flowers of Chinese thunder god vine, Tripterygium wilfordii, have been used for centuries as part of traditional Chinese medicine, as well as an agricultural insecticide. Pharmacologic preparations have been developed and numerous Chinese publications have documented the use of Tripterygium derivatives for a host of rheumatic disorders, including RA, systemic lupus erythematosus, Henoch-Schönlein purpura, Sweet's syndrome, systemic sclerosis (scleroderma), Behçet's syndrome, and psoriatic arthritis.

Pharmacologic, toxicologic, and chemical analyses suggest that the therapeutic activity of Tripterygium derives from the diterpenoid components with epoxide structures. T2, a chloroform-methanol extract, and EA, an ethyl acetate extract, have been shown to have a number of antiinflammatory and immunosuppressive effects. In-vitro and in-vivo studies have demonstrated inhibition of the production of proinflammatory cytokines (interleukin-2, interferon-γ) and inflammatory mediators, such as prostaglandin E$_2$ and nitric oxide. The mechanism may include the suppression of the transcription of genes for inflammatory mediators. Animal studies have shown efficacy in the adjuvant arthritis model that is comparable to immunosuppressive drugs, such as azathioprine and corticosteroids.

Most information about the use of Tripterygium comes from uncontrolled clinical trials and retrospective reports, but some reports have detailed observations in patients treated for up to a decade. One prospective, randomized, double-blind study of T2 in RA patients showed significant improvements in joint-tenderness scores, as well as in physician and patient global assessment. Erythrocyte sedimentation rate, C-reactive protein levels, and levels of rheumatoid factor fell in actively treated patients; however, considerable toxicity was documented as well. Up to one-third of patients had gastrointestinal side effects and many patients experienced amenorrhea. Other studies have suggested that amenorrhea may be irreversible in perimenopausal women exposed to Tripterygium and that exposed men may experience azoospermia. Treatment-related deaths have occurred as a result of myocardial damage, renal failure, and hypotensive episodes related to severe gastrointestinal side effects (31,32).

Avocado Soybean Unsaponifiables

A preparation made from the unsaponifiable fractions of avocado and soybean oils remains a popular remedy for OA pain in Western Europe.

A substantial body of in-vitro and animal studies suggest a variety of potentially relevant effects of avocado soybean unsaponifiables (ASU). Laboratory studies have shown that interleukin-1–mediated events may be affected by ASU and that collagen synthesis may be stimulated in articular chondrocyte culture. Additional cytokine levels and prostaglandin production may be altered as well. Reduction in cartilage lesions was seen in a rabbit model of OA. Clinical trials in humans have given discordant results with short-term trials in OA suggesting symptomatic improvement but a longer-term study showing none (33).

BUYER BEWARE

Patients and physicians interested in taking or prescribing over-the-counter dietary supplements should be aware of the provisions of the Dietary Supplement and Health Education Act passed by Congress in 1994. This legislation permits the over-the-counter sale of numerous herbal and other preparations, exempting them from documentation requirements for efficacy and safety that are required for prescription medications. Unfortunately, under this law, consumers cannot be assured of the purity or dosage of the herb or presumed active ingredient in over-the-counter "natural" products. Nor do manufacturers have any incentive to participate in clinical trials to further evaluate such products, since they may be sold for a variety of indications without demonstration of efficacy. This state of affairs has clearly impeded progress in establishing evidence-based guidelines for the use of herbal medications.

Adverse Effects of Dietary Supplements

The long-term adverse effects of herbal preparations and other dietary supplements are not well studied, although patients clearly expect their physicians to be aware of and advise them about potential side effects. Case reports have documented several instances of marked toxicity due to Chinese herbal preparations. These preparations generally contain multiple ingredients, which may vary between batches. Gastrointestinal bleeding due to the adulteration of Chinese herbs by NSAIDs has been well documented. It has been estimated that up to one-third of imported Chinese patent medicines may be adulterated with undeclared pharmaceuticals, including corticosteroids, hypoglycemics, and warfarin, as well as heavy metals. Contamination during the manufacturing process has been reported. A batch of Chinese herbs used for weight reduction and imported into Belgium was tainted by the nephrotoxic herb, *Aristolochia fangchi*. This supplement was subsequently implicated in the development of rapidly progressive renal failure resulting in end-stage renal disease and the appearance of urothelial carcinoma in almost half of those patients with renal failure. The US Food and Drug Administration (FDA) issues consumer alerts and warnings as information regarding problems with dietary supplements becomes available. This information is available on the FDA Web site under the Center for Food Safety and Applied Nutrition (www.cfsan.fda.gov).

Caution should be exercised when herbal preparations are used in combination with prescription medications. In particular, the potential for increased bleeding risk should be appreciated in patients taking antiplatelet therapy or anticoagulants who are also taking feverfew, devil's claw, ginseng, garlic, or gingko. Postoperative hemorrhage in patients taking dietary supplements has been reported. It has also been suggested that willow bark could increase plasma levels of methotrexate and that Echinacea should not be used in combination with methotrexate due to the risk of increased hepatoxicity. Theoretically,

the use of "immune boosters" such as Echinacea, *Astragalus*, licorice root, and alfalfa sprouts could interfere with the action of immunosuppressive medications. Recent surveys suggest that ~10% of patients taking dietary supplements are at risk for serious interactions with medications (34,35).

PHYSICAL INTERVENTIONS

Acupuncture

Acupuncture is an ancient Chinese technique traditionally indicated for redressing imbalances of *chi*, or energy. Needles placed along a series of meridians, or pathways, could be used to therapeutically direct the flow of chi in the body. More recent Western explanations of the analgesic efficacy of acupuncture invoke various alterations in the neurochemical microenvironment. Some observations suggest that stimulation of high-threshold, small-diameter nerve fibers occurs, which leads to specific blockage of pain messages in higher centers of the brain. At least part of the analgesic effect of acupuncture can be blocked by naloxone, suggesting a role for endogenous opioids. However, the absence of a clear understanding of the mechanism of action has led to debate about what the appropriate placebo control should be in clinical trials. Some studies have used no treatment as a control, whereas others have used needle placement in nonmeridian locations. However, it is known that even sham acupuncture can have analgesic effects.

Pain relief has been demonstrated in a few small and brief trials of patients with OA as well as in other clinical pain models. A meta-analysis of acupuncture used for the treatment of low back pain showed that acupuncture was superior to a variety of control interventions, although not clearly better than placebo (36). Similarly, a systematic review of acupuncture for OA of the knee revealed strong evidence to support the use of acupuncture for pain control, although its role in improving function was less clear (37). A subsequent, well-designed trial of acupuncture as adjunctive therapy in a group of individuals with moderate-to-severe pain due to knee OA was positive (38). This study randomly assigned 570 participants to receive either true or sham acupuncture or an education control. Those who completed the trial attended a mean of 23 sessions and the group treated with true acupuncture showed significant improvements in WOMAC pain, WOMAC function, and patient global assessment compared with controls. The most important limitation of the trial was the high attrition rate of 43% in the education control group and 25% in the 2 acupuncture groups.

Tai Chi

Tai Chi is an ancient Chinese practice that incorporates cognitive, cardiovascular, and musculoskeletal responses. This classic conditioning exercise has been performed for centuries to promote health and to be used in self-defense. It has been suggested that Tai Chi might maintain flexibility and mobility in arthritis patients after investigations showed improvements in muscle strength and aerobic efficiency. One prospective, randomized, controlled study demonstrated enhanced self-efficacy, quality of life, and functional mobility among older adults with OA who practiced Tai Chi for 12 weeks (39). Another suggested that Tai Chi enhanced bone mineral density and neuromuscular functioning in a group of 99 postmenopausal women (40). Many have suggested that the beneficial effect of Tai Chi on balance might reduce the risk of falls in the elderly.

Nursing and Rehabilitation Considerations for CAM

- Be aware of the complementary and alternative therapies taken by your patients and keep current on potential drug interactions and side effects.
- Patients with motor control and stability deficits may benefit from therapy augmented with Tai Chi and yoga.

Yoga

Yoga derives from writings dating back 2 millennia detailing the practice of postures or asanas as part of the path to achieving harmony of body, mind, and spirit. In Western practice, emphasis has often been placed on the ability of yoga to enhance strength and flexibility, as well as beneficial effects on cardiovascular functioning. A number of small studies have suggested that yoga may be of benefit in managing symptoms of carpal tunnel syndrome and osteoarthritis of the hands and knees (41).

ADVISING PATIENTS

The rigors of evidence-based medicine are only beginning to be applied to the vast and diverse practices encompassed by complementary and alternative medicine. However, epidemiologic data suggest that CAM use is increasing. Patients will continue to expect physicians to understand potential medication interactions, as well as other risks and benefits of seeking alternative approaches. As the field of CAM grows, one of the most useful interventions physicians can make is to ask their patients what alternative therapies they are using and why. A number of authors have suggested guidelines for practitioners that have wide applicability and, as health care providers, we must continue to inform ourselves as research results become available. The NIH also maintains important credible and timely resources for clinicians and the public at large (including a database of NIH-sponsored CAM clinical trials currently accepting patients) at their Web site (http://nccam.nih.gov). In the meantime, patients will continue to gather information from family, friends, and the Internet (see Chapter 48 for Web sites of interest).

REFERENCES

1. Committee on Rheumatologic Care. American College of Rheumatology position statement: complementary and alternative medicine for rheumatic diseases. Accessed July 21, 2006. URL: http://www.rheumatology.org/publications/position/complementary.asp.
2. Eisenberg DM, Kessler RC, Foster C, Norlock FE, Calkins DR, Delbanco TL. Unconventional medicine in the United States: prevalence, costs, and patterns of use. N Engl J Med 1993;328:246–52.
3. Eisenberg DM, Davis RB, Ettner SL, Appel S, Wilkey S, Van Rompay M, et al. Trends in alternative medicine use in the United States, 1990–1997: results of a follow-up national survey. JAMA 1998;280:1569–75.
4. Kolasinski SL. The use of alternative therapies by patients with rheumatic diseases. J Clin Rheum 1999;5:253–4.
5. Kolasinski SL. Complementary and alternative therapies for rheumatic disease. Hosp Pract 2001;36:31–6, 39.
6. Rao JK, Mihaliak K, Kroenke K, Bradley J, Tierney WM, Weinberger M. Use of complementary therapies for arthritis among patients of rheumatologists. Ann Intern Med 1999;131:409–16.
7. Quandt SA, Chen H, Grzywacz JG, Bell RA, Lang W, Arcury TA. Use of complementary and alternative medicine by persons with arthritis: results of the National Health Interview Study. Arthritis Rheum 2005;53:748–55.
8. Panush RS, Stroud RM, Webster EM. Food-induced (allergic) arthritis. Inflammatory arthritis exacerbated by milk. Arthritis Rheum 1986;29:220–6.
9. Ernst E, Chrubasik S. Phyto-anti-inflammatories: a systematic review of randomized, placebo-controlled, double-blind trials. Rheum Dis Clin North Am 2000;26:13–27, vii.
10. Henderson CJ, Panush RS. Diets, dietary supplements, and nutritional therapies in rheumatic diseases. Rheum Dis Clin North Am 1999;25:937–68, ix.
11. McAlindon TE, Felson DT, Zhang Y, Hannan MT, Aliabadi P, Weissman B, et al. Relation of dietary intake and serum levels of vitamin D to progression of osteoarthritis of the knee among participants in the Framingham Study. Ann Intern Med 1996;125:353–9.
12. Lane NE, Gore LR, Cummings SR, Hochberg MC, Scott JC, Williams EN, et al, Study of Osteoporotic Fractures Research Group. Serum vitamin D levels and incident changes of radiographic hip osteoarthritis: a longitudinal study. Arthritis Rheum 1999;42:854–60.
13. Bischoff-Ferrari HA, Zhang Y, Kiel DP, Felson DT. Positive association between serum 25-hydroxyvitamin D level and bone density in osteoarthritis. Arthritis Rheum 2005;53:821–6.
14. Merlino LA, Curtis J, Mikuls TR, Cerhan JR, Criswell LA, Saag KG. Vitamin D intake is inversely associated with rheumatoid arthritis. Arthritis Rheum 2004;50:72–7.
15. McAlindon TE, Jacques P, Zhang Y, Hannan MT, Aliabadi P, Weissman B, et al. Do antioxidant micronutrients protect against the development and progression of knee osteoarthritis? Arthritis Rheum 1996;39:648–56.
16. De Bandt M, Grossin M, Driss F, Pincemail J, Babin-Chevaye C, Pasquier C. Vitamin E uncouples joint destruction and clinical inflammation in a transgenic mouse model of rheumatoid arthritis. Arthritis Rheum 2002;46:522–32.
17. Edmonds SE, Winyard PG, Guo R, Kidd B, Merry P, Langrish-Smith A. Putative analgesic activity of repeated oral doses of vitamin E in the treatment of rheumatoid arthritis: results of a prospective placebo controlled double blind trial. Ann Rheum Dis 1997;56:649–55.
18. Band C, Snaddon J, Bailey M, Cicuttini F. Vitamin E is ineffective for symptomatic relief of knee osteoarthritis: a six month double blind, randomised, placebo controlled study. Ann Rheum Dis 2001;60: 946–9.
19. Wluka AE, Stuckey S, Brand C, Cicuttini FM. Supplementary vitamin E does not affect the loss of cartilage volume in knee osteoarthritis: a 2 year double blind randomized placebo controlled study. J Rheumatol 2002;29:2585–91.
20. Theodosakis J, Adderly B, Fox F. The arthritis cure: the medical miracle that can halt, reverse, and may even cure osteoarthritis. New York: St Martin's Press; 1997.
21. Deal CL, Moskowitz RW. Nutraceuticals as therapeutic agents in osteoarthritis: the role of glucosamine, chondroitin sulfate, and collagen hydrolysate. Rheum Dis Clin North Am 1999;25:379–95.
22. Delafuente JC. Glucosamine in the treatment of osteoarthritis. Rheum Dis Clin North Am 2000;26:1–11, vii.
23. Reginster JY, Deroisy R, Rovati LC, Lee RL, Lejeune E, Bruyere O, et al. Long-term effects of glucosamine sulphate on osteoarthritis progression: a randomised, placebo-controlled clinical trial. Lancet 2001;357:251–6.
24. Pavelka K, Gatterova J, Olejarova M, Machacek S, Giacovelli G, Rovati LC. Gulcosamine sulfate use and delay of progression of knee osteoarthritis. Arch Intern Med 2002;162:2113–23.
25. Towheed TE, Maxwell L, Anastassiades TP, Shea B, Houpt J, Robinson V, et al. Glucosamine therapy for treating osteoarthritis (review). Cochrane Database Syst Rev 2005;(2):CD002946.
26. Michel BA, Stucki G, Frey D, De Vathaire F, Vignon E, Bruehlmann P, et al. Chondroitins 4 and 6 sulfate in osteoarthritis of the knee. Arthritis Rheum 2005;52:779–86.
27. Clegg DO, Reda DJ, Harris CL, Klein MA, O'Dell JR, Hooper MM, et al. Glucosamine, chondrotin sulfate, and the two in conmbination for painful knee osteoarthritis. N Engl J Med 2006;354:795–808.
28. McAlindon TE, LaValley MP, Gulin JP, Felson DT. Glucosamine and chondroitin for treatment of osteoarthritis: a systematic quality assessment and meta-analysis. JAMA 2000;283:1469–75.
29. Chrubasik S, Eisenberg E, Balan E, Weinberger T, Luzzati R, Conradt C. Treatment of low back pain exacerbations with willow bark extract: a randomized double-blind study. Am J Med 2000;109:9–14.
30. Biegert C, Wagner I, Ludtke R, Kotter I, Lohmuller C, Gunaydin I, et al. Efficacy and safety of willow bark extract in the treatment of osteoarthritis and rheumatoid arthritis: results of 2 randomized double-blind controlled trials. J Rheumatol 2004;31:2121–30.
31. Tao X, Younger J, Fan FZ, Wang B, Lipsky PE. Benefits of an extract of *Tripterygium Wilfordii Hook F* in patients with rheumatoid arthritis: a double-blind, placebo-controlled study. Arthritis Rheum 2002;46:1735–43.
32. Wang B, Ma L, Tao X, Lipsky PE. Triptolide, an active component of the Chinese herbal remedy *Tripterygium Wilfordii Hook F*, in hibits

production of nitric oxide by decreasing nitric oxide synthetase gene transcription. Arthritis Rheum 2004;50:2995–303.

33. Ernst E. Avocado-soybean unsaponifiables (ASU) for osteoarthritis—a systemic review. Clin Rheumatol 2003;22:285–8.

34. Peng CC, Glassman PA, Trilli LE, Hayes-Hunter J, Good CB. Incidence and severity of potential drug-dietary supplement interactions in primary care patients: an exploratory study of 2 outpatient practices. Arch Intern Med 2004;164:630–6.

35. Holden W, Joseph J, Williamson L. Use of herbal remedies and potential drug interactions in rheumatology outpatients. Ann Rheum Dis 2005;64:790.

36. Ernst E, White AR. Acupuncture for back pain: a meta-analysis of randomized controlled trials. Arch Intern Med 1998;58:2235–41.

37. Ezzo J, Hadhazy V, Birch S, Lao L, Kaplan G, Hochberg M, et al. Acupuncture for osteoarthritis of the knee: a systematic review. Arthritis Rheum 2001;44:819–25.

38. Berman BM, Lao L, Langenberg P, Lee WL, Gilpin AMK, Hochberg MC. Effectiveness of acupuncture as adjunctive therapy in osteoarthritis of the knee. Ann Intern Med 2004;141:901–10.

39. Hartman CA, Manos TM, Winter C, Hartman DM, Li B, Smith JC. Effects of T'ai Chi training on function and quality of life indicators in older adults with osteoarthritis. J Am Geriatr Soc 2000;48:1553–9.

40. Qin L, Choy W, Leung K, Leung PC, Au S, Hung W, et al. Beneficial effects of regular tai chi exercise on musculoskeletal system. J Bone Miner Metab 2005;23:186–90.

41. Kolasinski SL, Garfinkel M, Gilden Tsai A, Matz W, Van Dyke A, Schumacher HR. Iyengar yoga for treating symptoms of osteoarthritis of the knees: a pilot study. J Altern Complementary Med 2005;11:689–93.

Recommended Reading

Hu Z, Yang X, Ho PC, Chan SY, Heng PW, Chan E, et al. Herb-drug interactions: a literature review. Drugs 2005;65:1239–82.

Institute of Medicine, Committee on the Use of Complementary and Alternative Medicine by the American Public. Complementary and alternative medicine in the United States. Washington (DC): National Academies Press, 2005.

Setty AR, Sigal LH. Herbal medications commonly used in the practice of rheumatology: mechanisms of action, efficacy, and side effects. Semin Arthritis Rheum 2005;34:773.

Stamp LK, James MJ, Cleland LG. Diet and rheumatoid arthritis: a review of the literature. Semin Arthritis Rheum 2005;35:77–94.

CHAPTER 37

Mobilization and Manipulation

MICHAEL S. PUNIELLO, DPT, MS, OCS, FAAOMPT

Joint mobilization and manipulation techniques are used to increase extensibility of joint tissues, improve joint alignment, and enhance mobility. These techniques can also decrease pain and muscle spasm, which in turn, increase joint range of motion (ROM). Clinicians in various specialties, including physical therapy, chiropractic, osteopathic medicine, and general medicine, incorporate joint mobilization and manipulation techniques to address these impairments.

The American Physical Therapy Association's *Guide to Physical Therapy Practice* defines mobilization and manipulation as "a manual therapy technique comprising a continuum of skilled passive movements to the joints and/or related soft tissues that are applied at varying speeds and amplitudes, including a small amplitude/high velocity therapeutic movement." The guide defines manual therapy techniques as "skilled hand movements to improve soft tissue extensibility; increase ROM; induce relaxation; mobilize or manipulate soft tissue and joints; modulate pain; and reduce soft tissue swelling, inflammation, or restriction" (1). The American Academy of Orthopaedic Manual Physical Therapists describes mobilization and manipulation techniques as part of a scope of practice that includes pain modulation; restoration of mobility of soft tissues, joints, and neural tissue; control of movement, muscle strengthening, and stabilization; and functional reablement (2).

The American Chiropractic Association (ACA) has similar definitions and defines the chiropractic adjustment as "any therapeutic procedure that utilizes controlled force, leverage, direction, amplitude and velocity which is directed at specific joints or anatomical region." The ACA defines manipulation as "a manual procedure that involves a directed thrust to move a joint past the physiological ROM, without exceeding the anatomical limit." Manual therapy is defined as "procedures by which the hands directly contact the body to treat the articulations and/or soft tissues." The ACA defines mobilization as "movement applied singularly or repetitively within or at the physiological range of joint motion, without imparting a thrust or impulse, with the goal of restoring joint mobility" (3).

The clinician performs a thorough examination of the neuromusculoskeletal system to formulate a diagnosis (1,4–6). The examination includes patient history and systems review, specific tests, and measures. The clinician then assesses the data to form a biomechanical diagnosis and a prognosis that directs specific interventions. The examination would 1) identify impairments contributing to the patient's dysfunction that would benefit from manual therapy treatment and 2) identify contraindications to treatment.

CONCEPTS OF MOBILIZATION AND MANIPULATION

Osteokinematic and Arthrokinematic Motions

Osteokinematic motion refers to movements of joints over which the person has conscious neuromuscular control. For example, raising the arm overhead encompasses the osteokinematic motion of shoulder flexion. *Arthrokinematic* motion consists of specific joint motions that the person cannot consciously control. These motions include translation, roll,

spin, and distraction of specific joint partners. For example, shoulder flexion requires the arthrokinematic motion of posterior-inferior translation with superior roll of the humeral head in the glenoid cavity. The joint capsule and ligaments stabilize this motion. If there is traumatic injury to the ligaments, allowing excessive translation, the joint becomes unstable. If the joint is immobilized, or not moved through full available ranges of motion, the joint capsule and ligaments can shorten and limit arthrokinematic movements. This results in loss of osteokinematic motion. The physical therapist examination includes manual assessment of joint translation and distraction (joint play). If the patient has decreased joint play resulting in loss of osteokinematic motion, treatment, including joint mobilization or manipulation, is indicated. Mobilization and manipulation techniques usually are performed in directions of translation or distraction (traction), however they are also performed in straight plane and combined osteokinematic motions as well. This is dependent on the type of limitation of a specific joint movement, patient comfort, and skill and preference of the clinician.

Effects of Mobilization and Manipulation

There are mechanical effects as well as neurophysiologic effects of joint mobilization and manipulation techniques.

Mechanical Effects. All tissues and structures undergo mechanical deformation with movement and stress. The *elastic phase of deformation* describes stretching the tissue to within normal limits, enabling the tissue to rebound to its original length. If the tissue is stressed beyond the limits of the elastic phase, failure of the tissue occurs and the tissue is lengthened. This is termed the *plastic phase of deformation* (7). If the tissue is stressed beyond its maximal structural capabilities, the tissue will tear completely. Healthy joint tissue normally functions in the elastic phase of tissue deformation, which is essential for normal tissue homeostasis. If tissue is not undergoing deformation in the healthy ranges because of lack of use or immobilization, it will not regenerate at a normal rate. The consequence is collagen crossbridging, lack of water in the tissue matrix, and tissue thickening, resulting in loss of tissue elasticity and tissue shortening (7). The patient will experience loss of joint ROM involving both osteokinematic and arthrokinematic motions. Joint mobilization techniques (consisting of oscillating movements at the end range of joint-play motions) or joint manipulation techniques (consisting of high-velocity, low-amplitude movements at the end of available joint-play movement), which exceed the motion barrier, submaximally stress the tissues in the plastic phase of deformation (7). Tissue length increases, resulting in increased arthrokinematic and osteokinematic movements.

Neurophysiologic Effects. There are nerve mechanoreceptors in the joint tissues, capsule, and ligaments that are stimulated by active and passive movements of the joints (8–11). When joint tissue is strained at the limits of normal tissue extensibility, nociceptors (pain nerve receptors) are activated, causing a pain response. Small nerve fibers from nociceptors and large nerve fibers from articular mechanoreceptors enter the spinal cord at the same area. Wyke (12) identified 4 types of joint mechanoreceptors. Types I and II mechanoreceptors can be stimulated by joint mobilization techniques in ranges of available joint-play motions. Mechanoreceptor stimulation activates the large nerve fibers, which presynaptically inhibits some of the input from the small nerve fibers at the spinal cord level; inhibition of small nerve fibers decreases pain perception (9). Type III mechanoreceptors found in ligaments can be stimulated by sustained distraction or spinal manipulation and cause muscle inhibition. Type IV receptors in Wyke's classification are nociceptors that are stimulated by injury (12). Recent studies on animals and humans show neurophysiologic changes with mobilization and manipulation (13–16).

Mobilization and manipulation techniques can be used to emphasize mechanical effects that will in turn improve extensibility of joint tissues, improve joint alignment, and enhance mobility. These techniques can also target neurophysiologic effects to decrease pain and muscle spasm, which can also improve joint ROM. The emphasis often changes from mechanical effects to neurophysiologic effects in one treatment session to attain the desired result. However, one cannot move a joint either actively or passively without engaging both systems.

EVIDENCE FOR MOBILIZATION AND MANIPULATION

Spine

There is varying evidence to support utilizing mobilization and manipulation procedures for the cervical, thoracic, and lumbar spine and sacroiliac joints. The emphasis is to treat mechanical dysfunction of the spine that results in pain and movement abnormalities. There is some evidence that manual therapy treatment for disc and nerve involvement is advantageous in some cases (17). A number of systematic reviews identified benefits of spinal mobilization and manipulation for acute episodes. There is less evidence of benefit for patients with chronic pain, and some reviews did not identify sufficient evidence for manipulation. A major problem with research methodology is in classifying which patients would benefit from spinal manipulation (18–23).

Flynn et al (18) developed a clinical prediction rule to identify patients with low back pain who would benefit from spinal manipulation. Five factors were identified to classify patients who improved at least 50% in pain on a numerical rating scale and on an Oswestry Low Back Pain Disability Scale. The factors were as follows:

1. Onset of pain less than 16 days;
2. No pain experienced below the knee;
3. Score on a Fear Avoidance Beliefs Questionnaire of <19 points, suggesting low fear avoidance response;
4. At least one lumbar spine segment assessed to be hypomobile; and
5. At least one hip with >35° of motion in internal rotation.

The authors calculated likelihood ratios and reported that if the patient exhibited at least 4 of the 5 factors, the probability of responding to 1 session of spinal manipulation treatment was 95%. If the patient exhibited 3 of the variables, the probability of improvement was 65%. With 2 of the variables present, the probability was 45% of improving with spinal manipulation.

Childs et al (24) conducted a multicenter randomized controlled trial utilizing the clinical prediction rule. They compared 131 subjects randomized into 2 groups of patients with low back pain. One group received spinal manipulation and range-of-motion exercise and the other group received an exercise program consisting of low-stress aerobic and lumbar strengthening exercises. Both groups received 5 treatment sessions, however, spinal manipulation was performed on only the first 2 treatment sessions. Post-treatment analysis revealed that patients who were positive on the prediction rule (4 of 5 factors present) had a 92% chance of improvement in outcome measures. Improvement was noted at the 1-week, 4-week, and 6-month followup exams. This study validates the clinical prediction rule developed by Flynn et al (18).

Santilli, et al (17) conducted a randomized double-blind study to compare the effects of spinal manipulation and simulated manipulation in patients with acute back pain and sciatica with disc protrusion. There were 102 patients from 2 hospitals in Rome, Italy, with at least 5 of 10 on a pain-rating numerical scale, indicating at least moderate pain. The manipulation group consisted of 53 patients and the simulation group, 49 patients. Treatment with thrust manipulation (same technique for every patient) was administered by experienced chiropractors and was performed 5 days per week. The simulated manipulation used the same patient position and clinician hand position, but did not include a thrust manipulation. The treatment duration was dependent on resolution of symptoms or until 20 treatment sessions were completed. The average number of treatment sessions was 12.8 for the active manipulation group and 13.0 for the simulated manipulation group. The active manipulation group had significantly more improvement in pain intensity, number of days with severe pain, and percentage of patients becoming pain-free.

Physical examination procedures are important in clinical decision making and the above studies rely on assessment of mobility of the spine and hip joints. Some studies report on the reliability of examination procedures to help classify patients with low back pain. As research methodology evolves, more studies validate the classification of patients to receive direct intervention strategies (25–27).

There is varying evidence for utilizing spinal mobilization and manipulation for patients complaining of neck pain. At this time, a clinical prediction rule has not been developed for cervical spine dysfunction. There is evidence that manual therapy is effective for this population. Hoving et al (28) compared manual physical therapy and exercise, exercise alone, and continued care by a general practitioner. Patients were treated for 6 weeks, with number of visits decided by the clinician based on the examination. At 7 weeks, the manual therapy group had significantly improved results for all outcome measures compared with the other groups. This corroborates the results of previous studies that report improvement with manual therapy and exercise (29,30). Other studies showed effectiveness of manual physical therapy treatment for cervical spine dysfunction. Giles and Muller (31) found cervical spine manipulation more effective than acupuncture and medication in improving pain and perceived disability. A Cochrane review concluded that spinal mobilization or manipulation alone was not effective in treating patients with persistent mechanical neck pain; however, combined with exercise, this treatment is beneficial. When compared with each other, neither mobilization nor manipulation was superior (32). Manual therapy treatment and exercise improved symptoms and function in patients with cervicogenic headaches in a randomized, controlled clinical trial (33). Cleland et al reported on improved outcomes with treatment to the cervical spine in patients with lateral epicondylitis (34). In another study, they reported improvement in neck pain after treatment with manipulation to the thoracic spine (35). De las Penas et al found a significant relationship between myofascial trigger points in the upper trapezius muscle and presence of mechanical dysfunction at the C3 and C4 vertebral segments (36). These studies suggest that there are many related factors in upper-quarter pain. The clinician must assess all areas in the upper and lower quadrant to identify related areas of mechanical dysfunction.

Lower Extremity

Recent studies provide evidence for manual therapy treatment for hip and knee osteoarthritis (OA) and ankle sprains. Hoeksma et al (37) compared manual therapy to exercise in people with hip OA in a randomized clinical trial. Eighty percent of subjects had moderate to severe OA based on the Kellgren-Lawrence rating system. In the manual therapy group, the mean age was 72 years. Duration of complaints ranged from 1 month to 1 year (n=22); 1 to 2 years (n=12); 2 to 5 years (n=9); 5 to 10 years (n=10); and >10 years (n=3). In the exercise therapy group, the mean age was 71 years. Duration of complaints ranged from 1 month to 1 year (n=15); 1 to 2 years (n=13); 2 to 5 years (n=15); 5 to 10 years (n=8); and >10 years (n=2). The manual therapy group received traction manipulation to the hip preceded by hip muscle stretching. The exercise group received joint mobility, muscle length, and function exercises as well as gait training. Subjects in both groups significantly improved on a 6-point Likert scale, with 81% in the manual therapy group and 50% in the exercise group reporting improvement. The manual therapy group also showed more improvement in the Harris Hip Score and in a pain-with-walking test. They had more improvement in reported pain and stiffness and in measured range of hip motion.

Deyle et al (38) conducted a randomized, controlled trial of manual therapy and exercise in patients with OA of the knee. Knee OA was diagnosed using the American College of Rheumatology (formerly American Rheumatism Association) criteria (39). The manual therapy group received mobilization treatment to the knee, hip, ankle, or lumbar spine, as indicated on initial examination. The placebo group received subtherapeutic ultrasound treatment to the knee. The manual therapy group had statistically significant improvement in walking distance in 6 minutes and improved score on the Western Ontario and McMaster Universities Osteoarthritis Index (WOMAC). Improvements were seen at 4 and 8 weeks after treatment and at 1 year after treatment. Deyle et al (40) conducted a similar study in 3 clinical settings and compared 1 group that received manual therapy and exercise with a group that completed a home exercise program. Subjects in both groups had significantly improved WOMAC scores, however the manual therapy group had 52% and the home exercise group had 26% improvement. This improvement was seen at 4- and 8-weeks' followup. At 1-year

followup, both groups reported similar improvement with continued home exercise. Cilborne et al (41) assessed the response of hip joint mobilization on pain and mobility for 3 clinical tests of the hip and one functional test in patients with knee OA. Subjects with knee OA had pain on the clinical tests compared with asymptomatic subjects who had no pain. Following treatment, the subjects with knee joint OA had improvement in all clinical tests, indicating at least short-term improvement with hip joint mobilization.

Green et al (42) reported in a randomized, controlled trial that patients with acute ankle sprains (within 72 hours of injury) had significant improvements in ankle dorsiflexion ROM and stride speed as a result of treatment with ankle joint mobilization. Subjects with knee OA in the study by Deyle et al also received ankle joint mobilization if indicated.

Upper Extremity

Some studies provide evidence for manual therapy treatment in the upper extremity. Bang and Deyle (43) compared manual physical therapy and exercise for flexibility and strength with exercise alone in patients with impingement syndrome of the shoulder. Posterior translation of the humeral head is reported to be limited in this patient population (44). Both groups in the Bang study (43) improved in pain and function, however there was considerably more improvement in pain in the manual therapy group. Strength measures improved significantly for the manual physical therapy group but not for the exercise group. A Cochrane review of physiotherapy interventions for shoulder pain found exercise to be beneficial for rotator cuff disease, and additional benefit was reported when mobilization treatment was combined with exercise (45). Another study compared high- and low-grade mobilization techniques in patients with adhesive capsulitis of the shoulder. Both types of mobilization procedures were reported to be beneficial in this patient population (46).

Mobilization with movement of the elbow for lateral epicondylalgia was reported to have similar physiologic effects to those reported with spinal manipulation (47). In a study consisting of an experimental group, a control group, and a placebo group, only the experimental group had improvement in pain-free grip force and pressure pain

Table 1. Indications and contraindications for manual therapy in select forms of arthritis*

Diagnosis	Indications	Contraindications	Comments
OA	Decreased ROM (with or without pain) with joint accessory motion or limitation of the involved joint or distant joints that effects the condition	Osteoporosis, nonhealed fracture or dislocation, bone tumor, bone infection or septic arthritis, instability, and severe joint deformity; vertebrobasilar insufficiency is contraindication for cervical spine	Often joint restrictions proximal or distal to the involved joint contribute to abnormal stress and require manual therapy treatment to correct the dysfunction.
RA	Same as OA; early disease without joint destruction, joint accessory motion limitation	Same as OA; cervical spine (especially with instability), joint destruction with instability	Low grades of mobilization are sometimes helpful for pain control, emphasizing the neurophysiologic effects.
Fibromyalgia	Same as OA	Same as OA; pain of psychological origin	Painful stimuli from joint dysfunction might increase the fibromyalgia pain response. Manual therapy treatment could help decrease this condition. Repeated manipulation for short-term pain relief is not recommended in long-term management.
Spinal stenosis	Same as OA	Same as OA	Improving lower extremity joint and muscle limitations could decrease abnormal stress to the lumbar spine.

* OA = osteoarthritis; RA = rheumatoid arthritis.

threshold from the mobilization technique. In addition, the experimental group had changes in sympathetic nervous system-related measures, indicating a neurophysiologic response to the joint mobilization technique (47).

CLINICAL MANAGEMENT

This section will address certain aspects of treatment for specific body regions and types of arthritis. The major areas will include the spine and the lower extremity. Patients with OA are most likely to benefit from mobilization and manipulation procedures. However, patients with early rheumatoid arthritis (RA), without joint destruction, would benefit from these procedures to improve pain and joint mobility. Mobilization and manipulation treatment is contraindicated in patients in the later stages of RA who exhibit joint deformity and instability.

A typical complaint in patients with spondylosis involving the lumbar and cervical spine is pain and stiffness, worse in the morning. Patients often report decreased functional status and endurance, sometimes resulting in limited recreational activities. These patients usually present with joint restrictions involving the spine as well as the peripheral joints, along with accompanying muscle and soft-tissue shortening. Treatment with mobilization should address the identified joint restrictions of the spine and extremities, and concentrate on specific muscle stretching. It is important to recognize that treatment is focused on improving the patient's ability to compensate for the structural deficits, thereby improving pain and function. Mobilization treatment should be combined with therapeutic exercise to improve mobility and functional stability. Mobilization techniques are graded I–IV, where Grade I = small amplitude movement at beginning of available joint play range; Grade II = large amplitude movement from beginning to mid range of available joint play range; Grade III = large amplitude movement from mid to end range of available joint play range; and Grade IV = small amplitude movement at the end of available joint play range. Mobilization techniques could utilize Grades I and II to stimulate joint mechanoreceptors to decrease pain (neurophysiologic effect), and Grades III and IV to stretch the joint tissue (mechanical effect). Sustained joint distraction or thrust manipulation could also create a neurophysiologic response, decreasing pain and causing muscle inhibition (9).

In patients with spinal stenosis, the typical finding is bilateral leg pain with walking. They usually are able to walk further with the trunk bent, such as when leaning on a shopping cart. In spinal extension, the spinal canal is narrowed, blocking the flow of cerebrospinal fluid, which results in leg pain (48). In spinal flexion, the spinal canal is wider, allowing better flow of spinal fluid, which allows the person to walk further with less leg pain. These patients typically present with hip joint hypomobility and shortening of the hip flexor muscles. In standing, there is anterior tilt of the pelvis, which moves the spine into extension, thereby narrowing the spinal canal. Stretching the hip flexor muscles and performing hip joint mobilization promotes improved posture, which may reduce pain and increase walking distance.

Patients with fibromyalgia often present with joint restrictions and muscle shortening that contributes to the pain response. Treatment with mobilization to the spine and extremities might be indicated to improve these areas so the patient can participate in an exercise program to improve their functional status. Manual therapy could be one component of clinical management in this patient population.

Safety is the main concern with any manual therapy procedure. The clinician should conduct a thorough history and physical examination to rule out problems that might be contraindications to mobilization or manipulation. In the cervical spine, vertebrobasilar insufficiency is a definite contraindication to treatment (see Table 1). Clinicians should be aware that instability at the C2 segment is a potential problem in patients with RA. There are many aspects to clinical management of any disorder of the neuromusculoskeletal system. Treatment with mobilization and manipulation should be considered as one component of an entire treatment plan.

REFERENCES

1. American Physical Therapy Association. Guide to physical therapy practice. Second edition. Phys Ther 2001;81:9–746.
2. Journal of Manual and Manipulative Therapy. 1993;Spring:73–4.
3. American Chiropractic Association Web site. Accessed June 14, 2006. URL: www.amerchiro.org/index.cfm.
4. Rothstein JM, Echternach JL. Hypothesis oriented algorithm for clinicians: a method for evaluation and treatment planning. Phys Ther 1986;66:1388–94.
5. Sahrmann SA. Diagnosis by the physical therapist: a prerequisite for treatment, a special communication. Phys Ther 1988;69:525–34.
6. Guccione A. Physical therapy diagnosis and the relationship between impairments and function. Phys Ther 1991;71:190–202.
7. Threlkeld JA. The effects of manual therapy on connective tissue. Phys Ther 1992;72:893–902.
8. Sluka KA. Pain mechanisms involved in musculoskeletal disorders. J Orthop Sports Phys Ther 1996;24:240–54.
9. Dutton M. Manual therapy of the spine: an integrated approach. New York: McGraw Hill; 2002. p. 20.
10. Grigg P. Articular neurophysiology. In: Zachazewski JE, Magee DJ, Quillen WS, editors. Athletic injuries and rehabilitation. Philadelphia: Saunders; 1996. p. 152–85.
11. Solomon OW, Guanche CA. Mechanoreceptors and reflex arc in the feline shoulder. J Shoulder Elbow Surg 1996;5:139–46.
12. Wyke BD. Articular neurology: a review. Physiotherapy 1972;58:94–9.
13. Malisza KL, Stroman PW, Turner A, Gregorash L, Foniok T, Wright A. Functional MRI of the rat lumbar spinal cord involving painful stimulation and effect of peripheral joint mobilization. J Magn Reson Imaging 2003;18:152–9.
14. Malisza KL, Gregorash L, Foniok T, Stroman PW, Allman AA, et al. Functional MRI involving painful stimulation of the ankle and the effect of physiotherapy joint mobilization. Magn Reson Imaging 2003;21:489–96.
15. Dishman JD, Bulbulian R. Spinal reflex attenuation associated with spinal manipulation. Spine 2000;25:2519–24.
16. Dishman JD, Dougherty PE, Burke JR. Evaluation of the effect of postural perturbation on motoneuronal activity following various methods of lumbar spinal manipulation. Spine J 2005;5:650–9.
17. Santilli V, Beghi E, Funucci S. Chiropractic manipulation in the treatment of acute back pain and sciatica with disc protrusion: a randomized double-blind clinical trial of active and simulated spinal manipulation. Spine J 2006;6:131–7.
18. Flynn T, Fritz J, Whitman J, Wainner R, Magel J, Rendeiro D, et al. A clinical prediction rule for classifying patients with low back pain who demonstrate short-term improvement with spinal manipulation. Spine 2002;27:2835–43.
19. Hurwitz EL, Morgenstern H, Kominski GF, Yu F, Chiang LM. A randomized trial of chiropractic and medical care for patients with low back pain: eighteen-month follow-up outcomes from the UCLA low back pain study. Spine 2006;31:611–21.
20. Wand BM, Bird C, McAuley JH, Dore CJ, MacDowell M, De Souza LH. Early intervention for the management of acute low back pain: a single-blind randomized controlled trial of biopsychosocial education, manual therapy, and exercise. Spine 2004;29:2350–6.
21. Hurley DA, McDonough SM, Dempster M, Moore AP, Baxter GD. A randomized clinical trial of manipulative therapy and interferential therapy for low back pain. Spine 2004;29:2207–16.
22. Koes BW, van Tulder MW, Ostelo R, Kim Burton A, Waddell G. Clinical guidelines for the management of low back pain in primary care: an international comparison. Spine 2001;26:2504–13.
23. Bouter LM, vanTulder MW, Koes BW. Methodological issues in low back pain research in primary care. Spine 1998;23:2014–20.
24. Childs JD, Fritz JM, Flynn TW, Irrgang JJ, Johnson KK, Majkowski GR, et al. A clinical prediction rule to identify patients with low back pain most likely to benefit from spinal manipulation: a validation study. Ann Intern Med 2004;141:920–8.
25. Fritz JM, Brennan GP, Clifford SN, Hunter SJ, Thackeray A. An examination of the reliability of a classification algorithm for subgrouping patients with low back pain. Spine 2006;31:77–82.

26. Fritz JM, Whitman JM, Childs JD. Lumbar spine segmental mobility assessment: an examination of validity for determining intervention strategies in patients with low back pain. Arch Phys Med Rehab 2005; 86:1745–52.

27. Brennan GP, Fritz JM, Hunter SJ, Thackeray A, Delitto A, Erhard RE. Identifying subgroups of patients with acute/subacute "nonspecific" low back pain: results of a randomized clinical trial. Spine 2006;31:623–31.

28. Hoving JL, Koes BW, de Vet HC, van der Windt DA, Assendelft WJ, van Mameren H, et al. Manual therapy, physical therapy, or continued care by a general practitioner for patients with neck pain: a randomized controlled trial. Ann Intern Med 2002;136:713–22.

29. Koes BW, Bouter LM, van Mameren H, Essers AH, Verstegen GM, Hofhuizen DM, et al. The effectiveness of manual therapy, physiotherapy, and treatment by the general practitioner for nonspecific back and neck complaints: a randomized clinical trial. Spine 1992;17:28–35.

30. Koes BW, Bouter LM, van Mameren H, Essers AH, Verstegen GJ, Hofhuizen DM, et al. A randomized clinical trial of manual therapy and physiotherapy for persistent back and neck complaints: subgroup analysis and relationship between outcome measures. J Manipulative Physiol Ther 1993;16:211–9.

31. Giles LGF, Muller R. Chronic spinal pain: a randomized trial comparing medication, acupuncture, and spinal manipulation. Spine 2003;28:1490–1502.

32. Gross AR, Hoving JL, Haines TA, Goldsmith CH, Kay T, Aker P, et al, and the Cervical Overview Group. A Cochrane review of manipulation and mobilization for mechanical neck disorders. Spine 2004;29:1541–8.

33. Jull G, Trott P, Potter H, Zito G, Niere K, Shirley D, et al. A randomized controlled trial of exercise and manipulative therapy for cervicogenic headache. Spine 2002;27:1835–43.

34. Cleland JA, Whitman JM, Fritz JM. Effectiveness of manual physical therapy to the cervical spine in the management of lateral epicondylalgia: a retrospective analysis. J Orthop Sport Phys Ther 2004;34:713–24.

35. Cleland JA, Childs JD, McRae M, Palmer JA, Stowell T. Immediate effects of thoracic manipulation in patients with neck pain: a randomized clinical trial. Man Ther 2005;10:127–35.

36. de las Penas C, Fernandez Carnero J, Miangolarra Page JC. Musculoskeletal disorders in mechanical neck pain: myofascial trigger points versus cervical joint dysfunction: a clinical study. J Musculoskel Pain 2005;13:27–35.

37. Hoeksma HL, Dekker J, Ronday HK, Heering A, van der Lubbe N, Vel C, et al. Comparison of manual therapy and exercise therapy in osteoarthritis of the hip: a randomized clinical trial. Arthritis Rheum 2004;51:722–9.

38. Deyle GD, Henderson NE, Matekel RL, Ryder MG, Garber MB, Allison SC. Effectiveness of manual physical therapy and exercise in osteoarthritis of the knee. Ann Intern Med 2000;132:173–81.

39. Altman R, Asch E, Bloch D, Bole G, Borenstein D, Brandt K, et al, and the Diagnostic and Therapeutic Criteria Committee of the American Rheumatism Association. Development of criteria for the classification and reporting of osteoarthritis: classification of osteoarthritis of the knee. Arthritis Rheum 1986;29:1039–49.

40. Deyle GD, Allison SC, Matekel RL, Ryder MG, Stang JM, Gohdes DD, et al. Physical therapy treatment effectiveness for osteoarthritis of the knee: a randomized comparison of supervised clinical exercise and manual therapy procedures versus a home exercise program. Phys Ther 2005;85:1301–17.

41. Cliborne AV, Wainner RS, Rhon DI, Judd CD, Fee TT, Matekel RL, et al. Clinical hip tests and functional squat test in patients with knee osteoarthritis: reliability, prevalence of positive test findings, and short-term response to hip mobilization. J Orthop Sports Phys Ther 2004;34:676–85.

42. Green T, Refshauge K, Crosbie J, Adams R. A randomized controlled trial of a passive accessory joint mobilization on acute ankle inversion sprains. Phys Ther 2001;81:984–94.

43. Bang MD, Deyle GD. Comparison of supervised exercise with and without manual physical therapy for patients with shoulder impingement syndrome. J Orthop Sports Phys Ther 2000;30:126–37.

44. Ludewig PM, Cook TM. Translation of the humerus in persons with shoulder impingement symptoms. J Orthop Sports Phys Ther 2002;32:248–59.

45. Green S, Buchbinder R, Hetrick S. Physiotherapy interventions for shoulder pain. Cochrane Database Syst Rev 2003;(2):CD004258.

46. van den Hout WB, Vermeulen HM, Rozing PM, Vliet Vlieland TP. Impact of adhesive capsulitis and economic evaluation of high-grade and low-grade mobilisation techniques. Aust J Physiother 2005;51:141–9.

47. Paungmali A, O'Leary S, Souvlis T, Vicenzino B. Hypoalgesic and sympathoexcitatory effects of mobilization with movement for lateral epicondylalgia. Phys Ther 2003;83:374–83.

48. White AA, Panjabi MM. Clinical biomechanics of the spine. Philadelphia: Lippincott; 1978.

CHAPTER 38

Thermal and Electrical Agents Used to Manage Arthritis Symptoms

KAREN W. HAYES, PT, PhD, FAPTA

Physical agents of heat, cold, and electricity are often used to alleviate the symptoms of rheumatic disease. Although no agent is capable of curing arthritis, amelioration of symptoms may lead to improved function. Overall function depends on freedom from impairments, such as weakness, limitation of motion, and pain. Specific treatment goals may include decreasing pain, increasing flexibility, and decreasing swelling. Heat, cold, and electrical stimulation are often used to produce improvement in these impairments in the interest of improving function.

SUPERFICIAL AND DEEP HEAT

Superficial- and deep-heat treatments are used primarily to decrease pain and improve flexibility. Heat contributes to pain relief by increasing the pain threshold, increasing blood flow (1), and washing out pain-producing metabolites. Heat also decreases muscle guarding through its effects on the muscle spindle and Golgi tendon organs (2). It may improve flexibility by reducing pain or by increasing the extensibility of connective tissue (3). The use of heat allows collagen to deform more readily, leading to increased range of motion, especially when combined with low-load, prolonged stretching (4).

Application of Superficial Heat

Superficial heat can be applied by using hot packs, paraffin wax baths, Fluidotherapy (a bath of small solid particles suspended in a stream of warmed air), infrared radiation (heat lamps), or hydrotherapy. Recently, chemical heat wraps that become warm when exposed to the air have come on the market. These continuous low-level heat wraps warm to 104°F in about 30 minutes and stay warm for at least 8 hours (5). Heat-retaining sleeves that reflect the infrared radiation emitted by the body have also been tested (6). Regardless of the source, superficial heat is in the infrared portion of the electromagnetic spectrum. Although it penetrates the skin only a few millimeters, superficial heat application increases skin and core temperature (1). With the exception of the continuous low-level heat wraps and heat-retaining sleeves, superficial heat should be applied for about 20 minutes to elevate skin temperature and activate optimal heat loss responses by the body. Physiologic effects occur through these reflex vascular and neural responses. Superficial heat can be used as needed up to twice daily.

Superficial heat is among the most commonly used methods of self-management by people with osteoarthritis (OA) and rheumatoid arthritis (RA) (7). It is convenient and safe for home use if patients have received proper instruction. Instructions should include the purpose of the treatment; the method of application; the duration, intensity, and frequency of the application; precautions for use; and a telephone number for the patient to contact a professional practitioner with questions and concerns. The practitioner should demonstrate the treatment and watch the patient perform it to ensure proper administration of the procedure.

Application of Deep Heat

Deep heat is provided through short-wave diathermy and ultrasound. Like superficial heat, deep heating elevates temperature, but it reaches deeper tissues, such as muscle and connective tissue. Deep heat is generally used 2–3 times per week. Short-wave diathermy is usually applied for 20 minutes to fairly large areas of the body. Ultrasound, on the other hand, may be focused on very small areas and is applied for shorter periods of time (5–10 minutes) (8). The heat from short-wave diathermy and ultrasound is produced by conversion of electrical or sound energy into heat energy below the level of the skin heat receptors. Consequently, people perceive the warmth from deep-heat sources to be much milder. Deep heat should be used under the supervision of a physical therapist. Sources for providing deep heat usually are not portable, and they are too expensive and hazardous for home use.

Contraindications and Precautions

Because of the mechanisms of heat production and the milder but deceptive heat perception, deep-heat sources can be hazardous. With short-wave diathermy, any condition that concentrates the electric field, such as metal and perspiration, can produce a burn. Ultrasound, if focused too long at a particular site, can also produce burning. Heat applications to large areas of the body, producing systemic heat loss responses, are contraindicated for people with conditions that prevent adequate thermoregulatory responses (such as cardiac insufficiency or impaired peripheral circulation). They are also contraindicated in conditions that could be aggravated or spread, such as swelling, fever, infection, hemorrhage, or malignancy (2). Short-wave diathermy is contraindicated for any patient with a pacemaker or electromedical device (internal defibrillators). Local heat applications to small areas may be safely used in stable cardiac conditions or when applied to areas of the body at a distance from areas of swelling, infection, hemorrhage, or malignancy. Because the amount of heat applied depends on the patient's perception, it should not be applied with people who have impaired sensation or impaired judgment or cognition.

In addition to these contraindications and precautions, there are special precautions associated with the use of heat in persons with acute, inflammatory arthritis. Heat may increase inflammation, thus increasing swelling of the synovial membrane (9). Increasing the intraarticular temperature could damage joint surfaces due to increased activity of collagenolytic enzymes (10). Both joint and skin temperature elevate following superficial heating, especially with the treatment times used in clinical practice (20 minutes) (11,12). Short-wave diathermy also heats the interior of the joint along with the skin, although not as much as superficial heat (12). There is no clinical evidence that heat affects long-term progression of RA as evidenced by elevations in erythrocyte sedimentation rate (13), white blood cell count and phagocytosis (14), or radiography (15); nonetheless, the use of heat in people with acute inflammatory arthritis is best avoided. People with RA often have

255

Use of Thermal and Electrical Agents

- Superficial heat treatments are safe and inexpensive; patients who feel better or are more active following heat treatments may be encouraged to use them.
- Deep-heat treatments can be hazardous and are expensive; when exercise or superficial heat can accomplish the same goals, there is little rationale for using deep heat.
- Cold treatments are effective in improving range of motion, pain, function, and swelling.
- Transcutaneous electrical nerve stimulation is safe and useful for decreasing pain and stiffness.
- Education by a knowledgeable professional is crucial for correct and safe application.

unstable vascular reactions following exposure to heat. Vasodilation may occur more slowly, causing them to retain heat (16). People with vasculitis associated with RA also may have impaired vasomotor heat-loss responses (17). Therefore, people with RA should be monitored carefully for susceptibility to heat stress when heat is used in their management.

Effectiveness

Some investigators have shown that superficial heat can decrease pain and increase range of motion for patients with RA (18–22) and OA (5,23), but others have found that superficial heat is not effective (10,13,24,25). The new continuous low-level heat wraps have been shown to be effective for pain relief (5,23), improvement in range of motion, and reduced disability in patients with OA as compared with placebo and with nonsteroidal antiinflammatory medications (23). When superficial heat combined with exercise is compared with exercise alone, heat produces no greater effect than that produced by the exercises alone (26,27), except in grip function (18). A systematic review of 7 randomized, controlled trials recently concluded that there are no positive or detrimental effects of superficial heat therapy for patients with RA and recommended that heat can be used in palliative care (28).

Many patients report global improvement following superficial heat treatments, despite lack of clinical evidence for improvement (20). People with RA find heat to be among the most effective means of self-management (7). If the appropriate contraindications or precautions are observed, patients who feel better or are more inclined to be active following heat treatments may be encouraged to use them. There is little danger or cost associated with superficial heat, and no apparent negative effects.

Deep heat appears to be capable of decreasing pain in patients with OA (29) and RA (30); it also has been found to decrease stiffness and increase grip strength, especially in younger patients and those with less severe RA (30). Repeated applications of short-wave diathermy (30 20-minute sessions) have recently been shown to reduce synovial sac thickness and pain in patients with knee OA, an indication of reduced chronic synovial inflammation (31). Repeated applications of continuous and pulsed ultrasound have been shown recently to enhance the effect of isokinetic exercise (32). Three groups of patients with knee OA received exercises 3 times a week for 8 weeks, with one group also receiving pulsed ultrasound and one group also receiving continuous ultrasound. All groups experienced improvement in pain, disability, and peak torque production, but both ultrasound groups achieved increased range of motion and ambulation speed as well. The group that received pulsed ultrasound experienced greater improvements in pain, range of motion, ambulation speed, disability, and torque production at

180°/second than those who received continuous ultrasound. The improvements were retained for the 1-year followup period.

Other investigators have found that deep heat is not effective for patients with OA or RA (33,34), and when combined with exercises, deep heat appears to be no more effective than exercise alone (24,29,35,36). In one study, the only people whose symptoms worsened were those who received short-wave diathermy (29).

Ultrasound is often used for patients with soft-tissue inflammatory conditions, such as tendinitis, bursitis, or epicondylitis. Investigators have shown that ultrasound reduces pain and pressure sensitivity in patients with a variety of periarticular inflammatory conditions (37–39) and contributes to increased range of motion (40). Successful treatment is not universal, however, as other investigators have found no evidence for effectiveness (33,34,41–43). Use of ultrasound in the management of calcific bursitis has been of particular interest. Improvements in pain and function, as well as resolution of calcium deposits, have been demonstrated with ultrasound treatment (44–47), with deposits in the resorptive stage decreasing more than those in the formative stage (48).

Patients who received deep-heat treatment have been shown to perceive a more satisfactory outcome than those who received placebo treatments, even when they have persistent disability (30). However, deep heat must be applied in a clinical setting. Such treatments are expensive and may be hazardous. When exercise or superficial heat can accomplish the same goals, there is little rationale for using deep heat.

There have been 3 recent systematic reviews of randomized controlled trials investigating the use of ultrasound in patients with OA of the knee or RA. Casimiro and colleagues (49) concluded that ultrasound might be useful in increasing grip strength for patients with RA, but noted the poor quality of the 2 trials they located. Similarly, based on a single trial, the Philadelphia Panel (50) concluded that there is insufficient evidence to recommend inclusion or exclusion of ultrasound in the management of OA of the knee. Welch and colleagues (51) reviewed 3 trials (not including a trial by Huang and colleagues [32]) and concluded that there was no evidence of benefit of ultrasound for OA of the knee.

COLD

The primary reasons for using cold applications are to decrease pain, swelling, and inflammation. Pain is decreased by slowing or blocking nerve conduction, decreasing activity of the muscle spindle (2), or releasing endorphins (19). Swelling is decreased through vasoconstriction, which decreases blood flow and capillary pressure. Gentle cooling also blocks histamine release, decreasing inflammation. The intraarticular temperature decreases as skin temperature decreases (12), perhaps reducing collagenolytic enzyme activity and inflammation in the joint.

Application

Cold is applied to the skin through ice or cold packs, ice massage, cold baths, or vapocoolant sprays. It usually is applied for 10–30 minutes, depending on the intensity of the cold source and the depth of the tissue to be reached. Deeper tissues require longer treatment times. Milder cold sources are more appropriate for swelling; very cold sources, capable of producing skin anesthesia, are more appropriate for pain reduction. Care should be taken not to frost the skin. Cold treatments can be used at home with proper instruction. Ice packs, ice massage, and cold baths can be used as needed up to twice daily.

Contraindications and Precautions

Patients who do not have sufficient vasoconstriction capabilities to conserve heat should not use cold treatments. In addition, because cold causes vasoconstriction, its use may delay healing.

Several precautions must be taken when using cold treatments. Cold produces stiffness in connective tissues in laboratory studies (3), but the stiffness does not necessarily manifest clinically in decreased range of motion. Nonetheless, caution must be exercised to move cooled joints more slowly. Force generation also may be affected by cold treatments. After using a cold treatment that is sufficient to cool the motor neurons and block nerve conduction, entire motor units may temporarily cease to function, with resulting weakness.

Some people are hypersensitive to cold; others actually exhibit cold allergy manifested as urticaria. People with RA have been shown to experience increased pain with cold exposure (52), especially if they smoke (53). Patients with RA have more vasomotor instability and get colder and stiffer in response to cold exposure. They also have been shown to cool and rewarm more slowly (16). Raynaud's phenomenon, a condition aggravated by cold exposure, is associated with a history of joint pain (54) and systemic sclerosis (55).

Effectiveness

Cold treatments can be effective in decreasing pain, improving function, and decreasing stiffness (19,20,56). The effect of cold on swelling in patients with arthritis has not been extensively studied. Repeated treatments with cold packs have been effective in reducing swelling in knee OA (27). One small-sample study showed that postsurgical hand volume and pain decreased, but not significantly, following cold treatments (57). A larger study demonstrated that ice massage to acupuncture points for 20 minutes produced significant improvement in pain, stiffness, walking time, and muscle strength of patients with OA of the knee when compared with placebo, although the change in walking time and range of motion was small (58). A systematic review of 3 randomized controlled trials recently concluded that ice massage is effective in improving range of motion, pain, and function in knee OA, while cold packs are effective in reducing swelling but are ineffective for reducing pain (59).

Heat and cold appear to be about equally effective for managing pain, stiffness, and limitation of motion (19,20). Cold has been shown to produce earlier decreases in pain and stiffness than short-wave diathermy or placebo treatments (56). Heat appears to be better for improving motion, whereas cold may be better for reducing pain (20). Patients often have no clear preference for heat or cold (19,21), although in some cases, patients continue to prefer heat even when cold has yielded greater improvement (20).

TRANSCUTANEOUS ELECTRICAL NERVE STIMULATION

Treatment with transcutaneous electrical nerve stimulation (TENS) may decrease pain and inflammation. Stiffness may decrease as well (60,61). The use of TENS was originally based on the gate control theory of pain advanced by Melzack and Wall (62). Stimulation of the large sensory fibers is thought to prevent impulses from the smaller pain fibers from being transmitted in the ascending tracks in the spinal cord. Theoretically, impulses from C fibers are blocked better than impulses from other fiber types. Because C fibers innervate the synovium and joint capsule, TENS could prove useful in the treatment

of arthritis (61). In addition, most forms of TENS have been shown to cause the release of various endogenous opioids in the midbrain (63,64).

Use of TENS has been shown to raise intraarticular temperature about 0.5°C in rabbits after a 5-minute treatment, but it also decreased inflammatory exudate and joint pressure and volume (65). The decreased inflammation and joint volume may help relieve pain in inflammatory arthritis.

Application

There are several modes of TENS, but the 3 most common are high-frequency TENS, low-frequency or acupuncture-like TENS, and burst-mode TENS. High-frequency TENS stimulates only the sensory nerve endings, using a continuous train of 50–125 μsec pulses in a frequency range of 50–110 Hz (66). High-frequency TENS theoretically works through the gate control mechanism as well as through the release of dynorphin (64). The usual electrode placement for people with arthritis is around the involved joint (61,67–71). Single-treatment duration varies, but a recent study showed that pain relief for patients with knee OA lasted longer and accumulated over several treatment sessions if those sessions were 40 minutes in length (72). Pain relief, if it occurs, has a rapid onset. High-frequency TENS is often used up to 3 times per day and may be used for several weeks.

Low-frequency TENS stimulates the motor endplates of muscles using wider, 250 μsec or longer pulses at a frequency of 1–4 Hz. This mode of TENS has been shown to cause an increase in cerebrospinal fluid levels of metenkephalin (64). Electrodes are placed over acupuncture points or motor points of muscles in the myotomes related to the painful joint.

Burst-mode TENS combines elements of both the high- and low-frequency modes. In burst mode, the carrier frequency of the current is high (70–100 Hz), but it is delivered in small bursts at a low rate (3–4 bursts per second). Burst mode also uses motor-level stimulation with electrode placements similar to those used with low-frequency TENS. This method produces longer-lasting pain relief, apparently through the same mechanisms as low-frequency TENS (66). The advantage of burst-mode TENS is the greater comfort of the current as compared with low-frequency TENS. Low-frequency and burst-mode TENS usually are applied for about 30 minutes. Low-frequency and burst-mode TENS usually are used only once per day but may be used for several weeks.

Contraindications and Precautions

People with cardiac pacing problems, who use pacemakers, or who have internal defibrillators should not use TENS near the heart. Electrodes should not be placed over the carotid sinus or the laryngeal or pharyngeal muscles (66). In addition, TENS should not be used during the first trimester of pregnancy, because the effect on the fetus is unknown.

As with the thermal agents, there are precautions associated with the use of TENS. Persons using TENS should use the joint carefully while being treated. Some people receiving TENS treatments find them uncomfortable. Discomfort may arise from skin irritation from the electrode couplant or adhesion system as much as from the electricity itself.

In a case report, 1 patient with RA reportedly developed paresthesias and increased pain following heat and TENS. These effects were delayed, so patients should be monitored closely by a qualified therapist (73).

Effectiveness

Pain relief from TENS has been found to be 50–90% (58,61,68–70,74). In some studies, pain relief was significantly greater than relief achieved from placebo treatments (58,67,70,71), while in others, both placebo and actual treatments produced similar amounts of relief (67,74–76). One difference in the effectiveness appears to be the number of treatments received, with more treatments being somewhat more effective than fewer treatments. The amount of pain relief attributed to placebo in studies with patients having RA or OA varies from 17% to 55% (71,75). Pain relief beyond that amount may be attributed to the TENS treatment (77). In addition to pain relief, TENS has been shown to contribute to decreased stiffness (58,60), as well as to improved 50-foot walk time, muscle strength, and knee flexion range of motion (58).

In people with rheumatic disease, pain relief from high-frequency and burst-mode TENS has been shown to last from 2.5 hours (70) to 18 hours (69), although patients may remain improved for days (68), weeks (72,74), or even months (78) following termination of treatment. The duration of pain relief from low-frequency TENS has not been reported extensively, but in 1 study, pain relief lasted 4 hours (69). Duration of pain relief appears to be related to duration of treatment, with 40-minute treatments producing longer relief than 20-minute treatments (72).

There is little evidence to favor one mode of TENS over another for patients with rheumatic disease. All 3 modes have been shown to be effective in some studies, with no one mode more effective than another (67,75,79). Other studies have shown that high-frequency and burst-mode TENS produce more and longer-lasting pain relief compared with low-frequency TENS (67,69). In a comparison of burst-mode TENS with high-frequency and placebo TENS in persons with OA, neither mode produced more pain relief than placebo, but the burst mode produced longer pain relief than placebo. High-frequency TENS decreased stiffness better than placebo, and both modes produced longer stiffness relief than placebo. High-frequency TENS reduced knee circumference better than burst mode, and burst mode was better than placebo for increasing range of motion (60). Burst-mode, low-frequency, and high-frequency TENS have all been effective in decreasing stiffness (58,60).

In comparing TENS with other treatments, pain relief produced by TENS has been shown to be longer lasting than that produced by analgesic medications (70). On the other hand, a nonsteroidal antiinflammatory medication was shown to be superior to TENS for patients with OA of the knee (76); however, less-than-optimal electrode placements were used in the study. In people with OA of the hip, electrical stimulation alone decreased pain as well as did ultrasound, short-wave diathermy, or ibuprofen (29). Appropriate use of TENS could decrease the need for pharmacologic interventions and would be superior to deep heat, which requires clinic-based application. TENS has also been shown to be comparable to ice treatments for reduction of pain in patients with knee OA (58).

Overall, TENS appears to be useful for decreasing pain and stiffness, and the symptomatic relief may last longer than relief produced by other treatments. Reviewing only randomized controlled trials, Osiri and colleagues (80) and the Philadelphia Panel (50) agreed that there is good evidence for including TENS in the management of pain for patients with knee OA. Because the patient controls TENS treatment, it is a good tool for home use when people are properly instructed and monitored.

SUMMARY

The therapeutic goals for people with arthritis include improved pain, stiffness, swelling, and function. Superficial heat is helpful in achieving these goals, but may not be necessary if patients exercise appropriately.

However, if patients who do not have acutely inflamed joints feel better after using superficial heat treatments, there appears to be no reason not to use them. Deep heat is costly, potentially hazardous, and requires clinic visits. Because other, safer means, such as exercise, can meet these goals without aggravating symptoms (especially in inflammatory arthritis), there is little reason to use deep heat in patients with arthritis.

In addition to the goals of symptomatic relief, it may be desirable to decrease the destructive inflammatory process for patients with inflammatory arthritis by cooling the joint. Cold treatments also promote improvement in pain, motion, and swelling. Cold treatments are not often considered for patients with arthritis, and patients may prefer heat, even when their symptoms are relieved better with cold (19,20). Patients should be encouraged to try cold treatments, especially when joints are acutely inflamed.

Use of TENS is effective for decreasing pain and stiffness without the potential hazard to the joint surfaces. The high-frequency and burst modes appear to work best for patients with arthritis. Patient improvement may be long lasting, and patients may be able to decrease medication use.

Appropriate professional supervision and instruction must accompany the use of any of the thermal and electrical agents for patients with rheumatic diseases. Any of these agents can be harmful if improperly applied. Education by a knowledgeable professional is crucial for correct and safe application.

REFERENCES

1. Berliner MN, Maurer AI. Effect of different methods of thermotherapy on skin microcirculation. Am J Phys Med Rehabil 2004;83:292–7.
2. Lehmann JF, DeLateur BJ. Therapeutic heat. In: Lehmann JF, ed. Therapeutic heat and cold. 3rd ed. Baltimore: Williams and Wilkins; 1982. p. 404–562.
3. Wright V, Johns RJ. Quantitative and qualitative analysis of joint stiffness in normal subjects and in patients with connective tissue diseases. Ann Rheum Dis 1961;20:36–46.
4. Lentell G, Heatherington T, Eagan J, Morgan M. The use of thermal agents to influence the effectiveness of a low-load prolonged stretch. J Orthop Sports Phys Ther 1992;16:200–7.
5. Michlovitz S, Hun L, Erasala GN, Hengehold DA, Weingand KW. Continuous low-level heat wrap therapy is effective for treating wrist pain. Arch Phys Med Rehabil 2004;85:1409–16.
6. Mazzuca SA, Page MC, Meldrum RD, Brandt KD, Petty-Saphon S. Pilot study of the effects of a heat-retaining knee sleeve on joint pain, stiffness, and function in patients with knee osteoarthritis. Arthritis Rheum 2004;51:716–21.
7. Veitiene D, Tamulaitiene M. Comparison of self-management methods for osteoarthritis and rheumatoid arthritis. J Rehabil Med 2005;37:58–60.
8. Hayes KW. Manual for physical agents. 5th ed. Norwalk (CT): Prentice-Hall; 2000.
9. Weinberger A, Fadilah R, Lev A, Levi A, Pinkhas J. Deep heat in the treatment of inflammatory joint disease. Med Hypotheses 1988;25:231–3.
10. Harris ED, McCroskery PA. The influence of temperature and fibril stability on degradation of cartilage collagen by rheumatoid synovial collagenase. N Engl J Med 1974;290:1–6.
11. Weinberger A, Fadilah R, Lev A, Pinkhas J. Intra-articular temperature measurements after superficial heating. Scand J Rehabil Med 1989;21:55–7.
12. Oosterveld FG, Rasker JJ, Jacobs JW, Overmars HJ. The effect of local heat and cold therapy on the intraarticular and skin surface temperature of the knee. Arthritis Rheum 1992;35:146–51.
13. Harris R, Millard JB. Paraffin-wax baths in the treatment of rheumatoid arthritis. Ann Rheum Dis 1955;14:278–82.
14. Dorwart BB, Hansell JR, Schumacher HR Jr. Effects of cold and heat on urate crystal-induced synovitis in the dog. Arthritis Rheum 1974;17:563–71.
15. Mainardi CL, Walter JM, Spiegel PK, Goldkamp OG, Harris ED Jr. Rheumatoid arthritis: failure of daily heat therapy to affect its progression. Arch Phys Med Rehabil 1979;60:390–3.
16. Martin GM, Roth GM, Elkins EC, Krusen FH. Cutaneous temperature of the extremities of normal subjects and of patients with rheumatoid arthritis. Arch Phys Med 1946;27:665–82.

17. Dyck PJ, Conn DL, Okazaki H. Necrotizing angiopathic neuropathy: three-dimensional morphology of fiber degeneration related to sites of occluded vessels. Mayo Clin Proc 1972;47:461–75.

18. Dellhag B, Wollersjö I, Bjelle A. Effect of active hand exercise and wax bath treatment in rheumatoid arthritis patients. Arthritis Care Res 1992;5:87–92.

19. Utsinger PD, Bonner F, Hogan N. Efficacy of cryotherapy and thermotherapy in the management of rheumatoid arthritis pain: evidence for an endorphin effect. Arthritis Rheum 1982;25 (suppl 9):S113.

20. Williams J, Harvey J, Tannenbaum H. Use of superficial heat versus ice for the rheumatoid arthritic shoulder: a pilot study. Physiother Can 1986;38:8–13.

21. Kirk JA, Kersley GD. Heat and cold in the physical treatment of rheumatoid arthritis of the knee: a controlled clinical trial. Ann Phys Med 1968;9:270–4.

22. Curkovic B, Vitulic V, Babic-Naglic D, Dürrigl T. The influence of heat and cold on the pain threshold in rheumatoid arthritis. Z Rheumatol 1993;52:289–91.

23. McCarberg W, Erasala G, Goodale M, Grender J, Hengehold D, Donikyan L. Therapeutic benefits of continuous low-level heat wrap therapy (CLHT) for osteoarthritis (OA) of the knee. 24th Annual Scientific Meeting of the American Pain Society. Boston (MA); 2005.

24. Hamilton DE, Bywaters EG, Please NW. A controlled trial of various forms of physiotherapy in arthritis. Br Med J 1959;1:542–4.

25. Bromley J, Unsworth A, Haslock I. Changes in stiffness following short- and long-term application of standard physiotherapeutic techniques. Br J Rheumatol 1994;33:555–61.

26. Green J, McKenna F, Redfern EJ, Chamberlain MA. Home exercises are as effective as outpatient hydrotherapy for osteoarthritis of the hip. Br J Rheumatol 1993;32:812–5.

27. Hecht PJ, Bachmann S, Booth RE Jr, Rothman RH. Effects of thermal therapy on rehabilitation after total knee arthroplasty. Clin Orthop Relat Res 1983;178:198–201.

28. Robinson VA, Brosseau L, Casimiro L Judd MG, Shea BJ, Tugwell P, et al. Thermotherapy for treating rheumatoid arthritis. The Cochrane Database Syst Rev. 2002;2:CD002826.

29. Svarcová J, Trnavsky K, Zvárová J. The influence of ultrasound, galvanic currents and shortwave diathermy on pain intensity in patients with osteoarthritis. Scand J Rheumatol Suppl 1987;67:83–5.

30. Konrad K. Randomized double blind placebo controlled study of ultrasonic treatment of the hands of rheumatoid arthritis patients. Eur J Phys Med Rehabil 1994;4:155–7.

31. Jan MH, Chai HM, Wang CL, Lin YF, Tsai LY. Effects of repetitive short-wave diathermy for reducing synovitis in patients with knee osteoarthritis: an ultrasonographic study. Phys Ther 2006;86:236–44.

32. Huang MH, Lin YS, Lee CL, Yang RC. Use of ultrasound to increase effectiveness of isokinetic exercise for knee osteoarthritis. Arch Phys Med Rehabil 2005;86:1545–51.

33. Mueller EE, Mead S, Schulz BF, Vaden MR. A placebo-controlled study of ultrasound treatment for periarthritis. Am J Phys Med 1954;33:31–5.

34. Hashish I, Harvey W, Harris M. Anti-inflammatory effects of ultrasound therapy: evidence for a major placebo effect. Br J Rheum 1986;25:77–81.

35. Falconer J, Hayes KW, Chang RW. Effect of ultrasound on mobility in osteoarthritis of the knee: a randomized clinical trial. Arthritis Care Res 1992;5:29–35.

36. Jan MH, Lai JS. The effects of physiotherapy on osteoarthritic knees of females. J Formos Med Assoc 1991;90:1008–13.

37. Klaiman MD, Shrader JA, Danoff JV, Hicks JE, Pesce WJ, Ferland J. Phonophoresis versus ultrasound in the treatment of common musculoskeletal conditions. MedSci Sports Exerc 1998;30:1349–55.

38. Halle JS, Franklin RJ, Karalfa BL. Comparison of four physical therapy modalitites in the treatment of lateral epicondylitis. J Orthop Sports Phys Ther 1986;8:62–70.

39. Binder A, Hodge G, Greenwood AM, Hazleman BL, Page Thomas DP. Is therapeutic ultrasound effective in treating soft tissue lesions? Br Med J (Clin Res Ed) 1985;290:512–4.

40. Lehmann JF, Erickson DJ, Martin GM, Krusen FH. Comparison of ultrasonic and microwave diathermy in the physical treatment of periarthritis of the shoulder; study of the effects of ultrasonic and microwave diathermy when employed in conjunction with massage and exercise. Arch Phys Med Rehabil 1954;35:627–34.

41. Nykänen M. Pulsed ultrasound treatment of the painful shoulder a randomized, double-blind, placebo-controlled study. Scand J Rehabil Med 1995;27:105–8.

42. Lundeberg T, Abrahamsson P, Haker E. A comparative study of continuous ultrasound, placebo ultrasound and rest in epicondylalgia. Scand J Rehabil Med 1988;20:99–101.

43. Downing DS, Weinstein A. Ultrasound therapy of subacromial bursitis: a double blind trial. Phys Ther 1986;66:194–9.

44. Ebenbichler GR, Erdogmus CB, Resch KL, Funovics MA, Kainberger F, Barisani G, et al. Ultrasound therapy for calcific tendinitis of the shoulder. N Engl J Med 1999;340:1533–8.

45. Flax HJ. Ultrasound treatment of peritendinitis calcarea of the shoulder. Am J Phys Med 1964;43:117–24.

46. Aldes JH, Klaras T. Use of ultrasonic radiation in the treatment of sub-deltoid bursitis with and without calcareous deposits. West J Surg Obstet Gynecol 1954;62:369–76.

47. Cline PD. Radiographic follow-up of ultrasound therapy in calcific bursitis. J Am Phys Ther Assoc 1963;43:659–60.

48. Perron M, Malouin F. Acetic acid iontophoresis and ultrasound for the treatment of calcifying tendinitis of the shoulder: a randomized control trial. Arch Phys Med Rehabil 1997;78:379–84.

49. Casimiro L, Brosseau L, Robinson V, Milne S, Judd MG, Wells G, et al. Therapeutic ultrasound for the treatment of rheumatoid arthritis. Cochrane Database Syst Rev 2002;(3):CD003787.

50. Philadelphia Panel. Philadelphia panel evidence-based clinical practice guidelines on selected rehabilitation interventions for knee pain. Phys Ther 2001;81:1675–700.

51. Welch V, Brosseau L, Peterson J, Shea B, Tugwell P, Wells G. Therapeutic ultrasound for osteoarthritis of the knee. Cochrane Database Syst Rev 2001;3:CD003132.

52. Jahanshahi M, Pitt P, Williams I. Pain avoidance in rheumatoid arthritis. J Psychom Res 1989;33:579–89.

53. Helliwell P. Smoking and ice therapy in rheumatoid arthritis. Physiotherapy 1989;75:551–2.

54. Leppert J, Åberg H, Ringqvist I, Sörensson S. Raynaud's phenomenon in a female population: prevalence and association with other conditions. Angiology 1987;38:871–7.

55. Medsger TA, Steen V. Systemic sclerosis and related syndromes. B. Clinical features and treatment. In: Schumacher HR, Klippel JH, Koopman WJ, eds. Primer on the rheumatic diseases. Atlanta: Arthritis Foundation; 1993. p. 120–7.

56. Clarke GR, Willis LA, Stenner L, Nichols PJ. Evaluation of physiotherapy in the treatment of osteoarthrosis of the knee. Rheumatol Rehabil 1974;13:190–7.

57. Rembe EC. Use of cryotherapy on the postsurgical rheumatoid hand. Phys Ther 1970;50:19–23.

58. Yurtkuran M, Kocagil T. TENS, electroacupuncture and ice massage: comparison of treatment for osteoarthritis of the knee. Am J Acupunct 1999;27:133–40.

59. Brosseau L, Yonge KA, Robinson V, Marchand S, Judd MG, Wells G, et al. Thermotherapy for treatment of osteoarthritis. Cochran Database Syst Rev. 2003;4:CD004522.

60. Grimmer K. A controlled double blind study comparing the effects of strong burst mode TENS and high rate TENS on painful osteoarthritic knees. Aust J Physiother 1992;38:49–56.

61. Kumar VN, Redford JB. Transcutaneous nerve stimulation in rheumatoid arthritis. Arch Phys Med Rehabil 1982;63:595–6.

62. Melzack R, Wall PD. Pain mechanisms: a new theory. Science. 1965;150:971–9.

63. Sjolund BH, Ericksson MBE. Endorphins and analgesia produced by peripheral conditioning stimulation. In: Bonica JJ, Liebeskind J, Albe-Fessard DG, eds. Advances in pain research and therapy. Vol 3. New York: Raven Press; 1979. p. 587–92.

64. Han JS, Chen XH, Sun SL, Xu XJ, Yuan Y, Hao JX, et al. Effect of low- and high-frequency TENS on Met-enkephalin-Arg-Phe and dynorphin A immunoreactivity in human lumbar CSF. Pain 1991;47:295–8.

65. Levy A, Dalith M, Abramovici A, Pinkhas J, Weinberger A. Transcutaneous electrical nerve stimulation in experimental acute arthritis. Arch Phys Med Rehabil 1987;68:75–8.

66. Foley RA. Transcutaneous electrical nerve stimulation. In: Hayes KW, ed. Manual for physical agents. Upper Saddle River (NJ): Prentice Hall; 2000. p. 121–47.

67. Møystad A, Krogstad BS, Larheim TA. Transcutaneous nerve stimulation in a group of patients with rheumatic disease involving the temporomandibular joint. J Prosth Dent 1990;64:596–600.

68. Mannheimer C, Lund S, Carlsson CA. The effect of transcutaneous electrical nerve stimulation (TNS) on joint pain in patients with rheumatoid arthritis. Scand J Rheumatol 1978;7:13–6.

69. Mannheimer C, Carlsson CA. The analgesic effect of transcutaneous electrical nerve stimulation (TNS) in patients with rheumatoid arthritis: a comparative study of different pulse patterns. Pain 1979;6:329–34.

70. Lewis D, Lewis B, Sturrock RD. Transcutaneous electrical nerve stimulation in osteoarthrosis: a therapeutic alternative? Ann Rheum Dis 1984;43:47–9.

71. Abelson K, Langley GB, Sheppeard H, Vlieg M, Wigley RD. Transcutaneous electrical nerve stimulation in rheumatoid arthritis. N Z Med J 1983;96:156–8.

72. Cheing GLY, Tsui AY, Lo SK, Hui-Chan CW. Optimal stimulation duration of tens in the management of osteoarthritic knee pain. J Rehabil Med 2003;35:62–8.

73. Griffin JW, McClure M. Adverse responses to transcutaneous electrical nerve stimulation in a patient with rheumatoid arthritis. Phys Ther 1981;61:354–5.

74. Smith CR, Lewith GT, Machin D. TNS and osteo-arthritic pain: preliminary study to establish a controlled method of assessing transcutaneous nerve stimulation as a treatment for the pain caused by osteo-arthritis of the knee. Physiotherapy 1983;69:266–8.

75. Langley GB, Sheppeard H, Johnson M, Wigley RD. The analgesic effects of transcutaneous electrical nerve stimulation and placebo in chronic pain patients: a double-blind non-crossover comparison. Rheumatol Int 1984;4:119–23.

76. Lewis B, Lewis D, Cumming G. The comparative analgesic efficacy of transcutaneous electrical nerve stimulation and a non-steroidal anti-inflammatory drug for painful osteoarthritis. Br J Rheumatol 1994;33: 455–60.

77. Hoffman GA, Harrington A, Fields HL. Pain and the placebo: what we have learned. Perspect Biol Med 2005;48:248–65.

78. Fargas-Babjak A, Rooney P, Gerecz E. Randomized trial of Codetron for pain control in osteoarthritis of the hip/knee. Clin J Pain 1989;5:137–41.

79. Law PP, Cheing GL. Optimal stimulation frequency of transcutaneous electrical nerve stimulation on people with knee osteoarthritis. J Rehabil Med 2004;36:220–5.

80. Osiri M, Welch V, Brosseau L, McGowan J, et al. Transcutaneous electrical nerve stimulation for knee osteoarthritis (Cochrane Review). Cochrane Database Syst Rev 2000;4:CD002823.

Splinting of the Hand

PAMELA B. HARRELL, OTR, CHT

Splints have been used throughout history to protect, immobilize, or mobilize various parts of the body. A splint may be defined as "a rigid or flexible appliance used for the prevention of movement of a joint or for the fixation of displaced or moveable parts." In current practice, splints are used to maintain and enhance motion, as well as to prevent it. Splints serve various purposes in the management of the hand with rheumatic disease; however, some controversy exists over the roles and benefits of splinting. Studies have supported the use of splints to reduce pain and inflammation, but additional studies are indicated to determine the outcome of splinting to prevent and correct deformity. Although indications for and use of splints vary widely among practitioners, most agree that splinting plays an important role in the overall management of rheumatic disease.

The use of splints should be based on knowledge of rheumatic disease, mechanisms of joint inflammation, and pathomechanics of joint deformity. The type of arthritis and stage of joint involvement should influence the treatment program, which may include splinting. How the joint has been affected by arthritis, and more importantly, how joint involvement has affected the person's ability to function should also be considered.

EVALUATION

A complete hand evaluation and functional assessment is necessary prior to establishing goals for a splinting program. An evaluation should include the following components.

Interview and Subjective Assessment

Obtain a clear history of the disease, including duration, medical management, functional performance, and effect of the arthritis on a person's lifestyle. Subjective assessment of pain, stiffness, and fatigue should include such information as intensity, duration, and activities that increase or decrease symptoms. Functional assessment can be performed through patient self-report measures, observation of functional activities, or standardized hand functional assessment tools.

Objective Measurements

Assessment of range of motion, both passively and actively; grip and pinch strength; and sensation will also provide input into splint design. Observation skills should be used to aid objective measurements. For example, during grip and pinch strength testing, observe the stability of the metacarpophalangeal (MCP) joints. Is there an increase in ulnar deviation during gripping activities? Observe metacarpal/interphalangeal joint motion during lateral pinch. Is there hyperextension? Is there a complaint of pain at the carpometacarpal (CMC) joint during pinch activities?

Visual Inspection and Manual Assessment

Through observation of swelling, joint alignment, and tendon and ligament integrity, articular and nonarticular manifestations of disease can be identified. Manual assessment of joint stability and ligamentous laxity should be performed. These manifestations should be addressed in the splinting process. For example, a splint may be utilized to provide external support for ligamentous laxity of proximal interphalangeal (PIP) joints, which may in turn reduce pain and improve function.

ESTABLISHING SPLINTING GOALS

An individualized approach should be used in establishing splinting program goals, based on problems identified through the evaluation. For example, in the case of a patient with rheumatoid arthritis (RA) who has MCP ulnar drift, goals for splinting should be established as follows: 1) the splint will place the fingers in a more functional position for hand use; 2) the splint will rest the MCP joints to reduce pain and inflammation; and 3) the splint will reduce intraarticular forces on supporting structures. Caution should be utilized in the application of splints. They should only be implemented after fully evaluating the patient's functional ability and establishing goals of splinting. Table 1 lists questions that may help define the parameters of a splinting program for the specific problems identified on the hand evaluation.

PURPOSES OF SPLINTING

Reducing Pain

Splints reduce pain by immobilizing or supporting painful joints and periarticular structures (1–4). Immobilization reduces stress on the joint capsule and synovial lining, thereby reducing pain. Supporting a painful joint with a splint allows improved functional use through reduction of pain. By reducing joint pain, reflexive muscle spasm is also reduced, which further reduces joint pain (3). Splints can reduce pain in such periarticular structures as tendons and ligaments by restricting full excursion and overstretching. The benefits of splinting in terms of pain reduction are well documented (2–8). One study found that more than 60% of patients had moderate to great pain relief by using splints (6,9). Another study showed that patients with splints achieved greater relief from pain than relief from morning stiffness (10). The same study also found that patients continued to wear splints because of the benefits of pain reduction.

Decreasing Inflammation

Splints reduce joint and tendon inflammation by restricting motion. Inflammation is also reduced by decreasing external forces on the inflamed tissues. Several studies have demonstrated reduction in joint

Table 1. Questions to aid in establishing the parameters of a splinting program for the hand.

- **What is the goal of the splint?** Is the splint being used to reduce pain and inflammation or to support an unstable joint? Is the splint being used to prevent or possibly correct deformity? Will the splint improve or hinder the functional use of the hand?
- **What is the best splint design for this particular person?** Which joint or joints need to be supported or immobilized to achieve the goal? Should the splint be dorsal or volar? Which materials will best achieve the goals of the splint?
- **When should the splint be worn?** Is the splint a resting splint for night wear or a functional daytime splint? How long should the splint be worn?

inflammation through splinting and rest (1,2,4,7,8,10). Consensus has not been reached on how much rest is necessary to reduce inflammation. It has been suggested, however, that splints used for the purpose of reducing inflammation be continued at night for several weeks after acute inflammation has resolved (6,11,12). Patients can be taught to monitor their inflammation and adjust their use of splints accordingly.

Preventing Deformity

Splints are often used to support joints in an attempt to prevent deformity. Controversy exists in this area, as there is a lack of outcome data supporting the use of splints for this purpose. Despite this, splints are often prescribed for patients with early signs of malalignment to hopefully delay progression, and for patients with more advanced deformity to prevent further deterioration.

Wrist involvement in juvenile arthritis is common, and wrist splints are often prescribed to prevent deformities of subluxation and ulnar deviation (13,14). Wrist splints have been shown to improve writing skills in more than 60% of children with arthritis; however, prevention of deformity has not been documented.

Hand deformity, particularly MCP ulnar deviation, is a common finding in RA (5,15). Resting hand splints and other ulnar deviation supports are commonly used to prevent or delay progression of malalignment. Few studies have addressed the role of splinting in preventing or correcting deformity. The use of a resting splint at night for at least 1 year was not found to delay the progression of ulnar deviation in 1 controlled study (5). However, the study suggested that dynamic splints could reduce ulnar deviation of MCP joints. Splints used for the purpose of preventing a deformity should be monitored closely.

Correcting Deformity

Splints may be used to correct flexion deformities of the fingers and wrist. Splinting for this purpose can be static (using serial, progressive splinting or casting) or dynamic. Whichever method is used, joint inflammation should be closely monitored, because dynamic forces may exacerbate inflammation. One study evaluated the effect of splinting on flexion contractures of fingers with RA. A comparison was performed between dynamic finger-based splints and static finger-based splints. Both splint groups showed significant improvement in correction of the contracture and also demonstrated improved grip strength and hand function scores. There was no difference in the amount of extension motion gained with the static or dynamic splints; however, patients who wore the dynamic splints demonstrated better flexion motion (16).

Supporting Function

Hand function can be decreased by painful, inflamed, poorly positioned, or unstable joints. Splinting may improve function by reducing pain and inflammation and by supporting joints in a more stable and functional position. Wrist supports, both commercial and custom, reduce forces on the wrist and protect the joint during daily activities, allowing for function of the distal joints. Finger and thumb splints place the joints in positions of function and support weakened ligaments, allowing for pinching and gripping with improved dexterity and strength.

The impact of an MCP ulnar deviation splint on pain, function, grip strength, and passive correction of the deformity was evaluated in a study by Rennie (17). Results showed significantly improved alignment in all fingers, with the exception of the index finger, as well as radiolgraphically observed correction of subluxation. The use of this MCP ulnar deviation splint also revealed a statistically significant improvement in 3-point pinch strength; however, there was no change in scores for hand function, pain, grip strength, or lateral pinch.

Postoperative Management

Dynamic and static splints are used in postoperative rehabilitation of the hand with rheumatic disease. Dynamic splints allow early postoperative motion in controlled ranges and planes, assist weakened muscles, and protect reconstructed joints and periarticular structures. Dynamic splints also assist in scar formation for stability and motion. Static splints immobilize surgical repairs and stabilize joints in proper alignment. In the case of MCP joint arthroplasty, a dorsal dynamic MCP extension outrigger is used continuously for the first 6–8 weeks postoperatively to maintain alignment of the joints and to allow exercise in a controlled range of motion. This type of splint may also be used for the same purposes in an extensor tendon repair or transfer. Postoperative splinting for repair of a boutonniere deformity is usually static, maintaining the extended position of the PIP joint while allowing the soft tissues to heal. Depending on the surgical technique and postoperative protocol, initiation of motion should be performed by removing the splint for intermittent periods of exercise. Proper use of splinting postoperatively requires a preoperative knowledge of the hand, an understanding of operative procedures, established postoperative goals, and a concerted team effort among the surgeon, therapist, and patient.

TYPES OF SPLINTS

Resting Splints

Resting splints are used primarily to reduce joint inflammation and pain. They may be used during the day as well as at night. Resting splints may also be used to reduce symptoms of nerve entrapment or tendon irritation, such as triggering and tenosynovitis. Caution should be used when determining the wearing time for resting splints to maintain joint motion and muscle strength. For this reason, resting splints may be worn at night and intermittently during the day during periods of active synovitis or tenosynovitis, alternating with gentle range of motion and functional activities.

Functional Splints

Functional splints are worn to improve hand function by reducing pain, improving joint alignment, or providing stability to weakened periarticular structures. Functional splints support or immobilize the minimum number of joints, thereby allowing all other joints to move freely. Functional splints may be static (to support weakened or painful joints) or dynamic (to gently realign joint deformity).

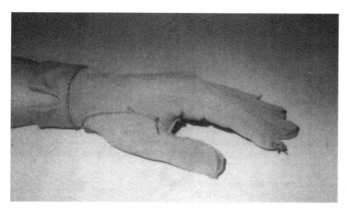

Figure 1. Stretch gloves can be used at night to help decrease morning stiffness and pain.

Corrective Splints

After a complete hand evaluation, it may be determined that a joint contracture is the result of shortening of periarticular structures. If the joint space is preserved, inflammation is at a minimum, and a "soft" end feel is present, splinting may be used to gently correct the contracture. Splints indicated for this purpose may be dynamic or static. Dynamic splinting should be approached cautiously in patients with rheumatic disease. Inflammation and pain may be exacerbated by excessive force on the joint. Static splints that are progressively molded to increase range of motion are often better tolerated due to a lesser amount of force being placed on the joint.

Soft Splints

Support can be provided to joints with gloves, wraps, and soft splints. Soft splints are often more comfortable to patients and may provide as much symptom relief as rigid splints. Using stretch gloves at night has been shown to decrease morning stiffness and pain, allowing for improved hand function (Figure 1) (18). These gloves work by providing gentle compression and neutral warmth to involved joints. Stretch gloves may be contraindicated if carpal tunnel syndrome is present, due to reports of exacerbation of paresthesia. Compressive wraps (such as Coban, Ace, and Tubigrip) also provide support and neutral warmth to joints while allowing joint motion.

Circumferential sleeves and tubes (such as Digisleeve, Digitube, and Compressogrip) can be used as soft splints for joint support. These splints only slightly limit joint mobility. In addition to cushioning and protecting the joint, individual finger wraps and sleeves also act as reminders to protect inflamed finger joints. Soft splints made of neoprene provide joint support and gently assist in realigning joints. Neoprene can be trimmed to fit the patient; however, it does not breathe and may be difficult to put on and wear. Neoprene wraps are often easier to don than tubes, especially when hand weakness is present. Another type of soft splint is fabricated from strapping material to support or realign joints (19). Strapping may be used to reposition ulnar-deviated fingers or to block full motion of interphalangeal joints.

FABRICATED VERSUS PREFABRICATED SPLINTS

A multitude of prefabricated splints, custom-ordered splints, and splinting materials exist. It is often difficult to determine whether it is best to custom fabricate a splint or to use a prefabricated design. There are several advantages of using custom-fabricated splints. The splint is molded to the patient, allowing for conformity to joint surfaces. The materials can be selected according to each individual's needs. In addition, a splint can be designed to support certain joints and allow for movement of others. Finally, modifications in the fit and design are easily made as needed.

The main disadvantage of custom-fabricated splints is the cost. Custom-fabricated splints are usually the most costly type of splint, due to fabrication time and materials used. Also, making these splints requires a skill that not all therapists possess. The time needed to fabricate a splint is often longer than fitting time of a prefabricated splint.

Prefabricated splints also have advantages and disadvantages. They are usually less expensive than custom-fabricated splints; however, they may not have the desired fit or provide as much support or immobilization. Prefabricated splints are usually available in only 3 or 4 basic sizes. Achieving a good fit may be problematic due to deformity, size of the forearm in relation to the hand, or general design of the splint. Some prefabricated splints allow for customization by molding of a metal bar or thermoplastic insert, trimming of splint edges, or adjustment of strapping.

One study compared a custom-fabricated thermoplastic splint versus a prefabricated neoprene splint for stage I and II osteoarthritis of the basal joint of the thumb (20). Both types of splints were shown to improve pain and function; however, the effect was greater with the neoprene splint, which was also shown to be the splint of preference for patients in the study. Both splints reduced subluxation of the first carpometacarpal joint; however, the custom fabricated splint demonstrated greater reduction.

PROBLEM IDENTIFICATION AND SPLINT SOLUTION

Identification of the problem through evaluation is the first step toward determining the best type of splint. Some of the more common hand joint problems associated with rheumatic disease are listed in Table 2, along with suggested splinting solutions.

Wrist Splints

A wrist support splint provides support for the wrist while allowing motion of the thumb and fingers (Figure 2). Indications for a wrist splint include wrist pain, synovitis, tenosynovitis, subluxation, nerve entrapment, and epicondylitis. A wrist support splint may be *dorsal*, which allows for sensation on the volar surface of the hand but does not support volar subluxation; *volar*, which supports volar subluxation but is often difficult to wear with activities that require resting the forearm on a surface; or *circumferential*, which may provide the greatest amount of immobilization. Custom-fabricated wrist splints are more likely to restrict motion, whereas prefabricated wrist supports tend to allow more midrange motion. One study demonstrated a reduction in finger dexterity with commercially available wrist splints and suggested that when commercial wrist orthoses are used during tasks that require maximum dexterity, this reduction should be weighed against the benefits of splinting (21). Another study found wrist splints significantly reduced pain and perceived difficulty during task performance and did not interfere with work performance or increase task difficulty (22).

A functional position of 20–30° of extension is advocated for most conditions; however, in the case of carpal tunnel syndrome, 10° of extension maximizes the carpal tunnel. Special care should be taken when fitting a wrist support for a patient with RA. If the MCP joints

Table 2. Problem identification and suggested splinting solution in the hand with rheumatic disease.*

Problem Identified on Evaluation	Splint Solution
Wrist joint Synovitis, tenosynovitis Pain Instability, subluxation Nerve entrapment, carpal tunnel syndrome	**Wrist support splint** Dorsal, volar, or circumferential Worn at rest and/or with activity Removed for range of motion Positioned in neutral to 10° extension
Wrist/thumb Synovitis of wrist and thumb Tenosynovitis of first dorsal compartment Pain in wrist and thumb	**Thumb spica splint** Volar design for greater immobilization Radial design to limit thumb motions and allow midrange wrist motion C-bar necessary for CMC joint; thumb IP may/may not be included depending on functional needs
Wrist/hand Synovitis of multiple joints Flexor/extensor tenosynovitis Pain at rest Changes in joint alignment	**Resting hand splint** Full resting splint for immobilization of multiple joints/tendons Modified resting splint for immobilization of wrist/MCPs
MCP joint Synovitis Ulnar deviation, subluxation Ligamentous laxity	**MCP ulnar deviation support** Built into resting hand splint Hand-based for functional activities May be static or dynamic for function
Finger Boutonniere deformity Swan neck deformity Lateral instability Flexion deformity	**Finger splints** PIP extension with DIP free to stretch oblique retinacular ligament PIP hyperextension block Lateral support for deviation Static progressive or dynamic Serial casts for PIP flexion deformities
Thumb CMC pain and/or subluxation MCP instability/deformity IP hyperextension IP lateral instability	**Thumb splints** Hand-based CMC support with C-bar Figure-eight MCP support IP hyperextension block Lateral support for deviation

* CMC = carpometacarpal; MCP = metacarpophalangeal; PIP = proximal interphalangeal; DIP = distal interphalangeal; IP = interphalangeal.

are involved, restricting wrist motion may place excess stress on these joints, possibly increasing ulnar deviating or subluxing forces. A position of wrist ulnar deviation is advocated to reduce ulnar deviating forces on the MCP joints.

Combination Wrist/Thumb Splints

Indications for combination wrist/thumb splints include synovitis of the wrist and thumb joints, tenosynovitis of the wrist and thumb tendons, deQuervain's tenosynovitis, wrist and thumb pain, and instability limiting functional use. Types of wrist and thumb supports include a volar-based thumb spica, a radial-based thumb spica with a C-bar for carpometacarpal involvement, and a thumb spica without a C-bar (Figure 3).

Combination Wrist/Hand Splints

Indications for combination wrist/hand splints include pain or synovitis in multiple joints, tenosynovitis in flexor/extensor tendons, pain or stiffness at night or in the morning, and complaints of waking with the hand in a fist. A full resting hand splint immobilizes the wrist and fingers to promote relief of pain and inflammation. Studies have shown these splints to be cumbersome to wear, leading to varying rates of use (23). An alternative to a full resting hand splint is the modified resting hand splint, which supports the wrist and MCP joints while allowing interphalangeal movement (Figure 4). The modified resting splint often results in better patient adherence and comfort, with less pain and stiffness related to splint wear. If a patient requires bilateral resting hand splints, an alternating schedule of night wear may improve adherence.

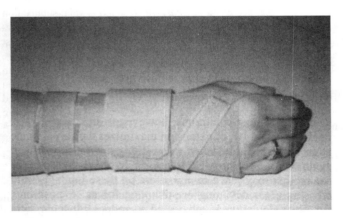

Figure 2. Wrist support splint.

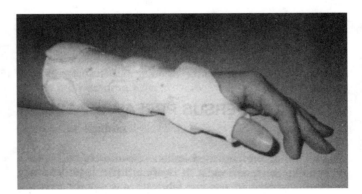

Figure 3. Thumb spica splint.

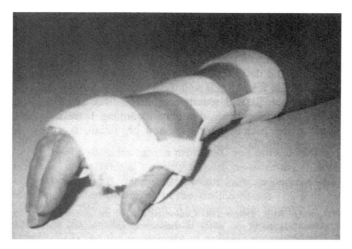

Figure 4. Modified resting hand splint.

Finger Splints

Splints for ulnar deviation of the MCP joints may be used to place the fingers in a more functional position or to possibly delay progression of deformity (Figure 5). Ulnar deviation splints may also lessen joint pain by supporting weakened ligaments and by resting the joint. Dynamic ulnar-deviation splints apply a gentle force to realign the joints in a more radial direction. Static splints hold the MCP joint in a more radial direction. These splints must be fitted carefully so that they do not interfere with function.

Proximal and Distal Interphalangeal Joint Splints

Splints for the PIP and distal interphalangeal (DIP) joints are used for synovitis, deformity, instability, pain, and tendon/ligament involvement. A volar- or dorsal-resting splint may reduce pain and inflammation. For the distal joint, a volar splint is often more supportive, but it may limit functional use by restricting sensation on the pad of the fingertip. A boutonniere splint (Figure 6) places the PIP joint in extension while allowing flexion of the DIP joint. A swan neck splint (Figure 7) supports the volar surface of the PIP joint from hyperextension, but allows flexion of the joint. Lateral instability of the PIP and DIP joints limits functional abilities of pinch and fine precision activities. A splint to

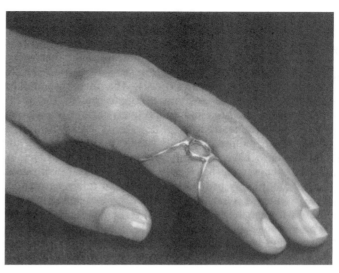

Figure 6. Ring splint for boutonniere deformity (photo courtesy of the Silver Ring Splint Company).

address lateral instability should provide support in the direction of the instability while allowing motions needed to perform daily hand tasks.

Silver Ring Splints have been shown to improve dexterity in patients with RA in a study looking at their effect on hand function (24). Grip strength scores, hand function self-report scores, and pain levels showed no significant change with the use of these splints.

Thumb Splints

The thumb accounts for 60% of hand function. When limited by pain, instability, or deformity, hand function is greatly reduced. Osteoarthritis of the CMC joint of the thumb is a common problem encountered in clinical practice. A hand- or forearm-based thumb support can improve function by reducing pain and supporting ligamentous laxity and joint subluxation (25). Patients may prefer a short hand-based splint over a forearm-based splint, and both types have been found to be effective in decreasing pain and reducing subluxation of the CMC joint (26–28). The splint should be fitted carefully to address an adequate C-bar for

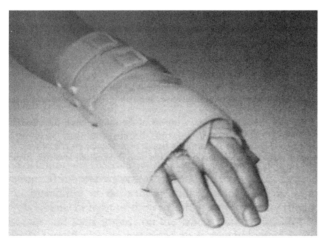

Figure 5. Metacarpophalangeal ulnar deviation splint.

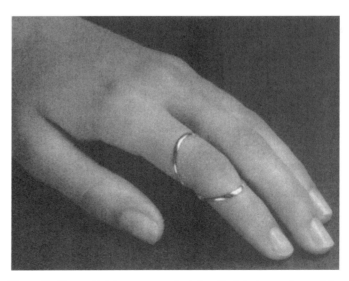

Figure 7. Ring splint for swan neck deformity (photo courtesy of the Silver Ring Splint Company).

maintenance of the web space (29). The thumb should be placed in a functional position of opposition to the index finger. In addition, wrist and thumb interphalangeal joint motion should not be restricted.

Splinting for osteoarthritis of the first carpometacarpal joint should be attempted prior to consideration of surgical intervention, and in one study was found to significantly reduce the need for surgery (30). These patients had a 7-month trial of conservative management, including splinting and activity modification, at the end of which 70% no longer required surgical intervention. At a 7-year followup evaluation, only an additional 10% required surgery.

An unstable, painful, or poorly positioned MCP joint of the thumb can also have a negative influence on hand function. Splints to support the MCP joint of the thumb can improve pinching abilities by providing support and relieving pain. A "figure 8" splint for this joint allows movement of the CMC and interphalangeal joints while providing volar and lateral support of the MCP joint for function. Splints for hyperextension and lateral instability of the interphalangeal joint of the thumb follow the same guidelines as for the PIP joints of the fingers.

SPECIAL CONSIDERATIONS

There are several special considerations in splinting the hand with rheumatic disease to ensure that goals of the splinting program and patient satisfaction are achieved. Patients who become involved in a splinting program should be willing to participate and should be educated as to the benefits of wearing the splint. Those who are not interested in wearing splints and who do not understand the purposes of splinting are less likely to adhere to this type of intervention.

Materials used to fabricate splints range from rigid to soft and should be selected according to the type of splint and the purpose of its use. Strapping materials can be integral in fitting the splint, ensuring proper support and joint alignment. Different strapping materials, ranging from elastic to cushioned to neoprene, may help in achieving the best fit. Precautions for joint position, skin integrity, effect on other joints, and wearing times should be communicated clearly to patients. Persons with arthritis may have more fragile skin due to their disease or to medications used to treat the disease. Splint fitting, padding, and lining can address this issue. Effects of immobilization on the targeted joint, as well as on adjacent joints, should be addressed when developing a schedule for splint wear. Splints should be removed periodically for range-of-motion exercise and to allow for skin care.

PATIENT EDUCATION

Principles of patient education should be applied in teaching patients about their splinting program (see Chapter 31, Self Management Education and Support). Patients who learn the purposes of splint use, expectations of splint use, and precautions for splint wear have improved adherence to splint regimens (31). Use of a positive affective tone and encouragement were shown in one study to positively influence splint wearing (31). Results from studies assessing adherence to splinting programs vary widely, ranging from 25% to 82.5% (26). When patients are better educated about their splinting program, adherence rates should increase. Contracting, written directions, and daily reports are some of the methods used to teach patients about their splints. Regular followup visits to ensure proper fit and wearing of the splints are crucial in meeting treatment goals. Partnership among team members, including the patient, therapist, and physician, is crucial in managing arthritis.

REFERENCES

1. Partridge REH, Duthie JJR. Controlled trial of the effect of complete immobilization of the joints in rheumatoid arthritis. Ann Rheum Dis 1963;22:91.
2. Gault SJ, Spyker MJ. Beneficial effect of immobilization of joints in rheumatoid and related arthritides: a splint study using sequential analysis. Arthritis Rheum 1969;12:34–44.
3. Melvin JL. Rheumatic disease in the adult and child: occupational therapy and rehabilitation 3rd ed. Philadelphia PA: FA Davis; 1982.
4. Feinberg J, Brandt KD. Use of resting splints by patients with rheumatoid arthritis. Am J Occup Ther 1981;35:173–8.
5. Malcus Johnson P, Sandkvist G, Ederhardt K, Liang B, Herrlin K. The usefulness of nocturnal resting splints in the treatment of ulnar deviation of the rheumatoid hand. Clin Rheumatol 1992;11:72–5.
6. Philips CA. Management of the patient with rheumatoid arthritis. The role of the hand therapist. Hand Clin 1989;5:291–309.
7. Ellis M. Splinting the rheumatoid hand. Clin Rheum Dis 1984;10:673–96.
8. Fred DM. Rest versus activity in arthritis and physical medicine. In: Licht E, editor. Arthritis and physical medicine. Baltimore: Waverly Press; 1969.
9. Zoeckler AA, Nicholas JJ. Prenyl hand splints for rheumatoid arthritis. Phys Ther 1969;49:377–9.
10. Nicholas JJ, Gruen H, Weiner G, Crawshaw C, Taylor F. Splinting in rheumatoid arthritis: I. Factors affecting patient compliance. Arch Phys Med Rehabil 1982;63:92–4.
11. Philips CA. Rehabilitation of the patient with rheumatoid hand involvement. Phys Ther 1989;69:1091–8.
12. Flatt AE. Care of the rheumatoid hand. 3rd ed. St. Louis MO: CV Mosby; 1974.
13. Eberhard BA, Sylvester KL, Ansell BM. A comparative study of orthoplast cock-up splints versus ready-made Droitwich work splints in juvenile chronic arthritis. Disabil Rehabil 1993;15:41–3.
14. Findley TW, Halpern D, Easton JK. Wrist subluxation in juvenile rheumatoid arthritis: pathophysiology and management. Arch Phys Med Rehabil 1983;64:69–74.
15. Overton J, Wolcott LE. The role of splints in prevention deformity in the rheumatoid hand and wrist. Mo Med 1966;63:423–7.
16. Li-Tsang CW, Hung LK, Mak AF. The effect of corrective splinting on flexion contracture of rheumatoid fingers. J Hand Ther 2002;15:185–91.
17. Rennie HJ. Evaluation of the effectiveness of a metacarpophalangeal ulnar deviation orthosis. J Hand Ther 1996; 9:371–7.
18. Ehrlich GE, DiPiero AM. Stretch gloves: nocturnal use to ameliorate morning stiffness in arthritic hands. Arch Phys Med Rehabil 1971;52:479–80.
19. Byron P. Splinting the arthritis hand. J Hand Ther 1994;7:29–30.
20. Weiss S, Lastayo P, Mills A, Bramlet D. Splinting the degenerative basal joint: custom-made or prefabricated neoprene? J Hand Ther 2004;17:401–6.
21. Stern EB, Ytterberg SR, Krug HE, Mahowald ML. Finger dexterity and hand function: effect of three commercial wrist extensor orthoses on patients with rheumatoid arthritis. Arthritis Care Res 1996;9:197–205.
22. Pagnotta A, Korner-Bitensky N, Mazer B, Baron M, Wood-Dauphinee S. Static wrist splint use in the performance of daily activities by individuals with rheumatoid arthritis. J Rheumatol 2005;32:2136–43.
23. King JW. Splinting the arthritic hand. J Hand Ther 1993;6:46–8.
24. Zijlstra TR, Heijnsdijk-Rouwenhorst L, Rasker JJ. Silver ring splints improve dexterity in patients with rheumatoid arthritis. Arthritis Rheum 2004;51:947–51.
25. Wolock BS, Moore JR, Weiland AJ. Arthritis of the basal joint of the thumb: a critical analysis of treatment options. J Arthroplasty 1989;4:65–78.
26. Weiss S, LaStayo P, Mills A, Bramlet D. Prospective analysis of splinting the first carpometacarpal joint: an objective, subjective, and radiographic assessment. J Hand Ther 2000;13:218–26.
27. Swigart CR, Eaton RG, Glickel SZ, Johnson C. Splinting in the treatment of arthritis of the first carpometacarpal joint. J Hand Surg [Am] 1999;24:86–91.
28. Weiss S, Lastayo P, Mills A, Bramlet D. Prospective analysis of splinting the first carpometacarpal joint: an objective, subjective, and radiographic assessment. J Hand Ther 2000; 13:218–26.
29. Poole JU, Pellegrini VD Jr. Arthritis of the thumb basal joint complex. J Hand Ther 2000;13:91–107.
30. Berggren M, Joost-Davidson A, Lindstrand J, Nylander G, Povlsen B. Reduction in the need for operation after conservative treatment of osteoarthritis of the first carpometacarpal joint: a seven year prospective study. Scand J Plast Reconstr Surg Hand Surg 2001;35:415–7.
31. Feinberg J. Effect of the arthritis health professional on compliance with use of resting hand splints by patients with rheumatoid arthritis. Arthritis Care Res 1992;5:17–23.

CHAPTER 40

Conservative and Surgical Management of the Foot and Ankle

H. J. HILLSTROM, PhD, K. WHITNEY, DPM, J. McGUIRE, DPM, PT, K. T. MAHAN, DPM, MS, and H. LEMONT, DPM

When examining and treating the foot and ankle, it is important to recognize that in a closed-chain system, each segment is interrelated and interdependent. Controlling the alignment of the foot and ankle with orthotic devices and footwear can prevent painful complications by reducing unwanted correlated motions and the need for compensation. In the severe stages of degenerative joint disease within the foot and ankle, surgical management may be needed.

CONSERVATIVE THERAPIES

Orthoses

Many posture and gait patterns associated with osseous and soft-tissue malalignments of the foot may be eliminated or minimized with correctly balanced *orthoses*, devices that correct maladjustments of the body. By modifying foot alignment and gait, orthoses can relieve symptomatic stress on the lower extremities through control of excessive or inadequate motion at specific joints.

Foot orthoses can be categorized as rigid, semirigid, or flexible and are selected based on the patient's needs. Rigid orthoses should be considered for patients requiring greater biomechanical control, because they reduce unwanted motion and help maintain the desired alignment. For patients who require improved foot alignment but want to maintain some degree of motion, the use of a semirigid device may be warranted. Patients who need protective accommodation for osseous deformity or lesions will generally do best with flexible orthoses.

The primary goals of orthosis management should be to reduce pain; limit motion of painful, inflamed, or unstable joints; and slow or arrest progression of deformity. Orthoses may also help to redistribute forces from high- to low-pressure areas, reduce shock and shear loading, correct positional (flexible) joint malalignments, accommodate fixed (rigid) deformities, and reduce abnormal shoe wear.

The type and shape of the orthosis and the degree of posting necessary is based on clinical measurements of the foot, postural and gait assessment, and the severity of radiographic changes. Patients with changes in the ankles and feet due to osteoarthritis (OA) will generally demonstrate numerous joint malalignments associated with pathologic pronation. For example, increased stress in the medial column of the foot with pronation may lead to continuous jamming of the first metatarsophalangeal (MTP) joint during the propulsive phase of gait. For this reason, orthosis management must restore both rearfoot alignment and first ray function. Specific features of orthoses for pronatory patients with OA changes in the feet are illustrated in Figure 1.

For patients with rheumatic disease associated with significant foot deformity, orthoses should provide stability to unstable or inflamed joints and should also address accommodative or protective needs for osseous deformity, nodules, and splayed metatarsals with associated bunion deformities. In addition to the features mentioned in Figure 1, the orthosis prescription should include a cushioned top liner material

to protect lesions and inflamed or irritated areas, as well as accommodative submetatarsal head apertures to off-load prominent or plantar-flexed metatarsals.

When complete resolution of symptoms may not be possible, the outcome measure should reflect the patient's expectations within the constraints of a realistic prognosis. For example, a realistic goal of orthotic therapy in a patient with chronic OA may be to reduce foot pain by 30–50%.

The extent to which correlated and compensatory motions (supinatory or pronatory) will occur depend on the severity and type of foot or limb deformity and the specific joint axis orientations. Several studies have demonstrated an association between foot and ankle malalignment and lower-extremity pathology. For example, excessive foot pronation may be associated the development of patellofemoral syndrome (1). Studies also have demonstrated that people with excessively pronated or supinated foot types are more susceptible to knee pain than those with neutral foot types (2). Fewer studies, however, have demonstrated the relationship between improved foot and ankle realignment therapies and reduction of foot or limb pathology. A double-blind, randomized clinical trial of people with recently diagnosed rheumatoid arthritis (RA) found that subjects who used a neutral-positioned foot orthosis were 73% less likely to develop hallux valgus deformity than those who used a placebo orthosis (3).

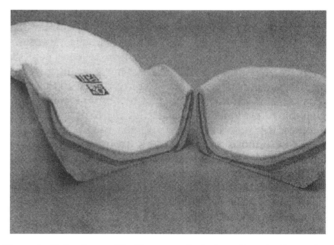

Figure 1. Orthosis modifications may include a deep heel cup, heel elevation, and medial skive technique for enhanced balance and foot alignment.
- Neutral subtalar frontal plane posting (when possible)
- Extended flanges for greater transverse plane stability
- Modest heel elevation to reduce ankle equinus stress
- First metatarsal head cut-out with kinetic wedge to improve first ray function associated with functional hallux limitus
- Deep heel cup with medial (Kirby) heel skive technique for cases with hyperpronation

Treatment of hallux abductovalgus deformity should be based on an evaluation of the pattern, degree, and reducibility of deformity. Mild deformities that are minimally deviated with a hallux abductovalgus angle of 15–25° and easily reducible should be treated conservatively. Moderate deformities demonstrating a malalignment angle of 25–35°, mild subluxation, or mild-to-moderate tracking of the joint will generally require a combined orthodigital and surgical (soft-tissue rebalancing) approach. Advanced-to-severe hallux abductovalgus deformities of ≥35°, with a nonreducible trackbound first MTP joint, will usually require soft-tissue and osseous reconstructive surgery. Following surgery, orthosis management and retentive orthodigital measures should be employed to maintain correction and prevent future recurrence. When surgical intervention is not an option, accommodative shoe prescription and protective shielding may be used (4).

FOOTWEAR CONSIDERATIONS

Many people with arthritis have some type of foot problem during their lives. RA and the connective tissue diseases affect the forefoot more frequently than the rearfoot. The loss of connective tissue strength produced by repetitive inflammation of the periarticular structures can result in the development of a number of malalignments, deformities, and mechanical problems. Feet affected in this manner need a wide, high toe box with soft compliant material that does not irritate the toes and can accommodate deformities, such as bunions or splayed feet. A loss of plantar fat, which protects the metatarsal heads, requires the use of soft protective inserts or orthotics specifically designed to shift weight from the forefoot to the midfoot. Proper shoe sizing, including adequate heel width, instep height, toe box depth, and forefoot width, is essential for a good clinical outcome. Orthotics or inserts take up significant space in the shoe and should always be worn when trying on new shoes to ensure a proper fit.

OA affects the first MTP joint and rearfoot most often. Inherent skeletal malalignments or secondary OA in the presence of repetitive microtrauma produce joint restriction, periarticular hypertrophy, and destruction of articular cartilage. This tends to restrict motion at the involved joint or produce pain with range of motion that will require foot orthoses, sole modifications to alter gait, or restrictive bracing to prevent motion and the resultant pain. Shoes must accommodate orthoses and have the appropriate sole design to facilitate a smooth, pain-free gait.

When considering footwear for patients with arthritis, one typically chooses boxy, in-depth shoes. However, a number of choices exist depending on the degree of foot deformity and the specific goals of therapy. Shoe choices are also restricted by nonmedical considerations, such as style, color, and feel of the shoe. Men's shoes are roomier and closer in style to the shoes commonly prescribed for moderate-to-severe foot deformity. Women often have to sacrifice a great deal of style to have a shoe with a firm supportive heel counter, reinforced midfoot, and wide roomy toe box (Figure 2). If a prescription orthotic or a cushioned inner sole is added to a narrow, high-heeled woman's shoe, such as a pump, it will often make the toe box tight and the shoe so bulky that the patient is unable to wear it. Women with a wide or splayed foot, or those who are developing bunions or hammer toe, have a difficult time finding shoes that will accommodate their condition.

The key to foot comfort is preventing the development of stress or irritation. Shoes need to support areas of instability and protect areas of deformity. The back or heel of the shoe is often reinforced by stiff leather or cardboard-like materials and is referred to as the *counter*. The counter helps keep the heel bone vertical and resist the tendency to roll inward with weight bearing. The *collar* of the shoe extends forward along the top of the counter to the laces and is often padded to

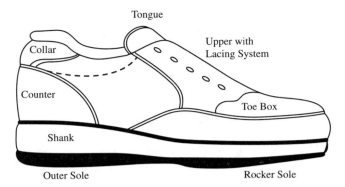

Figure 2. Foot segments and shoe design.

help protect the ankle bone from irritation. The sole of the shoe should be reinforced in the back by a stiff piece of plastic or metal referred to as the *shank*. This keeps the shoe from bending in the middle and provides most of the shoe's midfoot or arch support.

The remaining support for the midfoot comes from the lacing or fastening system of the shoe. Laces are the best way to adjust the shoe to allow for swelling and achieve a snug fit. Velcro closure or elastic laces are acceptable alternatives if the patient has hand involvement that prevents lacing. These features are important because they help the shoe contain or restrain a foot that often wants to deform and produce pain.

The front of the shoe is called the *toe box* and must be sufficiently flexible to allow for toe movement. It should be roomy enough to prevent crowding of the digits. Insufficient toe box room cannot only affect circulation, but can also lead to nail pathology and hard callus or corns forming on the toes.

The shoe should be constructed of good quality leather or soft breathable material to allow it to stretch easily around digital deformities. Patients with arthritis need extra padding or cushioning for the ball or widest part of the foot. It is often best to purchase a shoe with a removable innersole, so that a softer or more supportive orthosis may be easily incorporated.

Patients should be provided with all the information necessary to make an informed choice about their shoes. The individual is usually the best judge of whether something hurts or not. Every patient with developing arthritis should be seen by a podiatrist or other foot health professional to determine their foot type and advise them on any potential problems facing them in the future. People with existing foot pain may also benefit from a discussion about footwear options to help them function with less discomfort. If a clinician is not comfortable recommending shoes for patients, it is appropriate to refer them to a podiatric physician or pedorthist specially trained to help with the decision.

SURGICAL TREATMENT

Rheumatoid Arthritis (RA)

RA is the most common inflammatory arthropathy that leads to foot and ankle problems. In one study, 93 of 99 patients had foot and ankle involvement at some time since their diagnosis, and >50% of the patients had foot and ankle problems at any given time (5). The most common problematic areas for patients with RA are the forefoot, ankle, and rearfoot. In the forefoot, subluxation of the MTP joints with prominence of the metatarsal heads is the primary problem (Figure 3). Surgical treatment involves resection arthroplasty with excision of metatarsal heads 2–5. The base of the proximal phalanx is maintained, and severe digital deformities should be corrected (6). For the first MTP joint, the options are arthrodesis, implant arthroplasty, or resection of the first

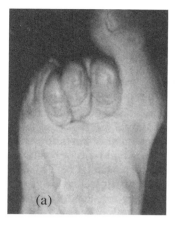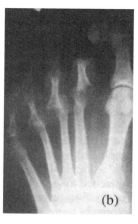

Figure 3. Forefoot deformities associated with rheumatoid arthritis. **a,** Clinical photo demonstrating dorsal contracture of toes 2,3, and 4 and hallux valgus. **b,** Anteroposterior radiograph demonstrating dislocation of the 2nd, 3rd, and 4th metatarsal proximal phalangeal joints.

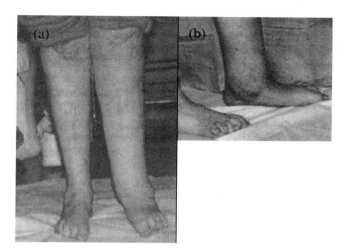

Figure 4. Rheumatoid arthritis patient with left foot valgus deformity. **a,** Note valgus malalignment at the knee as well. **b,** Medial view demonstrates medial column collapse.

metatarsal head. The choice of procedure depends on the overall foot structure, location of the pain, and extent of deformity. Improvement with respect to shoe wear, pain, and the ability to stand and walk are typical goals for this surgery. Because the MTP joints are lost with this surgery, the procedure is limited to patients who have significant, advanced disease and are already apropulsive.

Valgus foot deformities can occur in the rearfoot, often in conjunction with failure of the tibialis posterior tendon, resulting in severe abduction of the midtarsal joint and severe calcaneal eversion (Figure 4). Patients with RA are best treated with some combination of fusion procedures, such as double arthrodesis of the midtarsal joint or triple arthrodesis (7).

The ankle is frequently a site of severe pain in patients with RA. Surgical stabilization by means of fusion can restore alignment and significantly reduce pain. Frequently, because of the deterioration of the rearfoot joints, a pantalar fusion may be necessary.

Osteoarthritis (OA)

For OA, a broader array of options is available. The first MTP joint is frequently involved, resulting in hallux limitus. Treatment choices include simple resection of hypertrophic bone; reconstruction by means of shortening or plantar flexor osteotomy; resection arthroplasty, such as the Keller procedure for resection of the base of the proximal phalanx, single- or double-sided implant arthroplasty; or arthrodesis. Single-sided silicone implant arthroplasty is no longer recommended. Although a number of dual-component implants are now available, the long-term efficacy remains to be seen. For OA in other areas of the foot, such as the tarsometatarsal joints or the midtarsal or subtalar joints, fusion is the usual procedure if there is significant loss of cartilage. Debridement of hypertrophic bone formation may occasionally be adequate.

The ankle may be surgically treated by resection arthroplasty of the hypertrophic bone, mosaic plasty for replacement of deteriorated cartilage with autologous cartilage grafts, or arthrodesis. Recently, implant arthroplasty has become popular again. Although these implants have been used in Europe for some time, the long-term efficacy remains to be seen (8).

MECHANICALLY INDUCED SKIN AND SOFT-TISSUE CHANGES

Patients with RA, partially as a result of interosseous muscle atrophy, lose their ability to plantar flex the proximal phalanges of the toes, allowing the long extensors to dominate and causing hammered digits. As a

sequela of this deformity, the metatarsal fat pad frequently becomes displaced distally under the toes, allowing the metatarsals and interdigital nerves to be subjected to increased contact stress during locomotion. Interdigital neuralgia or Morton's neuroma and metatarsalgia frequently develop as a consequence.

As a protective mechanism to diminish the loading on skin, soft tissue, and bone, adventitial bursae may develop as a soft tissue replacement for the loss of the metatarsal fat pad. Most bursae develop around the head of the first metatarsal medially to protect the soft tissue structures associated with rheumatoid bunion deformity. These lesions also develop beneath the heads of the lesser metatarsals.

In addition, as a consequence of retrograde metatarsal loading to the plantar skin, the patient may develop painful corns and calluses over the ball of the foot. *Corns* are characterized by a sharply circumscribed keratinous, funnel-shaped plug that extends through most of the underlying dermis. *Calluses*, in contrast, lack a central plug and have a more even appearance. Corns are usually the more painful, because the plug pressure induces the formation of fibrous scarring within the dermis, dermal nerve thickening, and at times mild inflammation within the dermis. The latter occurs when the plug ruptures and evokes a foreign-body tissue response. Calluses do not exhibit the severity of dermal changes and therefore tend to be less symptomatic. The presence of dried blood or old hemorrhage within callus is seen on occasion in patients with RA. These collections of dried blood usually suggest the presence of associated angiitis seen in late-stage RA. Precipitated by increased metatarsal pressure on an underlying fragile inflamed vasculature (angiitis), these vessels rupture and extravasate blood within the overlying callus. These patients frequently exhibit associated vasculitic skin change around the digits, called *Bywaters lesions*.

Treatment

Conservative treatment options of these structural alterations consist of the use of accommodative foot orthoses. Because 90% of these alterations affect the forefoot, biomechanical off-loading to this area is the focus. Orthoses are modified to provide a substitute for loss of the plantar fat pad by using a combination of materials that exhibit shock attenuation and energy return. Decreasing interdigital nerve contact stress, metatarsal callus, and adventitial metatarsal bursa formation is accomplished by prescribing in-shoe build-ups or orthoses that include a longitudinal arch with a metatarsal bar. Metatarsal bars attached to the soles of shoes redistribute the load from the ball of the foot toward the toes. They are also used to relieve symptoms in more severe cases, but a rocker sole is preferred when cosmetically acceptable to the patient. Painful callus caused by hammer toe and bunion deformities requires shoes with a large toe box. A shoe that has a super wide shank with depth inlay, depth inlay (contour last), or a custom-molded shoe should be prescribed to accommodate severely deformed feet. Use of latex or silicone toe shields is helpful in reducing pain from severe deformities. Intermetatarsal joint corticosteroid injections using a combination of soluble and insoluble steroids should be used judiciously when dealing with inflammatory metatarsal joint synovitis, bursitis, or interdigital neuralgia. These injections are best given dorsally, parallel to the metatarsal heads at approximately a 45° angle, with the needle gradually inserted plantar and distally. Triamcinolone acetonide (5–10 mg) and dexamethasone phosphate (2 mg) mixed with lidocaine 2% (30 mg) per interspace helps relieve these symptoms. In advanced recalcitrant deformity, surgery may provide dramatic relief.

REFERENCES

1. Bennett P. A randomised clinical assessment of foot pronation and its relationship to patello-femoral syndrome. Aus Pod 1988:6–9.
2. Dahle L, Mueller M, Delitto A, Diamond J. Visual assessment of foot type and lower extremity injury. J Orthop Sports Phys Ther 1991;14: 70–4.
3. Budiman-Mak E, Conrad K, Roach K, et al. Can orthoses prevent hallux valgus deformity in rheumatoid arthritis? A randomized clinical trial. J Clin Rheumatol 1995;1:313–21.
4. Whitney A, Whitney K. Orthodigital evaluation and therapeutic management of digital deformity. In: Hallux valgus surgery. New York: Churchill Livingstone; 1993.
5. Michelson J, Easley M, Wigley FM, et al. Foot and ankle problems in rheumatoid arthritis. Foot Ankle Int 1994;15:608–13.
6. Coughlin MJ. Rheumatoid forefoot reconstruction. A long-term follow-up study. J Bone Joint Surg Am 2000;82:322–41.
7. Schuberth JM. Pedal fusions in the rheumatoid patient. Clin Podiatr Med Surg 1988;5:227–47.
8. Kofoed H, Sorensen TS. Ankle arthroplasty for rheumatoid arthritis and osteoarthritis: prospective long-term study of cemented replacements. J Bone Joint Surg Br 1998;80:328–32.

Lower Extremity Conservative Realignment Therapies and Ambulatory Aids

H. J. HILLSTROM, PhD, K. WHITNEY, DPM, J. McGUIRE, DPM, PT, D. J. BROWER, BA, DPM, PhD, C. RIEGGER-KRUGH, ScD, PT, and H. RALPH SCHUMACHER, MD

When treating patients with rheumatic disease that involves the load-bearing joints, a thorough assessment of lower extremity alignment is an important component of the clinical exam. Before selecting a conservative therapy or ambulatory aid for the patient, determining the biomechanical integrity of the lower extremity is imperative for successful treatment.

GENERAL EVALUATION

The condition of a joint depends upon structural (alignment, deformity, flexibility), functional (limitations in posture, locomotion, and activities of daily living), immunologic, and biochemical factors as well as a history of trauma. The biomechanical integrity of a joint includes assessment of stability, alignment, deformity, and movement performance. *Stability* refers to the quality of a joint's flexibility in rotation and translation (e.g., anterior drawer indicative of anterior cruciate ligament pathology). *Alignment* refers to the relative osseous positioning of a joint, which may be modifiable by soft-tissue contracture or laxity (e.g., genu varum). *Deformity*, often occurring at the extremes of malalignment, refers to a fixed osseous malposition (e.g., coxa vara). *Movement performance* is assessed through clinical observation or computerized analysis.

CONSERVATIVE THERAPIES

Neoprene Sleeves

Neoprene sleeves have provided some pain relief for mild knee osteoarthritis (OA) (1). When used alone, they provide warmth and mild compression to control edema. Neoprene sleeves may also reinforce joint proprioception by providing constant external stimulation to the skin. They do not provide structural support or realignment of the lower extremity.

Knee Braces

Outcome studies for a limited number of OA knee brace designs have demonstrated reduced pain (1–10) and improved function (1,3–7). Knee braces are available in both over-the-counter and custom-molded (or custom fit) designs. The advantage to over-the-counter designs is primarily in cost savings. The key disadvantage is the lack of a full range of sizes. Custom-molded or custom-fit braces have several advantages: 1) the device is fabricated either from a plaster cylinder cast of the patient's lower extremity or a set of pertinent anthropometric measurements obtained from the patient, 2) the materials employed within the shell and hinges are often of higher quality, and 3) in some custom braces it is possible to adjust the amount of correction. The primary

disadvantage is the additional cost compared with the cost of over-the-counter designs. The treatment goals, hinge designs, shell designs, materials employed, and fabrication techniques vary considerably from one manufacturer to another. Because few of the braces have clinical outcome studies to support their efficacy, it is difficult to determine the relative effectiveness of each design.

Currently available braces meet 4 basic treatment goals: ligament protection, tibiofemoral realignment, patellofemoral realignment, and bicompartmental realignment. Ligament protection braces have the primary goal of increasing sagittal plane stability (11,12). They are designed to augment or replace the role of the anterior cruciate ligament and posterior cruciate ligament. Many of the patients who benefit from this therapy are between 20–50 years of age and have injured a ligament as a result of overuse or trauma during sports activities.

Tibiofemoral OA braces have the primary goals of stabilizing and realigning the knee in the frontal plane. The mechanism of action for each brace varies according to design features, but the general aim is to reduce the load to the narrowed region of the joint space via a corrective moment. The single upright hinge designs offer an alternative.

Most braces have flat hinges that are constrained to planar function. These planar hinges may be uniaxial, biaxial, or exhibit a coupled planar motion about 2 axes. Two of the commercially available braces have hinges that move in a triplanar manner, which could be an advantage for preserving coupled motions, such as the screw home mechanism. The majority of knee braces have double upright hinges that are parallel to one another, which may be beneficial for enhanced stability but cause constraint in the transverse plane.

Also of interest is the amount of realignment. Some braces offer no realignment (only a restraint for further dynamic malalignment), some offer a fixed amount of realignment, and other braces offer adjustable correction. At this point, there has not been enough investigation into the subtleties of knee brace design to know which ones are preferred or perform best for a specific type of patient.

OA knee braces can have a variety of hinge designs (e.g., adjustable or fixed alignment, single or double upright, polyaxial or monaxial), shell designs (carbon graphite fibers or polypropylene), and fitting methods (custom-molded or off-the-shelf).

Patellofemoral braces have the primary goal of improving patellar tracking about the femoral condyles. Malpositioning or dysfunctional tracking of the patella has been suspected to be at least a component of patellofemoral OA pathogenesis. Devices for conservative therapy range from simple neoprene sleeves with a cutout for the patella to more complex bracing systems affording adjustable amounts of corrective load. Clinical outcome studies with objective biomechanical data are scarce.

Caution is necessary when prescribing and fitting knee braces for patients with rheumatic disease. If the prescribing physician's experience with these technologies is limited, it may be best to refer to a professional such as a certified orthotist who has the training and experience needed. In addition, followup care is necessary to check the patient's sensation, local swelling, and proper use of the brace.

Site-Specific Stability Orthoses

Lower extremity site-specific stability orthoses are often utilized in the management of malalignments and weakness of the leg in patients with rheumatic disease. Contrary to the perception that "braces" are only used to manage weakness or paralysis caused by neuromuscular disease, these devices are used to unload painful joints, stabilize joints with poor ligamentous or muscular support, and prevent deformity when extreme weakness has developed from disuse atrophy in the presence of marked dyskinesia.

Ankle-Foot Orthoses. Several different orthoses have been developed for either temporary or permanent control of the foot and ankle (13). When patients experience a simple drop foot due to pain or weakness of the anterior muscles and do not require medial or lateral support, a relatively inexpensive, easily dispensed, custom-fitted or off-the-shelf molded plastic orthosis may suffice.

The classic double-upright ankle-foot orthosis with fixed or moveable ankle joints has long been considered the workhorse of lower extremity bracing. Two metal uprights attached to a calf cuff are joined to the patient's shoe. The brace uses these uprights to establish medial/lateral support for the ankle and subtalar joints and relies on fixed or mobile articulations at the ankle to control pedal motions in the sagittal plane. Several types of ankle joints are available (e.g., solid, simple hinge, Klenzak, and double-action). These joints use adjustable stops or pins or a posterior spring insert to provide a dorsiflexion assist.

The most common use of the ankle-foot orthosis in patients with arthritis is for control of hyperpronating feet resulting from a partial or complete rupture of the tibialis posterior tendon. The patient's ankle motion is restricted, and the valgus attitude of the rear foot is realigned with the use of a leather T-strap attached to the lateral upright. Additional support is provided by an in-shoe foot orthosis posted in varus. Another use for the ankle-foot orthosis is to provide knee control for the patient with weak or absent quadriceps. Alteration of the ankle joint stop to lock the brace in 5–10° of plantar flexion tends to cause the knee to hyperextend slightly during midstance, preventing buckling and falls. Setting the brace in 5–10° of dorsiflexion induces slight flexion in midstance and can be used to prevent genu recurvatum or back knee in gait (13).

The plastic or molded ankle-foot orthosis is replacing the double-upright brace as the modality of choice in lower-extremity bracing (13). Because the device uses a molded foot section as its base, the patient has the freedom to change shoe styles without having to modify each one. The close contact of the polypropylene allows for excellent medial-lateral stability. Innovations in ankle joint and spring-assist technology allow versatility in application. One can use a molded, posted insert in the foot section of a polypropylene ankle-foot orthosis for added control and pedal realignment. It is possible to utilize the offset-varus heel seat in the Kirby-Skive orthosis to manage posterior tibial tendon dysfunction (13). However, cuneo-navicular pressure and breakdown can occur, where the foot collapses against the medial longitudinal arch of the brace.

Two types of molded ankle-foot orthoses are commonly utilized: the inexpensive, readily available custom-fitted or off-the-shelf device, and the custom-made or custom-molded device. Whenever fixed-ankle braces are used, the clinician should consider the addition of a rounded heel and rocker sole to promote a more fluid gait. Custom-molded devices are more expensive but can provide greater stability via their more precise fit. Customized padding, positioning, or angulation can be incorporated during the casting and fabrication of the device. Components such as ankle joints, stops, or spring assists can be easily incorporated as well.

Patellar Tendon Bearing Braces. The patellar tendon bearing brace consists of a standard double-upright or molded orthosis construction. It incorporates a molded leg section designed to provide cylindrical support for the limb, thus reducing weight on the foot and ankle. The leg section is constructed in 2 parts, either hinged or secured with Velcro, and designed to resemble the below-knee patellar tendon bearing prosthetic socket. With this modification, the physician can expect a 10–40% reduction in stress applied to the foot and ankle. Patellar tendon bearing braces are most commonly used for severely painful joints with collapse of the articular surfaces from OA, trauma, or rheumatoid arthritis. Although bulky, the patellar tendon bearing brace is sometimes the only way to unload a painful joint in a patient with a complicated medical history who cannot undergo joint fusion or replacement surgery.

Knee-Ankle-Foot Orthoses. Knee orthoses, in combination with ankle-foot orthoses, are occasionally used in the management of more involved lower-extremity neurologic or muscular conditions. The knee joint provides stability in the sagittal and frontal planes, preventing buckling in the weak limb. This stability is largely dependent on the integrity of the hip joint and the strength of the thigh, hip, and pelvic girdle musculature. When hip stability is compromised, use of a hip-knee-ankle-foot orthosis with a pelvic band and articulating hip joint may be required.

Foot Orthoses. Foot orthoses can realign and protect the arthritic foot as well as incorporate a correction for limb length discrepancy.

Ambulatory Aids

Ambulatory aids can be divided into those that increase stability by increasing the patient's base of support, or those that serve to unload painful or unstable joints. No ambulatory aid should be dispensed to a patient without a consultation with a physical therapist for proper fitting and, if needed, preambulatory conditioning to make sure the patient is capable of safely using the device. The physical therapist is specially trained to evaluate patients for balance and coordination, and is best suited to decide which of the various devices is most appropriate for a given patient.

Canes. In the arthritic hip, joint loading may be reduced by using a cane in the hand opposite to the involved hip. Canes come in many designs ranging from the simple wooden cane (adjusted by sawing off a portion of the base to achieve the proper height) to the aluminum adjustable cane that can be fit to the patient immediately by choosing one of several predetermined built-in heights.

Wider, flatter handgrips, compared with the standard narrow cane handle, provide a more comfortable resting surface for the hand while allowing the patient to produce greater grip strength. These improved grips can have a cone shape, narrower at the thenar border and wider at the ulnar side of the hand, which aids in improving grip strength of the ulnar digits and resists the tendency toward ulnar drift seen with the rheumatoid arthritis hand. When greater stability is needed due to a lack of wrist strength, a Canadian or forearm crutch with or without a platform addition can be substituted for a cane. Although these devices are technically considered crutches, when used singly they provide no weight reduction for an involved extremity and function as a cane.

The last feature of a cane is its base. Most canes use a simple wide rubber tip to provide stability on a variety of surfaces. Metal-spiked tips can be used for ice or when walking off paved surfaces. When a patient's balance is severely compromised, a tripod or quad base can be added to the cane to increase the base of support. However, this adds more weight to the cane—a factor that must be considered when ordering for your patients.

Crutches. Crutches come in a variety of designs and can utilize the wider handgrips described previously. The standard axillary crutch comes with sponge rubber pads over the tops to protect the patient's ribs and upper arms from irritation during use. The hand pieces are also padded to increase the grip size and protect the hands from irritation during ambulation. The tips of the crutches are covered with a wide rubber base and may be ordered with metal tips for ice or unpaved surfaces.

Crutches both increase the base of support and significantly reduce the weight carried by an involved extremity depending on the type of crutch gait used. Weight can be borne on a single uninvolved extremity utilizing a non–weight-bearing 3-point gait, or distributed between the 2 extremities using a partial weight-bearing 3-point or 4-point gait.

Crutches are measured to allow the patient's weight to be borne on the hands and wrists, and should never touch the skin under the axilla. Weight bearing through the axilla may result in serious damage to the nerves of the arm and hand. Crutch tops should be 2–3 inches below the axilla when the crutch tips are 6 inches in front of and 6 inches lateral to the ends of the toes. The hand pieces should be positioned with the arm bent at a 15–20° angle when standing. When a patient needs crutches for an extended period of time and has excellent hand, arm, and shoulder strength, forearm crutches should be considered. These crutches increase the base of support and reduce loading without putting pressure on the upper arm and chest wall, and are therefore more comfortable to use. If the patient has a painful hand, wrist, or elbow and limited arm strength, a platform crutch may be a better choice.

Walkers. Walkers provide the greatest stability of all the ambulatory aides but are the most cumbersome to use and provide the most storage problems when traveling in a car or on public transportation. It is impossible to climb stairs with a walker, and negotiating curbs is a difficult and often dangerous task. Walkers are well suited for patients who need to ambulate limited distances and have significant balance or muscle control problems that make them highly unstable.

The standard walker has 4 legs, each fitted with a large rubber tip for stability on smooth surfaces. The patient has to lift the walker, move it forward, and step up to it to ambulate. Wheeled walkers have wheels on the front 2 legs to make it easier for patients who find it difficult to lift the walker to move. Patients who have pain or weakness of the hands, wrists, or elbows can have their walkers fitted with a platform attachment that allows them to bear weight on their forearms and use their shoulders to move the walker. Bags or baskets can be attached to the walker to allow patients to carry things when both their hands are occupied manipulating the walker.

REFERENCES

1. Kirkley A, Webster-Bogaert S, Litchfield R, Amendola A, MacDonald S, McCalden R, et al. The effect of bracing on varus gonarthrosis. J Bone Joint Surg Am 1999;81:539–548.
2. Pollo FE, Otis JC, Wickiewicz TL, Warren RF. Biomechanical analysis of valgus bracing for the osteoarthritic knee. Paper presented at: North American Clinical Gait Laboratory Conference; April 9, 1994. Portland, OR.
3. Pollo FE, Otis JC, Wickiewicz TL, Warren RF. Biomechanical analysis of valgus bracing for the osteoarthritic knee. Arthritis Rheum 1995;38: p. S241.
4. Matsuno H, Kadowaki KM, Tsuji H, Generation II knee bracing for severe medial compartment osteoarthritis of the knee. Arch Phys Med Rehabil 1997;78:745–749.
5. Otis JC, Backus SI, Polle FE, Wickiewicz TL, Warren RF and et al. Load sharing at the knee during valgus bracing for medial compartment osteoarthritis. Gait Posture 1996;4:189.
6. Lindenfeld TN, Hewett TE, Andriacchi TP. Joint loading with valgus bracing in patients with varus gonarthrosis. Clin Orthop 1997;344: 290–297.
7. Otis J, Backus SI, Campbell DA, Furman GL, Montalvo E, Warren RF, et al. Valgus knee bracing for knee osteoarthritis: a biomechanical and clinical outcome study. Gait Posture 2000;11:116.
8. Horlick SG, Loomer RL. Valgus knee bracing for medical gonarthrosis. Clin J Sports Med 1993;3:251–255.
9. Hillstrom H, Brower DJ, Bhimji S, McGuire J, Whitney K, Snyder H, et al. Assessment of conservative realignment therapies for the treatment of varus knee osteoarthritis: biomechanics and joint pathophysiology. Gait Posture 2000;11:170–171.
10. Hewett TE, Noyes FR, Barber-Westin SD, Heckmann TP. Decrease in knee joint pain and increase in function in patients with medial compartment arthrosis: a prospective analysis of valgus bracing. Orthopedics 1998;21:131–138.
11. Liu SH, Mirzayan R. Current review. Functional knee bracing. Clin Orthop 1995;317:273–281.
12. Beynnon BD, Johnson RJ, Fleming BC, Peura GD, Renstrom PA, Nichols CE, et al. The effect of functional knee bracing on the anterior cruciate ligament in the weightbearing and nonweightbearing knee. Am J Sports Med 1997;25:353–359.
13. Braddom RL. Physical medicine and rehabilitation. Philadelphia: WB Saunders; 1996.

Sexual Intimacy

VICTORIA RUFFING, RN

"Sexuality is an integral part of human life. It carries the awesome potential to create new life. It can foster intimacy and bonding as well as shared pleasure in our relationships. It fulfills a number of personal and social needs, and we value the sexual part of our being for the pleasures and benefits it affords us….Sexuality encompasses more than sexual behavior…not only the physical, but the mental and spiritual as well."

David Satcher, MD, PhD
Surgeon General (1)

The fatigue and pain from arthritis, the limitations put on movement, and the damage or disfigurement caused to joints often create difficulties in a sexual relationship. Without prompting from the health professional, it is unlikely that clinicians will be aware of their patients' sexual issues. This chapter begins with an overview of why these important discussions may not be taking place. Next, the prevalence and potential causes of sexual dysfunction among rheumatic disease patients are discussed. Finally, strategies to encourage open discussion between health care providers and their patients, as well as suggestions to address sexual difficulties are also included.

THE ELEPHANT IN THE CLOSET

There is general agreement that patients' sexual interests should be addressed when providing health services (2). Nevertheless, discussions of sex and sexuality are frequently neglected in the health care system. A recent poll of 500 US adults age 25 and older found that 71% felt their doctor would dismiss any concerns about sexual problems they might bring up (3). And 68% expressed concern that discussing sexual problems would embarrass their physicians. Three-quarters believed there would be no medical treatment for their problems.

Health professionals are equally reticent to discuss sexual issues with their patients. Among rehabilitation specialists in the UK, 80% agreed that sexual adjustment was important for patients, yet only 9% felt comfortable discussing these issues with patients (2). The majority had never been asked by patients, and had not initiated discussion about sexual issues. Most (86%) said they were poorly trained in this area and nearly all (94%) said they were unlikely to discuss sexual issues with their patients. Clearly, training in human sexuality and sexual counseling needs to be integrated into the training of health care professionals.

Concerns about sexual relationships and activity are common among adolescents with rheumatic diseases as well. Like adults, pain and physical limitations account for much of the problem (4). However, adolescents may have additional concerns. The development of a healthy body image, which is important to all adolescents, may be hindered by problems with growth, use of corticosteroids (which alters fat deposition and can cause acne and hirsutism), or scars from orthopedic surgeries (4). In a study of 246 adults with juvenile idiopathic arthritis, Packham and Hall noted that about 7% reported being sexually active before age 16, and 38% were sexually active before the transfer to adult rheumatology care at age 18 (4). This suggests that discussion about

sexuality needs to begin in adolescent rheumatology clinics. Because of concerns about teratogenicity associated with use of antirheumatic drugs, there is a need to address contraception with adolescents.

PREVALENCE OF SEXUAL DYSFUNCTION

Sexual problems are common among patients with rheumatic diseases. For example, a recent study of rheumatoid arthritis (RA) patients reported more than half (56%) of the patients found that their arthritis placed limitations on sexual intercourse; the principal reasons cited were fatigue and pain (5). Sexual dysfunction appears to be equal among male and female patients with RA (5,6), though it may cause more overall distress among men. Overall, sexual ability is important to the majority of patients with rheumatic diseases, although up to half may lose interest during the course of their disease (5,6). About 60% of RA patients reported being dissatisfied with the quality of their sex lives (5). Men with RA often have reduced levels of testosterone (7). However, in younger patients with inactive or less active disease, sexual activity and frequency does not appear to differ from healthy age-matched controls (6,8).

In primary Sjögren's syndrome, dyspareunia (difficult or painful intercourse) occurs in up to 50% of women (9). Gynecologic problems including endometriosis occurs more frequently (10). Vaginal dryness and dyspareunia are also frequent among women with systemic lupus erythematosus. Up to one-third of men with ankylosing spondylitis report decreased libido, erectile dysfunction, and difficulty ejaculating (11). Systemic sclerosis can result in a range of sexual problems in women; in men, erectile dysfunction is often the result of small vessel disease, which affects the quality of erections (12).

Although the majority of sexual problems appear to be related to pain and disability, psychological issues also may play an important role (4,6,8,13). Many patients report that their disease has had a negative effect on their body image and self-confidence (4,13). Functional limitations may limit opportunities for socializing to form relationships, especially in adolescence. Relationships may be complicated by the fact that one's partner also becomes the caregiver at times. Depression and anxiety disorders are more common among rheumatic patients than the general population (13–19).

MEDICATIONS

Fortunately, most of the drugs used in the treatment of RA do not appear to affect libido or sexual functioning. However, Ostensen notes that there are reports of impotence in patients treated with methotrexate (6). Many RA drugs, however, are not compatible with pregnancy or are known teratogens (e.g., methotrexate, cyclophosphamide, chlorambucil, leflunomide), making the use of effective contraceptives mandatory. Cyclophosphamide may cause long-term ovarian failure such that consideration of egg harvest is sometimes indicated prior to the use of this medication. Additional administration of cholestyramine is needed to wash out leflunomide and its long-lived metabolites before considering conception.

The safety of other medications, including biological therapies, in pregnancy is less clear. Hydroxychloroquine is often continued during pregnancy and corticosteroids are also used.

Several drugs used for RA or medication side effects can be especially problematic in men, and sometimes interfere with libido (e.g., citmetidine, diclofenac, misoprostol, naproxen), erection (e.g., methotrexate, sulfasalazine, hydroxychloroquine), and ejaculation (e.g., methotrexate, naproxen) (13). Of some consideration as well is reversible azoospermia that may occur with sulfasalazine.

Up to 40% of persons with RA have clinically significant levels of depression (14,20–22). Clinical depression is frequently associated with loss of interest in sex (23). However, sexual dysfunction is also a common side effect of antidepressant medications. Loss of desire and difficulty with orgasm occur in up to 30–60% of individuals who use a selective serotonin reuptake inhibitor or a serotonin-norepinephrine reuptake inhibitor (24).

In summary, sexual problems are common among patients with rheumatic diseases. Reasons for this are multifactorial and include disease-related issues, psychosocial concerns, and medications. Nevertheless, Ostensen (6) notes that most problems related to sexual functioning do respond to treatment and, as a result, should be addressed as part of routine rheumatic care. A review of factors that can facilitate discussion about problems with sexual function is offered below.

COMMUNICATION

The comfort level of the professional in addressing sexual functioning can enhance the comfort with which the patient or couple can express concerns. Obtaining a sexual history may be an easy way to broach the subject. Opening this door gives the patient "professional permission" to discuss sexual functioning and intimacy (25).

Human sexuality has many more dimensions to it than mere physiological functioning. Sex involves 2 people whose feelings must be recognized. However, when chronic illness is involved and one's sex life changes, it can be even more difficult to raise concerns with a health care provider. There are a variety of reasons for this, including embarrassment or frustration, even fear. When sexual activity diminishes or stops completely, emotional estrangement can quickly occur. Encouraging patients to confront the issue of sex, in all its complexity, is the first step to ensuring that the problem is addressed to the mutual satisfaction of both partners (26).

Clinicians can help couples to navigate the difficulties of dealing with the persistent and invisible nature of chronic pain and the relationship patterns that emerge. Open communication can dispel myths and allay fears. Communication also will help to lessen the need to guess what others feel and need, and it will help to clarify boundaries (27). Questions regarding a patient's sexual relationship should be direct and general, and integrated into the routine care of all patients (see Table 1). It is often helpful to reassure patients that this is not an uncommon issue. Statements like "Many people with arthritis mention changes in their intimate physical relationship. Have you had any

Table 1. Strategies for opening the lines of communication with patients

Try the following prompts:
  • Has arthritis put a strain on your relationship?
  • Has arthritis put a strain on you sexual relationship?
  • Does your arthritis interfere with sexual intercourse?
  • Do you and your partner ever discuss the effects arthritis has on your relationship sexual or otherwise?

Table 2. Selected patient education materials

The Arthritis Foundation offers "Guide to Intimacy with Arthritis," available through local chapters, on the Web at www.arthritis.org, or by calling 800-568-4045.

The Scleroderma Foundation offers a brochure on sexuality in scleroderma through their Web site (www.scleroderma.org) or by calling 800-722-4673.

The National Institutes of Health (NIAMS) offers a patient information sheet and patient care guide for health professional entitled "Sexuality and Lupus" at http://www.niams.nih.gov/hi/topics/lupus/lupusguide/chppis10.htm.

The Center for Research on Women with Disabilities has made available the National Study of Women with Physical Disabilities—Executive Summary at http://www.bcm.edu/crowd/?pmid=1407.

difficulty with pain affecting your sexual relationship?" can help to normalize the patient's experience and decrease self-consciousness and embarrassment (25). Once the lines of communication have been established, strategies to improve or renew physical intimacy can take place. Before beginning any discussion about sexual intimacy, it is important to first examine your own beliefs and potential biases about the topic. Personal views on homosexuality, sex in the elderly population, between unmarried couples, the use of sexual aids, etc., should never be imposed (27).

Sex re-education is a critically important yet missing component in the arthritis education that is offered for the patient (Table 2). It is important to convey to patients that an active and satisfying sex life is possible, and indeed important to the overall health and well being. Most importantly, patients need to be aware that help is available by identifying and addressing problems directly and creatively.

PAIN MANAGMENT

Pain management goes hand in hand with time management in the setting of sexual intimacy. In order to maximize comfort, planning will be key (Table 3).

• Pain medications should be taken 30 to 60 minutes before engaging in sexual activity.
• Pillows and/or rolled sheets should be on hand to support joints.
• Avoid cold temperatures.
• Vaginal dryness is often a major issue. Petroleum-based products should never be used. Popular water-based lubricants include Astroglide, K-Y jelly, Replens, and Wet Original. These lubricants work well for partner sex, manual masturbation, and sex-toy play.

ALTERNATIVE POSITIONS

The sex positions people typically used before arthritis may no longer be possible because of the stress that is now placed on affected joints. Modification of these positions or trying completely new positions may help rejuvenate the patient's sex life.

Before going on, remember that if excessive movement triggers arthritis pain, encourage the patient's partner be the one who provides the movement during sex. Also, if arousal is now more difficult because of arthritis, consider the use of a water-based lubricant and a vibrator to enhance arousal.

Although there are many sex positions, most are variants of a few basic positions. Everyone's needs are different, so when reviewing

Table 3. A patient's guide to improving sexual function

1. **Open communication between partners**
   - Be honest with your partner about feelings, desires, and sexual needs.
   - Address each other's fears of physical harm.
   - Discuss each other's willingness to redefine intimacy through new positions, sexual aids, different techniques.
2. **Use tactile communication**
   - Kissing, caressing, petting, or massage may help restore lost intimacy and assist in helping both partners relax.
   - Some couples may want to try using the hands or mouth to help achieve orgasm.
3. **Environmental factors**
   - Plan blocks of time, within your regular schedule, when both of you are relaxed and comfortable.
   - Make sure that you get rest ahead of time.
   - Avoid cold temperatures by taking a warm bath or shower before sex.
   - Warm the bed by replacing cotton sheets with flannel sheets or turn on an electric blanket for a few minutes before getting into bed.
4. **Medications**
   - Take pain medication at least 30 minutes before sexual activity.
   - Discuss any possible sexual side effects of medications with your pharmacist.
   - Water-based lubricants may be helpful in the presence of vaginal dryness. Some common brands are Astroglide, K-Y jelly, Replens, and Wet Original. Never use petroleum-based products.
5. **Sexual Positions**
   - *The modified missionary position.* The woman—who is unable to move her legs apart, has stiff knees, or has had a hip replacement—is to lie on her back with a pillow supporting her hips and thighs. The man can then lie on top of her, supporting his own weight on his elbows, hands, and knees.
   - *Spoon position.* When the woman has painful hips or has had a hip replacement, she can lie on her side with her partner lying closely behind her. Imagine spoons stacked side by side in your silverware drawer. With a pillow between her knees, the man can enter her vagina from behind.
   - *Standing.* This position is a good one, especially when both partners are bothered by stiff or aching hips and knees. Both partners stand, with the woman using a tabletop or other piece of furniture for support. The man stands behind the woman and can enter her vagina from behind.
   - *Kneeling.* When the woman has hip stiffness or has had a hip replacement, she can kneel on a pillow, supporting her arms and chest on a low piece of furniture. The man kneels behind the woman and can enter her vagina from behind.
   - *Sitting.* For women with back or hip stiffness and pain, this is a good position that will offer support without any weight on top. With the man sitting in a comfortable chair, the woman sits in his lap. Many find this position to be more comfortable than sitting in bed.
   - *Lying down.* When a man has painful hips, back, or knees, or when he has had a knee or hip replacement, he can lie on his back, using a pillow under his neck for support. The woman straddles him, supporting herself on her knees or leaning forward and supporting herself on her elbows.

sexual positions with a patient, let him or her decide which will work best. Patients should take the following into consideration:

- comfort level
- personal inhibitions
- overall sexual satisfaction

The missionary position, with the man on top, offers problems for many people with arthritis, especially if the person has pain in his or her hips or knees. Having the woman sitting on top of the man may not work well if her hips and other large joints are affected.

There are pleasurable ways to achieve sexual satisfaction other than through intercourse. Many couples may be unfamiliar with oral sex but may want to explore this possibility. A comfortable position may be easier to find than with intercourse. Foreplay may become of greater importance.

Encourage creativity: For example, if hands are painful use the backs of the hands to caress the partner's breasts or genitals. Sexual aids from massage oils to vibrators may be suggested.

SUMMARY

A healthy active sexual life is important to overall wellbeing, self-confidence, self-esteem and general wellbeing. Unfortunately, sexual problems are common among persons with rheumatic illnesses. Discussions about sex and sexuality continue to be absent from most health care relationships. A major barrier has been lack of training of health care professionals about sex and sexuality. Though pain, fatigue, and limited mobility may interfere with sexual functioning, improved communication with the health care provider and partner can enhance understanding, identify new options for intimacy, and even improve the relationship through increased closeness.

REFERENCES

1. Satcher D. The Surgeon General's call to action to promote sexual health and responsible sexual behavior. Accessed June 8, 2006. URL: http://www.surgeongeneral.gov/library/sexualhealth/call.htm.
2. Haboubi NHJ, Lincoln N. Views of health professionals on discussing sexual issues with patients. Disabil Rehabil 2003;25:291–6.
3. Marwick C. Survey says patients expect little physician help on sex. JAMA 1999;281:2173–4.
4. Packham JC, Hall MA. Long-term follow-up of 246 adults with juvenile idiopathic arthritis: social function, relationships and sexual activity. Rheumatology (Oxford) 2002;41:1440–3.
5. Hill J, Bird H, Thorpe R. Effects of rheumatoid arthritis on sexual activity and relationships. Rheumatology (Oxford) 2003;42:280–6.
6. Ostensen M. New insights into sexual functioning and fertility in rheumatic diseases. Best Pract Res Clin Rheumatol 2004;18:219–32.
7. Tengstrand B, Carlstrom K, Hafstrom I. Bioavailable testosterone in men with rheumatoid arthritis-high frequency of hypogonadism. Rheumatology (Oxford) 2002;41:285–9.
8. Ostensen M, Almberg K, Koksvik HS. Sex, reproduction, and gynecological disease in young adults with a history of juvenile chronic arthritis. J Rheumatol 2000;27:1783–7.
9. Skopouli FN, Papanikolaou S, Malamou-Mitsi V, Papanikolaou N, Moutsopoulos HM. Obstetric and gynaecological profile in patients with primary Sjogren's syndrome. Ann Rheum Dis 1994;53:569–73.
10. Haga HJ, Gjesdal CG, Irgens LM, Ostensen M. Reproduction and gynaecological manifestations in women with primary Sjogren's syndrome: a case-control study. Scand J Rheumatol 2005;34:45–8.
11. Sant SM, O'Connell D. Cauda equina syndrome in ankylosing spondylitis: a case report and review of the literature. Clin Rheumatol 1995;14:224–6.
12. Nowlin NS, Brick JE, Weaver DJ, Wilson DA, Judd HL, Lu JK, et al. Impotence in scleroderma. Ann Intern Med 1986;104:794–8.
13. van Berlo WT, van de Wiel HB, Taal E, Rasker JJ, Weijmar Schultz WC, van Rijswijk MH. Sexual functioning of people with rheumatoid arthritis: a multicenter study. Clin Rheumatol. In press.
14. Covic T, Tyson G, Spencer D, Howe G. Depression in rheumatoid arthritis patients: demographic, clinical, and psychological predictors. J Psychosom Res 2006;60:469–76.
15. Brown GK, Nicassio PM, Wallston KA. Pain coping strategies and depression in rheumatoid arthritis. J Consult Clin Psychol 1989;57:652–7.

16. Katz PP, Yelin EH. Prevalence and correlates of depressive symptoms among persons with rheumatoid arthritis. J Rheumatol 1993;20:790–6.

17. Katz PP, Yelin EH. The development of depressive symptoms among women with rheumatoid arthritis: the role of function. Arthritis Rheum 1995;38:49–56.

18. El Miedany YM, Rasheed AHE. Is anxiety a more common disorder than depression in rheumatoid arthritis? Joint Bone Spine 2002;69:300–6.

19. VanDyke MM, Parker JC, Smarr KL, Hewett JE, Johnson GE, Slaughter JR, et al. Anxiety in rheumatoid arthritis. Arthritis Rheum 2004;51:408–12.

20. Bartlett SJ, Piedmont RL, Bilderback A, Matsumoto A, Bathon JM. Spirituality, well being and quality of life in persons with rheumatoid arthritis. Arthritis Rheum 2003;49:778–83.

21. Dickens C, Mcgowan L, Clark-Carter D, Creed F. Depression in rheumatoid arthritis: a systematic review of the literature with meta-analysis. Psychosom Med 2002;64:52–60.

22. Smarr KL, Parker JC, Kosciulek JF, Buchholz JL, Multon KD, Hewett JE, et al. Implications of depression in rheumatoid arthritis: do subtypes really matter? Arthritis Care Res 2000;13:23–32.

23. American Psychiatric Association. Diagnostic and statistical manual of mental disorders: DSM-IV. 4th ed. Washington, DC: American Psychiatric Association; 1994.

24. Gregorian RS, Golden KA, Bahce A, Goodman C, Kwong WJ, Khan ZM. Antidepressant-induced sexual dysfunction. Ann Pharmacother 2002;36: 1577–89.

25. Nusbaum MR, Hamilton C, Lenahan P. Chronic illness and sexual functioning. Am Fam Physician 2003;67:347–54.

26. Smith AA. Intimacy and family relationships of women with chronic pain. Pain Manag Nurs 2003;4:134–42.

27. Steinke EE. Intimacy needs and chronic illness: strategies for sexual counseling and self-management. J Gerontol Nurs 2005;31:40–50.

CHAPTER

43

Adherence in Children and Adults

MICHAEL A. RAPOFF, PhD, and SUSAN J. BARTLETT, PhD

Children and adults with rheumatic diseases are often asked to adhere consistently and over long periods of time to medical treatment, exercise programs, and self-management regimens. Treatments are complex, demanding, and costly; the benefits are often delayed, though side effects may arise quickly (1–3). These factors characterize regimens that are likely to result in nonadherence (4–6).

Adherence is now the preferred term, replacing compliance, because it more accurately reflects an active role of patients in consenting to and following prescribed treatments (7,8). Adherence has been defined as "...the extent to which a person's behavior (in terms of medications, following diets, or executing lifestyle changes) coincides with medical or health advice." (4). This definition has heuristic value because it: 1) specifies the range of adherence behaviors required for various regimens (such as medications, therapeutic exercises, and splinting in rheumatic diseases); 2) requires an evaluation of the "extent" of adherence, emphasizing that adherence is relative and can vary within persons over time, between persons, and across different regimen requirements; and 3) implies there is a standard (that coincides with medical advice) for determining acceptable adherence. Although many factors that influence adherence are common to both children and adults, with children the involvement of patients' families adds another dimension (6,7). The unique needs of each group will be addressed in this chapter.

ADHERENCE MEASURES

A variety of methods have been used to measure adherence, including drug assays, behavioral observations, electronic monitoring, pill counts, provider estimates, and patient report (6,7,9). As shown in Table 1, each of these methods has both assets and liabilities.

Drug Assays

The detection of drug levels, metabolites, or pharmacologically inert substances added to drugs as tracers can be detected in blood, urine, and, in rare cases, saliva (6). They are quantifiable, useful for dosing adjustments, and do not rely on patient or provider estimates. However, assays can be expensive, invasive (particularly relevant for children), and intermittently obtained, thereby reflecting more recent ingestion. In addition, drug levels may reflect factors other than patient adherence, such as inadequate dosing; non–steady-state concentrations in patients taking medications with long half-lives over a short period of time; pharmacokinetic variations due to the type of medication preparations (e.g., enteric coating); physiologic factors, such as gastric pH; interactions with other medications or foods; patient age; or patient behaviors, such as smoking (10,11).

Behavioral Observations

Observing patients is the most direct way of assessing adherence because the provider can evaluate how patients are carrying out treatments and provide corrective feedback as needed (2,6). A major drawback of observation is the limited access providers have to observe patients. However, family members can provide reliable observations of adherence if they are provided with a specific and relatively simple observational strategy and are adequately trained (12).

Electronic Monitoring

Microelectronic monitors are now available for recording, storing, and downloading information on medication removal (9). Electronic monitoring allows for continuous (real-time) and long-term assessment of medication adherence. These devices record and store several months of information regarding the date and time of medication use. Data can then be downloaded into a computer for analysis. Packaging equipped with electronic monitors can reveal a spectrum of adherence problems, including underdosing, overdosing, delayed dosing, drug "holidays" (omitting doses for several days in succession without provider authorization), and "white-coat" adherence (giving the appearance of adequate adherence by dumping medications or taking medications consistently several days before clinic visits) (13).

These devices present an exciting new avenue for adherence assessment, leading some to call electronic monitoring the new gold standard (7). The major drawback is that opening vials or removing medication from a blister pack does not guarantee ingestion. It seems unlikely that patients would deliberately dispense but fail to ingest medications; furthermore, it seems especially unlikely to continue over time because patients would have to do this at the precise times when medications are to be taken (7). The cost of these monitoring devices often prohibits routine clinical use.

> "Doctors do not treat chronic illnesses. The chronically ill treat themselves with the help of their physicians; the physician is part of the treatment. Patients are in charge of themselves. They determine their food, activity, medications, visits to their doctor—most of the details of their own treatment." (59)

Pharmacy Refill Data

Pharmacy databases can also provide a measure of presumed use based on refill patterns. These databases are increasingly used in population

Table 1. Assets and liabilities of adherence measures*

Measure	Assets	Liabilities
Assays	• Can adjust drug dosage • Objective; only way to know if medications have been ingested	• Pharmacokinetics may affect absorption and excretion rates. • Short-term, invasive, and expensive
Observation	• Direct measure of nonmedication regimen adherence • Can measure adherence on repeated occasions	• Obtrusive and reactive
Electronic monitoring	• Precise frequency and time of dosing obtained • Continuous and long-term measures	• Does not guarantee medications were ingested • Mechanical failures
Pharmacy refill data	• Unobtrusive measure of refill activity • Nonreactive • Provides long-term information	• Reliant on a current, well-integrated database • Invalid if prescriptions are refilled out of database network • Does not guarantee medications were ingested
Pill counts	• Easily obtained • Inexpensive	• Does not guarantee medications were ingested • Overestimates adherence
Provider estimates	• Clinically feasible • Generally more accurate than global patient estimates	• Physician experience or familiarity with patient unrelated to accuracy • Overestimates adherence
Patient report	• Clinically feasible • More accurate when patients report they are mostly nonadherent	• Overestimates adherence • Subject to reporting bias—"faking good"

* Adapted from reference 7.

and individual clinical monitoring situations. This approach is unobtrusive, nonreactive, and can be used for long-term monitoring. However, information is lost if patients refill their medication out of the database system and this method does not provide evidence of ingestion.

Pill Counts

Pill counts or volume measurements have been used extensively in adherence research. They are simple and can be routinely done during clinic visits or by phone. As with automated measures, the major liability is that medications removed are not necessarily ingested (6) and no information is available about the timing of daily doses (7).

Provider Estimates

Provider estimates generally involve a global rating of the degree to which patients are adherent to a regimen (6). Busy providers may find this the most feasible way to assess adherence. However, provider estimates consistently underestimate levels of nonadherence (6). This may be due to reliance on treatment outcomes for estimating adherence (e.g., viewing a lower active joint count as confirmation of adherence) and positive bias or expectancies, such as wanting to believe patients are adhering to recommendations.

Patient Report

Consistent with the emphasis on history taking in clinical practice, it is not surprising that patients are queried about their adherence. Family reports are often relied upon to assess pediatric adherence (6). These reports are often obtained by structured interviews or questionnaires (14,15). However, patient (or caregiver) ratings tend to overestimate the degree of adherence (2,7). This may be due to social desirability

effects whereby patients and families may want to preserve their relationships with their providers by reporting that they are behaving in socially approved ways.

How patients or family members are questioned about adherence may be critical in the quality of data obtained by reports. Questions that are nonjudgmental, specific, and time limited are likely to yield more accurate information about adherence because they are less likely to generate evasive and defensive reactions and are less subject to recall errors or misunderstanding. For example, questions about medication adherence can be prefaced by stating, "Most people—including the interviewer—miss doses of their medication for one reason or another," (16). In contrast, a judgmental and/or global approach (i.e., "You're taking your medicines like I told you, right?") without time referents can be useless or may induce deception (17).

An alternative is to have patients or family members monitor and record specific adherence behaviors. This can even be done using computerized diaries (9). The accuracy of such records can be improved by clearly specifying target behaviors, using simple monitoring strategies, emphasizing the importance of accuracy and honesty, demonstrating and having patients practice using the monitoring strategy, and periodic and independent checks on accuracy (6).

ADHERENCE RATES

Adherence rates vary depending on how adherence is assessed and what regimen has been prescribed. Among adults with rheumatoid arthritis (RA), medication adherence rates range from 16% to 84% (1,18–21). A European study evaluated adherence with electronic monitoring in persons with RA, polymyalgia rheumatica (PMR), and gout (22). RA patients took no medication 10% of the days and extra doses on 3% of days. In PMR and gout, no use occurred on 10% and 4% of days and overuse occurred on 15% and 7% of days, respectively. One study evaluated adherence of women who had had systemic lupus erythematosus (SLE) an average of 10 years using self reports. Among African Americans, 30.8%—versus 23.4% of whites—reported always taking their medications (p = not significant); 10% of both groups reported never taking their medication (23). In women with fibromyalgia, about half (47–54%) are nonadherent to medications, one-third of whom are intentionally nonadherent, 40.0% of whom are unintentionally nonadherent, and the remaining women were both (24,25). McElhorne et al

> "Many studies have shown that patients who are confident in their ability to manage are the ones who have the best health outcomes. Health professionals are instrumental in helping patients gain this confidence. Professionals must make it clear that they want patients to become expert patients." (63)

noted that rates of perfect adherence among white women with SLE varied by class of medication, ranging from 100% for azathioprine and 94% for oral steroids to 68% for nonsteroidal antiinflammatory drugs (NSAIDs) and 61% for bone-protective medications (26).

Few studies have directly addressed adherence in pediatric patients. Rates of adherence among children with of juvenile rheumatoid arthritis (JRA) range from 38% to 59% (2,6,7). A recent study, which used electronic monitoring over 28 days, among 48 children newly diagnosed with JRA showed full adherence 70% of days, partial adherence 14%, and nonadherence 7% (27).

Adherence rates for nonpharmacologic regimens (e.g., therapeutic exercises) are also highly variable, ranging from 25% to 65% in the treatment of RA (1,21). Iversen et al evaluated adherence to exercise in 132 RA patients 6 months after a visit with their rheumatologist; the percentage of individuals exercising decreased by 10%, from 37% to 27% (28). The ADAPT Trial recently evaluated the effectiveness of weight loss and exercise in 206 overweight and obese persons aged ≥60 years with knee OA (29). Over the 18 months of the study, participants attended 60.7% of diet and 53.2% of exercise sessions. In trials of children with JRA, exercise adherence has ranged from 25% to 65% (19,30).

Taken together, these studies suggest that adherence to medication and exercise recommendations are suboptimal in general, and highly variable among children and adults. What remains unknown at this time is the optimal level of adherence necessary to achieve adequate health and quality-of-life outcomes (7,31).

CONSEQUENCES OF NONADHERENCE

The consequences of nonadherence include compromised efficacy, increased health care costs and utilization, unnecessary escalation of therapy, and compromised clinical trials (6,31). Increased morbidity and possibly mortality (such as with abrupt discontinuation of corticosteroids) can be attributed to nonadherence (32). The cost-effectiveness of health care also may be adversely affected (33). Money may be wasted on treatments that are not followed, or families may incur the costs of additional but unnecessary diagnostic and treatment procedures (34). These unnecessary costs may further burden society in the form of increased insurance premiums and taxes. Treatment nonadherence can also interfere with clinical trials of therapeutic regimens by complicating judgments of efficacy and adding to the sample sizes needed to detect clinical effects (6).

> "Drugs don't work in patients who don't take them."
> C. Everett Koop, MD

FACTORS RELATED TO ADHERENCE

Because many children and adults are adherent to therapy, understanding factors that identify those at risk for suboptimal adherence would be useful (7). In a meta-analysis of 50 years of adherence research in chronic diseases, DiMatteo found that higher levels of adherence were achieved with more circumscribed regimens (i.e., medication use versus pervasive health behaviors) as well as in situations in which patients have greater resources (education, income, and practical and emotional support) (35). Adherence does not appear to be a function of illness type, severity, age, or sex in adults (31,35). There is a trend,

Table 2. Patient, family, disease, and regimen factors associated with nonadherence to medical regimens*

Patient and family factors
    Dissatisfaction with medical care
    Limited financial and social resources
    Lack of knowledge
    Low self-esteem
    Learned helplessness and pessimism
    Negative overall adjustment
    Poor coping strategies
    Family dysfunction

Disease factors
    Decrements in compliance over time
    Patient asymptomatic or in remission
    Increased number of symptoms
    Younger age at disease onset
    Disease not perceived as severe by patient and/or family

Medication and regimen factors
    Complex and demanding regimens
    Costly regimens
    Questionable efficacy
    Lack of continuity of care
    Limited provider supervision of regimen
    Shorter duration of subspecialty care
    Negative regimen side effects

* Adapted from references 2, 6, and 7.

however, for adolescents to be less adherent than younger children (35). Depression (36,37), comorbidity (38), substance abuse (39), and psychosocial factors (such as health distress, use of avoidant coping strategies, and greater impairments in physical and role functioning) also have been associated with lower adherence (40).

Much of the adherence literature has focused on identifying factors that promote or impede adherence. Typically this is done by correlating various factors with adherence or contrasting adherent and nonadherent patients along factorial dimensions (7). As shown in Table 2, patient, family, disease, and regimen factors have been most frequently studied as correlates of adherence. These studies can help determine risk profiles for adherence problems. Additionally, they can assist in formulating or augmenting theoretical models and suggest potentially modifiable variables for adherence intervention trials (6).

Patient and Family Factors

Adherence is likely to be compromised when patients and their families are not well informed, are dissatisfied with care, lack financial and social resources, and experience such adjustment problems as low self-esteem, decreased self-efficacy, and family disharmony. The search for a "typical" nonadherent patient has not been particularly fruitful (5,31); therefore, providers are cautioned to examine these potential patient and family factors in terms of their relevance for specific patients.

Disease Factors

Persons with rheumatic diseases are prime candidates for adherence problems due to the chronicity and fluctuations in their disease activity. This is particularly troublesome when adherence is found to be inconsistently related to disease activity (19). Patients may have few natural incentives, such as symptom relief or improved function, to adhere to prescribed regimens.

Medication and Regimen Factors

Treatments for rheumatic diseases may induce nonadherence for several reasons. Treatment often includes use of NSAIDs and disease-modifying antirheumatic drugs (DMARDs), and sometimes biologic therapies. Regimens are complex (e.g., up to 70 pills per week for RA) and costly. Medications must be used in the long term, even though for many they bring only partial relief and provide delayed benefits. Delayed benefits may particularly undermine patient adherence, as in the case of treating JRA with NSAIDs, which requires at least an 8-week trial (41). Medication side effects also play a role in adherence among RA patients taking DMARDs and anti-tumor necrosis factor therapy (8,42,43). Patients also may conceal symptoms or side effects out of fear of stopping biologic treatment (43).

Medication beliefs may be especially important in rheumatic diseases and are a more robust predictor of adherence than demographic characteristics (44). For example, most people with RA have positive beliefs about the necessity of their medication, however levels of concern are high and generally revolve around potential toxicity and long-term effects (17,42,44). Barber et al noted that a significant proportion of patients were nonadherent, many deliberately so, soon after new medications are prescribed (45); however, the longer patients remain on long-term medication, the poorer the adherence overall. There is also a significant emotional impact to being withdrawn from DMARD medication that appears to increase with DMARD exposure (42).

Dosing frequency is also inversely related to adherence. A review of studies that used electronic monitoring to assess adherence showed that adherence is inversely related to number of doses per day (46). Data from large studies of women receiving a new prescription (weekly versus daily dosing) for osteoporosis treatment confirmed that adherence was significantly greater in the weekly group (although suboptimal in all) (47,48).

IMPROVING ADHERENCE

Several theories of health behavior have been used to enhance understanding of adherence behaviors and to develop effective interventions.

Table 3. Self-management tasks for patients with chronic diseases*

- Medical management, such as taking medicines and exercising
- Maintaining and adapting important life roles, such as those of mother or worker
- Managing the anger, fear, frustration, or depression that come, singly or together, with having an uncertain future

* Adapted from reference 64.

Social cognitive theories suggest that 4 key factors determine an individual's adherence to treatment: threat of the illness (perceived severity and susceptibility), positive outcome expectancy (perceived benefits from treatment), barriers to using the treatment (e.g., expected disadvantages of treatment) and intent (intention to adhere to the treatment regimen) (49). Self-management theories emphasize the active role of patients (and their families) in achieving optimal health outcomes and acknowledge that only patients can assume responsibility for the day-to-day management of their disease (Table 3) (50). Self-efficacy, which is the individual's confidence in his or her capacity to undertake a behavior or behaviors that may lead to desired outcomes, may be a key determinant of outcomes associated with self-management programs (50). The best known example is the Arthritis Self-Management Program developed by Kate Lorig (also known as the Arthritis Self-Help Course and Challenging Arthritis), which is now more than 25 years old. It is used in the United States, Great Britain, Australia, New Zealand, and Canada. Notably, the 2010 Health Care Objectives for the US includes goals of increasing the number of patients receiving self-management education (51). Self-regulatory theory is also gaining favor in developing adherence interventions. Self-regulatory theory posits that treatment perceptions and illness representations have an important influence on medication adherence (52).

There is a paucity of adherence intervention studies in the rheumatology literature (see references 6–8, 18, and 30 for reviews). In general, adherence interventions can be broadly classified as educational, organizational, or behavioral (6,7).

Educational strategies rely on verbal and written instructions designed to inform patients and their families about the illness, regimen

Table 4. Adherence improvement strategies for rheumatic disease regimens in adults and children*

Educational strategies
- Educate early and often about their disease, treatment options, and benefits of consistent adherence
- Teach proven self-management strategies (e.g., monitoring adherence, problem solving around barriers)
- Emphasize the importance of adherence, especially when patients are asymptomatic or in remission
- Increase education about rheumatic diseases in the community to foster early diagnosis and referral for subspecialty care

Organizational strategies
- Minimize costs of treatments (e.g., use generic medications)
- Keep regimens as simple as possible (e.g., reduce number of exercises)
- Integrate regimens into daily/family routines
- Prevent or minimize negative side effects (e.g., gastrointestinal upset associated with NSAIDs by using proton-pump inhibitors)
- Anticipate problems with adherence, discuss nonjudgmentally, and problem solve around barriers.
- Incorporate discussions about adherence routine into clinic encounters
- Address barriers to adherence and sources of patient/family dissatisfaction on a continuing basis
- Link families to resources that can reduce financial and service accessibility barriers to adherence
- Refer patients or families to psychologists or other qualified mental health professionals if more serious problems exist concurrently with nonadherence or directly interfere with adherence

Behavioral strategies
- Make sure patients and families have the skills to carry out regimens. Rehearse these skills in the clinic (e.g., demonstrate exercises, splinting techniques, injection of biologic agents)
- Use skills learned in self-management training to encourage autonomy and self-esteem; in children, encourage patients and caregivers to supervise and monitor adherence (e.g., use an adherence chart or modified calendar posted in a prominent place in the home)
- Consider use of devices (e.g., watches, PDAs, cellphones, pillboxes, etc. with alarms that can be set) to prompt medication ingestion
- Provide social and tangible reinforcers to increase adherence, especially when treatment benefits are delayed
- With children, teach caregivers positive reinforcement strategies for promoting adherence (e.g., token reward systems); review discipline strategies with caregivers for children who are oppositional (e.g., time-out for younger child who refuses to take medications)

* Adapted from reference 7.

requirements, and the importance of consistent adherence. The strategies are necessary, but not sufficient to improve adherence.

Organizational strategies address the delivery of health care, including increasing accessibility to health care services, tailoring and simplifying regimens, and increasing provider supervision and feedback. Organization strategies are promising, particularly those that emphasize greater supervision and feedback to patients and their families. Emerging data suggest that disease-specific programs provide better outcomes than generic chronic disease approaches when resources and participants are sufficient to justify this approach (53).

Behavioral strategies refer to procedures designed to alter specific adherence behaviors by monitoring adherence, providing feedback and positive reinforcement, and soliciting social support from family members. These behavioral strategies, such as teaching patients and their families to monitor, prompt, and reward themselves for adherence, seem to be the most effective (2,5–7). Behavioral strategies are often combined with educational strategies and can be effectively merged with organizational strategies. For example, token-system programs combined with educational strategies can significantly increase adherence in children (2,7,12,54,55).

Table 4 provides specific recommendations for improving adherence by type of strategy. Clearly, providers can have a substantial impact on patient adherence. However, adherence does not occur in a clinical or social vacuum. Patients may experience personal and family adjustment problems that need to be addressed in addition or prior to addressing adherence problems (56).

Interventions also need to be tailored to individual patients and families based on their unique circumstances, barriers, and resources as revealed by an individualized assessment (55,57). One approach is to obtain information about adherence barriers through structured interviews or questionnaires. This information can be used to problem solve with the patient or caregivers on ways to overcome specific barriers (55).

CONCLUSIONS

Rheumatology providers play an important role in identifying, assessing, and managing adherence problems. Potentially the most important benefit is that patient care and outcomes will be enhanced. Providers will also be able to more accurately evaluate the efficacy and cost-effectiveness of their therapeutic endeavors.

However, as health care providers, we must only ask patients to adhere to regimens that are likely to be efficacious, congruent with the Hippocratic Oath: "I will follow that system of regimen which, according to my ability and judgment, I consider for the benefit of my patients, and abstain from whatever is deleterious and mischievous." (58).

Patients and their families demand and deserve an active role in their health care. The term "compliance" has lost favor because it implies an authoritative approach to health care that requires unquestioned obedience by patients to providers' recommendations (7,8). It has been replaced by the term "adherence," which implies a cooperative partnership between patients and providers as reflected in the following perspective by Cassell: "Doctors do not treat chronic illnesses. The chronically ill treat themselves with the help of their physicians; the physician is part of the treatment. Patients are in charge of themselves. They determine their food, ac.tivity, medications, visits to their doctor—most of the details of their own treatment." (59).

Finally, as rheumatology health care providers, we may need to entertain the possibility that failing to adhere to prescribed regimens may be strategic, rational, and adaptive in selected cases (60,61). As noted by Cousins, "The history of medicine is replete with accounts of drugs and modes of treatment that were in use for many years before it was recognized that they did more harm than good." (62). Patients also have the right to determine whether or not they will follow recommended therapies (61). Perhaps when our patients are nonadherent, we need to closely examine what we are recommending and why. This examination may lead us to evaluate the goals and methods for reaching treatment objectives that more appropriately address the day-to-day quality of life for our patients and their families.

REFERENCES

1. Bradley LA. Adherence with treatment regimens among adult rheumatoid arthritis patients: current status and future directions. Arthritis Care Res 1989;2:S33–9.
2. Rapoff MA. Compliance with treatment regimens for pediatric rheumatic diseases. Arthritis Care Res 1989;2:S40–7.
3. Thompson SM, Dahlquist LM, Koenning GM, Bartholomew LK. Brief report: adherence-facilitating behaviors of a multidisciplinary pediatric rheumatology staff. J Pediatr Psychol 1995;20:291–7.
4. Haynes RB, Taylor DW, Sackett DL. Compliance in health care. Baltimore: Johns Hopkins University Press; 1979.
5. Meichenbaum D, Turk DC. Facilitating treatment adherence: a practitioner's guide. New York: Plenum; 1987.
6. Rapoff MA. Adherence to pediatric regimens. New York: Kluwer Academic/ Plenum; 1999.
7. Rapoff MA. Management of adherence and chronic rheumatic disease in children and adolescents. Best Pract Res Clin Rheumatol 2006;20:301–14.
8. Treharne GJ, Lyons AC, Hale ED, Douglas KMJ, Kitas GD. 'Compliance' is futile but is 'concordance' between rheumatology patients and health professionals attainable? Rheumatology 2006;45:1–5.
9. Cramer JA. Microelectronic systems for monitoring and enhancing patient compliance with medication regimens. Drugs 1995;49:321–7.
10. Backes JM, Schentag JJ. Partial compliance as a source of variance in phyarmacokinetics and therapeutic drug monitoring. In: Cramer JA, Spilker B, editors. Patient compliance in medical practice and clinical trials. New York: Raven; 1991.
11. Bardare M, Cislaghi GU, Mandelli M, Sereni F. Value of monitoring plasma salicylate levels in treating juvenile rheumatoid arthritis: observations in 42 cases. Arch Dis Child 1978;53:381–5.
12. Rapoff MA, Lindsley CB, Christophersen ER. Improving compliance with medical regimens: case study with juvenile rheumatoid arthritis. Arch Phys Med Rehabil 1984;65:267–9.
13. Urquhart J. Role of patient compliance in clinical pharmacokinetics: a review of recent research. Clin Pharmacokinet 1994;27:202–15.
14. De Klerk E, Van Der HD, Landewe R, Van Der TH, Van Der LS. The compliance-questionnaire-rheumatology compared with electronic medication event monitoring: a validation study. J Rheumatol 2003;30:2469–75.
15. De Civita M, Dobkin PL, Ehrmann-Feldman D, Karp I, Duffy CM. Development and preliminary reproducibility and validity of the parent adherence report questionnaire: a measure of adherence in juvenile idiopathic arthritis. J Clin Psychol Med Settings 2005;12:1–12.
16. Lorish CD, Richards B, Brown S. Missed medication doses in rheumatic arthritis patients: intentional and unintentional reasons. Arthritis Care Res 1989;2:3–9.
17. Berry D, Bradlow A, Bersellini E. Perceptions of the risks and benefits of medicines in patients with rheumatoid arthritis and other painful musculoskeletal conditions. Rheumatology 2004;43:901–5.
18. Brus H, van de Laar M, Taal E, Rasker J, Wiegman O. Determinants of compliance with medication in patients with rheumatoid arthritis: the importance of self-efficacy expectations. Pat Educ Counsel 1999;36: 57–64.
19. Belcon MC, Haynes RB, Tugwell P. A critical review of compliance studies in rheumatoid arthritis. Arthritis Rheum 1984;27:1227–33.
20. Litt IF, Cuskey WR, Rosenberg A. Role of self-esteem and autonomy in determining medication compliance among adolescents with juvenile rheumatoid arthritis. Pediatrics 1982;69:15–17.
21. Litt IF, Cuskey WR. Compliance with salicylate therapy in adolescents with juvenile rheumatoid arthritis. Am J Dis Child 1981;135:434–6.
22. De Klerk E, van der HD, Landewe R, van der TH, Urquhart J, van der LS. Patient compliance in rheumatoid arthritis, polymyalgia rheumatica, and gout. J Rheumatol 2003;30:44–54.
23. Mosley-Williams A, Lumley MA, Gillis M, Leisen J, Guice D. Barriers to treatment adherence among African American and white women with systemic lupus erythematosus. Arthritis Rheum 2002;47:630–8.

24. Dobkin PL, Sita A, Sewitch MJ. Predictors of adherence to treatment in women with fibromyalgia. Clin J Pain 2006;22:286–94.

25. Sewitch MJ, Dobkin PL, Bernatsky S, Baron M, Starr M, Cohen M, et al. Medication non-adherence in women with fibromyalgia. Rheumatology (Oxford) 2004;43:648–54.

26. McElhone K, Teh LS, Walker J, Abbott J. Treatment adherence in systemic lupus erythematosus (SLE). Rheumatology 2005;44:I141.

27. Rapoff MA, Belmont JM, Lindsley CB, Olson NY. Electronically monitored adherence to medications by newly diagnosed patients with juvenile rheumatoid arthritis. Arthritis Rheum 2005;53:905–10.

28. Iversen MD, Fossel AH, Ayers K, Palmsten A, Wang HW, Daltroy LH. Predictors of exercise behavior in patients with rheumatoid arthritis 6 months following a visit with their rheumatologist. Phys Ther 2004; 84:706–16.

29. van Gool CH, Penninx BWJH, Kempen GIJM, Miller GD, van Eijk JT, Pahor M, et al. Determinants of high and low attendance to diet and exercise interventions among overweight and obese older adults: results from the arthritis, diet, and activity promotion trial. Contemp Clin Trials 2006;27:227–37.

30. Kroll T, Barlow JH, Shaw K. Treatment adherence in juvenile rheumatoid arthritis—a review. Scand J Rheumatol 1999;28:10–8.

31. Osterberg L, Blaschke T. Adherence to medication. N Engl J Med 2005;353:487–97.

32. Ruley EJ. Compliance in young hypertensive patients. Pediatr Clin North Am 1978;25:175–82.

33. Elliott RA, Barber N, Horne R. Cost-effectiveness of adherence-enhancing interventions: a quality assessment of the evidence. Ann Pharmacother 2005;39:508–15.

34. Smith M. The cost of noncompliance and the capacity of improved compliance to reduce health care expenditures. Improving mediation compliance. Proceedings of a symposium. Washington, DC: National Pharmaceutical Council; 1985. p. 35–42.

35. DiMatteo MR. Variations in patients' adherence to medical recommendations: a quantitative review of 50 years of research. Med Care 2004; 42:200–9.

36. Carney RM, Freedland KE, Eisen SA, Rich MW, Jaffe AS. Major depression and medication adherence in elderly patients with coronary artery disease. Health Psychol 1995;14:88–90.

37. DiMatteo MR, Lepper HS, Croghan TW. Depression is a risk factor for noncompliance with medical treatment: meta-analysis of the effects of anxiety and depression on patient adherence. Arch Intern Med 2000;160:2101–7.

38. DiMatteo MR, Giordani PJ, Lepper HS, Croghan TW. Patient adherence and medical treatment outcomes: a meta-analysis. Med Care 2002;40: 794–811.

39. Lucas GM, Gebo KA, Chaisson RE, Moore RD. Longitudinal assessment of the effects of drug and alcohol abuse on HIV-1 treatment outcomes in an urban clinic. AIDS 2002;16:767–74.

40. Sherbourne CD, Hays RD, Ordway L, DiMatteo MR, Kravitz RL. Antecedents of adherence to medical recommendations: results from the medical outcomes study. J Behav Med 1992;15:447–68.

41. Lovell DJ, Giannini EH, Brewer EJ Jr. Time course of response to nonsteroidal antiinflammatory drugs in juvenile rheumatoid arthritis. Arthritis Rheum 1984;27:1433–7.

42. Goodacre LJ, Goodacre JA. Factors influencing the beliefs of patients with rheumatoid arthritis regarding disease-modifying medication. Rheumatology (Oxford) 2004;43:583–6.

43. Kiely PD. Symptom concealment—a new phenomenon in patients treated with biological therapies? Rheumatology 2004;43:114–5.

44. Neame R, Hammond A. Beliefs about medications: a questionnaire survey of people with rheumatoid arthritis. Rheumatology 2005;44:762–7.

45. Barber N, Parsons J, Clifford S, Darracott R, Horne R. Patients' problems with new medication for chronic conditions. Qual Saf Health Care 2004;13:172–5.

46. Claxton AJ, Cramer J, Pierce C. A systematic review of the associations between dose regimens and medication compliance. Clin Ther 2001; 23:1296–1310.

47. Reginster JY, Rabenda V, Neuprez A. Adherence, patient preference and dosing frequency: understanding the relationship. Bone 2006;38(4 Suppl 1): S2–6.

48. Recker RR, Gallagher R, MacCosbe PE. Effect of dosing frequency on bisphosphonate medication adherence in a large longitudinal cohort of women. Mayo Clin Proc 2005;80:856–61.

49. Riekert KA, Drotar D. The beliefs about medication scale: development, reliability, and validity. J Clin Psychol Med Settings 2002;9:177–84.

50. Lorig KR, Holman H. Self-management education: history, definition, outcomes, and mechanisms. Ann Behav Med 2003;26:1–7.

51. Centers for Disease Control and Prevention. Healthy People 2010. Washington, DC: US Government Printing Office; 2000.

52. Horne R, Weinman J. Patients' beliefs about prescribed medicines and their role in adherence to treatment in chronic physical illness. J Psychosom Res 1999;47:555–67.

53. Lorig K, Ritter PL, Plant K. A disease-specific self-help program compared with a generalized chronic disease self-help program for arthritis patients. Arthritis Rheum 2005;53:950–7.

54. Pieper KB, Rapoff MA, Purviance MR, Lindsley CB. Improving compliance with prednisone therapy in pediatric patients with rheumatic disease. Arthritis Care Res 1989;2:132–5.

55. Bartlett SJ, Lukk P, Butz A, Lampros-Klein F, Rand CS. Enhancing medication adherence among inner-city children with asthma: results from pilot studies. J Asthma 2002;39:47–54.

56. Rapoff MA, Barnard MU. Compliance with pediatric medical regimens. In: Cramer JA, Spilker B, editors. Patient compliance in medical practice and clinical trials. New York: Raven; 1991. p. 73–98.

57. Kreuter MW, Strecher VJ, Glassman B. One size does not fit all: the case for tailoring print materials. Ann Behav Med 1999;21:276–83.

58. The Oath. In: Adams, translator, editor. The genuine works of Hippocrates. New York: William Wood; 1886.

59. Cassell EJ. The nature of suffering and the goals of medicine. New York: Oxford University Press; 1991.

60. Deaton AV. Adaptive noncompliance in pediatric asthma: the parent as expert. J Pediatr Psychol 1985;10:1–14.

61. Rand CS, Sevick MA. Ethics in adherence promotion and monitoring. Control Clin Trials 2000;21(5 Suppl 1):S241–7.

62. Cousins N. Anatomy of an illness as perceived by the patient. New York: Bantam; 1979.

63. Lorig K. Partnerships between expert patients and physicians. Lancet 2002;359:814–5.

64. Corbin J, Strauss A, editors. Unending work and care: managing chronic illness at home. San Francisco: Jossey-Bass; 1988.

Additional Recommended Reading

Rapoff MA. Adherence to pediatric medical regimens. New York: Kluwer Academic/Plenum; 1999.

Drotar D, editor. Promoting adherence to medical treatment in childhood chronic illness: concepts, methods, and interventions. Mahwah (NJ): Lawrence Erlbaum Associates; 2000.

Haynes RB, McDonald HP, Garg AX. Helping patients follow prescribed treatment: clinical applications. JAMA 2002;288:2880–3.

Sabate E. Adherence to long-term therapies: evidence for action. Geneva: World Health Organization, 2003. Accessed June 16, 2006. URL: http://www.who.int/chronic_conditions/en/adherence_report.pdf.

Shumaker SA, Schron EB, Ockene JK, McBee WL, editors. The handbook of health behavior change. 2nd ed. New York: Springer; 1998.

Fatigue

BASIA BELZA, PhD, RN, and KORI DEWING, MN, ARNP

Fatigue is a frequent, intrusive, and overwhelming problem for individuals with rheumatic disease (1). The purpose of this chapter is to examine the impact and prevalence of fatigue, describe its etiology, identify instruments that measure fatigue, and suggest management strategies to reduce fatigue in rheumatic diseases. The ability to effectively manage fatigue has important implications in the overall efforts of treating the disease process. Fatigue contributes to a sedentary lifestyle, may be a factor in discontinuing or not fully participating in rehabilitation, reduces quality of life, and impairs functional status.

Health professionals share responsibility for addressing fatigue. Whereas physicians' expertise lies in managing the medical aspects of illness, symptom management is shared by all rheumatology health professionals. Pain, fatigue, depressed mood, and disability are consequences of the illness. Health professionals are skilled in helping patients better understand and adjust to the consequences of disease. Collaborative efforts can lead to better utilization of the expertise of our colleagues and improved outcomes. Such disciplines as nursing, physical therapy, occupational therapy, vocational rehabilitation, and mental health care play pivotal roles in the management of fatigue.

DEFINITION AND IMPACT

Fatigue is a perception arising from the complex interplay of biologic processes, psychosocial phenomena, and behavioral manifestations (2). To some, fatigue may be the end result of excessive energy consumption, decreased oxygen carrying capacity (i.e., anemia), depleted hormones or neurotransmitters, or the diminished ability of muscle cells to contract (3). To others, fatigue is the subjective state of weariness related to reduced motivation, prolonged mental activity, or boredom. Fatigue can also be the awareness of a decreased capacity for physical or mental activity due to an imbalance in the availability, utilization, or restoration of resources needed to perform an activity (2). Chronic and pervasive feelings of overwhelming fatigue can also be an important indicator of psychological problems, such as anxiety and depression.

Fatigue permeates every sphere of life (1). Fatigue is associated with moderate impairment in functional capacity and reduced productivity. One patient with rheumatoid arthritis (RA) described the impact of fatigue as follows: "When I am fatigued everything is too great an effort. Ordinary tasks loom as overwhelming. Feelings of helplessness and hopelessness dominate." (4). Fatigue makes the management of associated symptoms, such as pain, more challenging. It may also be related to increased human error and associated with increased falls (5). The nature of fatigue restricts one's ability to fulfill normal roles in one's family and society (1). Fatigue is a persistent threat to continued employment (6). It has been associated with decreased work capacity, working fewer hours, and decreased work accuracy (7). The precise mechanism of how fatigue affects these areas is not known.

PREVALENCE

The prevalence and severity of fatigue vary by type of rheumatic disease. Although the diagnostic criteria for RA do not include fatigue,

one criterion for clinical remission is the absence of fatigue (8). In patients with RA, the presence of fatigue ranges from 88% to 100% (8–10). Although fatigue is highly prevalent in RA, one study found that fatigue ranked lower in importance when compared with functional disability, pain, and depression (11). The American College of Rheumatology 1990 Multicenter Study for Fibromyalgia, which defined fatigue as "usually or always being too tired to do what you want," found that 81% of persons with fibromyalgia reported fatigue (12). Fatigue is also present in 80–100% of patients with systemic lupus erythematosus and is one of the most disabling symptoms for patients (13,14). Levels of fatigue are higher in patients with active lupus than in patients with inactive disease (14). Fatigue has been found in at least 50% of patients with ankylosing spondylitis and has been found to be consistently associated with measures of mental health and disease activity (15,16). Disabling fatigue is a frequent extraglandular complaint in primary Sjögren's syndrome (17). The occurrence of fatigue across diagnostic categories at all phases of life underscores the need for empirically based interventions.

ETIOLOGY

Fatigue is a complex phenomenon with multiple causes and contributors that include physiological, psychological, and environmental factors. Components of the inflammatory process may contribute to fatigue. The level of fatigue in RA is strongly associated with pain, sleep disturbance, inactivity, comorbid conditions, poorer functional status, and newly diagnosed disease (7,9,18). Other factors associated with fatigue are depressive symptoms, female sex, and self-efficacy toward coping with RA (18,19). When in pain, people expend more energy to complete even the simplest tasks. Disturbed sleep leads to daytime fatigue. Inactivity leads to deconditioning and muscle atrophy.

As a result of disuse or reduced use, changes in the cardiorespiratory system reduce the body's energy-producing capacity and mechanical efficiency, contributing to decreased endurance. Muscle function may be impaired due to accumulation of metabolic products, which in turn leads to impaired muscle contractility. Functional impairment is associated with less efficient use of the musculoskeletal system or use of less-developed muscle groups to minimize pain. Disabilities associated with arthritis often cause fatigue, long task times, and pain (20).

Potential psychological causes of fatigue, such as depression and anxiety, have been noted in patients with rheumatic disease. The diagnostic criteria for depression include the presence of fatigue. Impairment in cognitive function, including decreased attention and impaired perception and thinking, has been associated with fatigue. Individuals with rheumatic diseases have reported cognitive changes, such as difficulty in thinking and inability to concentrate (13).

Unfortunately, treatments used to manage rheumatic conditions may worsen symptoms of fatigue. Most medications used to treat rheumatic conditions list fatigue as a potential side effect. Certain disease-modifying antirheumatic drugs, such as methotrexate or leflunamide, are more commonly implicated in worsening symptoms of fatigue than others. Yet, when inflammation comes under control, symptoms of fatigue often improve. Some would argue that the change in fatigue levels reflects general improvement in pain, function, and psychological status rather than any direct interference with cytokines controlling fatigue (11). Medications used to treat comorbidities of rheumatic conditions (i.e., depression, sleep disturbance) may worsen fatigue due to their mechanisms of action. And lastly, too much exercise can lead to a phenomenon called overtraining, which may lead to an increase in fatigue.

MEASUREMENT

Accurate measurement of fatigue is important for several reasons: 1) to understand the relationship of fatigue with other symptoms, such as pain and depression, 2) to monitor its natural history over time, 3) to screen or classify, 4) to assess individual health status, 5) to distinguish between disease conditions, 6) to guide management decisions, and 7) to evaluate the magnitude of change in response to treatment. Furthermore, it is often the most difficult symptom to control and most bothersome to our patients. In addition to assessing degree, duration, and severity of fatigue, several related areas need to be analyzed. Key questions to ask patients presenting with fatigue are: "What is the status of your rheumatic disease? Do you have any associated disorder(s), such as hypothyroidism? How well do you sleep?" Other factors to be assessed include minor or major mood disturbance, psychosocial stressors, and exercise and physical activity levels.

Familiarity with the several different fatigue measurement tools allows clinicians and researchers to select the scale that best meets their and their patients' needs (21,22). Table 1 includes a listing of published instruments used to measure fatigue that have been developed and tested in the rheumatic diseases. Resources exist such as the *Arthritis and Rheumatism (Arthritis Care and Research)* special issue "Patient Outcomes in Rheumatology: A Review of Measures," which provides a review of instruments that purport to measure fatigue and similar constructs (23). Instruments with multiple items typically measure different dimensions of fatigue, such as severity, intensity, distress, and impact. Single-item measures have also been used to assess fatigue in rheumatic diseases and are suitable for routine use in clinical care. One question frequently used to evaluate outcomes in clinical trials is how many hours elapse from the time of arising to the time of fatigue onset. Various scales have been used to measure fatigue or energy, such as determining energy level on an 11-point scale ranging from "not at all" to "a lot" or a 0 (none) to 10 (most) scale, or by determining fatigue intensity on a 4-point scale from "none" to "severe." Single-item visual analog scales

perform as well as or better than longer scales in respect to sensitivity to change, and are as correlated with clinical variables as longer scales (24). The overall purpose of the investigation should drive the selection of using a single- or multiple-item instrument to measure fatigue.

MANAGEMENT STRATEGIES

Treatment goals for the management of fatigue include resolving the underlying problem(s), helping the patient better understand fatigue, and reducing or alleviating the fatigue. If there is a single underlying problem causing fatigue, such as hypothyroidism, sleep disturbance/apnea, or anemia, it should be diagnosed and treated. If there is a component of depression, the patient should receive counseling and, if appropriate, antidepressant medication. The clinician and patient need to develop mutually agreed-upon treatment goals and identify strategies to reduce or alleviate fatigue. Strategies to reduce fatigue are listed.

Increasing Physical Activity Levels

Individuals with rheumatic disease who are involved in aerobic exercise of moderate intensity notice improvements in pain and fatigue. Additionally, improvements have been noted in muscle strength and functional status. Providers should encourage patients with arthritis to safely increase their activity level. The level of aerobic conditioning also has a significant influence on performance capability. Individuals with limited aerobic capacity due to pathologic state or a sedentary lifestyle can increase their endurance through training. After evaluation of the cardiorespiratory and musculoskeletal systems, and with consultation from an exercise specialist, patients can start a training program. Training produces improved heart rate, ventilation, and oxygen transport and utilization. Specific improvements in coordination and functional efficiency also occur, depending on type of activity and muscle groups trained. Endurance training lowers energy expenditure for a given effort, resulting in reduced fatigue and enhanced performance.

Participation in a Self-Help Program

Patients with arthritis who participate in the Arthritis Self-Management Program or a Chronic Disease Self-Management Program report positive outcomes, including reduced fatigue, compared with those

Table 1. Instruments that measure fatigue in the rheumatic diseases

Instrument	Description	Number and type of items	Comments
Multidimensional Assessment of Fatigue (9)	Measures 5 dimensions of fatigue: degree, severity, distress, impact on daily activities, and frequency	16-item instrument that uses numerical rating scales with endpoints of 1 (not at all) to 10 (a great deal)	Developed in RA and healthy adults; tested in other chronic conditions; translated into 25 languages.
Fatigue Severity Scale (13)	Measures symptoms associated with fatigue and its impact on work, family, and social life	9-item instrument that uses numerical rating scales with endpoints of 1 (low) to 7 (high)	Based on the characteristics of fatigue in systemic lupus erythematosus and multiple sclerosis.
Fatigue subscale; Profile of Mood States (POMS) (33)	Measures fatigue severity; the fatigue subscale is one of the 6 POMS subscales	7-item subscale that uses numerical rating scales with endpoints of 1 (not at all) to 5 (all the time)	Tested in a variety of clinical populations and healthy adults.
Fatigue Scale (34)	Measures physical and mental symptoms associated with the presentation of fatigue	14-item instrument that uses numerical rating scales on a continuum with 1 (better than usual) to 4 (much worse than usual)	Developed in chronic fatigue syndrome and patients attending a medical clinic
Profile of Fatigue-Related Symptoms (35)	Assesses the severity and pattern of illness and evaluates the effects of treatment	96-item multidimensional illness-specific instrument	Developed for use in chronic fatigue syndrome

who receive usual care (25). Programs are community-based and can be identified by contacting local chapters of the Arthritis Foundation or other similar organizations.

Self-Appraisal

Monitoring changes in one's own body is a basic activity of self-care (26). Completing a fatigue care wheel (Figure 1) may help a person see the relationship between specific causes of and solutions to fatigue. Using standardized measures to assess fatigue or maintaining a log may help identify patterns of, variations of, and contributors to fatigue. Suggesting that patients read the story "My Bowl of Marbles" (sidebar) may serve as a starting point for discussion about their own energy level.

Optimal Control of Inflammation

Although the mechanism is unknown, it is speculated that the release of interleukin-1, associated with the body's immune response, contributes to fatigue. Whatever the contributing factors, inflammation has been associated with fatigue. Appropriate type and amount of pharmacologic agents must be taken to control the inflammatory process. Some biologic response modifiers have been shown to reduce fatigue in patients with recent-onset and established RA (27).

Optimal Control of Pain

Next to fatigue, pain is one of the most frequently described symptoms reported by patients with a rheumatic disease. Providing adequate control of pain is essential. Only through effective treatment of pain can

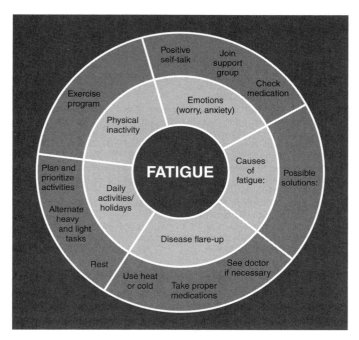

Figure 1. Example of fatigue care wheel*

*Fatigue is a frequent and bothersome symptom associated with many of the systemic rheumatic diseases. Patients can learn new self-management skills by identifying the causes of fatigue and using effective fatigue management strategies. Using a fatigue care wheel, instruct patients in identifying factors that bring on fatigue (inner circle) and strategies that decrease fatigue (outer circle). Encourage patients to post the fatigue care wheel in a prominent place at home or work to serve as a reminder. Reproduced, with permission, from Arthritis Foundation. Coping with fatigue. Atlanta: Arthritis Foundation; 1991.

My Bowl of Marbles
By Linda Jean Frame

I begin by thinking of energy as marbles. Each small, expendable amount of energy becomes a marble. I have a limited number of marbles to use each day and while the number of marbles may vary from day to day, I can pretty well judge each morning just how many marbles I will have to use that day. I then place my day's supply in an imaginary fish bowl and begin my day.

With each activity, such as washing my face or combing my hair, I use energy. When I expend one marble's worth of energy, I extract one marble from the bowl. I value each marble at a certain amount and can judge when I use that amount of energy. You might give a different value to each of your marbles, but it will all work out the same way in the end. Bigger projects require more marbles; however, on bad days you will find that even small activities will demand the use of more marbles than those same activities will require on good days. There are times when it is very frustrating to have so little energy and to have to use so much of it to do even simple things, but that's the way it is.

Starting each day with an awareness of your energy supply will enable you to choose what is really important to you, and you can plan accordingly. Try to avoid frustration by accepting your limitations. Frustration is a form of stress and stress is a marble user. Comfort yourself with the thought that you won't always have so few marbles to use. Tomorrow may be a better day. Remember to remove marbles during the day for any type of stress. Remove marbles for anything that causes tension or fear. I throw out a couple of marbles every time I have to drive in rush-hour traffic; not because the traffic bothers me, but because I know that I must be a little more alert and stressed than when I drive at other times of the day. If something really big happens, and I am really stressed or shocked, I may throw away the whole bowl and give myself the rest of the day off.

If you should see me or phone me at one of those times, when I have resigned from the human race, you might say, "Linda has lost her marbles," and you would be exactly right!

Arthritis Foundation. SLE self-help course leader's manual. Atlanta: Arthritis Foundation; 1994. p. 58. Reprinted with permission from TALS, the San Diego Chapter Newsletter.

---

there be hope for managing fatigue. Symptom clusters are common in rheumatic diseases. Pain and fatigue are closely related. With increased pain comes increased fatigue, and vice versa. This may be a function of disease activity (i.e., inflammation) or it may be related to interruption of sleep due to pain, leading to morning fatigue. Specific pain management strategies are presented in Chapters 33 and 38.

Symptom Reinterpretation

One strategy for improving self-efficacy—the belief in one's capability to exercise control over motivation and environmental demands—is reinterpretation of symptoms. This allows an individual to reconceptualize what he or she thinks about fatigue and to redefine physiologic symptoms and signs. For example, fatigue may be a warning sign of an impending increase in disease activity, and that warning should stimulate a patient to seek earlier medical treatment. People with high self-efficacy approach difficult tasks as challenges, set challenging goals, increase effort in face of difficulties, and experience low stress and depression. Improving self-efficacy is critical because it is strongly related to fatigue (19).

Energy Conservation

Energy conservation is the process of saving energy and improving the distribution of energy over time. Proper body positioning conserves energy. Energy is used when the body is in poor posture, such as with using incorrect work height, slumping, or hunching shoulders. Rest breaks reduce pain and stress to damaged joints (see Chapter 32, Exercise and Physical Activity). Activity analysis allows the examination of activities that might drain excessive time and energy. Strategies to alter work patterns include pacing, planning ahead, prioritizing, using adaptive equipment, and job simplification.

Sleep and Rest Behaviors

Obtaining adequate rest and sleep is an intuitively logical approach to managing fatigue. Principles of sleep hygiene are discussed in Chapter 45, Sleep Disturbances. For fatigue resulting from sleep apnea, myoclonus (restless leg syndrome), or other suspected sleep disturbances, refer the patient to a sleep clinic for evaluation and treatment.

Ease Psychological Distress

Overwhelming fatigue is often one of the primary symptoms associated with high levels of anxiety and depression. In patients with RA, fatigue, pain and disability are the strongest predictors of clinically significant levels of depressive symptoms (28). Beyond fatigue, depression and anxiety are associated with higher levels of stress, pain, and maladaptive coping in patients with rheumatic conditions (29–31). Depression and anxiety may also independently contribute to disability (29,32). Because effective treatments exist for anxiety and depression, clinicians should consider whether referral to a mental health specialist is indicated. (See also Chapter 33 Cognitive-Behavior Therapy.)

SUMMARY

Effective management of fatigue is a goal to strive toward. Consideration should be given to the multiple causes of fatigue and varied management strategies. More research is needed on factors that contribute to fatigue, and interventions must be tested to determine those most effective in alleviating or reducing fatigue. Treating fatigue requires an understanding of the inflammatory process, the impact of the rheumatic disease on the psychological system, and the personal attributes and motivations of the individual with arthritis.

REFERENCES

1. Hewlett S, Cockshott Z, Byron M, Kitchen K, Tipler S, Pope D, et al. Patients' perceptions of fatigue in rheumatoid arthritis: overwhelming, uncontrollable, and ignored. Arthritis Rheum 2005;53:697–702.
2. Aaronson JS, Teel CS, Cassmeyer V, Neuberger GB, Pallikkathayil L, Pierce J, et al. Defining and managing fatigue. Image J Nurs Sch 1999;31:45–50.
3. Poteliakhoff, A. Adrenocortical activity and some clinical findings in acute and chronic fatigue. J Psychosom Res 1981;25:91–5.
4. Tack B. Fatigue in rheumatoid arthritis: conditions, strategies, and consequences. Arthritis Care Res 1990;3:65–70.
5. Fessel KD. Fear of falling and activity limitation among persons with rheumatoid arthritis [abstract]. Arthritis Rheum 1995;38(Suppl 9):S305.
6. Mancuso CA, Paget SA, Charlson ME. Adaptations made by rheumatoid arthritis patients to continue working: a pilot study of workplace challenges and successful adaptations. Arthritis Care and Res 2000;13:89–99.
7. Wolfe F, Hawley D, Wilson K. The prevalence and meaning of fatigue in rheumatic diseases. J Rheumatol 1996;23:1407–17.
8. Pinals RS, Masi AT, Larsen RA, and the Subcommittee for Criteria of Remission in Rheumatoid Arthritis of the American Rheumatism Association Diagnostic and Therapeutic Criteria Committee. Preliminary criteria for clinical remission in rheumatoid arthritis. Arthritis Rheum 1981;24:1308–15.
9. Belza B, Henke C, Yelin E, Epstein W, Gilliss C. Correlates of fatigue in older adults with rheumatoid arthritis. Nurs Res 1993;42:93–9.
10. Neuberger G, Press A, Lindsley H, Hinton R, Cagle P, Carlson K, et al. Effects of exercise on fatigue, aerobic fitness, and disease activity measures in persons with rheumatoid arthritis. Res Nurs Health 1997;20:195–204.
11. Wolfe F, Michaud K, Pincus T. Fatigue, rheumatoid arthritis, and anti-tumor necrosis factor therapy: an investigation in 24,831 patients. J Rheumatol 2004;31:2115–20.
12. Wolfe F, Smythe HA, Yunus MB, Bennett RM, Bombardier C, Goldenberg DL, et al. The American College of Rheumatology 1990 criteria for the classification of fibromyalgia: report of the Multicenter Criteria Committee. Arthritis Rheum 1990;33:160–72.
13. Krupp L, LaRocca N, Muir-Nash J, Steinberg A. A study of fatigue in systemic lupus erythematosus. J Rheumatol 1990;17:1450–2.
14. Tench CM, McCordie I, White PD, D'Cruz DP. The prevalence and associations of fatigue in SLE. Rheumatology (Oxford) 2000;39:1249–54.
15. Calin A, Edmunds L, Kennedy L. Fatigue in ankylosing spondylitis—why is it ignored? J Rheumatol 1993;20:991–5.
16. Dagfinrud H, Vollestad NK, Loge JH, Kvien, TK, Mengshoel AM. Fatigue in patients with ankylosing spondylitis: a comparison with the general population and associations with clinical and self-reported measures. Arthritis Rheum 2005;53:5–11.
17. Lwin C, Bishay M, Platts R, Booth D, Bowman S. The assessment of fatigue in primary Sjogren's syndrome. Scand J Rheumatol 2003;32:33–7.
18. Riemsma RP, Rasker JJ, Taal E, Griep EN, Wouters JM, Wiegman O. Fatigue in rheumatoid arthritis: the role of self-efficacy and problematic social support. Br J Rheumatol 1998;37:1042–6.
19. Huyser BA, Parker JC, Thoreson R, Smarr KL, Johnson JC, Hoffman, R. Predictors of subjective fatigue among individuals with rheumatoid arthritis. Arthritis Rheum 1998;41:2230–7.
20. Verbrugge L, Juarez L Profile of arthritis disability: II. Arthritis Rheum 2006;55:102–13.
21. Goldenberg D. Fatigue in rheumatic disease. Bull Rheum Dis 1995;44:4–8.
22. Hewlett S, Hehir M, Kirwan JR. Measuring fatigue in rheumatoid arthritis: a systematic review of scales in use. Arthritis Rheum (in press).
23. Katz P, editor. Patient outcomes in rheumatology: a review of measures. Arthritis Rheum 2003;49(5).
24. Wolfe F. Fatigue assessments in rheumatoid arthritis: comparative performance of visual analog scales and longer fatigue questionnaires in 7760 patients. J Rheumatol 2004;31:1896–902.
25. Lorig KR, Ritter P, Plant K. A disease specific self-help program compared with a generalized chronic disease self-help program for arthritis patients. Arthritis Rheum 2005;53:950–7.
26. Keller M, Ward S, Baumann L. Processes of self-care: monitoring sensations and symptoms. Adv Nurs Sci 1989;12:54–66.
27. Moreland L, Genovese M, Sato R, Singh A. Effect of etanercept on fatigue in patients with recent or established rheumatoid arthritis. Arthritis Rheum 2006;55:287–93.
28. Covic T, Tyson G, Spencer D, Howe G. Depression in rheumatoid arthritis patients: demographic, clinical, and psychological predictors. J Psychosom Res 2006;60:469–76.
29. Patten SB, Williams JV, Wang J. Mental disorders in a population sample with musculoskeletal disorders. BMC Musculoskelet Disord 2006;7:37.
30. Dickens C, Mcgowan L, Clark-Carter D, Creed F. Depression in rheumatoid arthritis: a systematic review of the literature with meta-analysis. Psychosom Med 2002;64:52–60.
31. Valtysdottir ST, Gudbjornsson B, Lindqvist U, Hallgren R, Hetta J. Anxiety and depression in patients with primary Sjogren's syndrome. J Rheumatol 2000;27:165–9.
32. Escalante A, del Rincon I. The disablement process in rheumatoid arthritis. Arthritis Rheum 2002;47:333–42.
33. McNair D, Lorr R, Dropplemen L. EdITS manual for the profile of mood states. San Diego: Education and Industrial Testing Service; 1992.
34. Chalder T, Berelowitz G, Pawlikowska T, Watts L, Wessely S, Wright D, et al. Development of a fatigue scale. J Psychosom Res 1993;37:147–53.
35. Ray C, Weir W, Phillips S, Cullen S. Development of a measure of symptoms in chronic fatigue syndrome: the Profile of Fatigue Related Symptoms (PFRS). Psychol Health 1992;7:27–43.

CHAPTER 45

Sleep Disturbances in Rheumatic Diseases

MICHAEL T. SMITH, PhD, and STEPHEN T. WEGENER, PhD

Research demonstrates the comorbidity of pain, fatigue, disease activity, mood, and sleep disturbance in persons with rheumatic disease. Sleep problems are common in this population and certain sleep disruptions are associated with specific rheumatic diseases. The clinician working with rheumatic disease patients will encounter a range of sleep problems requiring a basic knowledge of sleep physiology, cycles, and disturbances as well as fundamental assessment and intervention techniques. Aggressive management of sleep disturbance has the potential to improve functioning, pain severity, and quality of life for persons with rheumatic disease.

SLEEP PHYSIOLOGY AND FUNCTION

Normal human sleep is a complex and dynamic neurophysiologic process that evolves in a highly organized manner over the course of the night. The precise functions of sleep are only beginning to be understood. Several leading theories are that sleep serves a restorative and energy-conservation function (1), plays a role in neuroplasticity (2), consolidates procedural memory (3), and regulates mood (4). Although the functions of sleep are not definitively known, it is clear that poor sleep quality is an independent risk factor for medical and psychiatric comorbidity, including coronary artery disease (5,6), diabetes (7), widespread pain (8), and depression (9). Sleep deprivation or disruption is known to adversely alter metabolic function (10), impair immune function (11), increase daytime circulating proinflammatory cytokine levels (12,13), and elevate pain sensitivity (14–16). Therefore, optimizing sleep is a potentially critical goal in the management of rheumatic diseases.

Sleep Cycles and Architecture

Healthy adults cycle through a series of stages during the sleep period (17). These sleep stages are characterized by distinct behavioral and physiologic states measured by electroencephalography (EEG), electro-oculography, electromyography (EMG), and multiple biometric indices of respiratory function that are collectively referred to as polysomnography (PSG). A usual night's sleep is divided into 2 broad categories—rapid eye movement (REM) sleep and non-REM (NREM) sleep. NREM sleep is further subdivided into 4 stages. NREM Stage 1 (NREM S1) typically initiates with a waking EEG alpha wave pattern (8–13 Hz) and transitions to a preponderance of slower, relatively low-voltage theta wave activity (2–7 Hz). NREM S1 typically ranges from 30 seconds to 7 minutes in duration and is marked by decreased EEG and EMG activity. The individual may report being awake and is easily aroused by environmental stimuli. During NREM Stage 2 (NREM S2), theta waves predominate with the phasic appearance of hallmark wave forms known as sleep spindles (waxing and waning, 12–14-Hz bursts, >0.5 seconds, typically lasting 1–2 sec) and K-complexes (negative sharp waves followed by a slower positive wave, ≥0.5 seconds). Both researchers and subjects report that unequivocal sleep begins during NREMS 2. After 15–30 minutes, most adults enter NREM Stages 3

and 4. These stages are collectively referred to as slow-wave sleep (SWS) or delta sleep, due to the predominance of well-synchronized delta wave forms (high-amplitude [>0.75 μV], low frequency [0.5–2 Hz EEG] activity). There is little movement during SWS, global cerebral metabolic function at it lowest (18), and the person may be very difficult to awaken. The majority of growth hormone is secreted in a pulsitile fashion during SWS (19) and disruption of SWS may be associated with malaise and myofascial pain (15,20).

The healthy adult sleeper returns briefly to NREM S1–2 and then enters the first REM sleep period, typically 90 minutes after sleep onset. Vivid dreams are frequently reported upon waking from REM sleep. REM sleep is characterized by low-voltage, mixed EEG frequencies similar to waking levels. Increased regional cerebral metabolic function is observed in the limbic system, brainstem, and occipital cortices; relative deactivation is observed in the frontal cortices (21). EMG-measured muscle tone is at its lowest level, reflecting an active motor inhibition process. Recent work on REM sleep suggests it may play a role in procedural memory (3) and mood regulation (4,22).

The 4 NREM sleep stages and REM sleep are expressed in cycles each night. In the first third of the night, SWS is dominant within a cycle. As sleep progresses, REM periods increase in duration and slow-wave activity diminishes. The average adult has 4–6 cycles per night depending on age, previous sleep history, and medications. Typical adult (young) sleep is allocated: NREM S1, 2–5%; NREM S2, 45–55%; SWS (NREM 3 and 4), 13–23%; and REM, 20–25% (23).

Sleep Requirements

In the United States, adults average 7–8 hours of sleep per night; however, there are large variations in individual requirements (24). It is widely observed that our society has a significant sleep debt due to the lack of adequate sleep, particularly among school-age children and working adults (25). The endogenous sleep-wake cycle is ~24.3 hours long and is entrained and regulated within a 24-hour day by light input from the optic nerves. The circadian master clock, located in the hypothalamic, suprachiasmatic nuclei, promotes sleep during the dark hours of the day when melatonin is secreted and peak alertness during daylight hours when melatonin is suppressed.

Sleep Across the Life Span

As the individual ages, there is a growing variability in quality and quantity of sleep. Babies and young children have a higher percentage of NREM S3–4 and there is less interindividual variation in sleep patterns. As the individual ages, there is an increasing tendency to spend less time in SWS and to sleep for shorter periods. The adolescent experiences a dramatic drop in the amount of time asleep, which decreases further to the range of 7–8 hours for adults. With older age, there is a decrease in sleep efficiency. Sleep efficiency is the amount of time sleeping divided by the amount of time in bed. Older adults have greater variability in their sleep patterns, but often maintain their usual amount of sleep via daytime napping. The elderly are subject to more

Table 1. Six main categories of sleep disturbance based on the International Classification of Sleep Disorders, Second Edition (ICSD-2) (27).

I. **Insomnias:** disorders initiating and maintaining sleep, including psychophysiologic insomnia ("primary"), insomnia due to a mental or medical disorder, paradoxical insomnia, etc.*

II. **Sleep-related breathing disorders:** obstructive sleep apnea, central sleep apnea, etc.

III. **Hypersomnia of central origin not due to a circadian rhythm sleep disorder, sleep-related breathing disorder, or other cause of disturbed nocturnal sleep:** narcolepsy with or without cataplexy, idiopathic hypersomnia, etc.

IV. **Circadian rhythm sleep disorders:** sleep disturbances caused by alterations in the circadian time-keeping system or misalignment between the endogenous circadian rhythm and exogenous factors that effect the timing and duration of sleep, e.g., delayed or advanced sleep phase disorders, jet lag, shift-work disorder, etc.

V. **Parasomnias:** undesirable physical events or experiences that occur during entry into sleep, within sleep, or during arousals from sleep, e.g., rapid eye movement sleep behavior disorder, night terrors, nightmare disorder, confusional arousals

VI. **Sleep-related movement disorders:** periodic limb movement disorder, restless legs syndrome, sleep bruxism, sleep-related leg cramps, etc.

* Psychophysiologic insomnia can and should be diagnosed when occurring within the context of medical and psychiatric comorbidity, if the problem is maintained in part by factors not directly related to the medical or psychiatric condition.

frequent midsleep awakenings. It is unknown whether older adults need less sleep or are simply less able to achieve the same amount or consolidation of sleep relative to middle age. Factors contributing to the changes in sleep quality may include degeneration of the nervous system, increasing prevalence of physical illness, alteration in the chronobiologic system, reduced level of physical activity, and continued expectation of previous sleep patterns (23,26).

SLEEP DISTURBANCES

The clinician can observe a wide variety of sleep problems within the population of persons with rheumatic disease that may, or may not, be related to the rheumatic disease. The 6 main categories of sleep disturbances are listed in Table 1 (27). Different types of sleep disorders are often seen in various age groups. In children, common problems are parasomnias, such as night terrors and enuresis, and fears related to separation at bedtime. Adolescents tend to suffer from sleep deprivation related to chronobiologic factors (circadian rhythm disorders, i.e., delayed sleep phase disorder), which manifests as prolonged sleep onset latency, difficulty rising in the morning, daytime sleepiness, but normal sleep latency and sleep duration with ad libitum sleep on weekends. Clinicians should be aware that in older adults, there is increasing prevalence of insomnia (19–38%), sleep apnea (19.7%), periodic limb movement disorder (4–11%), and restless legs syndrome (RLS; 9–20%) (28–30).

Epidemiology of Insomnia

Insomnia is the most common sleep disorder and includes difficulty initiating sleep, frequent or prolonged midsleep awakenings, early morning awakenings, or nonrestorative sleep that impacts daytime function. Due to the various definitions used in epidemiologic studies of insomnia, the true incidence and prevalence of persistent insomnia is not known, although rates generally range between 10% and 15% and between 19% and 38% for older adults (28). Transient insomnia (lasting <1 month) is quite common, impacting approximately one-third of adults. In the United States, ~40 million Americans have chronic sleep disorders and most cases go undiagnosed (25). Individuals with serious sleep problems have an almost 50% percent comorbidity rate of psychologic distress, anxiety, depression, and medical illness (25). Chronic insomnia is more commonly symptomatic of medical or psychiatric disturbance, although in can be a free-standing, primary disorder. Even in the presence of contributing medical and psychopathology, chronic insomnia is often associated with perpetuating behavioral factors, such as poor sleep hygiene, keeping irregular bed and wake times, excessive napping, and the learned habit of problem solving or ruminating in bed (31). In this case, individuals may be diagnosed with primary or psychophysiologic insomnia, despite having a comorbid major medical/psychiatric condition. However, teasing apart relative contributions to symptom presentation is often difficult. Effective management of insomnia begins with accurate diagnosis of the underlying causes or illness, but often may require targeted therapy to address maintaining factors.

SLEEP PROBLEMS IN RHEUMATIC DISEASE

Individuals with rheumatic disease are at risk for sleep problems due to chronic pain and increased incidence of depression. Pain is the most commonly cited cause of sleep problems by patients (32). Although sleep disturbance is often a consequence of mood disorder, it is also a well-established risk factor for new-onset depressive epidodes (9,33,34). Certain sleep disruptions have been linked with specific rheumatic diseases.

Fibromyalgia (FM)

Fibromyalgia has the most consistent and well-replicated association with sleep disruptions. Although current data do not establish whether sleep disruptions are a cause or effect of FM, a convergence of experimental and clinical data suggest that the relationship is likely to be reciprocal (35). Replicated longitudinal studies document both self-report and PSG evidence of sleep disruptions in persons with FM. Frequently reported is a pattern of increased nocturnal vigilance, light nonrestorative sleep, and sleep maintenance difficulty (36). These sleep complaints and patterns are associated with stiffness, fatigue, and cognitive disturbances in persons with FM (37). In FM and other rheumatologic conditions, a night of poor sleep is associated with a following day of enhanced pain intensity, which in turn is followed by a night of poor sleep (38,39).

In FM, polysomnographic sleep studies have repeatedly documented the intrusion of alpha waves without frank waking during NREM sleep (alpha sleep) (36). Alpha waves are generally indicative of arousal. The intrusion of this pattern into sleep stages is related to poor sleep quality reported by persons with FM (36). Increased alpha sleep is associated with increased pain reports in people with FM (36,40), and inducing deep pain during sleep is associated with an increase in this anomaly in healthy controls (41). However, this NREM sleep anomaly is not found in all patients with FM, and was first reported in psychiatric disorders, indicting the marker may be sensitive for, but not specific to, the nonrestorative sleep pattern associated with FM (42,43). More recent work has identified 3 distinct patterns of alpha sleep activity in persons with fibromyalgia, only one of which (phasic) was related to clinical manifestations of FM (44). This suggests the relationship between the sleep disturbance and clinical symptoms in FM is more complex than originally thought.

Other documented PSG anomalies include delayed sleep onset (45), reduced SWS (46), greater number of arousals (37,46), reduced REM sleep (46), greater sleep fragmentation (47), and greater wake time after sleep onset (46). Recent work has also demonstrated that women with FM have reduced sleep spindle activity, suggesting an impairment in sensory motor gating thought to be permissive of sleep (48). Other sleep disorders have been noted in persons with FM, including sleep apnea, periodic limb movement disorder, and RLS (49). Although present in a subset of persons with FM, early work suggests that neither sleep apnea nor periodic limb movements were consistently associated with the musculoskeletal symptoms of FM. However, recent work that more sensitively quantifies upper airway resistance (inspiratory flow limitations) has found a positive association between sleep-disordered breathing (not frank apnea) and fibromyalgia symptomotology in women (50). Furthermore, daytime symptoms improved after continuous positive airway pressure therapy, which reverses flow limitations. Sleep disruptions—motor agitation, nocturnal awakening, and nonfreshing sleep—seem to be prominent in children with FM, but may be different than those seen in adults (51).

Studies do not consistently observe reduced sleep time in persons with FM, suggesting it is the quality of sleep, indicated by alterations in sleep stages or increased arousal, rather than absolute sleep time that may be critical. The mechanism(s) by which sleep anomalies develop and are related to the etiology or maintenance of FM remain unclear. One line of inquiry suggests low levels of serotonin are related to decreased SWS, which may lead to development of FM (52). Secondly, low levels of the growth hormone somatomedin C have been identified in some patients with FM and may serve as a potential link between disturbed sleep and muscle pain (53). Finally, reductions in regional cerebral blood flow (rCBF) to the thalamus and caudate nucleus have been correlated with laboratory pain sensitivity and may be related to disruption of the neuroendcrine system and sleep architecture (54). Interestingly, a neuroimaging study of NREM sleep in primary insomnia also observed reductions in rCBF in the basal ganglia compared with matched controls, suggesting that insomnia may share a similar neurobiologic dysregulation with chronic pain (55). Taken together, this literature along with several experimental studies indicating that sleep disturbance may directly cause hyperalgesia (14,16), argues that sleep disturbance should be aggressively treated in FM.

Rheumatoid Arthritis (RA)

Sleep fragmentation—light, easily disrupted sleep, with multiple mid-sleep awakenings—has been observed by EEG and by self-report in adults (56,57) and children with RA (58). In adults, sleep fragmentation has been associated with higher pain reports and morning stiffness (59). Decreased time awake after sleep onset and decreased SWS predict pain and disease severity at 6 months (60). Clinicians should be aware that persons with RA who have cervical instability may be at increased risk for sleep apnea (61). Several reports suggest an increased prevalence of RLS in RA (62–64). One study found the prevalence of RLS in RA to be 25% and that the RLS paresthesias were positively correlated with RA disease severity (64). The degree of comorbidity between RLS and RA, and the cause for this association is not well established, but clinicians should assess for the cardinal symptoms of RLS (urge to move legs, distressing paresthesias or dysethesias in legs, which are relieved by movement or externally applied somatosensory input to the affected regions). Symptoms follow a prototypical circadian pattern with manifestation or worsening in the late evening and night. RA patients with RLS symptoms should be evaluated for other causes of RLS, including anemia (a serum ferritin test should be conducted) and peripheral neuropathy. Symptoms should be distinguished from movement needed to relieve positional discomfort due to arthritic pain (63). Dopaminergic and opioid therapies are effective treatments for RLS.

Osteoarthritis (OA)

Epidemiologic surveys consistently report that at least 50% of patients with OA have significant disturbances initiating or maintaining sleep (65–70). OASIS, a large-scale study of people with OA, reported that 58% of knee OA patients complain of problems maintaining sleep at least 3 nights per week (66). A study of 48 hip arthroplasty candidates found significant presurgical sleep maintenance disturbance, with diary and actigraphy sleep efficiency estimates of ~78%, well below the widely accepted "normal" minimum of 85% (71,72). Many other studies have corroborated that prolonged middle-of-the-night awakening is the most common form of insomnia reported by pain patients (70,73). Although PSG data in OA are scarce, one small PSG study found that 14 OA patients demonstrated an increase in NREM Stage 1 sleep, a decrease in NREM Stage 2 sleep, and more wake-after-sleep-onset time compared with controls (74). A report comparing 10 FM to 10 OA patients found both groups demonstrated similar sleep disturbance profiles, including prolonged sleep latency, prolonged middle awakenings, and frequent alpha intrusion (microarousal) during NREM S2 (75). These small studies suggest that the sleep of OA patients may be "lighter" than normal. Age and obesity are major risk factors for both knee/hip OA and obstructive sleep apnea. At least one study of OA patients awaiting arthroplasty found PSG-documented rates of sleep apnea to be ~6.7%, and that cases could easily be detected based on simple screening questions pertaining to loud persistent snoring, waking up gasping for breath, the presence of significant excessive daytime sleepiness (not fatigue), and the consideration of body mass index (76).

Other Rheumatic Diseases

Persons with primary Sjögren's syndrome report a variety of sleep problems, including midsleep awakenings and less efficient sleep (77). Poor sleep has been reported as a quality-of-life concern by the majority of samples of persons with ankylosing spondylitis (78).

A recent cross-sectional study of 100 women with systemic lupus erythematosus (SLE) found the self-reported prevalence of moderate-to-severe sleep disturbance to be 56%, with depressed mood, prednisone use, and decreased exercise being the primary correlates of poor sleep (79). Other self-report studies highlight an association between pain, fatigue, and poor sleep in SLE (80,81).

In systemic sclerosis (scleroderma), although data are limited, a PSG study of 27 consecutive clinic patients found decreased sleep efficiency, decreased REM sleep, increased SWS, and increased arousals relative to normative data. This study also reported a high rate of periodic limb movement disorder and RLS, indicating clinicians should actively assess and consider referral for these disorders in scleroderma. Esophageal dyskinesia and dyspnea were associated with sleep disturbance in scleroderma (82).

The importance of these observations for the etiology, prognosis, and treatment of Sjögren's syndrome, SLE, and scleroderma is unknown. The incidence, prevalence, and consequences of sleep problems in other forms of rheumatic diseases remain largely uninvestigated.

ASSESSMENT OF SLEEP PROBLEMS

A review of sleep parameters should be included in all patients' initial history. Critical information for the diagnosis and treatment planning is provided by a thorough review of medical, psychiatric, and family history; evaluation of medication usage; and an environmental assessment. Sleep patterns may be affected by pain, respiratory problems, psychiatric or neurologic conditions, medications, or environmental stimuli. Short-term complaints and difficulties need to be distinguished from chronic problems. Inquiry regarding what steps the patient has taken to address the sleep problem will indicate the chronicity and severity of the symptom. A complete history is often enhanced by involving the patient's bed partner. Careful review of medications is necessary to identify pharmacologic agents that may be disrupting sleep patterns. Some medications disrupt sleep during active use and others during the withdrawal period. Over-the-counter (OTC) medication review should not be overlooked. OTC agents contain substances that disrupt sleep, such as alcohol, caffeine, or phenylpropanolamine.

As part of the history and physical, assess the patient's behavior in terms of eating, substance use/abuse, exercise habits, sleep schedule, and presleep activities. An assessment of the individual's sleep environment in light of sleep hygiene principles is indicated.

A full physical and neurological examination with emphasis on detecting disorders that can affect the nervous system is indicated for those with severe sleep problems. Evaluation of anxiety and depression are critical because psychiatric illness is common in persons with sleep problems. If a mood disturbance is suspected, referral for psychiatric or behavioral sleep medicine evaluation is strongly recommended.

Sleep diaries are an inexpensive and convenient tool for assessing sleep problems. A week-long daily record of the individual's sleep patterns (including bedtime, rising time, midsleep awakenings, pain, mood, and medication use) is essential. Review of the diary with the patient provides useful data for diagnosis and treatment. Subsequent weekly diaries are also critical for evaluating treatment response.

Several self-report functional measures for monitoring outcomes in rheumatic disease are available and clinicians are encouraged to incorporate one into their assessment (see Chapter 10, Functional Ability). Several of these measures assess sleep quality, e.g., Multidimensional Health Assessment Questionnaire (83) and Nottingham Health Profile (84). Routine use of a functional assessment measure that includes an assessment of sleep parameters will aid in identifying sleep problems and determining the effectiveness of any subsequent treatment. Table 2 summarizes and compares several relatively brief, sleep-specific instruments that have been validated or often used in rheumatic conditions (85).

WHEN TO REFER FOR SLEEP EVALUATION

Referral for a sleep medicine evaluation depends on a number of factors, including the individual's presenting symptoms, duration of the problem, and impact on daytime function. Due to the close association between excessive daytime sleepiness (fighting to stay awake versus fatigue—decreased physical and mental energy, malaise, etc.) and potentially serious organic pathology, individuals with this presenting problem (especially those falling asleep at inappropriate times or places) should be strongly considered for referral to a sleep medicine specialist. When patients present with clear signs, symptoms, or risk factors for primary sleep disorders, such as sleep apnea (obesity, persistent loud snoring, daytime sleepiness), periodic limb movement disorder (report of repetitive leg jerks, daytime fatigue or sleepiness), or narcolepsy (persistent, often life-long, unexplained excessive daytime sleepiness with or without cataplexy), then a sleep disorders center evaluation is appropriate.

When patients present with insomnia ≥3 nights per week, in the absence of other primary sleep disorder symptoms, that does remit with standard treatment(s) for the identified comorbid medical/psychiatric conditions, a specialty evaluation should be considered based on the duration of the complaint or the severity of associated daytime impairment. Transient or acute insomnia lasting <1 month can often be effectively treated with a course of benzodiazepine receptor agonists (eszopiclone, zaleplon, zopidem) and may not warrant a specialty referral. Entrenched symptomotology, persistent for several months with obvious behavioral, psychological, or psychiatric components, are cases generally best evaluated and treated by a behavioral sleep medicine (BSM) specialist. BSM specialists are typically members of a multidisciplinary treatment team at most American Academy of Sleep Medicine accredited sleep disorders centers (see Table 3 for links to lists of accredited sleep disorders centers and certified BSM specialists by state).

TREATMENT OF PERSISTENT INSOMNIA

In treating sleep initiation and maintenance problems in persons with rheumatic diseases, optimizing treatment of underlying disease is a necessary first step. Special attention should be given to maximizing pain control at night and considering the use of adjunctive, sedating tricyclic antidepressants for pain, as appropriate (see below). A review and modification of the timing of medications that may disrupt sleep is especially important (e.g., clonidine, beta blockers, sympathomimetics, and possibly opioids, etc.) (86). Treatment of other medical, psychiatric, or primary sleep problems (e.g., sleep apnea, RLS) are a necessary part of initial efforts to improve sleep parameters. After maximizing disease management and ruling out intrinsic sleep disorders other than insomnia, a hierarchical approach to the treatment of insomnia is recommended (Table 4).

A reasonable first approach would be to assess and address sleep hygiene practices before referring the patient for specialized cognitive-behavioral therapy or psychopharmacology for insomnia. The following treatment recommendations are based largely on studies in nonrheumatic disease populations; when available, specific data is presented on rheumatic disease patients.

Sleep Hygiene Education

Sleep hygiene education involves using motivational interviewing to teach subjects about environmental and behavioral factors (e.g., alcohol, exercise, light exposure, etc.) that may influence sleep (87,88). Poor sleep hygiene may be both a risk factor and a contributing factor for developing insomnia (89). Sleep hygiene recommendations provided in brief oral or written form are unlikely to change behavior or have any impact on the sleep problem. Effective sleep hygiene intervention requires ongoing counseling and contact with the patient to translate the advice into behavior change. Sleep hygiene principles are listed in Table 5. Because it is difficult to modify several habits at once, the clinician and patient should identify 1 or 2 initial habits to target, establish those new behaviors, and then address additional behaviors. For chronic insomnia that has multiple behavioral, medical, and psychosocial contributions, sleep hygiene education, although necessary, is often ineffective as a monotherapy and should not be considered full cognitive-behavior therapy for insomnia (CBT-I).

Exercise is one particularly beneficial sleep hygiene principle that should be emphasized in rheumatic disease (90). Exercise has been shown to an effective intervention for improving sleep parameters and other symptoms in persons with FM, but problems with compliance often undermine long-term benefits (91). The potential for improving sleep quality and quantity is one of many compelling reasons for including exercise in a self-management program for persons with rheumatic disease.

Table 2. Self-reported sleep measures*

Instrument	Content	Item formats	Response format	Method of administration	Time for administration	Primary scale outputs	Validated populations	Reliability	Validity	Responsiveness
								Psychometric properties		
PSQI	Sleep-wake patterns, sleep duration, sleep latency, frequency and severity of sleep disturbances, use of sleep medications, daytime consequences, overall and global sleep quality	19 items; questions pertaining to sleep continuity parameters and graded severity and frequency of common sleep disturbances and behaviors	Some free-entry and 4-point Likert scale items	Self	5–10 min	Global Sleep Quality Score with established cut-offs; 7 subscales	General sleep disorders; insomnia; breast cancer; transplant patients *Used in rheumatology?* chronic pain; fibromyalgia; TMD	Good	Good	Insufficient data
ISI	Severity of sleep onset, maintenance, and early morning awakening insomnia; sleep satisfaction; insomnia-related distress; daytime impairment	7 items; severity ratings of insomnia symptoms	5-point Likert scale	Self, clinician interview, and significant other report	5 min or less	Overall severity index with established cut-offs	Primary insomnia and medical or psychiatric insomnia *Used in rheumatology?* chronic pain	Good	Good	Good
PSD	Timing of meals, stimulants, medications, exercise, napping, bed and wake times, sleep continuity parameters, sleep quality, mood and alertness on waking	17 items; diary entries made twice a day (morning and night)	Free response to standard questions, some categorical and 6-point Likert scale items	Self	10 min	Sleep latency, number of awakenings, wake-after-sleep-onset time, total sleep time, sleep efficiency	Sleep disorders *Used in rheumatology?* similar diaries used in chronic pain and fibromyalgia	Good	Good	Good
MOS	Sleep initiation, quantity, maintenance, respiratory problems, perceived adequacy of sleep, somnolence	12 items; sleep continuity and graded severity of common sleep disturbances	Free response and 6-point Likert scale	Self, clinician interview	5 min or less	Overall sleep problem severity index	Primary care and multispecialty care patients *Used in rheumatology?* arthritis samples, back problems	Good	Fair	Insufficient data

* PSQI = Pittsburgh Sleep Quality Index; TMD = temporomandibular joint disorder; ISI = Insomnia Severity Index; PSD = Pittsburgh Sleep Diary; MOS = Medical Outcomes Study. Reprinted with permission from reference 85.

Table 3. Suggested sleep resources

- American Academy of Sleep Medicine (AASM); URL: http://www.aasmnet. org/
- List of AASM-accredited sleep disorders centers by state; URL: http://www. sleepcenters.org/
- List of AASM providers certified in behavioral sleep medicine by state; URL: http://www.aasmnet.org/BSME.aspx
- National Sleep Foundation; URL: http://www.sleepfoundation.org

Cognitive-Behavior Therapy for Insomnia

CBT-I alters maladaptive compensatory strategies (e.g., using alcohol, spending excessive time in bed) and cognitive processes (92) that play a maintaining role in sleep disturbance (93,94). It is typically conducted by a behavioral sleep medicine specialist in 4–8 sessions. CBT-I is a data-driven therapy comprised of a number of well-validated interventions, including stimulus control therapy (SCT) (95), sleep restriction therapy (SRT) (96), and cognitive therapies (71,97). Many of these procedures are effectively combined as multicomponent approaches (31). CBT-I that includes SCT is identified by the American Academy of Sleep Medicine as a "standard" treatment for primary insomnia (98,99), based on the strong evidence attesting to its efficacy (100–103). This evidence includes double-blind, randomized, placebo-controlled trials (104), a meta-analysis demonstrating comparable short-term efficacy to benzodiazepine receptor agonists (105), and a meta-analysis demonstrating that CBT-I is efficacious in older adults (106). As an additional benefit, in contrast to pharmacotherapy, the long-term effects of CBT-I are well maintained for as long as 2 years (102,107,108), even after discontinuation of treatment. Recent work has shown that CBT-I, which includes sleep restriction and stimulus control procedures, not only improves objective measures of sleep continuity (104,109), but it may also improve measures of rCBF (110) and sleep microstructure, notably increasing delta power and reducing faster frequency activity (alpha and beta) (111,112). This may be of particular benefit to rheumatic patients.

An accumulating literature base demonstrates the efficacy of CBT-I in psychiatric and medical disorders with generally large effect sizes (i.e., Cohen's $d \geq 0.8$ for wake-after-sleep-onset time) (35,113). Moreover, several recent studies of insomnia occurring in the context of medical disorders have included large samples of chronic pain patients (114–118). In a recent placebo-controlled study that included OA patients, improvement was found on multiple diary measures of sleep outcomes (119). To date, however, there have been only 2 studies of CBT-I exclusive to pain-related disorders. One showed significant posttreatment improvements in sleep continuity in the CBT-I group (120), with large effect sizes (0.80). The CBT-I group also showed a trend toward greater reductions in pain severity ($P = 0.12$; Currie SR: personal communication).

Table 4. Sleep management*

Sleep hygiene	Avoid over-the-counter sleep aids
	Avoid late meals
	Reduce caffeine and alcohol intake
	Exercise regularly
	Develop a regular sleep schedule
	Maintain a cool, well-ventilated, quiet room
Behavior therapy	Relaxation therapy
	Sleep habit training
Pharmacotherapy	Sedative and hypnotic agents
	Low-dose antidepressants

* Once rheumatic disease management is maximized these additional steps are taken to address sleep problems. Adapted from the ARHP Teaching Slide Collection for Clinicians and Educators, Assessment and Management of the Rheumatic Diseases, 3rd Edition.

Table 5. Sleep hygiene principles

Regular sleep patterns
  Go to bed and arise the same time each day
  Avoid naps, except for brief (<30 minutes) periods 8 hours after rising
  Take a hot (30-minute) bath to raise core body temperature 1.5–2 hours before bedtime
  Avoid bright light if you have to arise during the sleep period
  Ensure adequate light exposure in the morning and into the late evening

Environmental factors
  Avoid large meals 2–3 hours before bedtime
  Establish a bedtime ritual
  Keep clock face turned away
  Keep sleeping environment dark, quiet, and comfortable
  Consider using a white noise machine to screen out background noise

Exercise
  Regular exercise each day
  Avoid vigorous exercise 2 hours prior to bedtime

Drug effects
  Give up smoking entirely or avoid smoking several hours before bedtime
  Do not smoke if you have a midsleep awakening
  Limit use of alcoholic beverages because they fragment sleep
  Discontinue caffeine use–caffeinated coffee, tea, soft drinks
  Avoid use of over-the-counter sleep medications

Aging
  Educate patients regarding changes in sleep parameters that occur with age to reduce unrealistic expectations and anxiety

The pain-reduction effect size at 3 months for CBT-I was 0.56 (moderate) compared with 0.15 for the waitlist control group. A more recent study by Edinger and colleagues in patients with FM demonstrated the relative efficacy of CBT-I compared with either sleep hygiene or usual medical care (121). CBT-I produced a 50% reduction in wake-after-sleep-onset time, which was superior to usual care and sleep hygiene. This study also found a significant reduction in clinical pain at the end of treatment and at 6 months posttreatment, which was evident only for those who engaged in SCT and SRT. In pooled analyses, improvement in pain was associated with reductions in wake time (r = 0.34, P < 0.05). These 2 studies strongly suggest that standard CBT-I interventions are likely to produce significant reductions in clinical pain over long-term followup.

Pharmacologic Interventions

Optimal medical management of the rheumatic disease is the initial intervention for patients whose sleep problem is related to their primary disease process. Adequate dosing and optimal timing of nonsteroidal antiinflammatory drugs or analgesic medication may facilitate restful sleep. This section will focus specifically on medications to improve sleep parameters.

The most appropriate use of hypnotic medication is in individuals with sleep problems of recent onset. The role of hypnotics in chronic insomnia is less clear and should only be used as part of a coordinated clinical management strategy to address the underlying problems. If chronic use is anticipated and the sleep disturbance is related to pain or fibromyalgia, consider the use of a tricyclic antidepressant (122). Duration of action is the primary consideration in choosing a hypnotic agent. This duration is determined by rates of absorption, distribution, and elimination. The choice of hypnotic is based on whether the intended effect is to reduce time to sleep onset, midsleep awakenings, or anxiety related to sleep disturbance. If the main difficulty is falling asleep, rapidly eliminated agents, such as zaleplon or zolpidem (5–15 mg) or midazolam (7.5 mg) should be considered. Zolpidem (5–15 mg) has demonstrated efficacy in FM (123).

When frequent midsleep awakenings are the problem, hypnotics with moderate duration of action but rapid elimination may be helpful (e.g., zopiclone, 3.75–7.5 mg; eszopiclone, 1–3 mg; zolpidem, extended release 6.5 mg in the elderly or 12.5 mg; and brotizolam, 0.125–0.25 mg). In persons with RA, short-term zopiclone (7.5 mg) was effective in improving subjective sleep complaints (124). The clinician must be mindful of residual effects and inevitable accumulation that can occur with some longer-acting benzodiazepines, such as flurazepam and nitrazepam. Use the smallest dosage possible and avoid chronic use of hypnotic agents, particularly traditional benzodiazepine hypnotics. The newer benzodiazepine receptor agonists (zolpidem, zaleplon, eszopiclone, zopiclone) have better safety profiles and have been associated with minimal rebound insomnia or tolerance, even with relatively long-term nightly use (6 months) (125). Therefore, these agents are recommended before initiating benzodiazepines, which may also aggravate obstructive sleep apnea due to their myorelaxing properties. Special care must be taken in the elderly due to the slowing of metabolism, which may result in higher plasma levels and greater sensitivity of the central nervous system. Benzodiazepines and even some of the newer benzodiazepine receptor agonists have been associated with increased falls and hip fractures in the frail elderly (126,127). If sleep disturbance persists, further diagnostic evaluation and treatment of underlying causes is indicated.

As a group, sedating tricyclic (e.g., amitriptyline, nortriptyline) and tetracyclic (e.g., trazodone) antidepressants in less than antidepressant doses at bedtime can be effective in reducing sleep disturbances, particularly in persons with FM (122). Antidepressants as a group, both tricyclics and selective serotonin reuptake inhibitors (SSRIs), appear to improve self-reported sleep parameters, pain, fatigue, and wellbeing, but not trigger points. However, it is not clear if these improvements are independent of depression (128). In FM, the effectiveness of amitriptyline or fluoxetine alone to improve sleep quality may diminish over time (129–132). One study indicated a combination of fluoxetine (20 mg every morning) and amitriptyline (25 mg at bedtime) may be more effective than either agent alone (132). The effect of tricyclic antidepressants on the alpha EEG NREM sleep anomaly is unclear (52). The positive effect of these agents needs to be weighed against the side effects related to their anticholinergic activity and possible cardiotoxicity, particularly in the elderly. For a significant minority of patients, SSRIs have a negative effect on sleep (133). For those individuals with sleep disturbances and concomitant depression, agents that block the serotonin type 2 receptor (e.g., nefazodone) have demonstrated acute beneficial effects (133).

Cyclobenzaprine (10–40 mg/day) has also demonstrated improvement in total sleep time in persons with FM (129), although this may be contraindicated for individuals with sleep apnea. Alternative therapies for sleep and pain that should be considered experimental, requiring further study, are gamma-hydroxybutyrate (GHB) and melatonin. GHB is known to enhance SWS and preliminary work in FM suggests that it may improve sleep and daytime symptoms (134). Although the literature is mixed regarding whether FM patients may have underlying chronobiologic dysregulation and/or an abnormal melatonin profile (135–137), some uncontrolled work suggests that melatonin supplementation may be helpful for some patients (138,139).

REFERENCES

1. Siegel JM. Clues to the functions of mammalian sleep. Nature 2005;437:1264–71.
2. Steriade M, Timofeev I. Neuronal plasticity in thalamocortical networks during sleep and waking oscillations. Neuron 2003;37:563–76.
3. Stickgold R, Hobson JA, Fosse R, Fosse M. Sleep, learning, and dreams: off-line memory reprocessing. Science 2001;294:1052–7.
4. Cartwright RD, Luten A, Young M, Mercer P, Bears M. Role of REM sleep and dream affect in overnight mood regulation: a study of normal volunteers. Psych Res 1998;81:1–8.
5. Mallon L, Broman JE, Hetta J. Relationship between insomnia, depression, and mortality: a 12-year follow-up of older adults in the community. Int Psychogeriatr 2000;12:295–306.
6. Mallon L, Broman JE, Hetta J. Sleep complaints predict coronary artery disease mortality in males: a 12-year follow-up study of a middle-aged Swedish population. J Intern Med 2002;251:207–16.
7. Meisinger C, Heier M, Loewel H. Sleep disturbance as a predictor of type 2 diabetes mellitus in men and women from the general population. Diabetologia 2005;48:235–41.
8. Mikkelsson M, Sourander A, Salminen JJ, Kautiainen H, Piha J. Widespread pain and neck pain in schoolchildren: a prospective one-year follow-up study. Acta Paediatr 1999;88:1119–24.
9. Breslau N, Roth T, Rosenthal L, Andreski P. Sleep disturbance and psychiatric disorders: a longitudinal epidemiological study of young adults. Biol Psychiatry 1996;39:411–8.
10. Spiegel K, Leproult R, van Cauter E. Impact of sleep debt on metabolic and endocrine function. Lancet 1999;354:1435–9.
11. Irwin M, McClintick J, Costlow C, Fortner M, White J, Gillin JC. Partial night sleep deprivation reduces natural killer and cellular immune responses in humans. FASEB J 1996;10:643–53.
12. Vgontzas AN, Zoumakis E, Bixler EO, Lin HM, Follett H, Kales A, et al. Adverse effects of modest sleep restriction on sleepiness, performance, and inflammatory cytokines. J Clin Endocrinol Metab 2004;89:2119–26.
13. Vgontzas AN, Zoumakis M, Papanicolaou DA, Bixler EO, Prolo P, Lin HM, et al. Chronic insomnia is associated with a shift of interleukin-6 and tumor necrosis factor secretion from nighttime to daytime. Metabolism 2002;51:887–92.
14. Kundermann B, Spernal J, Huber MT, Krieg JC, Lautenbacher S. Sleep deprivation affects thermal pain thresholds but not somatosensory thresholds in healthy volunteers. Psychosom Med 2004;66:932–7.
15. Lentz MJ, Landis CA, Rothermel J, Shaver JL. Effects of selective slow wave sleep disruption on musculoskeletal pain and fatigue in middle aged women. J Rheumatol 1999;26:1586–92.
16. Roehrs TA, Hyde M, Blaisdell MS, Greenwald M, Roth T. Sleep loss and REM sleep loss are hyperalgesic. Sleep 2006;29:145–51.
17. Rechtschaffen A, Kales A. A manual of standardized terminology, techniques and scoring system for sleep stages of human subjects. Washington (DC): U.S. Government Printing Office; 1968.
18. Maquet P. Positron emission tomography studies of sleep and sleep disorders. J Neurol 1997;244(4 Suppl 1):S23–8.
19. van Cauter E, Latta F, Nedeltcheva A, Spiegel K, Leproult R, Vandenbril C, et al. Reciprocal interactions between the GH axis and sleep. Growth Horm IGF Res 2004;14 (Suppl A):S10–7.
20. Moldofsky H, Scarisbrick P. Induction of neurasthenic musculoskeletal pain syndrome by selective sleep stage deprivation. Psychosom Med 1976;38:35–44.
21. Braun AR, Balkin TJ, Wesenten NJ, Carson RE, Varga M, Baldwin P, et al. Regional cerebral blood flow throughout the sleep-wake cycle: an H2(15) O PET study. Brain 1997;120:1173–97.
22. Cartwright R, Agargun MY, Kirkby J, Friedman JK. Relation of dreams to waking concerns. Psychiatry Res 2006;141:261–70.
23. Carskadon M, Dement WC. Normal human sleep. In: Kryger M, Roth T, Dement WC, editors. Principles and practice of sleep medicine. Philadelphia: Elsevier Saunders; 2005. p. 13–23.
24. Gallup Organization. Sleep in america. Princeton (NJ): The Gallup Organization; 1995.
25. National Commission on Sleep Disorders Research. Wake up America a national sleep alert. Program 470-M. Washington (DC): Department of Health and Human Services; 1993.
26. Vitiello MV, Moe KE, Prinz PN. Sleep complaints cosegregate with illness in older adults: clinical research informed by and informing epidemiological studies of sleep. J Psychosom Res 2002;53:555–9.
27. American Academy of Sleep Medicine. The International Classification of Sleep Disorders: diagnostic and coding manual, 2nd ed. Westchester (IL): American Academy of Sleep Medicine; 2005.
28. Bliwise DL. Normal aging. In: Kryger MH, Roth T, Dement WC, editors. Principles and practice of sleep medicine. Philadelphia: Elsevier; 2006. p. 24–38.
29. Haas DC, Foster GL, Nieto FJ, Redline S, Resnick HE, Robbins JA, et al. Age-dependent associations between sleep-disordered breathing and hypertension: importance of discriminating between systolic/diastolic hypertension and isolated systolic hypertension in the Sleep Heart Health Study. Circulation 2005;111:614–21.
30. Hornyak M, Trenkwalder C. Restless legs syndrome and periodic limb movement disorder in the elderly. J Psychosom Res 2004;56:543–8.

31. Smith MT, Neubauer DN. Cognitive behavior therapy for chronic insomnia. Clin Cornerstone 2003;5:28–40.

32. Leigh TJ, Bird HA, Hindmarch I, Wright V. A comparison of sleep in rheumatic and non-rheumatic patients. Clin Exp Rheumatol 1987;5:363–5.

33. Ford DE, Kamerow DB. Epidemiologic study of sleep disturbances and psychiatric disorders: an opportunity for prevention? JAMA 1989;262:1479–84.

34. Dryman A, Eaton WW. Affective symptoms associated with the onset of major depression in the community: findings from the US National Institute of Mental Health Epidemiologic Catchment Area Program. Acta Psychiatr Scand 1991;84:1–5.

35. Smith MT, Haythornthwaite JA. How do sleep disturbance and chronic pain inter-relate? Insights from the longitudinal and cognitive-behavioral clinical trials literature. Sleep Med Rev 2004;8:119–32.

36. Moldofsky H. Sleep and fibrositis syndrome. Rheum Dis Clin North Am 1989;15:91–103.

37. Jennum P, Drewes AM, Andreasen A, Nielsen KD. Sleep and other symptoms in primary fibromyalgia and in healthy controls. J Rheumatol 1993;20:1756–9.

38. Affleck G, Urrows S, Tennen H, Higgins P, Abeles M. Sequential daily relations of sleep, pain intensity, and attention to pain among women with fibromyalgia. Pain 1996;68:363–8.

39. Stone AA, Broderick JE, Porter LS, Kaell AT. The experience of rheumatoid arthritis pain and fatigue: examining momentary reports and correlates over one week. Arthritis Care Res 1997;10:185–93.

40. Drewes A, Nielsen K, Jennum P, Andreasen A. Alpha intrusion in fibromyalgia. J Musculoskel Pain 1993;3:223–8.

41. Drewes AM, Nielsen KD, Arendt-Nielsen L, Birket-Smith L, Hansen LM. The effect of cutaneous and deep pain on the electroencephalogram during sleep—an experimental study. Sleep 1997;20:632–40.

42. Mahowald ML, Mahowald MW. Nighttime sleep and daytime functioning (sleepiness and fatigue) in less well-defined chronic rheumatic diseases with particular reference to the 'alpha-delta NREM sleep anomaly'. Sleep Med 2000;1:195–207.

43. Rains JC, Penzien DB. Sleep and chronic pain: challenges to the alpha-EEG sleep pattern as a pain specific sleep anomaly. 1. J Psychosom Res 2003;54:77–83.

44. Roizenblatt S, Moldofsky H, Benedito-Silva AA, Tufik S. Alpha sleep characteristics in fibromyalgia. Arthritis Rheum 2001;44:222–30.

45. Horne J, Shackell B. Alpha-like EEG activity in non-REM sleep and the fibromyalgia (fibrositis) syndrome. Electroencephalogr Clin Neurophysiol 1991;79:271–6.

46. Branco J, Atalaia A, Paiva T. Sleep cycles and alpha-delta sleep in fibromyalgia syndrome. J Rheumatol 1994;21:1113–7.

47. Shaver JL, Lentz M, Landis CA, Heitkemper MM, Buchwald DS, Woods NF. Sleep, psychological distress, and stress arousal in women with fibromyalgia. Res Nurs Health 1997;20:247–57.

48. Landis CA, Lentz MJ, Rothermel J, Buchwald D, Shaver JL. Decreased sleep spindles and spindle activity in midlife women with fibromyalgia and pain. Sleep 2004;27:741–50.

49. Lario BA, Teran J, Alonso J, Arroyo I, Viejo JL. Lack of association between fibromyalgia and sleep apnea syndrome. Ann Rheum Disease 1992;51:108–111.

50. Gold AR, Dipalo F, Gold MS, Broderick J. Inspiratory airflow dynamics during sleep in women with fibromyalgia. Sleep 2004;27:459–66.

51. Kashikar-Zuck S, Graham TB, Huenefeld MD, Powers SW. A review of biobehavioral research in juvenile primary fibromyalgia syndrome. Arthritis Care Res 2000;13:388–97.

52. Carette S, Oakson G, Guimont C, Steriade M. Sleep electroencephalography and the clinical response to amitriptyline in patients with fibromyalgia. Arthritis Rheum 1995;38:1211–7.

53. Bennett RM, Clark SR, Campbell SM, Burckhardt CS. Low levels of somatomedin C in patients with the fibromyalgia syndrome: a possible link between sleep and muscle pain. Arthritis Rheum 1992;35:1113–6.

54. Mountz JM, Bradley LA, Modell JG, Alexander RW, Triana-Alexander M, Aaron LA, et al. Fibromyalgia in women: abnormalities of regional cerebral blood flow in the thalamus and the caudate-nucleus are associated with low pain threshold levels. Arthritis Rheum 1995;38:926–38.

55. Smith MT, Perlis ML, Chengazi VU, Pennington J, Soeffing J, Ryan JM, et al. Neuroimaging of NREM sleep in primary insomnia: a Tc-99-HMPAO single photon emission computed tomography study. Sleep 2002;25:325–35.

56. Mahowald MW, Mahowald ML, Bundlie SR, Ytterberg SR. Sleep fragmentation in rheumatoid arthritis. Arthritis Rheum 1989;32:974–83.

57. Hirsch M, Carlander B, Verge M, Tafti M, Anaya J, Billiard M, et al. Objective and subjective sleep disturbances in patients with rheumatoid arthritis. Arthritis Rheum 1994;37:41–9.

58. Zamir G, Press J, Tal A, Tarasiuk A. Sleep fragmentation in children with juvenile rheumatoid arthritis. J Rheumatol 1998;25:1191–7.

59. Drewes AM, Svendsen L, Taagholt SJ, Bjerregard K, Nielsen KD, Hansen B. Sleep in rheumatoid arthritis: a comparison with healthy subjects and studies of sleep/wake interactions. Br J Rheumatol 1998;37:71–81.

60. Drewes AM, Nielsen KD, Hansen B, Taagholt SJ, Bjerregard K, Svendsen L. A longitudinal study of clinical symptoms and sleep parameters in rheumatoid arthritis. Rheumatology (Oxford) 2000;39:1287–9.

61. Drossaers-Bakker KW, Hamburger HL, Bongartz EB, Dijkmans BA, Van Soesbergen RM. Sleep apnoea caused by rheumatoid arthritis. Br J Rheumatol 1998;37:889–94.

62. O'Keeffe ST. Restless legs syndrome: a review. Arch Intern Med 1996;156:243–8.

63. Trenkwalder C, Paulus W, Walters AS. The restless legs syndrome. Lancet Neurol 2005;4:465–75.

64. Salih AM, Gray RE, Mills KR, Webley M. A clinical, serological and neurophysiological study of restless legs syndrome in rheumatoid arthritis. Br J Rheumatol 1994;33:60–3.

65. Leigh TJ, Bird HA, Hindmarch I, Wright V. A comparison of sleep in rheumatic and non-rheumatic patients. Clin Exp Rheumatol 1987;5:363–5.

66. Wilcox S, Brenes GA, Levine D, Sevick MA, Shumaker SA, Craven T. Factors related to sleep disturbance in older adults experiencing knee pain or knee pain with radiographic evidence of knee osteoarthritis. J Am Geriatr Soc 2000;48:1241–51.

67. Gallup Organization. Adult public's expereinces with nighttime pain. Washington (DC): National Sleep Foundation; 1997.

68. Davis GC. Improved sleep may reduce arthritis pain. Holist Nurs Pract 2003;17:128–35.

68. Gallup Organization. Sleep and aging. Washington (DC): National Sleep Foundation; 1996.

70. Ohayon MM. Relationship between chronic painful physical condition and insomnia. J Psychiatr Res 2005;39:151–9.

71. Morin CM. Insomnia: psychological assessment and management. New York: Guilford Press; 1993.

72. Edinger JD, Bonnet MH, Bootzin RR, Doghramji K, Dorsey CM, Espie CA, et al. Derivation of research diagnostic criteria for insomnia: report of an American Academy of Sleep Medicine Work Group. Sleep 2004;27:1567–96.

73. Smith MT, Perlis ML, Smith MS, Giles DE, Carmody TP. Sleep quality and presleep arousal in chronic pain. J Behav Med 2000;23:1–13.

74. Leigh TJ, Hindmarch I, Bird HA, Wright V. Comparison of sleep in osteoarthritic patients and age and sex matched healthy controls. Ann Rheum Dis 1988;47:40–2.

75. Doherty M, Smith J. Elusive 'alpha-delta' sleep in fibromyalgia and osteoarthritis. Ann Rheum Dis 1993;52:245.

76. Harrison MM, Childs A, Carson PE. Incidence of undiagnosed sleep apnea in patients scheduled for elective total joint arthroplasty. J Arthroplasty 2003;18:1044–7.

77. Tishler M, Barak Y, Paran D, Yaron M. Sleep disturbances, fibromyalgia and primary Sjogren's syndrome. Clin Exp Rheumatol 1997;15:71–4.

78. Ward MM. Health-related quality of life in ankylosing spondylitis: a survey of 175 patients. Arthritis Care Res 1999;12:247–55.

79. Costa DD, Bernatsky S, Dritsa M, Clarke AE, Dasgupta K, Keshani A, et al. Determinants of sleep quality in women with systemic lupus erythematosus. Arthritis Rheum 2005;53:272–8.

80. Gudbjornsson B, Hetta J. Sleep disturbances in patients with systemic lupus erythematosus: a questionnaire-based study. Clin Exp Rheumatol 2001;19:509–14.

81. Tench CM, McCurdie I, White PD, D'Cruz DP. The prevalence and associations of fatigue in systemic lupus erythematosus. Rheumatology (Oxford) 2000;39:1249–54.

82. Prado GF, Allen RP, Trevisani VM, Toscano VG, Earley CJ. Sleep disruption in systemic sclerosis (scleroderma) patients: clinical and polysomnographic findings. Sleep Med 2002;3:341–5.

83. Pincus T, Swearingen C, Wolfe F. Toward a multidimensional Health Assessment Questionnaire (MDHAQ): assessment of advanced activities of daily living and psychological status in the patient-friendly health assessment questionnaire format. Arthritis Rheum 1999;42:2220–30.

84. Houssien DA, McKenna SP, Scott DL. The Nottingham Health Profile as a measure of disease activity and outcome in rheumatoid arthritis. Br J Rheumatol 1997;36:69–73.

85. Smith MT, Wegener ST. Measures of sleep. Arthritis Rheum 2003;49 (5 suppl):S184–96.

86. Shaw IR, Lavigne G, Mayer P, Choiniere M. Acute intravenous administration of morphine perturbs sleep architecture in healthy pain-free young adults: a preliminary study. Sleep 2005;28:677–82.

87. Kleitman N. Sleep and wakefulness. Chicago: University of Chicago Press; 1987.

88. Zarcone VP. Sleep hygiene. In: Kryger MH, Roth T, Dement WC, editors. Principles and practice of sleep medicine. Philadelphia: Saunders; 1989.

89. Jefferson CD, Drake CL, Scofield HM, Myers E, McClure T, Roehrs T, et al. Sleep hygiene practices in a population-based sample of insomniacs. Sleep 2005;28:611–5.

90. Fontaine KR, Heo M, Bathon J. Are US adults with arthritis meeting public health recommendations for physical activity? Arthritis Rheum 2004;50:624–8.

91. Wigers SH, Stiles TC, Vogel PA. Effects of aerobic exercise versus stress management treatment in fibromyalgia: A 4.5 year prospective study. Scand J Rheumatol 1996;25:77–86.

92. Smith MT, Perlis ML, Smith MS, Giles DE. Pre-sleep cognitions in patients with insomnia secondary to chronic pain. J Behav Med 2001;24:93–114.

93. Buysse DJ, Reynolds CF III, Kupfer DJ, Thorpy MJ, Bixler E, Manfredi R, et al. Clinical diagnoses in 216 insomnia patients using the International Classification of Sleep Disorders (ICDS), DSM-IV and ICD-10 categories: a report from the APA/NIMH DSV-IV field trial. Sleep 1994;17:630–7.

94. Spielman A, Caruso L, Glovinsky P. A behavioral perspective on insomnia treatment. Psychiatr Clin North Am 1987;10:541–53.

95. Bootzin RR. Stimulus control treatment for insomnia. Proceedings, 80th Annual Convention of the American Psychiatric Association 1972;395–6.

96. Spielman AJ, Saskin P, Thorpy MJ. Treatment of chronic insomnia by restriction of time in bed. Sleep 1987;10:45–56.

97. Harvey AG, Payne S. The management of unwanted pre-sleep thoughts in insomnia: distraction with imagery versus general distraction. Behav Res Ther 2002;40:267–77.

98. Chesson AL Jr, Anderson WM, Littner M, Davila D, Hartse K, Johnson S, et al. Practice parameters for the nonpharmacologic treatment of chronic insomnia: an American Academy of Sleep Medicine report. Sleep 1999;22:1128–33.

99. Morin CM, Bootzin RR, Buysee DJ, Edinger JD, Espie CA, Lichstein KL. Psychological and behavioral treatment of insomnia: an update of recent evidence (1998–2004). Sleep. In press.

100. Murtagh DR, Greenwood KM. Identifying effective psychological treatments for insomnia: a meta-analysis. J Consult Clin Psychol 1995;63:79–89.

101. Morin CM, Culbert JP, Schwartz SM. Nonpharmacological interventions for insomnia: a meta-analysis of treatment efficacy. Am J Psychiatry 1994;151:1172–80.

102. Morin CM, Colecchi C, Stone J, Sood R, Brink D. Behavioral and pharmacological therapies for late-life insomnia: a randomized controlled trial. JAMA 1999;281:991–9.

103. Riedel BW, Lichstein KL, Dwyer WO. Sleep compression and sleep education for older insomniacs: self- help versus therapist guidance. Psychol Aging 1995;10:54–63.

104. Edinger JD, Wohlgemuth WK, Radtke RA, Marsh GR, Quillian RE. Cognitive behavioral therapy for treatment of chronic primary insomnia: a randomized controlled trial. JAMA 2001;285:1856–64.

105. Smith MT, Perlis ML, Park A, Smith MS, Pennington JY, Giles DE, et al. Comparative meta-analysis of pharmacotherapy and behavior therapy for persistent insomnia. Am J Psychiatry 2002;159:5–11.

106. Irwin M, Cole JC, Nicassio PM. Comparative meta-analysis of behavioral interventions for insomnia and their efficacy in adults and in older adults 55+ years. Health Psychol 2006;25:3–14.

107. Milby JB, Williams V, Hall JN, Khuder S, McGill T, Wooten V. Effectiveness of combined triazolam-behavioral therapy for primary insomnia. Am J Psychiatry 1993;150:1259–60.

108. McClusky HY, Milby JB, Switzer PK, Williams V, Wooten V. Efficacy of behavioral versus triazolam treatment in persistent sleep-onset insomnia. Am J Psychiatry 1991;148:121–6.

109. Jacobs GD, Pace-Schott EF, Stickgold R, Otto MW. Cognitive behavior therapy and pharmacotherapy for insomnia: a randomized controlled trial and direct comparison. Arch Intern Med 2004;164:1888–96.

110. Smith MT, Perlis ML, Chengazi VU, Soeffing J, McCann U. NREM sleep cerebral blood flow before and after behavior therapy for chronic primary insomnia: preliminary single photon emission computed tomography (SPECT) data. Sleep Med 2005;6:93–4.

111. Cervena K, Dauvilliers Y, Espa F, Touchon J, Matousek M, Billiard M, et al. Effect of cognitive behavioural therapy for insomnia on sleep architecture and sleep EEG power spectra in psychophysiological insomnia. J Sleep Res 2004;13:385–93.

112. Besset A, Villemin E, Tafti M, Billiard M. Homeostatic process and sleep spindles in patients with sleep-maintenance insomnia: effect of partial (21 h) sleep deprivation. Electroencephalogr Clin Neurophysiol 1998;107:122–32.

113. Smith MT, Huang MI, Manber R. Cognitive behavior therapy for chronic insomnia occurring within the context of medical and psychiatric disorders. Clin Psychol Rev 2005;25:559–92.

114. Morin CM, Kowatch RA, O'Shanick G. Sleep restriction for the inpatient treatment of insomnia. Sleep 1990;13:183–6.

115. Morin CM, Stone J, McDonald K, Jones S. Psychological management of insomnia: a clinical replication series with 100 patients. Behav Ther 1994;25:291–309.

116. Lichstein KL, Wilson NM, Johnson CT. Psychological treatment of secondary insomnia. Psychol Aging 2000;15:232–40.

117. Perlis ML, Sharpe M, Smith MT, Greenblatt D, Giles D. Behavioral treatment of insomnia: treatment outcome and the relevance of medical and psychiatric morbidity. J Behav Med 2001;24:281–96.

118. Rybarczyk B, Lopez M, Benson R, Alsten C, Stepanski E. Efficacy of two behavioral treatment programs for comorbid geriatric inosmnia. Psychol Aging 2004;17:288–98.

119. Rybarczyk B, Stepanski E, Fogg L, Lopez M, Barry P, Davis A. A placebo-controlled test of cognitive-behavioral therapy for comorbid insomnia in older adults. J Consult Clin Psychol 2005;73:1164–74.

120. Currie SR, Wilson KG, Pontefract AJ, deLaplante L. Cognitive-behavioral treatment of insomnia secondary to chronic pain. J Consult Clin Psychol 2000;68:407–16.

121. Edinger JD, Wohlgemuth WK, Krystal AD, Rice JR. Behavioral insomnia therapy for fibromyalgia patients: a randomized clinical trial. Arch Intern Med 2005;165:2527–35.

122. Arnold LM, Keck PE Jr, Welge JA. Antidepressant treatment of fibromyalgia: a meta-analysis and review. Psychosomatics 2000;41:104–13.

123. Moldofsky H, Lue FA, Mously C, Roth-Schechter B, Reynolds WJ. The effect of zolpidem in patients with fibromyalgia: a dose ranging, double blind, placebo controlled, modified crossover study. J Rheumatol 1996;23:529–33.

124. Drewes AM, Bjerregard K, Taagholt SJ, Svendsen L, Nielsen KD. Zopiclone as night medication in rheumatoid arthritis. Scand J Rheumatol 1998;27:180–7.

125. Krystal AD, Walsh JK, Laska E, Caron J, Amato DA, Wessel TC, et al. Sustained efficacy of eszopiclone over 6 months of nightly treatment: results of a randomized, double-blind, placebo-controlled study in adults with chronic insomnia. Sleep 2003;26:793–9.

126. Allain H, Bentue-Ferrer D, Tarral A, Gandon JM. Effects on postural oscillation and memory functions of a single dose of zolpidem 5 mg, zopiclone 3.75 mg and lormetazepam 1 mg in elderly healthy subjects: a randomized, cross-over, double-blind study versus placebo. Eur J Clin Pharmacol 2003;59:179–88.

127. Allain H, Bentue-Ferrer D, Polard E, Akwa Y, Patat A. Postural instability and consequent falls and hip fractures associated with use of hypnotics in the elderly: a comparative review. Drugs Aging 2005;22:749–65.

128. O'Malley PG, Balden E, Tomkins G, Santoro J, Kroenke K, Jackson JL. Treatment of fibromyalgia with antidepressants: a meta-analysis. J Gen Intern Med 2000;15:659–66.

129. Carette S, Bell MJ, Reynolds WJ, Haraoui B, McCain GA, Bykerk VP, et al. Comparison of amitriptyline, cyclobenzaprine, and placebo in the treatment of fibromyalgia: a randomized, double-blind clinical trial. Arthritis Rheum 1994;37:32–40.

130. Wolfe F, Cathey MA, Hawley DJ. A double-blind placebo controlled trial of fluoxetine in fibromyalgia. Scand J Rheumatol 1994;23:255–9.

131. Wolfe F, Smythe HA, Yunus MB, Bennett RM, Bombardier C, Goldenberg DL, et al. The American College of Rheumatology 1990 criteria for the classification of fibromyalgia: report of the Multicenter Criteria Committee. Arthritis Rheum 1990;33:160–72.

132. Goldenberg D, Mayskiy M, Mossey C, Ruthazer R, Schmid C. A randomized, double-blind crossover trial of fluoxetine and amitriptyline in the treatment of fibromyalgia. Arthritis Rheum 1996;39:1852–9.

133. Thase ME. Treatment issues related to sleep and depression. J Clin Psychiatry 2000;61(Suppl 11):46–50.

134. Scharf MB, Baumann M, Berkowitz DV. The effects of sodium oxybate on clinical symptoms and sleep patterns in patients with fibromyalgia. J Rheumatol 2003;30:1070–4.

135. Wikner J, Hirsch U, Wetterberg L, Rojdmark S. Fibromyalgia—a syndrome associated with decreased nocturnal melatonin secretion. Clin Endocrinol (Oxford) 1998;49:179–83.

136. Korszun A. Sleep and circadian rhythm disorders in fibromyalgia. Curr Rheumatol Rep 2000;2:124–30.

137. Klerman EB, Goldenberg DL, Brown EN, Maliszewski AM, Adler GK. Circadian rhythms of women with fibromyalgia. J Clin Endocrinol Metab 2001;86:1034–9.

138. Acuna-Castroviejo D, Escames G, Reiter RJ. Melatonin therapy in fibromyalgia. J Pineal Res 2006;40:98–9.

139. Citera G, Arias MA, Maldonado-Cocco JA, Lazaro MA, Rosemffet MG, Brusco LI, et al. The effect of melatonin in patients with fibromyalgia: a pilot study. Clin Rheumatol 2000;19:9–13.

CHAPTER 46

Obtaining Disability Benefits

DAVID WAYNE SMITH, DEd

One of the most difficult issues faced by practitioners in the field of rheumatic diseases today is determining the degree to which their patients are disabled related to their capacity to perform work in the competitive labor market. Requests for such information come not only from patients, but from the programs that deal with determining disability and provide financial assistance for those who qualify.

The issue is surrounded by numerous and often very perplexing questions, e.g., "Can my patient perform work on a regular or part-time basis?" "Could he or she perform work if it were modified to accommodate existing physical restrictions and limitations?" "Is there any work situation in which my patient would not be placed at risk?"

If the answer to all these questions is "No," and if it is obvious that the patient will require some type of financial assistance to get on with his or her life, the next difficult and perplexing question is, "How can I help my patient obtain that assistance?"

This chapter is written with the hope that it will provide answers to those, as well as other, questions related to obtaining disability benefits for your patient. The author is with the Disability Assessment Research Clinic, University of Arizona College of Medicine, and has >50 years' experience in Social Security Disability and is a Diplomat of the American College of Forensic Examiners. The Clinic sees ~500 patients and clients annually in Tucson, Phoenix, and several other cities in southern Arizona. The staff, which has >150 years combined experience, is comprised of physicians, psychologists, and vocational evaluators who conduct comprehensive, integrated medical, psychological, neuropsychological, cognitive, and functional capacity assessments.

The Clinic's primary goal is to return individuals to productive employment in the competitive labor market. However, when evidence indicates that individuals cannot return to work, the Clinic's goal then becomes assisting them to obtain disability benefits. At that point in the process, the Clinic becomes the individual's advocate. In the 10 years the Clinic has been in operation, it has been successful in obtaining disability benefits for 90% of its patients it determined were disabled. That success is based primarily on the Clinic's advocacy role in which it coordinates all patient, practitioner, and attorney input combined with its very close adherence to the steps outlined in this Chapter for obtaining disability benefits.

DETERMINING YOUR PATIENT'S DISABILITY

There are 3 very important factors for the practitioner to consider in the overall process of assisting patients in obtaining disability benefits: 1) determine, for yourself, that your patient is disabled; 2) determine that the disability is based on valid, objective evidence; and 3) determine that the evidence can be defended without question.

The importance of valid, objective information cannot be overemphasized. It is the basis for determining disability in the programs designed to provide financial assistance for their disabled clients. These programs include 1) Social Security Disability Insurance (SSDI), 2) Federal Supplementary Security Insurance (SSI), 3 and 4) Short and Long Term Disability Insurance (STDI; LTDI), and 5) Workers' Compensation Insurance (WCI). Although each program differs in its operation, each has its specific disability criteria, consultants (physicians, psychiatrists, psychologists, physical therapists, etc.), and review process. More importantly, all programs determine disability based primarily on the validity and objectivity of the evidence provided to its disability determination unit.

Consequently, the evidence you use to determine for yourself that your patient is disabled is the same as what you need to provide the program(s) from which he or she is seeking assistance. The general nature and type of evidence needed in determining disability in these programs is presented below.

Evidence of Disability

First and foremost, the evidence needs to include all available, objective data substantiating the patient's medical condition. That data should include the results of x-rays, laboratory work, magnetic resonance imaging, as well as results from any specific evaluations requested (e.g., neurological, psychological, vocational, functional capacities, etc.). No objective data that helps substantiate the practitioner's conclusions should be omitted.

Second, but as important, the evidence needs to substantiate the practitioner's interpretation of the impact of that medical condition upon the patient's functional capacities. For example, if the practitioner states that the patient's medical condition is such that it creates a substantial loss of hand function, the evidence needs to substantiate any resulting diminished functional capacity as well as how that diminished capacity affects the patient's ability to perform the physical tasks required in his or her job (current, last, future). In addition, evidence needs to substantiate the degree of risk the practitioner states can be created for the patient if he or she continues performing those required tasks.

Because the loss or diminishment of functional capacity of any body part is so critical in the ultimate decision of disability, it is extremely important for the practitioner to be aware that adjudicators in most disability programs look specifically for its impact related to 3 areas: 1) the performance of the physical demand factors required for performing jobs in the competitive labor market, 2) the performance of any number of additional physical activities related to the patient's daily living, and 3) the affect of pain or other symptoms on the performance of physical activities.

Physical demand factors can include the following: lifting and carrying, walking (ambulating), climbing, balancing, stooping, kneeling, crouching, crawling, pushing, and pulling. Specific attention is given to the ability to perform upper-extremity fine and gross movements effectively as they relate to reaching, grasping, and fingering.

Additional physical activities can include performing activities of daily living, such as the ability to prepare a simple meal, feed oneself, take care of personal hygiene, drive a car, ride a bus, and use a cane, walker, or wheelchair. Consequently, whatever statement the practitioner makes related to these and other physical functions, the evidence needs to support it.

If, in the practitioner's opinion, pain or other symptoms are affecting the patient's ability to perform specific tasks, objective medical evidence must show the existence of a medically determined impairment that could reasonably be expected to produce pain or other symptoms being experienced by the patient.

Evidence and Malingering

Another important, although disconcerting, reason for providing valid and objective data is the role it plays in the area of malingering. Related to that area, it's important for the practitioner to be aware of the fact that adjudicators are not advocates for the patient applying for benefits from their programs. In fact, experience dictates that in numerous cases, the opposite is often true. For example, an SSDI residual functional capacity form asks the practitioner whether or not the patient is a malingerer. Given that situation, the evidence provided to disability programs must not only support the practitioner's statements, it must also be strong enough to eliminate or neutralize the possibility of malingering. If questions remain, referral to a psychologist for an evaluation can be useful to assess potential malingering.

DISABILITY PROGRAMS

When the practitioner has gathered and reviewed all available data, and has made the decision that his or her patient is disabled, he or she is ready to assist the patient in obtaining disability benefits.

As stated above, there are 5 primary disability programs designed to provide financial assistance to qualified applicants: Social Security Disability Insurance, Federal Supplemental Security Insurance, Short and Long Term Disability Insurance, and Worker's Compensation Insurance.

Only the SSDI program will be reviewed in this Chapter. The reason for doing so is pragmatic in nature. The SSDI disability determination process is generally the most structured and demanding of all disability programs. If the evidence provided to SSDI determines disability for your patient, it will almost certainly suffice for determining disability in the remaining 4 programs including SSI, a federal program for welfare recipients who may be disabled. SSI patients are treated under Medicaid in most states and under the state's welfare health care program in others. For example, in Arizona, the program is the Arizona Health Care Cost Containment System. The disability criteria for SSI are the same as for SSDI.

Social Security Disability Insurance

SSDI is the most common, and most extensive of all disability programs. It is paid for by payroll taxes and is provided for all workers who have contributed enough to the system to qualify. Once the patient qualifies for SSDI, he or she receives monthly benefits, which may include payments for children under the age of 18. Actual benefits are determined by the amount of the patient's contributions to the Social Security system. The more the patient has paid into the system, the higher his or her benefit amount.

However, prior to qualifying for benefits, the patient must step through the disability determination process; the first step is to make an application. When a patient initiates an application for SSDI benefits, it is usually handled by a field office of the Social Security Administration (SSA). When that office has verified personal information, it sends the case to a State Disability Determination Services unit (DDS). DDS, which is usually funded by the federal government, is a state agency responsible for developing and reviewing medical evidence and making an initial disability determination.

If, upon review, it is determined that additional data are required, or that there are inconsistencies in the existing data, DDS refers claimants (your patients) to its consulting physicians and other specialists for additional evaluation.

When DDS has gathered all existing data, and all inconsistencies have been resolved, it determines disability based on the sequential process presented below:

- Step 1: Is the claimant currently engaging in substantial gainful activity?
- Step 2: Does the claimant possess a severe impairment?
- Step 3: Does the claimant possess one or more impairments that meet or exceed the listing of impairments?
- Step 4: Can the claimant perform past relevant work?
- Step 5: Can the claimant do any other work?

The steps in the determination process are sequential. For example, if the answer to the Step 1 question "no," the process proceeds to Step 2, and so forth. DDS answers question 3 based on Listings of Impairments found in *Disability Evaluation Under Social Security*, also known as the "Blue Book." It is a must-have resource for every practitioner attempting to assist patients in obtaining disability benefits. It is essentially a cookbook for determining disability and it is easily available in hard copy or on the Internet.

It's important for the practitioner to know that if the severity of the patient's condition meets or equals the level of severity described in the Listings, the patient will be determined to be disabled. If not, the process will continue and there must be an evaluation of whether or not the patient retains the residual functional capacity to do other work. Given that information, it makes some sense not only to know and understand the Listings, but also to present your evidence as it relates to their content.

Of some importance in providing evidence for SSDI is the practitioner knowing that the SSA reserves for itself the ultimate role of determining whether or not a patient is disabled. In that respect, the adjudicators look only for evidence to support disability, and dismiss any general statement by the practitioner indicating that the patient is disabled. Practitioners would be well advised to not make such a statement but to just present the evidence that confirms it.

If the patient is denied benefits based on the initial application, he or she can appeal by requesting the decision be reconsidered and can provide additional evidence at that time.

If the patient is denied again, he or she can request a hearing before an Administrative Law Judge (ALJ) in the SSA's Office of Hearings and Appeals. At each level of appeal, new evidence needs to be provided. In that respect, it becomes increasingly important that new evidence is as valid, objective, and directly related to the Listings as already provided (if not more so).

It is also important to know that at the initial level of review, 63% of cases are denied. Of much interest related to that rate is the fact that it almost matches the approval rate at the ALJ level. It's also important to know that with appropriate evidence, experienced disability attorneys are, more often than not, successful in obtaining benefits for patients at the ALJ level. Knowing that, it makes some sense for the practitioner to suggest that the patient obtain the services of a disability attorney, especially when the claim has been denied at the initial and reconsideration levels.

All the above information points to the fact that the practitioner needs to continue to provide valid, objective evidence for the patient as he or she moves through the disability determination process.

SSDI and Early Retirement Benefits

There is yet another important reason for providing evidence that assists your patient in obtaining SSDI benefits. That is the relationship between those benefits and early retirement benefits. Because of the severity of specific rheumatic diseases and their debilitating impact on functional capacities, many patients are forced to retire early from the work force. At that point in time, it is important for the practitioner to be aware of the possibility that the patient, regardless of his or her age, can combine early retirement benefits with SSDI benefits. For example, if, based on the evidence, you feel your patient's medical impairment is such that he or she could qualify for SSDI benefits, he or she should be encouraged to apply. If approved, the benefit would be the same as would have been awarded if the patient had continued to work until the graded age, which is based on date of birth.

ADDITIONAL STRATEGIES

As has been presented to this point, the number 1 strategy for obtaining disability benefits for your patient is providing valid, objective evidence in a manner that meets the criteria established by your patient's disability program. To do that, you need to know how that program works. For example, you need to 1) understand the SSDI, SSI, STDI, LTDI, and WCI programs, how their disability determination units function, and what evidence they look for; and 2) get that evidence and provide it the way the unit wants it.

The time has long past when a letter from the practitioner stating that the patient is disabled and cannot work will obtain disability benefits for that patient.

A second important strategy is to identify established, aggressive patient advocacy programs of which the practitioner can become an integral part. The reasons for this are twofold and not all that complicated. 1) Almost without exception, patients are not successful in getting on disability by themselves. The process is too complex, confusing, and demanding and it usually requires more knowledge and expertise than they possess. 2) Almost without exception, practitioners have neither the time nor resources required to establish or operate such a program.

The advocate can be a person, an agency, a program, or any resource that has an excellent working knowledge of the disability programs presented above and can do the following: 1) take the patient through all the steps (starting with the application) required to get on disability, 2) coordinate the efforts of the professionals involved with the patient's application (practitioner, specialists, attorney), and 3) protect the patient's rights in the disability process. Possible advocacy resources are presented in the next section.

Another important strategy is to establish a direct relationship with your patient's disability program. For example, in addition to having the "Blue Book" in house, request a meeting with, or talk with, the director of your state DDS or the manager of the DDS office handling your patient's claims to be certain you're providing the evidence the service needs in the format it can use. It takes time and resources to put the evidence package together. If it's not obtaining disability benefits for your patient, you need to know why.

ADVOCACY RESOURCES

Advocacy resources differ from city to city; however, most major population centers have voluntary agencies capable of assisting patients through the disability process, especially the application process. In Arizona, for example, an excellent program in the greater-Phoenix area is Arizona Bridge to Independent Living. Similar independent living programs, centers, and agencies are available in most cities. Additional resources include the Lupus Foundation and the United Way. Both organizations can either assist your patient directly or help you identify appropriate volunteer services.

If your patient has been denied benefits, and you feel that he or she is truly disabled, perhaps the most important advocate your patient can have at that point in the process is an experienced, knowledgeable disability attorney. It has been my experience, confirmed by the 63% denial rate of initial applications, that patients do not have the expertise required to deal successfully with the disability system. Using the objective evidence you provide them, disability attorneys can, more often than not, obtain the benefits you feel your patient deserves.

PROPOSED CHANGES IN THE SSDI PROGRAM

It's important for the practitioner to know that there are proposed changes in the SSDI system that could have a positive affect on your patient obtaining disability benefits. Currently, if an initial denial is appealed, DDS is responsible for reviewing the case at the reconsideration level. The proposed change would have those cases reviewed by a panel of experts, the makeup of which has not yet been determined but would certainly include physicians, psychiatrists, psychologists, etc. The primary reasons for the changes are to limit the number of cases that rise to the ALJ level and, in so doing, reduce the current 18-month waiting period. It is the general consensus among many prominent experts in the field that such a panel could work to the advantage of the patient, given the panel is provided with the evidence as has been discussed in this chapter.

SUMMARY

Helping your patient receive disability insurance is not an easy task. The system is difficult, demanding, and oftentimes adversarial. Getting through it requires a combination of tenacity, knowledge of the disability programs involved, and a commitment to the patient. However, if you are convinced your patient is, indeed, disabled, it's not an impossible task to overcome and is certainly more than worth the effort.

Special thanks to Mr. John Ellis for his review of the chapter's content related to the SSDI program.

Recommended Reading

Code of Federal Regulations, Title 20, Appendix 1 to Subpart P of Part 404– Listings of Impairments.

Disability Evaluation under Social Security, Social Security Administration, Office of Disability Programs, SSH Pub. No. 64-039, ICN 468600, January, 2005.

Federal Register, (Definition of Disability, 404.1505/1506/1508/1509/1510/ 1511) (Evaluation of Disability, 404.1520/1520a/1521/1522/1523) (Medical Considerations, 404.1525/1526/1527/1528/1529) (Residual Functional Capacity, 404.1545/1546)

Field J, Field T. The transitional classification of jobs. 6th ed. Athens (GA): Elliott & Fitzpatrick, Inc; 2004.

Social Security Forum, Volume 27, No. 4, April, 2005, Page 23.

Living with Rheumatoid Arthritis: Accepting the Diagnosis and Finding "Normal" Again

CHERYL L. KOEHN

When I was a kid, I used to love riding roller coasters with my mother. The bigger and scarier the ride, the better. I was thrilled at the uncertainty of the track's direction; how it would suddenly turn to the right or left, or unexpectedly plunge 100 feet or more, leaving my stomach feeling light and my spine tingly. I still love to ride on roller coasters, but 16 years ago, I got on one that frightened me to the core of my being—the rheumatoid arthritis roller coaster.

Unlike with the amusement park version, I quickly learned that the turns, ascents and drops of the rheumatoid arthritis (RA) roller coaster were significantly more daunting than any I had ever experienced at an amusement park. I also learned how it would profoundly affect every part of my life—work, home, and leisure. The onset of symptoms, a pain in the ball of my foot and an inexplicably swollen index finger one day to 35 affected joints 1 month later, was completely overwhelming. From the day I received my diagnosis and throughout the first year of living with the disease, I struggled even to understand the word "arthritis." I still remember (as though it were yesterday) the precise moment the rheumatologist spoke the words "rheumatoid arthritis." I reacted then the way society does today when it hears the word "arthritis"—I'm 30 years old, I can't have arthritis, I'm too young. I'm a former member of the United States Women's Volleyball team; I'm in excellent health and fit as a fiddle. This diagnosis can't possibly be correct.

The next thing that happened during that first visit was the rheumatologist told me I had a "different" type of arthritis, one that—whether mild, moderate, or severe—was likely not going away. After that, he told me about a few medications I should consider taking, one that had to be injected and one that I would take by mouth every day. Again, I reacted the way society tends to react when it comes to medications: I don't want to take medication every day—and certainly not by injection—to deal with something as innocuous as arthritis. After having been together for roughly 10 minutes discussing the findings of the lab tests and physical examination, the rheumatologist and I could not have been further apart in terms of a shared understanding of RA and the early steps I needed to take to deal with it.

The point I am trying to make is this: when a person finds out they have a disease called "arthritis"—something they thought they knew all about—try to give that person the key pieces of information he or she needs to arrive at diagnosis comprehension and disease acceptance. *And go slowly if at all possible.* It is important to take the time to explain that RA is one in a family of arthritides and an autoimmune disease, what the common symptoms are (including the ones the patient is actually experiencing), and what happens if the disease goes untreated. Share your confidence in the diagnosis, explaining what signs and symptoms led you to arrive at it. Acknowledge how difficult it may be for the person to hear and accept the diagnosis, and encourage and support him or her in appropriate ways to build their own unique, evidence-based treatment plan (see Table 1). *Most of all, given all of what I describe, try to understand that someone receiving a diagnosis of RA may not be ready to start medications the same day—or even weeks—after hearing the news.*

Had this type of approach been used with me, I may have avoided a year of non–evidence-based treatment failures, resulting in emotional and physical misery.

LEARNING TO MAKE HEALTHY, RESPONSIBLE CHOICES

As I mentioned, during the first year I lived with RA, I did not follow the rheumatologist's advice to initiate gold and methotrexate therapy. The only recommendation I followed was to attend a once-monthly appointment to check on my disease's progress. To the rheumatologist's credit, he stuck with me and patiently waited for me to acknowledge and accept that the noninstitutional medical approach I followed for a year was a failure.

When I look back now, I shake my head and wonder, "What was I thinking?" Without any evidence—scientific or otherwise—I chose to embark upon a "natural" healing path, knowing little about the approaches being recommended by friends, family, and alternative health care practitioners. I tried *everything* that first year: naturopathy, homeopathy, Chinese herb therapy, elimination diets, among other non–evidence-based approaches. All to no avail. And believe me, I followed each of these alternative treatment approaches to the letter. If any of them were going to work, it would have.

Along with not having any idea what RA was when I was diagnosed, society and its perception of arthritis had a profound (and mostly deleterious) effect on my health care choices. These included what types

Table 1. Helping your patients: Information to give and questions to ask on the first and second visits

- Provide an easy-to-understand definition of the disease—to both patient and family—and ask them to repeat it back to you when they are ready.
- Tell them about the basic treatment principles for the disease: education, exercise and rest, healthy living approaches, and medication therapy.
- Tell them about the importance of initiating a well-rounded treatment plan within the first 6 weeks of disease onset and how this approach delivers the best results and possibly prevents future irreparable damage.
- Let them know there are no "natural" cures for arthritis, but that if they are interested in trying a natural therapy, they should do so along with the medications being prescribed by the rheumatologist. Remind them to start the first natural therapy *three months after* they start the first medication prescribed by the doctor.
- Ask them if they would like to talk to another person living with the disease—one of a similar age and life experience.
- Encourage them to ask questions before they leave the visit. The questions they ask will give you a good idea where they are on the learning and acceptance curve. Stimulating dialogue will help to build good future communications between you, them, and their families.
- Give them homework to do before the next visit. This could be a Web site to review, another person with arthritis to speak with, pamphlets on their disease to read, etc.
- If they have not already done so, encourage the person with arthritis to bring a support person along with them to the next visit.

Table 2. Tips to help your patients with decision making

- Help the person with arthritis and family members to understand there will be many decisions to make around treating the disease, and that these decisions may have to be revisited frequently, particularly in the first few years.
- Remind them that every person with arthritis is unique and requires a customized treatment plan.
- Describe the principles of evidence-based medicine.
- Review the basic principles of risk–benefit analysis with them. This is particularly important when discussing medication treatment options.
- Describe to them the possible consequences (from most likely to happen to least) of untreated, or undertreated disease.
- Ask them what pieces of information they need (in addition to those already provided) to empower their decision-making process.

of practitioners I sought out, my attitude toward prescription medications, and my misplaced belief in natural remedies or cures. Like society's, my initial reaction was that arthritis was no big deal. I, like many others I have spoken with since and who live with RA, thought that I could deal with it myself, either by toughing it out until the pain subsided or by trying myriad over-the-counter or alternative medical treatments. After all, that is what my grandparents did, and they are the ones from whom I first learned about arthritis, as I imagine most do.

As part of a society of consumers, I was certainly influenced by the bombardment of advertisements in magazines, television, and on radio touting the latest "cures" for arthritis. In addition, my friends and family were either seeing naturopaths and taking all manner of herbal preparations for their minor ills or had heard about someone's aunt who drank only grapefruit juice for a month and was cured of her arthritis. When you are dealing with something as painful and debilitating as an aggressive onset of severe RA, you want to believe that these things being promoted to you by people you love and respect will work, to the degree that you take their advice over your doctor's.

The one thing I did do in that first year was carry on with my pre-RA fitness and strengthening exercise routine. Even on my worst days, I forced myself to the gym. For cardiovascular exercise, I literally crawled onto the stationary bike and worked my heart and lungs. I wore the largest sized weightlifting gloves I could find to hide the swelling in my fingers and hands, and cautiously worked my way around the gym, being extra careful to lift only the lightest weights possible and in ways that protected my joints. As a former Olympic-caliber volleyball player, keeping up with my exercise routine was the one thing I knew I could still do—even though it was with great difficulty due to unrelenting joint pain and stiffness.

In retrospect, what I needed to help me make better health care choices was a society informed about RA—one that included my family, friends, and coworkers. Then, I would have enjoyed the support of people who loved me and who understood the differences between RA and osteoarthritis, and the need to make evidence-based decisions about the medications I should have taken early on to gain control over the disease.

I also needed to understand that in chronic disease, a team of knowledgeable health care professionals was available to assist me with the myriad physical, emotional, and social challenges I faced. I learned over the course of the first 2 years how to access nurses, physiotherapists, occupational therapists, social workers, and counselors; found out what information they required to provide the services I needed; and worked hard at creating optimal channels of communication between myself and each of them, and among them.

At this point in my life with RA, I know which health care professionals can help me with which problems, but asking the person with 3–6 months' disease experience to figure it all out on their own is cruel. A simple, easy-to-read primer on all of this would save them countless days and months of frustration and health energy—a gift from the gods, really (see Table 2).

FINDING "NORMAL" AGAIN

For me, one of the more frustrating aspects of the earliest years of my disease was the time spent by the rheumatologist and other health care professionals collecting information on my function, pain, medication side effects, and other physical findings, with little or no time spent talking about aspects of RA that had as significant an impact on my life as the physical symptoms. Those critical aspects of life with chronic illness include fatigue, ability to sleep and sleep well, intimacy, sexuality, family understanding and support, participation (at home, leisure, and work), emotional and social difficulties, challenges in the workplace, among other topics. These are the things that for me, and I suspect for many others, make up a person's quality of life. These are the things that, when balanced, help make me feel "normal" again.

Finding "normal" again—in my personal relationships, work life, and society—was not easy. But as I worked with a counselor, I began to learn again how to make sense of my future, about new and shifted priorities in my life, and most importantly about love—of myself first, and then others. Not surprisingly, certain aspects of my life shifted dramatically: I changed careers; divorced and remarried; cowrote a book on rheumatoid arthritis; and founded a grass-roots arthritis organization that provides free evidence-based education to others with arthritis and their families, to name a few.

When I look back now, RA made me reexamine every aspect of my life, and it was only because I had the disease that I embarked on the journey. I decided that if I was going to have to live with such a crummy disease, I wanted the other parts of my life, at work, at home, and at leisure, to be as balanced and fulfilling as possible.

At this point in my life, I spend some time each summer thinking about what I want the following year to be and feel like for me. First, I think about my health and assess how well my RA treatment plan is working by looking at outcomes that are meaningful to me. Do I have a fulfilling life with my husband? Am I still able to work out and play tennis? Do I have kind, caring friends? Am I able to travel on my own without assistance? Am I financially independent? These are the outcomes I want to achieve with my well-rounded treatment plan. If I find myself saying "no" to even a few of these questions, I know I have to revisit some of my choices and possibly make some significant changes (Table 3).

CHANGING THE COURSE OF RHEUMATOID ARTHRITIS

Of all the lessons taught me by RA, the most important was around the need to self-advocate. Because of the chronic nature of the disease, I, like millions of others in North America, have unmet needs each day, month, and for years on end. Many of us have lost our ability to walk or

Table 3. Discussion points that may help people get back to "normal"

Although time in the clinic is limited, try to ensure that enough is allotted to the person with arthritis to talk about their "life stuff"

- Prompt the person with arthritis to tell you about fears they may have about the diagnosis. If a family member is present, be sure to include them in the discussion, if and when appropriate.
- Refer the person and their family to a counselor if you believe they could benefit from support and expertise outside of your professional scope of practice.
- Ask the person about any intimacy or sexuality issues they and their partner might be experiencing. This topic is seldom raised in clinic but is usually something people with arthritis want to talk about, but are shy about or embarrassed to discuss.

stand free of challenge or pain. Some of us cannot cope financially due to loss of employment or insurance benefits. Others of us lost marriages because spouses could not learn to adapt to the relationship changes as a result of RA coming into the home. I realized fairly soon after developing RA that I had to open my mouth and tell someone what I needed if I wanted to survive and thrive. I knew I had to do things—something, anything—to change the course of my disease.

I realized at the time of my diagnosis that I was blessed to have the education and communication skills to advocate for my own needs. What I did not realize was that the voice of one could have a profoundly positive effect for many others.

Today, I know that if people with RA and their health care providers speak with one large, loud voice, the course of RA can change. Health policy makers will see that innovative treatment interventions are worth paying for because they will understand their value to the person with RA and to society. There will be the recognition that early aggressive treatment limits the inexorable toll of RA, and the development of new agents and treatment protocols will continue to alter radically how consumers and health care providers think about the disease. People with RA will no longer have to give up work, as had been almost universal within 10 years of disease onset. Society will no longer believe that exercise is for other people. All of this because people living with RA and those they interact with will advocate changing the course of rheumatoid arthritis (Table 4).

Table 4. Connecting with others who work or volunteer in arthritis (listed alphabetically)

- Arthritis Care (United Kingdom) www.arthritiscare.org.uk
- Arthritis Foundation (United States) www.arthritis.org
- Arthritis Consumer Experts (Canada) www.arthritisconsumerexperts.org
- Arthritis Research Centre of Canada www.arthritisresearch.ca
- Canadian Arthritis Network www.arthritisnetwork.ca
- Canadian Arthritis Patient Alliance www.arthritis.ca/capa
- Cochrane Musculoskeletal Group (International) www.cochranemsk.org
- National Institute of Arthritis and Musculoskeletal and Skin Diseases, National Institutes of Health (United States) www.niams.nih.gov
- The Arthritis Society of Canada www.arthritis.ca
- The Missouri Arthritis Rehabilitation Research and Training Center www.marrtc.org

SECTION E: RESOURCES

CHAPTER

48

Online Resources for Rheumatology Care Providers and Their Patients

JANE McKENZIE-WHITE, MAS, and MARY BETH HANSEN, MA

Neilsen/Net Ratings reports that, as of February 2006, 74% of people in the United Sates have home Internet access, and about two-thirds of those with home access have a high-speed connection to the Internet (1). Based on a national survey conducted November 25 through December 22, 2002, 8 of 10 adult Internet users have sought health information online (2). Similarly, in a review of data from the Health Information National Trends Survey, Hess and colleagues (3) found that 64% of the online population had searched for health information at least once over the previous 12 months. Already an integral part of private and professional life for most of us, the Internet is an especially rich and powerful resource for health care providers and their patients. By providing ready, rapid, on-demand, and free or relatively low-cost access to the following 5 types of resources in particular, the Internet provides access to a wealth of materials that can enhance and enrich clinical care and disease management:

- Current information from reputable sources to inform and update professionals and patients;
- Online continuing professional education and development;
- Innovative tools that update and enhance clinical practice, provide decision support for both health care providers and patients, and assist with disease management;
- Communication and data exchange systems;
- Tools for searching and retrieving materials from the best medical libraries and databases in the world.

The Internet has already changed clinical practice in powerful ways by opening access to materials previously available only to professionals, by helping patients to be more informed, by opening new channels of communication, and by making it easier for care providers to stay up to date. An article in *Nursing Spectrum* states "technology has advanced even further this year and is being increasingly embraced by nursing. Some schools of nursing no longer use printed textbooks, relying instead on material housed on the Internet or downloaded to personal digital

assistants (PDAs) and MP3 players. The options for online classes have greatly expanded. Many scientific journals now publish online, and full articles can be accessed and downloaded through PubMed. PDAs and iPods are a requirement at some schools, and podcasting is becoming more common" (4).

What is the National Health Council?

The National Health Council has adopted a set of good operating practices to ensure that its voluntary health agency members maintain the highest standards of organizational effectiveness and public stewardship. For a complete checklist of their Standards of Excellence criteria, see www.nationalhealthcouncil.org/aboutus/stand-good_operating.htm

---

WHAT TO EXPECT IN THIS CHAPTER

In this chapter, we focus on presenting a broad array of resources in each of the 5 categories listed above. The best way to learn about what is on the Internet and how to use it is to pull up a chair, turn on your computer, open your browser, and head out onto the World Wide Web. We've identified some good online resources specific to rheumatology. They are just a start, though, and this is by no means an exhaustive review of Web sites (though we do provide links to such reviews). And while we have included a few of the obvious sites that anyone would think of or be able to find, we have put most of our efforts into finding sites that you may not find on your own if you are not a regular or dedicated Web user.

We worked from a few assumptions:
- We assumed that you already have some familiarity and experience using the Internet;
- We assumed that most of the sites listed here will be useful across rheumatology health professions.
- We assumed that your patients use the Internet and have interest in learning more from credible sources to which you can direct them.
- Since many of you also conduct research, we include some resources for this area as well.
- It is also not within the scope of this chapter to address topics such as electronic health records, e-prescribing, computerized ordering, billing, pharmacy, etc. We assumed you are learning about those

---

What is the HON Code?

The Internet's most widely recognized standard-setting organization for online medical and health information is the Geneva-based Health On the Net (HON) Foundation. Compliance is voluntary and approved sites adhere to a set of established principles outlined in their Code of Conduct, which can be found at www.hon.ch/HONcode/Conduct.html. Click on the HON code seal wherever you see it to verify that a Web site complies with HON principles.

issues elsewhere. Our focus is on Internet resources rather than the whole world of online medical practice support.

And finally, an important reminder: The World Wide Web is made up of links. Good sites tend to link to other good sites, so if you are using a good site from a reputable source, chances are that site is linked to others. Look for the links and follow them to a wealth of other resources.

Unless otherwise noted, all Web sites listed in this chapter were accessed and available on April 9, 2006.

RESOURCES AND TOOLS FOR HEALTH CARE PROVIDERS

Directories and Guides to Online Continuing Medical Education

Online continuing medical education (CME) has become a major advantage of the Internet for health care providers. The Internet offers an excellent opportunity for earning continuing education credits from the convenience of your office or home. In 2005, Fordis and colleagues found that evidenced-based, online CME programs were as effective or better than interactive live CME events in producing objective changes in physician knowledge and behavior (5). Some reliable sources for professionally oriented Web sites are listed (Table 1).

Annotated List of Online Continuing Medical Education. Compiled and updated by Bernard Sklar, MD, this annotated list (www.cmelist.com/list.htm) of online CME offerings has links to and descriptions of more than 275 online CME sites offering ~15,000 activities and >25,000 hours of American Medical Association (AMA) Category 1 CME credit. Don't miss Dr. Sklar's glossary and explanation of different types of online CME, or his

Introduction to Online CME, a slide presentation that describes how online CME works and encourages physicians to participate.

The Doctor's Guide. This site (www.docguide.com/news/content.nsf/) indexes and provides links to free, multimedia and text online CME from multiple sources, including the Cleveland Clinic, Cornell University, University of Florida, etc.

Resources for Staying Up to Date and Searching for Information

A major challenge of Internet Web sites is the ability to stay up to date in areas related to their field. By knowing where to turn, rheumatology heath care providers can find the latest information on clinical care, drug approvals, journal publications, professional conferences, clinical trials, and more. Many academic institutions, foundations, and independent Internet resources with provider-driven, evidence-based content are available. Indices and directories can save time searching by compiling and providing direct links to relevant resources. Tables 2–5 provide concise reliable Web sites to meet the demands of keeping current. Peer-reviewed articles from professional journals are readily

found on the Internet. If you are a member of the Association of Rheumatology Health Professionals or American College of Rheumatology, you will also have access to many pdf files of rheumatology journal articles at no cost. Peer-reviewed articles from professional journals are readily found on the Internet.

For late-breaking information and concise medical news, RSS feeds (see sidebar) are available. There are also dozens of Blogs (see sidebar), also called Web logs, about the practice of medicine written by doctors, scientists, and other health professionals. Table 6 can get you started on learning more about these Internet resources.

USEFUL TOOLS FOR HANDHELD COMPUTERS

The portability of handheld devices allows for an interactive, point-of-care decision support tool. Numerous applications, including treatment algorithms, news feeds, and CME activities can be downloaded directly to a handheld device. Dee and colleagues (6) conducted a study of 108 physicians and trainees and found that ~60% reporting occasional PDA use indicated that the PDA had influenced their overall clinical decision making, and 54% specifically mentioned a change to their patient's treatment plan. A survey of 946 physicians using ePocrates Rx on a handheld device found it "saves time during information retrieval, is easily incorporated into their usual workflow, and improves drug-related decision making." They also felt that it reduced the rate of preventable adverse drug events (7). Table 7 introduces some possibilities for your PDA.

Table 1. Sources of online CME for rheumatology*

Name of Web site: URL	Offerings	Method of certification	Cost
American Medical Association Online Series: www.ama-assn.org/ama/pub/category/5008.html	• Osteoporosis Management: 12 modules; 1.5 credits each • Pain Management: 12 modules, 1 credit each • JAMA CME (articles for CME): For subscribers and AMA members only	Automatically reports credit to AMA; online certificate	Online courses are free; journal CME requires subscription or AMA membership
JointandBone.org: www.jointandbone.org/viewArticle.do?primaryKey=618147	Variety of titles and formats, including satellite programs; credits vary by activity	Tracking unclear; online certificate	Free for health care providers
Cleveland Clinic Center for Continuing Education, Online CME: www.clevelandclinicmeded.com/online/topics.htm	Multiple offerings in rheumatology	Tracking unclear; online certificate	Free
Journal of Clinical and Experimental Rheumatology Online: www.clinexprheumatol.org	Title: Quantitative Assessment of Rheumatic Diseases; up to 20 Category 1 credits (each article is 0.5 credits)	Tracking unclear; online certificate	Free
CE Medicus: www.cemedicus.com	Online catalog of CME, searchable by topic, disease, type of activity, and profession; credits vary by activity; variety of sources/authors	Tracks usage; online certificate	Free
E-Medicine: www.emedicine.com/med/RHEUMATOLOGY.htm	More than 60 articles on topics in rheumatology; 1.5 hours of Category 1 CME per article	Tracks usage; online certificate	$7.50 per 1.5 hours; first 1.5 hours are free
FreeMedCME.com: www.freemedcme.com; See also: www.pain.com	Search by specialty; 2 titles in rheumatology; 1 CME credit each	Tracks usage; online certificate	Free
Harvard Medical School Online CME cmeonline.med.harvard.edu	Limited number of courses; 1 rheumatology-specific title	Certificates are mailed	$25 per credit
Hospital for Special Surgery Online CME: www.hss.edu/professionals/Professional-Education/CME-Programs	Several titles in rheumatology, including the Visiting Lecture Series; 1 credit each	Certificates are mailed	Free
Johns Hopkins Arthritis: www.hopkins-arthritis.org	CME credit offered for individual lectures in the *Rheumatology Rounds* series and the 2006 Rheumatology course	Tracks usage; online certificate	Both free and fee-based programs
Medpage Today CME: www.medpagetoday.com/cme.cfm	Real-time CME based on coverage of medical news, journal articles, meetings, and other sources of breaking news; >25 titles in rheumatology, including ACR conference coverage	Tracks usage; online certificate	Free
Medscape Rheumatology CME: Accessible through Medscape's rheumatology specialty homepage: www.Medscape.com/cmecenterdirectory/rheumatology?src=pdown	Variety of CME activities, including conference coverage, professional education activities developed by Medscape and its partners, case CME, journal CME, and medical news CME; credits vary by activity; optional CME alert for e-mail notice when new specialty area CME is posted	Tracks usage; online certificate	Free
Ohio State University Center for Continuing Medical Education: www.ccme.osu.edu/cmeactivities/	4 titles in rheumatology; 1 credit each; also offers live Web casts on multiple topics	Tracks usage; online certificate	$18 per program
Up-To-Date: www.uptodate.com	Subscription service delivering peer-reviewed content; tracks and awards CME credits for use; unlimited category 1 CME	Tracks usage; online certificate	$495 per year for individual.

* Information is current as of April 9, 2006. All continuing medical education (CME) programs listed in this table are American Academy for Continuing Medical Education accredited. Unless otherwise stated, credits are Category 1 credits. CME activities are available in multiple formats: text, video, audio, slide sets. JAMA = Journal of the American Medical Association; AMA = American Medical Association; ACR = American College of Rheumatology.

RESOURCES FOR PATIENTS

Patient Education Materials

In a review of data from the Health Information National Trends Survey, Hesse et al (3) noted that 64% of the online population had searched for health information at least once over the previous 12 months. Your patients are online—be proactive! Additionally, educated patients are more active participants in their health care and tend to be more adherent with disease management. Through a meta-analysis of 32 controlled clinical trials, Guevara et al (8) found that educational programs for the self-management of asthma in children and adolescents were associated with improved health outcomes, including

lung function, reduced absenteeism from school, and reduced number of visits to the emergency room.

Search Engines Promoting Trustworthy Health and Medical Web Sites
• www.Kosmix.com • www.Mamashealth.com • www.Healthline.com • www.Webmd.com

Table 2. Specialized search tools, indices, and directories*

Web site name: URL	Description
Entrez Pub Med: http://www.ncbi.nlm.nih.gov/entrez/query.fcgi?db=PubMed • Open access	National Library of Medicine's search service that provides access to >11 million citations in MEDLINE, PreMEDLINE, and other related databases, with links to participating online journals
Free Medical Journals: www.freemedicaljournals.com/ Free books for doctors: www.freebooks4doctors.com/ • Open access	• 1,450 journals sorted by specialty and title • 650 medical textbooks; 2 titles in rheumatology • Available in English, French, German, Spanish, Portuguese, and a variety of other languages
Genamics Journal Seek: http://www.journalseek.net • Open Access	From the Web site: "Largest completely categorized database of freely available journal information available on the Internet;" 91,118 titles; index includes 57 titles for rheumatology
Healthweb: www.healthweb.org/index.cfm • Open access	A collaborative project of >20 health science libraries; index of rheumatology sites and electronic texts
LLRX: www.llrx.com/features/medical2005.htm • Open access article	"Researching Medical Literature on the Internet—2005 Update," a guide to medical resources on the Web that includes lists of resources
MD Express: www.mdexpress.com • Open access	By doctors, for doctors: "Our primary goal at MDExpress is to make the Internet worth your while. Toward that end, we've developed great tools to find the '20%' that would be valuable to physicians. MDExpress transforms what can be an inefficient, unruly morass of information into a format that works smarter and faster for busy people."
MedBioWorld: www.sciencekomm.at/index.html • Open access	". . . the largest medical and bioscience resource directory on the Internet." Includes 8,697 journals within 80 medical specialties and 101 bioscience fields; 7,250 associations; 32,000 Reuters Health and Industry news articles; 3,100 medical and bioscience databases; >2,000 bioscience companies
Med Hunt: www.hon.ch/MedHunt/(Health On the Net Foundation) • Open access	Metasearch tool of the following types: • HON code sites: HON code accredited Web sites • All Web sites: all medical Web sites • HONselect combines 5 information types: MeSH terms, authoritative scientific articles, healthcare news, Web sites, and multimedia • News: Search 300 medical topics and themes in the news • Conferences: HON's d-base of medical meetings • Images: Repository of 6,800 medical images and videos • Available in 5 languages: English, French, Dutch, Spanish, and Portuguese
National Library of Medicine, National Institutes of Health: www.nlm.nih.gov/	Online access to the world's largest medical library; the collections stand at 5 million items: books, journals, technical reports, manuscripts, microfilms, photographs, and images
University of Maryland Center for Integrative Medicine Arthritis and Complementary Medicine Database: www.campain.umm.edu/ris/risweb.isa • Open access	ARCAM databases are compiled from regular, comprehensive electronic and hand searches of scientific literature sources world-wide

* HON = Health On the Net; MeSh = medical subject headings; ARCAM = arthritis and complementry medicine.

Table 3. Directories of images

Web site name: URL (all sites are open access)
Internet Pathology Laboratory for Medical Education, Florida State University College of Medicine: www-medlib.med.utah.edu/WebPath/webpath.html#MENU Bone and joint pathology index: www-medlib.med.utah.edu/WebPath/BONEHTML/BONEIDX.html
Medical Images on the Web: www.unmc.edu/library/reference/medimage.html University of Nebraska Medical Center's large collection of annotated links to online image collections
Hardin.MD: www.lib.uiowa.edu/hardin/md/ Skeletal system/bone disease: www.lib.uiowa.edu/hardin/md/ortho.html University of Iowa's index of medical and disease images, clustered by subject, system, and diseases.

Table 4. Peer-reviewed journals*

Web site or journal name: URL	Description
Annals of the Rheumatic Diseases: ard.bmjjournals.com • Some open access; subscription required for full access	Full text of editor's-choice articles and selected supplements offered for free; no registration required; RSS feeds: current issue, recent issues, and online first (articles published before inclusion in an issue)
Arthritis & Rheumatism: www.rheumatology.org/publications/ar/index.asp?aud=mem • Subscription required for online access	Only tables of content and abstracts available without subscription; sample issue maybe requested
Arthritis Care & Research: www3.interscience.wiley.com/cgi-bin/jhome/77005015 • Subscription required for online access	Only tables of content and abstracts available without subscription; sample issue maybe requested
Arthritis Research & Therapy: www.arthritis-research.com/home/ • Some open access; subscription required for full access	Full text of selected articles, reviews, features, and meeting reports available through open access; non—peer-reviewed research and paper reports available through open access
BioMed Central: www.biomedcentral.com/home/ • Open access	BioMed central "is an independent publishing house committed to providing immediate open access to peer-reviewed biomedical research that publishes 150+ peer-reviewed, open access journals. All original research articles published by BioMed Central are made freely and permanently accessible online immediately upon publication."
BMC Musculoskeletal Disorders: www.biomedcentral.com/1471-2474/ • Open access	Open-access journal publishing original peer-reviewed research articles
Clinical and Experimental Rheumatology: www.clinexprheumatol.org/ • Some open access; subscription required for full access	Subscription required to access current issue; free materials include any article published in 2000–2002, and all issues in the annual series "Contemporary Advances in Clinical Rheumatology;" RSS feed available
Lancet: www.thelancet.com	Online version allows free access only to tables of content and abstracts; subscription required for full access; online-only subscription available; discussion forum available
Nature Clinical Practice Rheumatology: www.nature.com/ncprheum/about_journal/index.html • Some open access with registration; subscription required for full access	One of Nature's specialty journals; no RSS feed for this journal, but the Nature Publishing group offers an extensive list of other Nature feeds: npg.nature.com/npg/servlet/Content?data=xml/02_newsfeed.xml&style=xml/02_newsfeed.xsl
Nature Medicine: www.nature.com/nm	Free access to current table of contents and article overview; subscription required for full access; RSS feeds and e-mail alerts available
New England Journal of Medicine: http://content.nejm.org	Free access to current table of contents and abstracts; subscription required for full access; online access is free with print subscription; PDA access, e-mail alerts, and free online CME exams available
PLoS Medicine: medicine.plosjournals.org • Open access	Multidisciplinary print and Web journal published by the Public Library of Science; RSS feed available

* RSS = really simple syndication; PDA = personal digital assistant; CME = continuing medical education.

Table 5. Medical news*

Web site name: URL	Description
Doctor's Lounge: www.thedoctorslounge.net/rheumatology/index.htm • Open access	Today's medical and rheumatology news (and other news by specialty); includes other disease-specific resources; RSS feed for headlines
Joint and Bone: www.jointandbone.org • Free registration required for full access	Focused on the musculoskeletal diseases; includes news, education, discussion forums, satellite programs, CME, etc.; owned by WebMD.
Medscape rheumatology newsletters and alerts: www.Medscape.com/rheumatology-home • Open access with registration	Medscape offers e-mail alerts and newsletters • MedPulse: Highlighting key medical news and features by specialty (weekly) • CME Alerts: e-mail notification of new CME programs • Medscape Best Evidence (HTML only): Key journal articles ranked for newsworthiness and clinical relevance in each specialty, linked to Medlineabstracts • Breaking Conference News: email notification of breaking conference news posts • Medsacpe Today: Breaking news by specialty, conference reports • RSS feed available
Rheuma21s: www.rheuma21st.com/ • Open access	Written by "academic and practicing rheumatologists and immunologists from every civilized continent who are among the world's leading teaching experts." Focused on reporting from "both large and closed or little-known meetings" on "the subjects we believe to have the most future potential. . . . [and] our reading on the meaning and importance of the material." Emphasizes critical analysis and distillation of meetings and what's new in the fields of rheumatology and immunology. "Our readers learn long before print journals of not only the content but also the meaning of what is presented throughout the world."
Rheumatology News: www.rheumatologynews.com/ • Open access for a limited time; subscription required for print	Independent monthly newspaper for rheumatologists, includes meeting coverage, expert opinion; e-mail alerts available; check out "PocketConsult" for free PDA downloads of RSS feeds, drug updates, medical calculators

* CME = continuing medical education; RSS = really simple syndication; PDA = personal digital assistant.

Table 6. Other useful sites, blogs, and RSS feeds*

Name of Web site: URL	Description
American College of Rheumatology: www.rheumatology.org/ • Open access	Official organization for doctors and health professionals who treat arthritis and other rheumatic diseases; education, research, publications, etc
Centers for Medicare & Medicaid Services: www.cms.hhs.gov/ • Open access	Quick access to accurate Medicare program information; "a resource focused on the informational needs and interests of Medicare Fee-for-Service (FFS) providers, including physicians, other practitioners and suppliers." Offers many e-mail newsletters related to Medicaid and Medicare, covering a variety of providers and settings
Healthcare Freeware–Medical Databases: www.healthcarefreeware.com/med_data.htm • Open access	A list of freeware that provides databases and electronic publications containing medical reference resources
MEDLOG: www.medlog.net • Open Access	This is a directory of medical blogs and medical news feeds that features blogs by physicians, nurses, other professionals, patients, etc.; includes an extensive list of other blogs by medical practitioners, with links
Medical Download.com: www.medicaldownload.com • Open access	A clearinghouse for medically related software ranging from medical billing to practice management tools
National Institute of Arthritis and Musculoskeletal and Skin Diseases: www.niams.nih.gov/ • Open access	Health information, research and training, news and events; available in Spanish
Johns Hopkins Medicine Podcasts: www.hopkinsmedicine.org/mediaII/Podcasts.html • Open access	Podcasts of the week's medical news and how it may affect the provider; Free service
Rss4medics.com: www.rss4medics.com/ www.rss4medics.com/rss_directory/rheumatology_feeds.html • Open access	Created by a doctor, for doctors, this directory of RSS feeds in medicine (and rheumatology) explains RSS and provides links to readers and discussion forums; "Set up by a surgical doctor who used RSS to help with his research once he realized that the technology would be extremely useful for his colleagues, many of whom have little time but need to keep up to date with all new medical developments related to their specialties and participate in medical research on an ongoing basis," explains RSS from a nontechnical medical user's point of view.
International Classification of Functioning (ICF): http://www3.who.int/icf/icftemplate.cfm	The World Health Organization provides all the materials needed for using their ICF

* RSS = really simple syndication (see sidebar).

How to tell a good site from a bad one. Many people find it difficult to distinguish the good from the bad on the Internet, often making the mistake of thinking that because a Web site looks good or sounds authoritative, the information it presents must be trustworthy. Without knowing how to choose reputable sources, your patients may be persuaded by a sales pitch made to sound like something different. Fortunately, there are many Web sites that explain how to tell the good from the bad, including the 4 listed in Table 8, which have published standards for reliable health information online.

Why Care Providers Have Web Sites

- Marketing and referrals
- Augment patient services
- Electronic communication, e.g., e-mail, labs, etc.
- Announcements
- Sharing information and data with other health care professionals
- Blogging

Table 7. Guides and links to downloads for your PDA*

Name of Web site: URL	Description (note: many downloads are free)
Ectopic Brain–Palm OS Handhelds in Clinical Medicine: www.medicalpda.net/ (great site!)	This Web site was created by Dr. Kent Willyard, a family practice physician, who finds PDAs valuable for "organization and efficiency, reducing errors, and improving patient care." The Web site includes the following extensive lists of annotated links, with archives that go back to 2001: • The basics: getting started, technical stuff, books, magazines, newsgroups, online forums, and newsgroups • Medical apps: A long list of tools to download for your Palm PDA, organized as tools for reference, calculators, patient tracking, and other applications • Medical links: Links to commercial, educational, and other sites • Other links: News, software, e-books, hardware, and miscellaneous **Don't miss**: "What's new" for cartoons and announcements about the release of new handhelds and software; RSS feed available
Epocrates: www.epocrates.com	Epocrates, a widely used drug reference and formulary, has been around for a long time and is very well regarded, which is why we include this individual software app in our list of resource sites; Epocrates has recently added the Medicare Part D formulary; some products are free, others must be purchased; Epocrates products are compatible with Palm OS and Pocket PC PDAs, and with Windows and Macintosh computers **Don't miss**: Epocrates has just launched a new mobile CME program for your handheld, a free download
MDTool.com: www.mdtool.com/	An excellent guide to medical resources on the net, with a good section on handheld computers, with links to free software downloads, other PDA resources on the net, and much more **Don't miss**: The "handheld buying guide" and the "Palm resources" section for links to other great sites
MedPD.net: www.medpda.net/	Reviews, guides, articles, and news about devices and medical applications for PDAs, including PalmOS and PocketPC **Don't miss**: "Getting RSS feeds for most medical journals" in the features section
Skyscape Rheumatology PDA References for Palm, Pocket PC PDA or Smartphone: www.skyscape.com/estore/store.aspx?category=14	From the Web site: "Gold standard PDA medical software for Rheumatology Specialists, including drug guides and practice manuals. Read customer reviews and download online for your Palm, Pocket PC, PDA or Smartphone." This software, which is not free, can be purchased from the Web site **Don't miss**: Browse "products by specialty" for tools for physicians, PAs, nurses, nurse practitioners, students and residents, pharmacists, EMS/paramedics, and vets
University of Tennessee Health Sciences Library and Biocommunications Center, Electronic Resources list: library.utmem.edu/HSLBC/eresources/SPT—BrowseResources.php	310 annotated links to medical electronic resources

* apps = applications; PDA = personal digital assistant; RSS = really simple syndication; CME = continuing medical education; PA = physician's assistant; EMS = emergency medical services.

What's a Blog?

Blogs (short for "web log") are open access, push-button publishing that come in many forms:

- Personal diary
- Pulpit or soapbox
- Political or other types of commentary
- Gossip
- Breaking news outlet
- Collection of links and recommended sites
- Anything the author(s) want it to be

Blogs have been around for about 5 years, and they have the changed the landscape of the World Wide Web, the news, and politics. For more information, links to sample blogs, and the tools to start your own blog, see the BLOGGER Web site: www.Blogger.com, and see MEDLOGS www.medlogs.com for medical news feeds and medical blogs.

All agree that the hallmarks of trustworthiness for healthcare-related sites are as follows:

- Authorship—does the Web site list the authors of material?
- The date of posting is included for all material;
- Material is based on referenced evidence;
- There is an editorial policy clearly stated;
- There is clear disclosure of support or advertising.

Finding credible patient information about rheumatology online. Keep in mind that reliable Web sites tend to link to other reliable Web sites. Table 9 provides some excellent choices to get patients started on their search for trustworthy content. Each site provides links to additional resources.

Advocacy

The Web sites of volunteer organizations that focus on patient advocacy are an excellent source of information and resources for patients to learn more, stay connected, and be involved (Table 10).

Table 8. Organizations that promote quality health care information

Name of organization and Web site: URL
Health On the Net: HON Code of Conduct: http://www.hon.ch/HONcode/Conduct.html
Internet Healthcare Coalition: IHC eHealth Code of Ethics: www.ihealthcoalition.org/ethics/ehcode.html
Hi-Ethics: Ethical Principles: www.hiethics.com/Principles/index.asp
National Health Council: Standards of Excellence: www.nationalhealthcouncil.org/aboutus/stand-good_operating.htm

Useful Tools and Other Helpful Web Sites for Your Patients

Athale and colleagues (9) demonstrated that when a patient self-assessment questionnaire is administered in 2 different formats, a computer version and a paper version, the scores from each correlated

Table 9. A sampling of resources for patient education*

Web site name: URL	Description
WebMD: www.webmd.com	An A-to-Z guide to health topics based on a comprehensive directory of >4,000 conditions, including major rheumatic diseases
National Institute of Health: www.nih.gov/	An alphabetical clearinghouse of disease information
MedlinePlus: www.medlineplus.org	An encyclopedia that discusses health conditions and includes medical illustrations
Wikipedia: wikipedia.org	This free encyclopedia has >1 million articles in multiple languages
Johns Hopkins Vasculitis Center: vasculitis.med.jhu.edu	Includes newsletters on a variety of vasculitides and treatments
Scleroderma from A to Z: www.sclero.org/index.html	In 22 languages, this site has a wealth of content, images, patient support, and links to outside resources
MayoClinic.com: www.mayoclinic.com	Diseases & Conditions A-Z: Use the alphabet links to search for disease conditions
The Arthritis Society: www.arthritis.ca	Tips for Living Well: In addition to disease content, the site offers information on QOL issues and a variety of discussion boards
Medem: www.medem.com	For Patients: The medical library provides content in some of the major rheumatic diseases
A.D.A.M. Healthcare Center: adam.about.com	Illustrated Health Encyclopedia: Includes discussions of the major rheumatic diseases, it also boasts an extensive library of excellent illustrations
Hospital for Special Surgery: www.hss.edu/Conditions	Conditions & Treatments: An index of orthopedic and rheumatologic discussions for patients in Q&A format
Johns Hopkins Arthritis Center www.hopkins-arthritis.org/corner/corner.html	Patients Corner: Although the overall site is geared to the provider, this section of the Web site is focused specifically on patient information
Stanford SOM Self-Management Programs http://patienteducation.stanford.edu/Internet/	Internet Self-Management Programs: Internet education programs for back pain and healthy living with arthritis

* QOL = quality of life; Q&A = question and answer

Table 10. A sampling of reputable patient advocacy Web sites*

Web site name: URL	Message board	Local resources	Free ed. materials	Member NHC	Current news	Other language
Scleroderma Foundation: www.scleroderma.org	X	X	X	X	X	X
Lupus Foundation of America: www.lupus.org		X	X	X	X	X
Arthritis Foundation: www.arthritis.org	X	X	X	X	X	X
Myositis Association: www.myositis.org	X	X	X			
Spondylitis Association of America: www.spondylitis.org/		X	X			
National Psoriasis Foundation: www.psoriasis.org	X	X	X	X	X	
Vasculitis Clinical Research Consortium: rarediseasesnetwork.epi.usf.edu/vcrc/index.htm		X	X			

* Local resources include chapters, support groups, etc. NHC = National Health Council.

well, implying that Internet-based self-assessments can facilitate a physician's ability to monitor a patient's disease activity. Some self-monitoring tools available to your patients are listed in Table 11.

E-MAIL

It is important to recognize that regular e-mail is not secure. The most common type of security risk is unauthorized interception of messages, which means that messages can be intercepted, read, and modified in transit. Guidelines for the use of e-mail with patients have been established by the AMA (10) (http://www.ama-assn.org/ama/pub/category/2386.html) and are useful for any provider considering establishing e-mail communication with their patients. Recommendations include the following:

- Establish turnaround time with patients;
- Establish permitted transactions (prescription refills, etc.);
- Instruct patients to use the subject line to categorize their request;

- Do not send group mailings to patients unless using blind copy feature;
- Send new message to inform patient of completed request;
- Print entire string of messages for paper record in chart.

What is RSS?

RSS stands for Really Simple Syndication. One of the best explanations we've seen comes from the RSS4Medics Web site (www.rss4medics.com), which explains it as follows: RSS is a tool for finding new information quickly and easily without having to search and read through hundreds of pages. Sites create RSS feeds "by publishing short headlines and summaries that say what is new on a Web site, with links to the full articles. These summaries (RSS files) are picked up and read by simplified Web browsers known as RSS Readers (or RSS Aggregators). RSS can also be used to announce your own news and publications to the world." Many leading online medical journals and news sources now offer RSS feeds. To take advantage of RSS, you can download a free RSS reader/aggregator, or you can buy one. The folks behind RSS4medics say they are campaigning for RSS in medicine, and consider it "the future." For more information and links to downloads and feeds, check out their Web site.

Table 11. Tools and useful sites for rheumatology patients*

Web site name: URL	Description
JHU Arthritis Center Rheumatoid Arthritis Activity Minder: www.hopkins-arthritis.org/arthritis_sa/home.cfm	This interactive tool for patients with rheumatoid arthritis helps them to monitor disease activity over time by completing online validated assessments; free registration required
My Exercise Plan: www.myexerciseplan.com	For a small fee, this site provides a personalized exercise program based on fitness level, goals, and available exercise equipment; includes animated demos of exercises, online diary for logging exercise, and nutrition analysis
iHealthRecord: www.ihealthrecord.org	This online tool allows patients to create and store an online comprehensive health record; no fee; can be printed, allowing patients to keep their health information on hand in case of emergency and for sharing with multiple providers
CalorieKing: www.calorieking.com	Nutrition and exercise management software designed to provide personalized weight loss management; graphic reports provide feedback over time
DisabilityInfo.gov: www.disabilityinfo.gov	From the Web site: "This site provides access to disability-related information and programs available across the government on numerous subjects, including civil rights, community life, education, employment, housing, health, income support, technology and transportation."
Informed Consumer's Guide for People with Arthritis: www.abledata.com/abledata_docs/arth_in.htm	A consumer guide to adaptive devices for arthritis patients; scroll down to "Starting Out": Helps patients assess how arthritis affects their ability to carry out ADLs and provides an assistive device identification worksheet; contains a list of numerous online catalogs

* JHU = Johns Hopkins University; ADLs = activities of daily living.

Table 12. Information and education resources on HIPAA compliance*

Web site name: URL	Description
HIPAA-REGS Listserv: www.aspe.hhs.gov/admnsimp/lsnotify.htm	Subscribe to be notified by e-mail when documents or events related to the HIPAA Administrative Simplification regulations are published or posted
HIPA Advisory: www.hipaadvisory.com/	A resource for HIPAA news, regulations, resources, and compliance tools, with specific information on technologies for electronic information security
U.S. Department of Health & Human Services: www.hhs.gov/ocr/hipaa:	The Office of Civil Rights provides helpful fact sheets for informing consumers about privacy policies
American Medical Association: www.ama-assn.org/ama/pub/category/4234.html	The AMA offers practice management tools and resources

* HIPAA = Health Insurance Portability & Accountability Act of 1996; AMA = American Medical Association.

What is a Metasearch Engine?

A metasearch engine searches other search engines instead of Web sites. A few good examples:

- www.dogpile.com
- www.Surfwax.com
- www.copernic.com (a desktop search tool that requires a free download and lets you specify which engines to search)
- www.Mamma.com ("the mother of all search engines")
- www.Vivisimo.com
- www.omnimedicalsearch.com/
- HON Foundation Med Hunt: www.hon.ch/MedHunt/
- Stanford's MedBot: www.medworld.stanford.edu/medbot/

For more information, see Search Engine Watch at www.searchenginewatch.com/links/article.php/2156241

HIPAA REGULATIONS

The Health Insurance Portability & Accountability Act of 1996 (HIPAA) is complicated and affects all health care organizations. Compliance is mandatory and calls for sweeping changes on most every level of health care administration. Electronic communication is specifically addressed and, as a provider, it is your responsibility to stay current with regulations (Table 12).

REFERENCES

1. Neilsen//Net Ratings. Accessed March 20, 2006. URL: http://www.nielsen-netratings.com/pr/pr_060314.pdf
2. Fox S, Fallows D. Internet health resources. Washington (DC): Pew Internet & American Life Project, 2003. Accessed March 20, 2006. URL: http://www.pewInternet.org/pdfs/PIP_Health_Report_July_2003.pdf
3. Hesse B, Nelson D, Kreps G, Croyle R, Arora N, Rimer B, et al. Trust and sources of health information. Arch Intern Med 2005;165:2618–24.
4. Ulrich, B. Looking back, looking forward. Nursing Spectrum April 1, 2006. Accessed July 10, 2006. URL: http://community.nursingspectrum.com/MagazineArticles/article.cfm?AID=20422
5. Fordis M, King J, Ballantyne C, Jones P, Schneider K, Spann S, et al. Comparison of the instructional efficacy of Internet-based CME with live interactive CME workshops. JAMA 2005;294:1043–51.
6. Dee C, Marilyn Teolis M, Todd A. Physicians' use of the personal digital assistant (PDA) in clinical decision making. J Med Libr Assoc 2005;93:480–6.
7. Rothschild J, Lee T, Bae T, Bates D. Clinician use of a palmtop drug reference guide. J Am Med Inform Assoc 2002;9:223–9.
8. Guevara J, Wolf F, Grum C, Clark N. Effects of educational interventions for self management of asthma in children and adolescents: systematic review and meta-analysis. BMJ 2003;326:1308–9.
9. Athale N, Sturley A, Skoczen S, Kavanaugh A, Lenert L. A web-compatible instrument for measuring self-reported disease activity in arthritis. J Rheumatol 2004;31:223–8.
10. Kane B, Sands DZ, The AMIA Internet Working Group, Task Force on Guidelines for the Use of Clinic–Patient Electronic Mail. Guidelines for the clinical use of electronic mail with patients. J Am Med Inform Assoc 1998;5:104–11. [look up]
11. Bennett N, Casebeer L, Kristofco R, Strasser S. Physicians' Internet information seeking behaviors. J Contin Educ Health Prof 2002;22:33–42.

Subject Index

ASSOCIATION OF RHEUMATOLOGY
HEALTH PROFESSIONALS
A DIVISION OF THE AMERICAN COLLEGE OF RHEUMATOLOGY

The Association of Rheumatology Health Professionals, a division of the American College of Rheumatology, is a professional membership society composed of non-physician health care professionals specializing in rheumatology, such as advanced practice nurses, nurses, occupational therapists, physical therapists, psychologists, social workers, epidemiologists, physician assistants, educators, clinicians and researchers.

ARHP Purpose
Using programs of education, practice, research, and advocacy, the Association of Rheumatology Health Professionals will advance the knowledge and skills of health professionals in the area of rheumatology and will improve their understanding and management of the physical, emotional, psychological, and cultural factors influencing health in order to improve the health outcomes for people with or at risk for rheumatic disease and musculoskeletal conditions.

Application Process

Please fill out all pages of the application for ARHP Membership and send it with your payment to the address or fax below. Check payments need to be made to the ACR.
Fax: (404) 633-1870
Mailing Address: ACR, PO Box 102295, Atlanta, GA 30368

>>> *For more information, go to the ARHP Web site at www.rheumatology.org/arhp*

ACR/ARHP Rules of Procedure
ACR/ARHP Rules of Procedure state that an applicant must have a recommendation from another ACR/ARHP member. Any applicant who is unable to get a recommendation may appeal to the ARHP by contacting the Program Services Specialist on staff at (404) 633-3777. Thereafter, a recommendation for approval will be forwarded to the ACR Board of Directors for Rheumatology Health Professional membership, Rheumatology Health Professional International membership and Emeritus membership who will make the final decision on the applicant. Election to membership will be made by an affirmative vote. If an applicant is not approved, the applicant may reapply as a member three years after the date of the adverse decision.

Associate and Student Member Applicants are approved by the ARHP Executive Committee and are considered members of the ARHP but not the ACR.

Membership Dues
Please pay membership dues in full. The ACR/ARHP does not prorate. Annual dues are due by December 31 each year.

Reinstatement
If a member resigns, reinstatement may be granted by filling out a new membership application and completing the election process. A resigned member reinstatement may also be granted by vote of the ACR Board of Directors if all arrears are paid in full prior to the end of the fiscal year of the ACR in which the termination occured.

>>> *Please keep the first and second page of the application for reference.* <<<

(Continued on the other side)

CATEGORIES OF MEMBERSHIP *(Please indicate the category of membership for which you are applying.)*

■ **RHEUMATOLOGY HEALTH PROFESSIONAL MEMBER - $125.00** *(a printed AC&R subscription is included in dues, and members may not deduct subscription price from dues)*

To qualify as a Rheumatology Health Professional Member, an applicant must:
· Be a citizen or resident of the United States, Canada or Mexico
· Be eligible for membership in his or her professional discipline's national association
· Have demonstrated an interest in rheumatology practice, research or education
· Be a degreed professional in fields including, but not limited to, physical therapy, social work, psychology, occupational therapy, pharmacy and nursing
· Obtain the signature of a current member of the ARHP or ACR who is familiar with the applicant's professional competence, ethics and moral standing

■ **INTERNATIONAL RHEUMATOLOGY HEALTH PROFESSIONAL MEMBER - $125.00** *($146 with printed AC&R subscription)*

To qualify as an International Rheumatology Health Professional Member, an applicant must:
· Reside out of the United States, Canada and Mexico
· Be eligible for membership in his or her professional discipline's national association
· Have demonstrated an interest in rheumatology practice, research or education
· Be a degreed professional in fields including, but not limited to, physical therapy, social work, psychology, occupational therapy, pharmacy and nursing
· Obtain the signature of a current member of the ARHP or ACR who is familiar with the applicant's professional competence, ethics and moral standing

■ **EMERITUS MEMBER - $25.00** *($50.00 with printed AC&R subscription)*

To qualify as an Emeritus Member, an applicant must be one of the following:
· A Member or International Member who has retired from active practice
· Permanently disabled
· Charter member (October 5, 1965- June 1, 1967), and elected by the ARHP Executive Committee

■ **ASSOCIATE RHEUMATOLOGY HEALTH PROFESSIONAL MEMBER - $75.00**

To qualify as an Associate Rheumatology Health Professional Member, an applicant must:
· Reside in the United States, Canada, or Mexico
· Have demonstrated an interest in and is employed in rheumatology practice, research or education. Examples include, but are not limited to, physical therapy assistants, occupational therapy assistants, nursing assistants, laboratory technicians, non-degreed clinical research coordinators, medical assistants, licensed vocational nurses, licensed practical nurses, radiology technicians and rheumatology office staff
· Obtain the signature of a current member of the ARHP or ACR who is familiar with the applicant's professional competence, ethics and moral standing
  > Registered nurses are not eligible for associate membership

■ **STUDENT MEMBERSHIP - $75.00**

To qualify as a Student Member, an applicant must:
· Be a citizen of or reside in the United States, Canada, or Mexico
· Have demonstrated an interest in rheumatology and shall be enrolled in a health professional program leading to a baccalaureate or graduate degree. Health professional programs may include nursing, physical therapy, occupational therapy, social work, psychology, laboratory sciences, physician assistant, health education and epidemiology
· Obtain the signature of their program director of faculty advisor and may be elected by the Executive Committee at any of its regular or special meetings

>>> Please keep the first and second page of the application for reference. <<<

ARHP Member ID _____

APPLICATION
FOR ARHP MEMBERSHIP

HOME ADDRESS

Preferred Mailing Address: ☐ Home   ☐ Office

Last Name _____ First Name _____ MI _____

Street _____

City _____ State/Province _____ Zip/Postal Code _____ Country _____

Telephone _____ Fax _____ E-mail _____

Demographic Information: ☐ Male ☐ Female   Date of Birth _____ / _____ / _____

☐ Do not rent my name to other organizations for promotional mailings

PROFESSIONAL ADDRESS *(for listing in Membership Directory)*

Last Name _____ First Name _____ MI _____

Department _____ Institution _____

Street _____

City _____ State/Province _____ Zip/Postal Code _____ Country _____

Telephone _____ Fax _____ E-mail _____

Degrees:

Undergraduate	Graduate	Professional Licence or Certification

Print name of current ACR/ARHP sponsor/member who recruited you _____

Signature of current ACR/ARHP sponsor/member _____

PAYMENT INFORMATION *(please print clearly)*

☐ Health Professional Member - $125.00   ☐ Emeritus - $25.00 *($50.00 with printed AC&R subscription)*   ☐ Associate - $75.00

☐ International Health Professional - $125.00 *($146 with printed AC&R subscription)*   ☐ Student - $75.00

☐ **Charge the following card:** ☐ AMEX ☐ MC ☐ VISA   **Amount $** _____

Card number ☐☐☐☐ ☐☐☐☐ ☐☐☐☐ ☐☐☐☐   Exp. date ☐☐ / ☐☐   MONTH/YEAR

Signature _____ Print name as it appears on card _____

☐ **Check enclosed $** _____

Checks must be made payable to the ACR in U.S. dollars drawn on U.S. banks. Transfers, cash or purchase orders will not be accepted.

ASSOCIATION OF RHEUMATOLOGY
HEALTH PROFESSIONALS
A DIVISION OF THE AMERICAN COLLEGE OF RHEUMATOLOGY

Send complete application form and payment to: ACR, PO Box 102295, Atlanta, GA 30368; or fax to the
ACR Accounting Department at (404) 633-1870 *(please include credit card number).*

ACR OFFICE USE ONLY						CCT06

Received _____ Dues Entered _____ New Member ID# _____ Receipt _____ Ack'd _____ Date Elected _____ Notified _____

(Continued on the other side)

APPLICATION FOR ARHP MEMBERSHIP

Disciplines/Specialties *(Select up to 3 disciplines. If other, write in name of other.)*

Primary: _____ **Secondary:** _____ **Tertiary :** _____

Administrator	Laboratory Technician	Pharmacist	Researcher-Clinical
Advanced Practice Nurse	Licensed Practical Nurse	Physiatrist	Researcher-Evaluation
Biostatistician	Medical Assistant	Physical Therapist	Researcher-Health Services
Clinical Nurse Specialist	Medical Librarian	Physician	Researcher-Population Health
Counselor	Nurse	Physician's Assistant	Retired
Dietician/Nutritionist	Nurse Practitioner	Podiatrist	Social Worker
Epidemiologist	Occupational Therapist	Psychologist	Sociologist
Hand Therapist	Office Manager	Registered Nurse	Statistician
Health Educator	Office Staff	Research Coordinator	Student
Health Service Researcher	Orthotist/Prosthetist	Researcher-Basic Science	Other _____

Professional Work Settings/Locations *(Select up to 3 locations. If other, write in name of other.)*

Primary: _____ **Secondary:** _____ **Tertiary:** _____

College or University	Industry-Pharmaceutical	Practice-Single Specialty Group	Retired
Government Agency	Long-Term Care Facility	Practice-Solo	Staff Model HMO
Home Health Agency	Medical School	Private/Public School	VA Hospital
Hospital	Practice-Multiple Specialty Group	Public Health Agency	Other _____
Industry	Practice-Partnership	Rehabilitation/Vocational Center	

Areas Where Time Is Spent *(Select 3 areas in which you spend time. If other, write in name of other.)*

Primary: _____ **Secondary:** _____ **Tertiary :** _____

Administration	Public Policy	Research-Health Services	Student
Clinical Practice	Research-Basic Science	Research-Population Health	Teaching
Consultation	Research-Clinical	Retired	Other _____
Counseling	Research-Evaluation		

Age Group Focus for Patients *(Choose all that apply.)*   ☐ Adult   ☐ Pediatric   ☐ Geriatric   ☐ All Ages

Diagnostic Focus *(Choose all that apply. If other, write in the name of the focus.)*

☐ Ankylosing Spondylitis /Spondylarthropathies	☐ Hypermobility syndromes	☐ Osteoporosis	☐ Scleroderma
	☐ Obesity	☐ Overuse syndromes	☐ Systemic Lupus Erythematosus
☐ Fibromyalgia	☐ Orthopedics	☐ Psoriatic Arthritis	☐ Vasculitis
☐ Gout	☐ Osteoarthritis	☐ Rheumatoid Arthritis	☐ Other_____

Practice Focus *(Choose all that apply. If other, write in the name of the focus.)*

☐ Advocacy/Public Policy	☐ Economics/Cost of Health Care	☐ Pain Management	☐ Psychosocial issues
☐ Assistive Devices/Orthoses	☐ Epidemiology	☐ Patient/Family Education & Counseling	☐ Public Health
☐ Behavioral approaches	☐ Fatigue		☐ Quality of Life
☐ Biologics	☐ Functional Status	☐ Physical Activity/Exercise	☐ Work Disability
☐ Biomechanics	☐ Nutrition	☐ Practice Management	☐ Other_____
☐ Developmental/Life Skills			

Research Methods *(Choose all that apply. If other, write in the name of the method.)*

☐ Biostatistics		☐ Qualitative methods & analysis
☐ Clinical Trials Design	☐ Meta-analyses	☐ Other _____
☐ Clinical Trials Management	☐ Outcomes/Evaluative research	

EVERY DAY. EVERYWHERE. PUTTING PATIENTS FIRST.

ACROSS AMERICA. For over 50 years, Merck has made its drugs available free to those who can least afford them. In 2005, we provided free medicines to fill nearly 7 million prescriptions for uninsured Americans in need. For a list of specific Merck medicines included in this program and to learn more, **call 1-800-506-3725 or visit merckhelps.com.**

AROUND THE WORLD. Merck strives to improve the world's health through its medicines and vaccines and to ensure that patients have access to them. We're working to combat disease in more than 140 countries. Merck not only provides free medicines, but is also helping to get them into the hands of the people who need them most.

IN THE LAB. Merck has invested billions to research heart disease, asthma, cholesterol, and blood pressure. Now, 8,000 Merck scientists are trying to make Alzheimer's, obesity, cancer, and other diseases history, too.

IN YOUR HANDS. Merck provides comprehensive and unbiased medical resources to help keep you informed and healthy, like *The Merck Manual*, free online at **mercksource.com.**

To learn more,
call 1-800-963-7257 or
visit merck.com/consumer.

Where patients come first 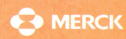 **MERCK**

WE MAKE OUR MEDICINES FOR EVERYONE WHO NEEDS THEM.

NOT JUST THOSE WHO CAN AFFORD THEM.

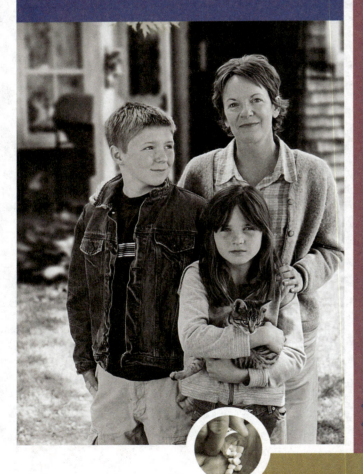

At Merck, we believe it's not enough to create medicines, we need to help get them to people. That's why we offer programs to do just that.

The Merck Patient Assistance Program.
For over 50 years, this program has provided Merck medicines free to millions of Americans who can't afford them. In 2005, we provided free medicines to fill nearly 7 million prescriptions for uninsured Americans in need.

You may be eligible for one of Merck's assistance programs. They are free to join and have no hidden charges. You can get a list of specific Merck medicines included in the programs by calling us. We'll also send you a free copy of Merck's *Guide to Affordable Medicine* and the latest issue of *Your Health Now* magazine.

Call 1-800-506-3725 or visit merckhelps.com.

Where patients come first 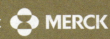 MERCK